TEXTBOOK OF

Physical Diagnosis

MARK H. SWARTZ

M.D., F.A.C.P.

Professor of Medicine
Marietta & Charles C. Morchand Professor of Medical Education
Director, The Morchand Center for Clinical Competence
Mount Sinai School of Medicine
New York, New York

THIRD EDITION

TEXTBOOK OF

Physical Diagnosis

HISTORY AND EXAMINATION

W.B. SAUNDERS COMPANY
A Division of Harcourt Brace & Company
Philadelphia   London   Toronto   Montreal   Sydney   Tokyo

W.B. SAUNDERS COMPANY
A Division of Harcourt Brace & Company

The Curtis Center
Independence Square West
Philadelphia, Pennsylvania 19106

Library of Congress Cataloging-in-Publication Data

Swartz, Mark H.
Textbook of physical diagnosis: history and examination / Mark H.
Swartz.—3rd ed.

p.   cm.

Includes bibliographical references and index.

ISBN 0–7216–7514–X

1. Physical diagnosis.   2. Medical history taking.
   [DNLM: 1. Diagnosis.   2. Medical History Taking.   3. Physical
   Examination.   WB 200 S973t 1998]

RC76.S95   1998   616.07′54—dc21

DNLM/DLC   97-12945

TEXTBOOK OF PHYSICAL DIAGNOSIS: History and Examination   ISBN 0–7216–7514–X

Printed in the United States of America

Last digit is the print number: 9   8   7   6   5   4   3   2   1

One of the essential qualities of the clinician
is interest in humanity,
*for the secret in the care **of** the patient*
*is in caring **for** the patient.*

FRANCIS WELD PEABODY
1881–1927

To **Vivian,**
my life's companion and best friend,
for her love, support, and understanding;

To **Talia,**
my wonderful and devoted daughter;

and

To my father, **Philip,** and in memory of my mother, **Hilda.**

Preface to the Third Edition

Although 9 years have passed since the publication of the first edition of *Textbook of Physical Diagnosis: History and Examination,* my feeling remains that this volume offers a new approach and presentation to physical diagnosis. By clearly discussing pathophysiology and emphasizing the humanistic element, I attempt to show the importance of the "old-fashioned" doctor's approach to the patient. "The *primary* aim of this textbook," as stated in the Preface to the First Edition, "is to provide a framework for the clinical assessment of the patient in a *humanistic* manner." The book, then and now, focuses on the patient: his/her needs, problems, and concerns. This philosophy remains unchanged since the first edition—perhaps now even more than ever, in our rapidly changing world of managed care. This book is designed for all students of health care, who are learning to communicate effectively with patients, to examine them, and to assess their medical problems.

From the very first edition, it is clearly stated that a health-care provider must have insight into his/her own feelings, attitudes, and vulnerabilities. The history and physical examination must not be seen simply as techniques performed by a robot but rather as a process that requires interpersonal awareness as well as technical skill. In this era of modern medical technology, there has been progressive subordination of the importance of the clinical history and physical examination to that of procedures and tests. While medical costs skyrocket, we must educate our medical personnel about two of the least costly, but most valuable, of all medical evaluations—the history and physical examination. This book continues with its primary-care orientation as its basis while it constantly emphasizes a holistic approach to the patient. At the same time, it focuses on patients who are persons suffering from disease as opposed to patients as entities manifesting disease.

In 1989, shortly after publication of the first edition, the book was cited in the *New England Journal of Medicine* as "the gold standard" and "well on its way to becoming the Gray's *Anatomy* of physical diagnosis." Within the past few years, there have been many excellent reviews of the book and a heartening acceptance of it both in the United States and abroad, where it has already been translated into many foreign languages. The *Journal of General Internal Medicine* in 1994 reviewed the second edition and stated that the ". . . organization, ample use of color illustrations, easy readability, a practical clinicopathologic approach, and a patient-centered philosophy make *Textbook of Physical Diagnosis* the premier book in the field." The *Annals of Internal Medicine* hailed the second edition as "the standard text for learning history taking and physical examination skills."

The fact that the book remains single-authored has been cited in numerous reviews as a notable strength when compared with the book's competition; it provides writing that is uniform, clear, and accurate. The illustrations and photographs have also been drawn or taken by a single illustrator or photographer, respectively; all illustrations have been clearly matched to the text. I have welcomed the many solicited and unsolicited criticisms of the book. I have been pleased to make changes where necessary in this new edition.

Two new chapters have been included in the volume. Cultural diversity has been an important part of the previous two editions, but this one recognizes its even broader significance. Students' awareness of the impact of culture within the context of illness is imperative in today's world. The new chapter on cultural diversity discusses ethnic differences in communication, diet, and family relationships as well as various health practices and beliefs.

A second new chapter in this book deals with the assessment of the acutely ill patient. The condition of these patients must be assessed expeditiously so that appropriate care can be provided for them. The chapter describes the emergency evaluation of patients with life-threatening conditions and includes two algorithms that should prove to be extremely useful.

The chapter on clinical decision-making has been completely rewritten to mirror our better understanding of this most important aspect of patient care.

All of the other chapters have been reviewed and modified where appropriate. As times change, so do standards of physical diagnosis. Therefore, several of the tests indicated in the previous editions have either been modified or eliminated.

Our awareness of the post-traumatic stress disorder and its many manifestations has increased enormously over the past decade. I have therefore given special emphasis to this pervasive problem. Abuse—physical, sexual, child, elder, domestic—continues to be on the rise, and failure to recognize it and help the victims is all too common. Chapter 2 includes essential tips to help the student recognize and deal with this major problem.

More than 170 new color photographs have been included to enhance the text. Since the AIDS pandemic was first recognized in 1981, our knowledge of the clinical expression of disease caused by the human immunodeficiency virus (HIV) has been considerably expanded. This volume includes a discussion and many photographs of the common oral, dermatologic, ophthalmologic, and pediatric clinical manifestations of the HIV infection.

The health-care provider of today must be able to synthesize basic pathophysiology and provide humane medical care. The medical profession continues to be under great scrutiny. We must place special emphasis on a more humanistic approach to patient care, recognizing the role of culture in illness, and use modern technology only to enhance our clinical assessment, *not* replace it. We must always remember that a patient is a *person* suffering from disease.

I hope that you will find this third edition of *Textbook of Physical Diagnosis: History and Examination* to be an easy-to-read, informative, and exciting addition to your library.

MARK H. SWARTZ, M.D.

Acknowledgments

I wish to acknowledge all of my colleagues and friends who have supported me in writing this third edition. I express my heartfelt thanks to the following people, without whose assistance I could not have brought this book from an idea to a reality:

To all my teachers, students, and patients who have taught me so much about medicine.

To Jerry A. Colliver, Ph.D., of Southern Illinois University School of Medicine, and Ethan D. Fried, M.D., of the State University of New York, Health Science Center at Brooklyn, for their invaluable help in writing the chapter entitled *Diagnostic Reasoning in Physical Diagnosis* and making it more relevant to today's students of medicine.

To Sheldon Jacobson, M.D., of Mount Sinai School of Medicine, for his many ideas and invaluable help in reviewing the new chapter entitled *The Critically Ill Patient*.

To Mark A. Kosinski, D.P.M., of the New York College of Podiatric Medicine, for his helpful suggestions for improving the chapter entitled *The Musculoskeletal System*.

To Peter B. Liebert, M.D., of Mount Sinai School of Medicine, for his expertise and excellent review of the chapter entitled *The Pregnant Patient*.

To James R. Bonner, M.D., and Dennis W. Boulware, M.D., of the University of Alabama School of Medicine at Birmingham, for their excellent suggestions for improving the text.

To Tracie L. DeMack, of the University of Chicago School of Medicine, for her suggestions for improving the chapter entitled *The Breast* by including the vertical strip/grid method.

To Meryl H. Mendelson, M.D., of Mount Sinai School of Medicine, for bringing me up to date with the current guidelines on precautions to take during the physical examination.

To Gabriele Chryssanthou, C.O., for her help in clarifying the examination and actions of the extraocular muscles.

To the individuals who critiqued the new chapter entitled *Caring for Patients in a Culturally Diverse Society*. I am indebted to all the health-care providers from around the country who have offered many suggestions. In particular, I would like to thank Edward J. Poliandro, Ph.D.; Carol Burnett, M.D.; Gladys M. Ayala, M.D.; Michael Diaz, M.D.; Paula Elbirt-Bender, M.D.; Unsup Kim, M.D.; Taj Mejai, M.D.; Jose Ramírez, Dr. P.H.; Hong-yen Li, Ph.D.; Angela Diaz, M.D.; Jeanet SooHoo; Yuan Ling-Hsu, M.D.; Joseph Goldfarb, Ph.D.; Thirispoon Chithiraporn, M.D.; and Hali Ajumobi, M.D. A special "thank you" to Michael Diaz, M.D., for also taking the time and interest to introduce me to a *botánica* in New York City.

To the many members of the W.B. Saunders Company for their expert assistance and cooperation. In particular, I would like to acknowledge the help of William R. Schmitt, Elizabeth A. Hatter, Scott Filderman, Michael Carcel, Laurie Sander, Pat Morrison, Tracy Baldwin, and Lisa Lambert.

And to my wife, Vivian Hirshaut, M.D., and our daughter, Talia Swartz, for their endless patience. The writing of this book occurred during so much valuable "family time." I am grateful to them for their efforts in reviewing the manuscript so meticulously to correct my grammar and syntax. With this edition, both my wife and daughter became my best critics, editors, and proofreaders. Without their boundless affection, indefatigable help, sustained devotion, and encouragement, this book could never have come to fruition.

MARK H. SWARTZ, M.D.

Photograph Credits

A photograph makes a concept or disease entity more understandable and easier to recognize. As the well-known proverb says, *"A picture is worth a thousand words."* I wish to acknowledge with deep gratitude the following physician colleagues who have graciously allowed me to use slides from their own teaching collections to help clarify the various disease states described in this edition.

Donald E. Hazelrigg, M.D.
Welborn Clinic
Evansville, Indiana
Figures 6–31, 6–47

Raul Fleischmajer, M.D.
Department of Dermatology
Mount Sinai Medical Center
Figure 6–34

Stephen A. Estes, M.D.
University of Cincinnati
Dept. of Dermatology
Cincinnati, Ohio
Figure 6–67

Joseph B. Walsh, M.D.
Department of Ophthalmology
New York Eye and Ear Infirmary
Figures 8–34, 8–41, 8–42, 8–43, 8–44, 8–46, 8–47, 8–49

Alan Friedman, M.D.
Department of Ophthalmology
Mount Sinai Medical Center
Figures 8–48, 8–50, 8–51, 8–52

Michael Hawke, M.D.
Department of Otolaryngology
University of Toronto
Figures 9–3, 9–4, 9–10, 9–15, 9–17, 9–18, 9–24, 9–25, 9–26, 9–27

Phillip A. Wackym, M.D.
Department of Otolaryngology
Mount Sinai Medical Center
Figures 9–30, 9–31, 9–33, 9–34

William Lawson, M.D.
Department of Otolaryngology
Mount Sinai Medical Center
Figures 10–11, 10–15, 10–16, 10–19, 10–22, 10–24C, 10–29, 10–32, 10–37, 10–40, 10–41, 10–42, 10–43, 10–48

Harry Lumerman, D.D.S.
Departments of Pathology and Dentistry
Division of Oral Pathology
Mount Sinai Medical Center
Figures 10–13, 10–14, 10–18, 10–20, 10–21, 10–23, 10–24B, 10–30, 10–33, 10–38, 10–39, 10–44, 10–45, 10–46, 10–49

Neil A. Fenske, M.D.
Dermatology and Cutaneous Surgery
University of South Florida
College of Medicine
Tampa, Florida
Figure 13–1

Mark A. Kosinski, D.P.M.
New York College of Podiatric Medicine
Figures 18–50, 18–51, 18–52, 18–53, 18–61, 18–63, 18–64, 18–67, 18–69A, 18–69B

Deborah L. Shapiro, M.D.
Department of Rheumatology
Mount Sinai Medical Center
Figure 18–59

Katherine Ward, D.P.M.
New York College of Podiatric Medicine
Figures 18–65A, 18–65B

Howard Fox, D.P.M.
New York College of Podiatric Medicine
Figures 18–66, 18–71

Arthur Steinhart, D.P.M.
New York College of Podiatric Medicine
Figure 18–68

Andrew H. Eichenfield, M.D.
Department of Pediatrics
Mount Sinai Medical Center
Figure 22–32

I wish to acknowledge with thanks the authors and publishers of the following books for permission to reprint figures from their texts:

Figure 3–16 from Wensel LO (ed): Acupuncture in Medical Practice. Reston, Reston Publishing Co., Appleton & Lange, 1980.

Figures 6–6, 6–14, 6–25, 6–29, 6–32, 6–38, 6–44, 6–50, 6–58, 6–59, 6–60, 6–70, 6–77, 6–79, 6–80, 6–81, 6–82, 9–19, 10–24A, 12–13, 13–15, 14–5, 14–13, 16–11, 16–14, 16–30, 16–31, and 22–31 from Callen JP, Greer KE, Hood AF, et al: Color Atlas of Dermatology. Philadelphia, W.B. Saunders Co., 1993.

Figures 6–68, 6–84, 6–85, 12–14, 15–5, 18–59, and 18–60 from Lebwohl MG (ed): Atlas of the Skin and Systemic Disease. New York, Churchill Livingstone, 1995.

Figures 6–55, 6–71, 6–72B, 6–72C, 6–72D, 6–72E, 6–73A, 6–73B, 6–78, and 8–15 from Friedman-Kien AE, Cockerell CJ (eds): Color Atlas of AIDS, 2nd ed. Philadelphia, W.B. Saunders Co., 1996.

Figure 7–14 from Wallace C, Siminoski K: The Pemberton sign. Ann Intern Med 125: 568, 1996.

Figures 8–16, 8–21, 8–22, 8–23, 8–25, 8–26, 8–28, 8–29, 11–7, 11–8, and 15–14 from Mir MA: Atlas of Clinical Diagnosis. London, W.B. Saunders Co. Ltd., 1995.

Figures 8–40 and 8–45 from Albert DM, Jakobiec FA: Atlas of Clinical Ophthalmology. Philadelphia, W.B. Saunders Co., 1996.

Figures 10–10, 22–6, 22–8, 22–16, 22–18, 22–29, and 22–30 from Cohen BA: Atlas of Pediatric Dermatology. London, Wolfe Publishing, 1993.

Figures 10–26 and 10–47 from Silverman S: Color Atlas of Oral Manifestations of AIDS, 2nd ed. St. Louis, Mosby–Year Book, 1996.

Figures 16–7, 16–8, 16–9, 16–29, 17–28, and 17–29 from Korting GW: Practical Dermatology of the Genital Region. Philadelphia, W.B. Saunders Co., 1980.

Figure 18–62 from Nzuzi SM: Common nail disorders. Clin Podiatr Med Surg 6:273, 1989.

Figure 18–70 from Kosinski MA, Stewart D: Nail changes associated with systemic disease and vascular insufficiency. Clin Podiatr Med Surg 6:295, 1989.

Figures 24–3A and 24–3B from Henry MC, Stapleton ER: EMT Prehospital Care, 2nd ed. Philadelphia, W.B. Saunders Co., 1997.

Figure 25–3 from Fagan TJ: Nomogram for Bayes' theorem. N Engl J Med 293:257, 1975. Copyright 1975 Massachusetts Medical Society. All rights reserved.

Figures 25–5 and 25–6 from Sackett DL, Haynes RB, Guyatt GH, et al (eds): Clinical Epidemiology: A Basic Science for Clinical Medicine, 2nd ed. New York, Little, Brown & Co., 1991.

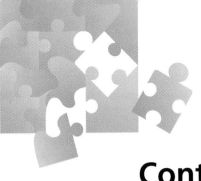

Contents

Epilogue

SECTION I

The Art of
Interviewing

CHAPTER 1

The Interviewer's Questions

What is spoken of as a "clinical picture" is not just a photograph of a man sick in bed; it is an impressionistic painting of the patient surrounded by his home, his work, his relations, his friends, his joys, sorrows, hopes and fears.

Francis Weld Peabody
1881–1927

Basic Principles

The main purpose of an interview is to gather all basic information pertinent to the patient's illness and the patient's adaptation to illness. An assessment of the patient's condition can then be made. An experienced interviewer considers all the aspects of the patient's presentation and then follows the leads that appear to deserve the most attention. The interviewer should also be aware of the influence of social, economic, and cultural factors in shaping the nature of the patient's problems.

Any patient who seeks consultation from a clinician needs to be evaluated in the broadest sense. The clinician must be keenly aware of all clues, subtle or obvious. Although body language is very important, the spoken word still remains the most important diagnostic tool in medicine. For this reason, the art of talking and listening continues to be the central part of the doctor-patient interaction. Once all the clues from the history have been gathered, the assimilation of the clues into an ultimate diagnosis is relatively easy.

Communication is the key to a successful interview. The interviewer must be able to ask questions of the patient freely. These questions must always be easily understood and keyed to the medical sophistication of the patient. If necessary, slang words describing certain conditions may be used in order to facilitate communication and avoid misunderstanding.

For any patient who speaks another language, it is important that the clinician seek the help of a trained medical *interpreter*. Unless fluent in the patient's language and culture, the clinician should always use an interpreter. The interpreter can be thought of as a bridge, spanning the ideas, mores, biases, emotions, and problems of the clinician and patient. The communication is very much influenced by the extent to which the patient, the interpreter, and the clinician share the same understanding and beliefs regarding the patient's problem. The best interpreters are those who are familiar with the patient's culture. The interpreter's presence, however, adds an additional variable in the clinician-patient relationship. For example, a family member who translates for the patient may alter the meaning of what has been said. When a family member is the interpreter, the patient may be reluctant to provide information about sensitive issues, such as sexual history or substance abuse. It would be advantageous, therefore, to have an objective observer act as an interpreter. On occasion, the patient may request that a family member be the interpreter. In such a case, respect the patient's wishes. Although they are helpful in times of emergency, friends and strangers should be avoided as their translation skills are unknown. Confidentiality is another concern. The clinician should, however, master a number of key words and phrases in several common languages in order to gain the respect and confidence of the patient. When using an interpreter, remember the following guidelines:

1. Choose an individual trained in medical terminology
2. Choose a person of the same sex as the patient and of comparable age
3. Talk with the interpreter beforehand to establish an approach
4. When speaking to the patient, watch the patient, not the interpreter
5. Do not expect a word-for-word translation
6. Ask the interpreter about the patient's fears and expectations
7. Use short questions

8. Use simple language
9. Keep your explanations brief
10. Avoid questions using "if," "would," and "could" because these require nuances of language
11. Avoid idiomatic expressions

When speaking with the patient, the interviewer must determine not only the main medical problems but also the patient's reaction to the illness. This is of great importance. How has the illness affected the patient? How has he or she reacted to it? What impact has it had on the family? work? social life?

The interview is best conducted when the interviewer is cheerful, friendly, and genuinely concerned about the patient. This type of approach is clearly better than that of the interviewer who acts like a nosy busybody shooting questions from a standard list at the poor defenseless patient. Bombarding patients with rapid-fire questions is a technique that should not be used.

In the beginning, the patient will bring up the subjects that are easiest to discuss. The more painful experiences can be elicited by tactful questioning. The novice interviewer needs to gain experience to feel comfortable asking questions about subjects that are more painful, delicate, or unpleasant. Timing of such questions is critical.

A cardinal principle of interviewing is to permit patients to express their story in their own words. The manner in which patients tell their story reveals much about the nature of the patient's illness. Careful observation of a patient's facial expressions as well as body movements may provide valuable nonverbal clues. The interviewer may also use body language such as a smile, nod, silence, hand gesture, or questioning look to encourage the patient to continue the story.

Listening without interruption is important and requires skill. If given the chance, patients often disclose their problems spontaneously. Interviewers need to *hear* what is being said. All too often, an interview may fail to reveal all the clues because the interviewer didn't listen to the patient. Several studies have shown that clinicians commonly do not listen to their patients. They are abrupt, appear uninterested in the patients' distress, and are prone to control the interview.

The best clinical interview focuses on the patient, not on the clinician's agenda. An important rule for improved interviewing is to *listen more, talk less, and interrupt infrequently.* Interrupting disrupts the patient's train of thought. Allow the patient, at least in part, to control the interview.

Interviewers should be attentive as to how patients use their words to conceal or reveal their thoughts and history. Interviewers should be wary of quick, very positive statements such as, "Everything's fine!," "I'm very happy," or "No problems." If interviewers have reason to doubt these statements, they may respond by saying, "Is everything really as fine as it could be?"

If the history given is vague, the interviewer may use direct questioning. Asking "how," "where," or "when" is generally more effective than "why," which tends to put patients on the defensive. The interviewer must be particularly careful not to disapprove of certain aspects of the patient's story. Different cultures have different mores, and the interviewer must listen without any suggestion of prejudice.

Always treat the patient with respect. Do not contradict or impose your moral standards on the patient. Knowledge of the patient's social and economic background will make the interview progress more smoothly.

The interviewer's appearance will influence the success of the interview. Patients have an image of clinicians. Neatness counts. A slovenly interviewer might be considered immature or careless, and his or her competence may be questioned from the start. Surveys of patients have indicated that patients prefer medical personnel to dress in white coats and to wear shoes instead of sneakers.

Clinicians must be compassionate and interested in the patient's story. They must create an atmosphere of openness in which the patient will feel comfortable and will be encouraged to describe the problem. These guidelines will set a foundation for effective interviewing.

As a rule, patients like to respond to questions in a way that will satisfy the clinician in order to gain approval. This may represent fear on the part of the patients. The clinician should be aware of this phenomenon.

The interviewer must be able to question the patient about subjects that may be distressing or embarrassing to the interviewer or the patient or both. Frequently, the interviewer may have more of a problem than the patient with questions related to sexuality, alcoholism, death, or secrets. Answers to many routine questions may cause embarrassment to interviewers and leave them speechless. Therefore, there is a tendency to avoid such questions. The interviewer's ability to be open and frank about such topics will promote the chances of discussion in these areas.

Very often, patients feel comfortable discussing what an interviewer would consider antisocial behavior. This may include drug addiction, unlawful actions, or "aberrations" of sexual behavior. Interviewers must be careful not to pass judgment on this "unusual" behavior. Should an interviewer pass judgment, the patient may reject him or her as an unsuitable listener. Acceptance, however, will indicate to the patient a feeling that the interviewer is sensitive. It may be appropriate for the interviewer to nod and say, "I understand." (Some patients might interpret the "I understand" statement as a signal that the interviewer has heard enough; it should be used with care.) It is also important not to imply approval of behavior; this may reinforce behavior that is actually destructive.

Follow the "rule of five vowels" when conducting an interview. The rule states that a good interview contains the elements of *a*udition, *e*valuation, *i*nquiry, *o*bservation, and *u*nderstanding. *Audition* reminds the interviewer to listen carefully to the patient's story. *Evaluation* refers to sorting out relevant from irrelevant data and to the importance of the data. *Inquiry* leads the interviewer to probe into significant areas requiring more clarification. *Observation* refers to the importance of nonverbal communication, regardless of what is said. *Understanding* the patient's concerns and apprehensions enables the interviewer to play a more empathetic role.

Speech patterns, referred to as paralanguage components, are relevant to the interview. By manipulating the intonation, rate, emphasis, and volume of speech, both the interviewer and the patient can convey significant emotional meaning to their dialogue. By controlling intonation, the interviewer or patient can change the entire meaning of words. Because many of these features are not under conscious control, they may provide an important statement about the patient's personal attributes. These audible parameters are useful in detecting a patient's anxiety or depression, as well as other affective and emotional states. The interviewer's use of a warm, soft tone is soothing to the patient and enhances the communication.

A broad interest in body language has evolved. This type of nonverbal communication, in association with spoken language, can provide a more total picture of the patient's behavior. It is well known that the interviewer may learn more about the patient from the way in which the patient tells the story than from the story itself. A patient who strikes a fist on a table while talking is dramatically emphasizing what has been said. A patient who moves about in a chair and looks embarrassed is uncomfortable. A frown indicates annoyance or disapproval. The patient who slips his wedding band on and off may be ambivalent about his marriage. A palm placed over the heart asserts sincerity or credibility. Many people rub or cover their eyes when they refuse to accept something that is pointed out. When patients disapprove of a statement made by the interviewer but restrain themselves from speaking, they may start to remove dust or lint from their clothing. Lack of comprehension is indicated by knitted brows.

Full interpretation of body language can be made only in the context of the patient's cultural and ethnic background, because different cultures have different standards of nonverbal behavior. Arabic and Asian patients often speak with dropped eyelids. This type of body language would indicate depression or lack of attentiveness in a patient from the United States. The interviewer may use facial expression to facilitate the interview. An appearance of attention demonstrates an interest in what the patient is describing. Attentiveness on the part of the interviewer is also indicated by leaning slightly forward toward the patient.

Touching the patient can also be very useful. Touch can communicate warmth, affection, caring, and understanding. Many factors, including gender and cultural background as well as the location of the touch, influence the response to the touch. Although there are wide variations within each cultural group, Latinos tend to be a contact group, whereas the British tend to be a noncontact group. Scandinavians and Anglo-Saxon Americans are in the middle of this spectrum. In general, the older the patient, the more important is touch. Appropriate placement of a hand on a patient's shoulder suggests support. The interviewer who walks with good posture to a patient's bedside can hope to gain the patient's respect and confidence. The interviewer who maintains eye contact with the patient conveys interest in the patient.

In this age of rapid scientific and biomedical advancements, a new problem has arisen. With the advent of the latest technology in the medical world, there has been a depersonalization of the doctor-patient relationship. Both doctor and patient may feel increasingly neglected, rejected, or abused. Patients may feel dehumanized upon admission to the hospital. Many find themselves in a strange environment. They may be apprehensive because they have a problem that their health-care provider considers too serious to be treated on an outpatient basis. The future is filled with uncertainty. The patient admitted to the hospital is stripped of clothing and many times, of dentures, glasses, hearing aids, and other personal belongings. This serves to lower the morale of the patient. At the same time, physicians may be pressed for time, overworked, and sometimes unable to cope with everyday pressures. They may become irritable and pay inadequate attention to the patient's story. They may eventually come to rely on the technical results and reports. This failure to communicate undermines the doctor-patient relationship.

Inexperienced interviewers not only must learn about the patient's problems but also must gain insight into their *own* feelings, attitudes, and vulnerabilities. Such introspection will enhance the self-image of the interviewer and will result in the interviewers being perceived by the patient as a more careful and compassionate human being to whom the patient can turn in time of crisis.

A good interviewing session will determine what patients comprehend about their own health problems. What do the *patients* think is wrong with them? Do not accept merely the diagnosis. Inquire specifically as to what the patients think is happening. What kind of impact does the illness bear on work, family, or financial situation? Is there a feeling of loss of control? Do the patients feel guilt about their own illness? Do the patients think they will die? By pondering these questions, you will learn much about patients, and the patients will realize that you have an interest in them as whole persons, not merely as statistics among the admissions to the hospital.

The literature indicates that malpractice suits have increased at an alarming rate. The good doctor-patient relationship is probably the most important factor in preventing malpractice claims. Most malpractice litigation is the result of a deterioration of the traditional doctor-patient relationship rather than the result of true medical negligence. The patient is dissatisfied with and may have lost respect for the physician. From the patient's point of view, the most serious barriers to a good relationship are the physician's lack of time, seeming lack of concern, and failure to inform the patient about what the patient needs to know about his or her illness. Failure to discuss the patient's illness and treatment in understandable terms is viewed as a rejection by the patient. A doctor-patient relationship based on honesty and understanding is thus recognized as essential for good medical practice and the well-being of the patient.

It is sometimes difficult for a novice interviewer to remember that there is no need to try to make a diagnosis out of every bit of information obtained from the interview. Accept all the clues and then later work with them in trying to establish a diagnosis.

If during the interview you cannot answer a question, do not. You can always act as the patient's advocate; listen to the question and later find someone who can provide an appropriate answer.

In summary, the medical interview is a blend of the cognitive and technical skills of the interviewer and the feelings and personalities of both the patient and the interviewer. The interview should be flexible and spontaneous and not interrogative. When utilized correctly, it is a powerful diagnostic tool.

Symptoms and Signs

The clinician must be able to elicit and recognize a wide variety of symptoms and signs. *Symptom* refers to what the patient feels. Symptoms are described by the patient to clarify the nature of the illness. Shortness of breath, chest pain, nausea, diarrhea, and double vision are all symptoms. These labels help the patient to describe the discomfort or distress that he or she is experiencing. Symptoms are *not* absolute; they are influenced by culture, intelligence, and socioeconomic background. As an example, consider the symptom of pain: patients have different thresholds of pain. This will be discussed further in Chapter 3.

Constitutional refers to those symptoms commonly occurring with problems in any of the body systems, such as fever, chills, weight loss, or excessive sweating.

Sign refers to that which the examiner finds. Signs can be observed and quantified. Certain signs are also symptoms. For example, a patient may describe episodes of wheezing; this is a symptom. In addition, an examiner may hear wheezing during a patient's physical examination; this is a sign.

The major task of the interviewer is to sort out the symptoms and signs associated with a specific illness. A major advantage that the seasoned interviewer has over the beginner is a better understanding of the pathophysiology of disease states. The novice operates under the limitation of not knowing all the signs and symptoms of the associated diseases. With experience and education, the novice will recognize the combination of symptoms and signs as they relate to the underlying illness. For any given disease, there is usually a clustering of symptoms and signs that tend to occur together. When there is only an isolated symptom, the interviewer must be careful in making a definitive assessment.

Conducting an Interview

Getting Started

The diagnostic process begins at the first moment of meeting. The interviewer should greet the patient by name, make eye contact, shake hands firmly, and smile. The interviewer may wish to say,

> *"Mr. Smith, I'm John Jones, a medical student (or student doctor) at this hospital. I've been asked to interview and examine you."*

It is appropriate to address the patient by his or her correct title, e.g., Mr., Mrs., Dr., Ms. A formal address clarifies the professional nature of the interview. Terms such as "dear" or "grandpa" are *not* to be used.

The patient may address the interviewer as Mr. Jones or could elect to call the interviewer by the first name. The interviewer now has two choices. The preferred choice would be to disregard the patient's casual form of address. It is not correct at this time for the interviewer to address the patient by his or her first name. Furthermore, the interviewer might say,

> *"I would prefer if you would call me Mr. Jones."*

This approach would tend to formalize the interview but might make the patient ill at ease.

If the patient is having a meal, ask if you may return when he or she has finished eating. If the patient is using a urinal or bedpan, allow privacy. Do not begin an interview in this setting. If the patient has a visitor, you may inquire whether the *patient* wishes the visitor to stay. Do not assume that the visitor is a family member. Allow the patient to introduce the person to you.

The interview can be helped or hindered by the physical setting in which the interview is conducted. If possible, the interview should take place in a quiet, well-lit room. Unfortunately, most hospital rooms do not afford such luxury. The teaching hospital with four patients in a room is rarely conducive for good human interactions. Therefore, make the best of the existing environment. The curtains should be drawn around the patient's bed to create privacy. You may request that the volume of neighboring patients' radios or televisions be turned down. Lights and window shades can be adjusted to eliminate excessive glare or shade. Arrange the patient's bed light so that the patient does not feel as if under interrogation.

You should make the patient as comfortable as possible. If the patient's eyeglasses, hearing aid, or dentures were removed, ask whether he or she would like to use them. It is often useful to use your stethoscope as a hearing aid for hearing-impaired patients without other devices. The eartips should be placed in the ears of the patient, and you can use the diaphragm as a microphone. The patient may be in a chair or lying in bed. Allow the patient the choice of position. This makes patients feel that you are interested and concerned about them, and it allows them some control over the interview. If the patient is in bed, it is a nice gesture to ask whether the pillows should be arranged to make him or her more comfortable.

Normally, the interviewer and patient should be seated comfortably at the same level. Sometimes, it is useful to have the patient sitting higher than the interviewer to allow the patient to have the visual advantage. In this position, the patient may find it easier to open up to questions. The interviewer should sit in a chair directly facing the patient in order to make good eye contact. Sitting on the bed is too familiar and not appropriate. It is generally preferred that the interviewer sit at a distance of about 3–4 feet from the patient. Distances greater than 5 feet are impersonal, and distances closer than 3 feet interfere with the patient's "private space." The interviewer should sit in a relaxed position without crossing arms across the chest. The crossed-arms position is not appropriate as this body language projects an attitude of superiority and may interfere with the progress of the interview.

Once the introduction has been made, you may begin the interview by asking a general, open-ended question such as "What problem has brought you to the hospital?" This type of opening remark allows the patient to speak first. The interviewer can then determine the patient's *chief complaint* or the problem that is regarded as paramount. If the patient says, "Haven't you read my records?" it is correct to say, "No, I've been asked to interview you without any prior information." Alternatively, the interviewer could say, "I would like to hear your story in your own words."

The Narrative

Novice interviewers are often worried about remembering the patient's history. It is poor form to write extensive notes during the interview. Attention should be focused more on what the person is saying and less on the written word. In addition, by taking notes, the interviewer cannot observe the facial expressions and body language that are so important to the patient's story. A pad of paper may be used to jot down important dates or names during the session.

After the introductory question, the interviewer should proceed to questions related to the chief complaint. These should naturally evolve into questions related to the other formal parts of the medical history, such as the present illness, past illnesses, social and educational history, and review of body systems. Patients should largely be allowed to conduct the narrative in their own way. The interviewer must select certain aspects about which further details must be explored and guide the patient toward them. Overdirection is to be avoided, because this will stifle the interview and prevent important points from being clarified.

"Small talk" is a very useful method of enhancing the narrative. Small talk is neither random nor pointless, and studies in conversation analysis have indicated that it is actually useful in communication. It has been shown that during conversations, the individual who tells a humorous anecdote is the one who is in "power." For example, if an interviewer interjects a humorous remark during an interview and the patient laughs, the interviewer is "in control." If the patient does not laugh, the patient may take control.

Be aware of the patient who asks, "Let me ask you a hypothetical question" or "I have a friend with _____, what do you think about _____?" In each case, the question is probably related to the patient's own concerns.

A patient often uses words such as "uh," "ah," and "well" to avoid unpleasant topics. It is natural for a patient to delay talking about an unpleasant situation or condition. Pauses between words as well as the use of the words cited provide a means for the patient to put off discussing a painful subject.

When patients use terms such as "somewhat," "a little," "fair," "reasonably well," "sometimes," "rarely," or "average," the interviewer must ask for clarification. Precise communication is always desirable, and these terms have been shown to have significant variations in meaning.

The interviewer should be alert for subtle clues from the patient to guide the interview further. There are a variety of techniques to encourage and sustain the narrative. These guidelines consist of verbal and nonverbal facilitation, reflection, confrontation, interpretation, and directed questioning. These techniques are discussed later in this chapter.

The Closing

It is important that the interviewer pace the interview so that adequate time will be left for any patient questions and the physical examination. About 5 minutes before the end of the interview, the interviewer should begin to close the important issues that were discussed.

By the conclusion of the interview, the interviewer should have a clear impression of the reason(s) why the patient sought medical help, the history of the present illness, the patient's past medical history, and an understanding of the patient's social and economic position. At this time, the interviewer may wish to say, "You've been very helpful. I would now like to take a few notes." If any part of the history needs clarification, this is the time to obtain it. The interviewer may wish to summarize for the patient the most important parts of the history to help illuminate the important points made.

If the patient asks for an opinion, it is prudent for the novice interviewer to answer, "I am a medical student. I think it would be best to ask your doctor that question." You have not provided the patient with the answer that he or she was seeking; however, you have not jeopardized the existing doctor-patient relationship by possibly giving either the wrong information or a different opinion.

At the conclusion, it is polite to encourage the patient to discuss any additional problems or ask any questions. "Is there anything else that you would like to tell me that I have not already asked?" "Are there any questions you might like to ask?" Usually, all possible avenues of discussion have been exhausted, but these remarks allow the patient "the final say." At this time, you, the interviewer, can thank the patient and tell him or her that you are ready to begin the physical examination.

Basic Interviewing Techniques

The successful interview is smooth and spontaneous. The interviewer must be aware of subtleties and be able to pick up on these clues. The successful interviewer sustains the interview. There are several techniques that are used every day to encourage someone to continue speaking. This section discusses those interviewing techniques. Each of them has its limitations, and not all of them are used in every interview.

Types of Questions

The secret of effective interviewing lies in the art of questioning. The wording of the question is often less important than the tone of voice used to ask it. In general, questions that stimulate the patient to talk freely are preferred.

Open-Ended Questions

Open-ended questions are used to ask the patient for general information. This type of question is most useful in opening up the interview or for changing the area to be discussed. An open-ended question allows the patient to tell his or her story spontaneously and does not presuppose a specific answer. It can be very useful to allow the patient to "ramble on." Too much rambling, however, must be controlled by the interviewer in a sensitive but firm manner. This freedom of speech should obviously be avoided with the overtalkative patient, whereas it should be utilized often with the silent patient. Examples of open-ended questions are the following:

> *"What kind of problem are you having?"*
> *"Are you having stomach pain? Tell me about it."*
> *"How was your health before your heart attack?"*
> *"Can you describe your feelings when you get the pain?"*

Direct Questions

After a period of open-ended questioning, the interviewer should direct the attention to specific facts learned during the open-ended questioning period. These *direct questions* serve to clarify the areas and add detail to the story. This type of question gives the patient little room for explanation or qualification. A direct question can usually be answered in one word or a brief sentence. For example:

> *"Where does it hurt?"*
> *"When do you get the burning?"*
> *"How do you compare this pain with your ulcer pain?"*

Care must be taken to avoid asking direct questions in a manner that might bias the response.

Symptoms are gathered into the classic seven elements: *bodily location, quality, quantity, chronology, setting, aggravating* (or *alleviating*) *factors,* and *associated manifestations.* These elements may be used as a framework to clarify the illness. Examples include the following:

Bodily Location

"Where in your back?"
"Can you tell me where you feel the pain?"
"Do you feel it anywhere else?"

Quality

"What does it feel like?"
"What do you mean by 'a sticking pain'?"
"Was it sharp, dull, or aching?"

Quantity

"How many sanitary napkins do you use?"
"What do you mean by 'a lot'?"
"What kind of effect does the pain have on your work?"
"How does the pain compare with the time you broke your leg?"
"How does it compare with childbirth?"

Chronology

"When did you first notice it?"
"How long did it last?"
"Have you had the pain since that time?"
"Then what happened?"
"Have you noticed that it is worse during your menstrual period?"
"When you get the pain, is it steady, or does it change?"

Setting

"Does it ever occur at rest?"
"Do you ever get the pain when you are emotionally upset?"
"Where were you when it occurred?"

Aggravating Factors

"What seems to bring on the pain?"
"Have you noticed that it occurs at a certain time of day?"
"Is there anything else besides exercise that makes it worse?"

Alleviating Factors

"What do you do to make it better?"
"Does lying quietly in bed help you?"

Associated Manifestations

"Do you ever have nausea with the pain?"
"Have you noticed other changes that happen when you start to sweat?"
"Before you get the headache, do you ever experience a strange taste or smell?"

■ Question Types to Avoid

There are several types of questions that are to be avoided. The *yes-no* question is one that when answered with a "yes" leaves the interviewer unsure of its true meaning. For example,

Interviewer "Have you been taking the medicine?"

Patient "Yes."

The "yes" can mean (1) the patient *is* taking the medicine, (2) the patient wants to please the interviewer even if he or she has not been taking the medicine, (3) the patient takes the medicine but not according to the directions, or (4) the patient wants to avoid the subject.

Another type of question to avoid is the *suggestive* one. This type provides the answer to the question. For example,

> *"Do you feel the pain in your left arm when you get it in your chest?"*

A better way to ask the same question would be,

> *"When you get the pain in your chest, do you notice it anywhere else?"*

The *why* question carries tones of accusation. This type of question almost always asks a patient to account for his or her behavior and tends to put him or her on the defensive. For example,

> *"Why haven't you taken the medication?"*
> *"Why did you wait so long to call me?"*

The use of the *multiple question* is likewise to be avoided. In this type of question, there is more than one point of inquiry. The patient can easily become confused and respond incorrectly. For example,

> *"How many brothers and sisters do you have, and has any one of them ever had asthma, pneumonia, or tuberculosis?"*

Questions should be concise and easily understandable. The context should be free of medical jargon. Frequently, novice interviewers try to use their new vocabulary of medicine. They may at times respond to the patient with technical terms, leaving the patient feeling confused or put down. This use of technical terms is sometimes called "doctorese." For example,

> *"You seem to have a homonymous hemianopsia."*
> *"We perform Papanicolaou smears to check for carcinoma in-situ."*

Medical terminology, as a rule, should not be used in conversations with patients. Technical terms scare patients. Every medical and nursing student understands the term *heart failure*. A patient might interpret this term as failure of the heart to pump: i.e., cardiac standstill, or death. Although patients should be given only as much information as they can handle, adequate explanations must always be given. A partial explanation will leave the patient confused and fearful.

A *leading* or *biased* question carries a suggestion of the kind of response the interviewer is looking for. For example, "You haven't used any types of drugs, have you?" suggests that the interviewer disapproves of the patient's use of drugs. If the patient has used drugs, he or she may not admit to it under this line of questioning. The leading question almost invites a particular answer. For example: "Did you notice that the pain came on after you vomited?"

In addition to avoiding certain types of questions, the interviewer should avoid certain situations. Patients may respond to a question in a manner not expected by the interviewer. This could potentially leave a period of unexpected silence. This "stumped silence" can be interpreted by the patient in a variety of ways. The interviewer must be able to respond quickly in such instances, even if it means broaching another topic.

False reassurances restore a patient's confidence but ignore the reality of the situation. Telling a patient that "surgery is always successful" clearly discounts the known morbidity and mortality rates associated with it. The patient *wants* to hear what has been said, but this may be a false reassurance.

If a patient suggests that a test not be performed, perhaps because of an underlying fear of the test, the interviewer should never respond by stating, "I'm the doctor. I'll make the decisions." The interviewer should recognize the anxiety and handle the response from that point of view.

Silence

This technique is most useful for silent patients. Silence should never be used with overtalkative patients, because letting them "have the floor" would not allow the interviewer to control the interview. This difficult type of communication, when used correctly, can indicate interest and support. Silence on the part of the patient can be related to hostility, shyness, or embarrassment. The interviewer should remain silent with direct eye contact and attentiveness. The interviewer may lean forward and even nod. After no more than 2 minutes of silence, the interviewer may say,

"What are you thinking about?"
"You were saying. . . ."
"These things are hard to talk about."
"You were about to say. . . ."

If the patient remains silent, another method of sustaining the interview must be chosen.

The interviewer must utilize silence when the patient becomes overwhelmed by emotion. This act allows the patient to release some of the tension evoked by the history and indicates to the patient that it is "OK" to cry. Handing the patient a box of tissues is a supportive gesture. It is inappropriate for the interviewer to say, "Don't cry" or "Pull yourself together," because these statements imply that the patient is wasting the interviewer's time or that it is shameful to show emotions.

It is important to use silence correctly. The interviewer who remains silent, becomes fidgety, reviews notes, or makes a facial expression of evaluation will inhibit the patient. The patient may perceive the frequent use of silence by the interviewer as aloofness or a lack of knowledge.

Facilitation

Facilitation is a technique of verbal or nonverbal communication that encourages a patient to continue speaking but does not direct him or her to a topic. A common verbal facilitation is "Uh huh." Other examples of verbal facilitations include "Go on," "Tell me more about that," "And then?," and "Mmmm."

An important nonverbal facilitation is nodding the head or a hand gesture to continue. Moving toward the patient connotes interest. Be careful not to nod too much as this may convey approval in situations in which approval may not be intended.

Often, a puzzled expression can be used as a nonverbal facilitation to indicate, "I don't understand."

Confrontation

Confrontation is a response based on an observation by the interviewer that points out to the patient something striking about the patient's behavior or previous statement. This interviewing technique directs the patient's attention to something of which he or she may or may not be aware. The confrontation may be either a statement or a question. For example,

"You look upset."
"Is there any reason why you always look away when you talk to me?"
"You're angry."
"You sound uncomfortable about it."
"Why are you so silent?"
"You look as though you are going to cry."

Confrontation is particularly useful in encouraging the patient to continue the narrative when there are subtle clues given. By confronting the patient, the interviewer may be able to permit the patient to explain the problem further. Confrontation is also useful to clarify discrepancies in the history.

Confrontation must be used with care; excessive use is considered impolite and overbearing. If correctly utilized, however, confrontation can be a very powerful technique. Suppose a patient is describing a symptom of chest pain. By observing the patient, you notice that there are now tears in his or her eyes. By saying sympathetically, "You look very upset," you are encouraging the patient to express emotions.

Interpretation

Interpretation is a type of confrontation that is based on inference rather than on observation. The interviewer "interprets" the patient's behavior, encouraging the patient to observe his or her own role in the problem. The interviewer must first fully understand the clues that the patient has given before he or she can offer an interpretation. The interviewer must look for signs of underlying fear or anxiety that may be indicated by other symptoms, such as recurrent pain, dizziness, headaches, or weakness. Once these underlying fears have been discovered the patient may be led to the recognition of the inciting event in future interviews. Interpretation frequently opens new lines of communication previously not recognized. Examples are the following:

"You seem to be quite happy about that."
"Sounds like you're scared."
"Are you afraid you've done something wrong?"
"Your dizziness appears to be aggravated by your arguments with your wife."

Interpretation can demonstrate support and understanding if used correctly.

Reflection

Reflection is a response that mirrors or echoes that which has just been expressed by the patient. The tone of the voice is important in reflection. The intonation of the words may indicate entirely different meanings. For example,

Patient: "I was so sick that I haven't worked since January 1996."

Response: "Haven't worked since *1996?*"

In this example, the emphasis should be on "1996?" This asks the patient to further describe the conditions that did not allow him or her to work. If the emphasis is incorrectly placed on "worked," the interviewer immediately puts the patient on the defensive, implying "What did you do with your time?" Although generally very useful, reflection can hamper the progress of the interview if used improperly.

Support

Support is a response that indicates an interest in or an understanding of the patient. Supportive remarks promote a feeling of security in the doctor-patient relationship. A supportive response might be, "I understand." An important time to use support is immediately after a patient has expressed strong feelings. The use of support when a patient suddenly begins to cry strengthens the doctor-patient relationship. Two important subgroups of support are *reassurance* and *empathy*.

■ Reassurance

Reassurance is a response that conveys to the patient that the interviewer understands what has been expressed. It may also indicate that the interviewer approves of something the patient has done or thought. It can be a powerful tool, but false reassurance can be devastating. Examples of reassurance are the following:

"That's wonderful. I'm delighted that you started in the rehabilitation program at the hospital!"
"You're improving steadily!"

The use of reassurance is particularly helpful when the patient seems upset or frightened. Reassurance must always be based on fact.

■ Empathy

Empathy is a response that recognizes the patient's feeling and does not criticize it. It is understanding, not an emotional state of sympathy. The empathetic response is saying, "I'm with you." The use of empathy can strengthen the doctor-patient relationship and allow for the interview to flow smoothly. Examples of empathy are the following:

"I'm sure your daughter's problem has given you much anxiety."
"The death of someone so close to you is hard to take."
"I guess that this has been kind of a silent fear all of your life."
"You must have been very sad."
"I know it's not easy for you . . . I'm delighted to see that you're trying to eat everything on your tray."

The last example illustrates an important point: giving credit to patients to encourage *their* role in their own improvement.

Empathetic responses can also be nonverbal. An understanding nod is an empathetic response. The interviewer who places a hand on the shoulder of an upset patient communicates support. The interviewer understands and appreciates how the patient feels without actually showing any emotion.

Format of the History

The information obtained by the interviewer is organized into a comprehensive statement about the patient's health. The interviewer should proceed through each of these major sections in a logical sequence and direct the questions relevantly to each area. The format of the history is as follows:

- Source and reliability
- Chief complaint
- History of the present illness
- Past medical history
- Occupational and environmental history
- Biographic information
- Family history
- Psychosocial history
- Sexual, reproductive, and gynecologic history
- Review of systems

Source and Reliability

The *source* is usually the patient. If the patient requires a translator, the source is the patient and the translator. If family members help in the interview, their names should be included in a single sentence statement. The reliability of the interview should be assessed.

Chief Complaint

The *chief complaint* is the patient's brief statement explaining why he or she sought medical attention. It is the answer to the question, "What is the problem that brought you to the hospital?" In the written history, it is frequently a quoted statement of the patient; for example,

> *"Chest pain for the past 5 hours"*
> *"Terrible nausea and vomiting for 2 days"*
> *"Headache for the last week, on and off"*
> *"Routine examination for school"*

Patients sometimes use medical terms. The interviewer must ask the patient to define such terms to ascertain what the patient means by them.

History of Present Illness

The *history of the present illness* refers to the recent changes in health that led the patient to seek medical attention at this time. It describes the information relevant to the chief complaint. It should answer the questions what, when, how, where, which, who, and why.

Chronology is the most practical framework within which to organize the history. It enables the interviewer to comprehend the sequence of the development of the underlying pathologic process easily. It is in this section that the interviewer gathers all necessary information, starting with the first symptoms of the present illness and following its progression to the present day. It is important to verify that the patient was entirely well before the earliest symptom to establish the beginning of the current illness clearly. Patients often do not remember when a symptom developed. If the patient is uncertain about the presence of a symptom at a certain time, the interviewer may be able to relate it to an important or memorable event. For example, "Did you have the pain during Christmas vacation?" In this part of the interview, mainly open-ended questions are asked of the patient, as these afford the greatest opportunity to describe the history.

Past Medical History

The *past medical history* consists of the overall assessment of the patient's health before the present illness. It includes all of the following:

- General state of health
- Past illnesses
- Injuries
- Hospitalizations
- Surgery
- Allergies
- Immunizations
- Substance abuse
- Diet
- Sleep patterns
- Current medications

As an introduction to the past medical history, the interviewer may ask, "How has your health been in the past?" If the patient doesn't elaborate about specific illnesses but says only, "Excellent" or "Fair," for example, the interviewer might ask, "What does excellent [fair] mean to you?" Direct questioning is appropriate and allows the interviewer to focus on pertinent points that need further elaboration.

The record of *past illnesses* should include a statement of childhood and adult problems. The recording of childhood illnesses is obviously more important for the pediatric and young adult interview. All patients should nevertheless be asked about measles, mumps, whooping cough, rheumatic fever, chickenpox, polio, and scarlet fever. Older patients may respond, "I really don't remember." It is important to remember that a "diagnosis" given to the interviewer by a patient should never be considered absolute. Even if the patient had been evaluated by a competent physician in a reputable medical center, the patient may have misunderstood the information given.

The patient should be asked about any prior *injuries* or accidents. The type of injury and the date are important to record.

All *hospitalizations* must be indicated, if not already described. These include admissions for both medical and psychiatric illnesses. The interviewer should not be embarrassed to ask specifically about psychiatric illness. Psychiatric illness *is* a medical problem. Interviewer embarrassment will inevitably lead to patient embarrassment and will reinforce the "shame" associated with a psychiatric illness. Students should learn to ask direct questions in a sensitive manner. The interviewer might ask, "Have you ever been in therapy or counseling?" or "What nervous or emotional problems have you had?"

All *surgical procedures* should be specified. The type of procedure, date, hospital, and surgeon's name should be obtained, if possible.

All *allergies* should be described. These include environmental, ingestible, or drug-related. The interviewer should seek specificity and verification of the patient's allergic response. "How do you know you're allergic?" "What kind of problem did you have when you took _____?" The symptoms of an allergy (e.g., rashes, itching, anaphylaxis) should be clearly indicated.

It is important to determine the *immunization history* of all patients. Tetanus-diphtheria immunity is present in fewer than 25% of adults, and fewer than 25% of targeted groups receive influenza vaccine yearly.

Tetanus and diphtheria are preventable, and the current recommendation is to use the combined toxoid whenever either immunization is considered. Any patient who has never received this toxoid receives an initial injection and follow-ups at 1 and 6 to 12 months. A booster dose is required every 10 years.

All patients with chronic cardiovascular, pulmonary, metabolic, renal, or hematologic disorders and patients with immunosuppression should be vaccinated yearly against influenza. Patients older than the age of 65 years should also receive the vaccine.

Indications for the pneumococcal polysaccharide vaccine are similar to those for the influenza vaccine. In addition, patients with multiple myeloma, lymphoma, alcoholism, cirrhosis, and functional or anatomic asplenia should receive the vaccine. This vaccine usually provides lifelong immunity. Revaccination every 6 years is necessary only in asplenic patients because they are at high risk for pneumococcal infection.

Hepatitis B vaccine should be given to all health-care providers, staff of institutions for the developmentally disabled, intravenous drug abusers, males with homosexual behavior, patients with multiple sexual partners, hemodialysis patients, sexual partners of hepatitis B carriers, and hemophiliacs. Complete immunization necessitates three injections: an initial one and follow-ups at 1 and 6 months. Booster doses are not required. For best results, high-risk patients (especially medical, dental, and nursing students) should receive immunization before possible exposure.

Haemophilus influenzae type B vaccine is now used routinely in children to prevent invasive *H. influenzae* diseases.

There was a 75% decrease in 1992 over 1991 in the number of cases of measles, mumps, and rubella (MMR), presumably because of the use of the MMR vaccine. This vaccine is now typically given in childhood, but it should be given to adult health-care providers who have not had the diseases. Because the vaccine is a live vaccine, it should not be given to pregnant patients, those with generalized malignancies, those receiving steroid therapy, those with active tuberculosis, or those receiving antimetabolites.

A careful review of any *substance abuse* by the patient is included in the past medical history. Substance abuse includes cigarette smoking and use of alcohol and "recreational drugs." The interviewer should determine whether the patient smokes and for how long. Ask "Do you use nicotine in any form: cigarettes, cigars, chewing tobacco?" A *pack-year* is the number of years a patient has smoked cigarettes multiplied by the number of packs per day. A patient who has smoked two packs of cigarettes a day for the past 25 years has a smoking history of 50 pack-years.

The history of alcohol consumption and dependency should be integrated into the history immediately after the interviewer inquires about less threatening subjects such as cigarettes. It is acceptable to broach the topic of alcoholism by asking directly, "Do you drink alcohol, including wine, wine coolers, beer, or distilled spirits?" The interviewer should focus not on the quantity of alcohol consumed but rather on the adverse effects of drinking. By asking, "How much do you drink?," the interviewer may put the patient on the defensive. This type of question may also create an unnecessary power struggle between patient and interviewer. Ask instead, "How much **can** you drink?" which puts the patient and interviewer in a position of alliance. Most individuals who drink also underestimate the quantities they consume. The interviewer will often learn more about the quantity of alcohol consumed by asking about the patient's feelings and interpersonal relationships than by asking directly about the amount. Determine whether the patient drives while intoxicated, has suffered amnesia of events while drinking, neglects or abuses his or her family, and has missed work as a result of alcohol consumption.

Ewing and Rouse (1970) suggested the CAGE questionnaire as a tool for helping to make the diagnosis of alcoholism. The acronym CAGE helps the interviewer to remember the four clinical interview questions. Once it is established that a patient drinks alcohol, the following questions should be asked:

"Have you ever felt the need to Cut down on your drinking?"
"Have people Annoyed you by criticizing your drinking?"
"Have you ever felt bad or Guilty about your drinking?"
"Have you ever taken a morning 'Eye-opener' to steady your nerves or get rid of a hangover?"

Since its introduction, the CAGE questionnaire has been shown to be one of the most efficient and effective screening devices for detecting alcoholism. Four affirmative responses are pathognomonic for alcoholism. Two or three affirmative answers should create a high level of suspicion. If neither the answers nor the nonverbal responses to these questions are affirmative, the diagnosis of alcoholism can be generally excluded. One study by Bush and associates (1987) indicated that one or more affirmative responses to these questions reflect a sensitivity of 85% and a specificity of 89%.

The history of alcoholic consumption and dependency can be further assessed by using the sets of questions referred to by the acronyms HALT, BUMP, and FATAL DT. The HALT questions are as follows:

"Do you usually drink to get High?"
"Do you drink Alone?"
"Do you ever find yourself Looking forward to drinking?"
"Have you noticed whether you seem to be becoming Tolerant of alcohol?"

The BUMP questions are as follows:

"Have you ever had Blackouts?"
"Have you ever used alcohol in an Unplanned* way?"
"Do you ever drink alcohol for Medicinal† reasons?"
"Do you find yourself Protecting‡ your supply of alcohol?"

The final acronym will remind the interviewer about other major associations with alcoholism. The FATAL DT questions are as follows:

"Is there a Family history of alcoholic problems?"
"Have you ever been a member of Alcoholics Anonymous?"
"Do you Think you are an alcoholic?"
"Have you ever Attempted or had thoughts of suicide?"
"Have you ever had any Legal problems related to alcohol consumption?"
"Do you ever Drive while intoxicated?"
"Do you ever use Tranquilizers to steady your nerves?"

These questions provide the interviewer with a useful, thoughtful, and organized approach to the interview strategy designed to identify the patient with a drinking problem.

In the late stages of alcoholism, a person may suffer delirium tremens, or "DTs." DTs are completely different from the hallucinations that occur in the earlier stages of alcoholism. During hallucinations, the patient may see or hear "things." DTs occur from 24 to 96 hours after withdrawal from alcohol; occasionally the patient may hallucinate, but the patient will always shake and possibly go into convulsions. DTs are the most severe form of withdrawal and are fatal in one of every four cases.

The interviewer must ask all patients about the use of other drugs. People who use recreational drugs often engender negative feelings or anger in their interviewer. These feelings are almost unavoidable. The interviewer must not allow these feelings to interfere with empathetic interviewing. A useful way of approaching the topic of recreational drugs is to ask,

"Have you ever used drugs other than those required for medical reasons?"
"Do you use drugs other than those prescribed by a physician?"
"Have you abused prescription drugs?"

If the answer to any one of these questions is affirmative, determine the types of drugs used, the route(s) of administration, and the frequency of use. In contrast to alcoholics, drug abusers are more likely to magnify their use. The interviewer must ask all patients with a history of drug abuse the following questions:

"What type of drugs do you use?"
"At what age did you start using drugs?"
"What was your period of heaviest use?"
"What is your recent pattern of use?"
"Are larger doses necessary to get the same effect now?"
"What do you feel when you take the drug?"
"Have you ever tried to quit? What happened?"
"Have you ever had any convulsions after taking the drug?"
"Do you use more than one drug at a time?"
"Do you use drugs on a continuous basis?"
"Have you been in trouble at work because of drug use?"
"Have you ever had withdrawal symptoms as a result of your use of drugs?"

It is important to use simple words and expressions when inquiring about recreational drugs. It may also be more appropriate to use the slang than to use the more

---

* Drink more than you intended or have an additional drink after you have decided you have had enough.
† As a cure for anxiety, depression, or the "shakes."
‡ Buying enough alcohol just in case "company" arrives.

formal terms. For example, "Do you ever shoot up or snort coke?" may be better understood than "Have you ever taken cocaine intravenously or by insufflation?" With experience, the interviewer will acquire relevant knowledge about recreational drugs. Knowing the local street names is often as important as knowing the pharmacology. The knowledge of these names may provide a means for better communication. It should be recognized that these street names are often different from place to place and change from time to time. Appendix A at the end of this book summarizes some commonly abused drugs, their street names, and the major symptoms and signs associated with each of them.

When questioning a patient about *diet*, it is useful to ask the patient to describe what he or she ate the day before, including all three meals plus any snacks. How many fish meals does he or she have each week? What is the proportion of red meat in the diet in comparison with fish or poultry? How much saturated fat is there in the diet? Does the patient add salt when he or she cooks, and does he or she add salt at the table? Has his or her diet changed recently? What kinds of foods does the patient like or dislike and why? Are there any food intolerances? Does the patient eat foods with high fiber content, such as whole grain breads and cereals, bran, fresh fruits, and vegetables? High fiber snack foods include sesame bread sticks, date nut bread, oatmeal cookies, fig bars, granola bars, and corn chips. What is the consumption of sodium? Pickled foods, cured meats, snack foods, and prepared soups have high sodium content. The interviewer should ascertain the amount of exercise the patient gets. The consumption of caffeine-containing products, such as coffee, tea, cola sodas, or chocolate, is important to determine. Caffeine ingestion may produce a variety of symptoms, including heart palpitations, fatigue, lightheadedness, headaches, irritability, and many gastrointestinal symptoms.

It is important to know a patient's *sleep patterns*, because this may provide information about the patient's psychological problems. When does the patient go to bed? Does he or she have trouble falling asleep? Does he or she stay asleep the whole night, or does he or she awaken in the middle of the night, unable to go back to sleep?

All *current medications* should be noted. If possible, ask the patient to show you the bottles and to tell you how the medications are taken. Note whether the patient is taking them according to the directions on the bottle. Ask the patient whether he or she is taking any other medicines. Frequently, patients consider over-the-counter medications such as vitamins, laxatives, antacids, or cold remedies not worth mentioning. Ask specifically about each of these types of drugs. Determine the type of contraception used, if any, and whether a woman has used or uses birth control pills.

Occupational and Environmental History

The *occupational and environmental history* concerns exposure to potential disease-producing substances or environments. Occupational exposures account for an estimated 50,000–70,000 deaths annually in the United States. There are more than 350,000 new cases of occupational disease recognized each year. These diseases can involve every organ system. Because these diseases often mimic other diseases, occupational disease may be incorrectly ascribed to some other cause. One of the important barriers to the accurate diagnosis of occupational and environmental diseases is the long latency between exposure and the appearance of the illness.

Many occupational diseases have been well described over the years, such as malignant mesothelioma in workers exposed to asbestos; cancer of the bladder in aniline dye workers; malignant neoplasms of the nasal cavities in woodworkers; pneumoconiosis in coal miners; silicosis in sandblasters and quarry workers; leukemia in those exposed to benzene; hepatic angiosarcoma in workers exposed to vinyl chloride; byssinosis in cotton industry workers; skin cancer in those chronically exposed to the sun, such as sailors; ornithosis in bird breeders; toxic hepatitis in solvent utilizers and workers in the plastics industry; and chronic bronchitis in individuals exposed to industrial dusts. It has been shown that there is an association of sterility in men and women exposed to certain pesticides and dementia in individuals exposed to certain solvents.

The environment is also responsible for significant morbidity and mortality rates. Lead, radon, pesticides, and air pollution cause illness and death. For example, recall

Chernobyl with its widespread high levels of radiation; Minamata Bay in Japan with its mercury poisoning; Hopewell, Virginia with its poisoning pesticide chlordecone; and Bhopal, India, where a leak at an industrial plant exposed hundreds of thousands of people to toxic methyl isocyanate gas. Thousands died shortly after exposure, and more than 200,000 people have suffered illness from the gas. The long-range effects of these agents have yet to be determined.

The careful occupational and environmental history is the most effective means for proper diagnosis of occupational and environmental disease. It is important to inquire about all occupations and the duration of each. The history should include more than just a listing of jobs. The duration and precise activities must be ascertained. The use of protective devices and cleanup practices as well as work in adjacent areas must also be determined. The job title (e.g., electrician, machine operator) is important, but actual exposure to hazardous materials may not be reflected in these descriptions. Industrial work areas are complex, and it is important to ascertain the actual location of work in relationship to other areas where hazardous materials are used. It is well known that just living near areas of industrial toxins is linked to the development of disease many years later. It is therefore relevant to inquire whether the patient resides or ever resided near mines, farms, factories, or shipyards. The following questions regarding occupational and environmental exposure should be asked of all patients:

> *"What type of work do you do?"*
> *"How long have you been doing this work?"*
> *"Describe your work."*
> *"Are you exposed to any hazardous materials? Do you ever use protective equipment?"*
> *"What kind of work did you do before you had your present job?"*
> *"What was your wartime employment, if any?"*
> *"Where do you live? For how long?"*
> *"Have you ever lived near any factories, shipyards, or other potentially hazardous facilities?"*
> *"Has anyone in your household ever worked with hazardous materials that could have been brought home?"*
> *"What type of hobbies do you have? What types of exposures are involved?"*
> *"Do you now or have you previously had environmental or occupational exposure to asbestos, lead, fumes, chemicals, dusts, loud noise, radiation, or other toxic factors?"*

Attention must be paid to any temporal relationship between the onset of illness and toxic exposure in the workplace. Did the symptoms start after the patient began a new job? Did the symptoms abate during a vacation and then recur when the patient resumed work? Were the symptoms related to the implementation of any new chemical or process? Is there anyone else at work or are there any neighbors with a similar illness?

Biographic Information

Biographic information includes the date and place of birth, sex, race, and ethnic background.

Family History

The *family history* provides information about the health of the entire family, living and dead. Pay particular attention to possible genetic and environmental aspects of disease that might have implications for the patient. The age and health of all the immediate family members should be determined. If a family member is deceased, the age of the person and the cause of death should be recorded. It is important to inquire how a family member's illness psychologically affects the patient.

It is important to inquire where the patient's parents were born. Where were the grandparents born? In what setting did the patient grow up? Urban? Rural? In what country did the parents grow up? If the patient was born in another country, at what age did he or she come to the United States? Does the patient maintain contact with other family members? Was the original family name changed? If the patient is married, is the spouse of the same ethnic background as the patient? What is the patient's native language?

The answers to these questions will provide valuable information as a heritage assessment.

Psychosocial History

The psychosocial history includes information on the education, life experiences, and personal relationships of the patient. This section should include the patient's lifestyle, other people living with the patient, schooling, military service, religious beliefs (in relation to the perceptions of health and treatment), and marital and/or significant-other relationships. A statement regarding the patient's knowledge of symptoms and illness is important. Has the illness caused the patient to lose time from work? What kind of insight does the patient have regarding the symptom? Does he or she think about the future? If so, how does it look? An excellent question that can elicit a vast amount of information is "What is your typical day like?"

Sexual, Reproductive, and Gynecologic History

The *sexual history* has traditionally been part of the psychosocial history or review of systems. However, because the sexual, reproductive, and gynecologic history is so vital for the complete evaluation of the patient, these histories are now considered a separate part of the interview.

There are several reasons for taking a sexual history. Sexual drive is a sensitive indicator of general well-being. Anxiety, depression, and anger may relate to sexual dysfunction; however, many physical symptoms may lead to sexual problems. In addition, it is critically important to identify risk behaviors. A well-taken sexual history enables the examiner to establish norms of sexuality for the patient. Opening up the interview about sexuality allows the interviewer to educate the patient about human immunodeficiency virus–related illnesses, sexually transmitted diseases, and ways to prevent pregnancies. It is an excellent opportunity to provide useful information to the patient.

It is as important to ask about sexual activity in children as it is in older adults. Child abuse is very common, and the interviewer must identify it as early as possible. Do not assume that a senior citizen is sexually inactive. Sexuality is a part of normal life, and many older adults enjoy sexual contact.

Tailor your questions to each specific interview.

The interviewer must inquire about sexual relationships in a nonjudgmental manner. Direct questions regarding oral and anal sex, sexual contacts, and sexual problems are very important. Patients are frequently less inhibited about discussing their sexual behavior than is the novice interviewer in asking about it. When a patient's sexual preference is in doubt, the term *partner* rather than a gender-specific term is appropriate. There is no easy way to ask about sexual preference, but it is vital to know. Allow the patient to tell you something about his or her partner(s). Asking the patient whether he or she has had any contact with individuals with acquired immunodeficiency syndrome (AIDS) or AIDS-related illness is appropriate. The term *homosexual* as an adjective for gender (e.g., homosexual male) should be avoided, as it is generally perceived to be demeaning. The term is acceptable, however, to describe the behavior (e.g., homosexual behavior).

There are several general questions that can help broach the topic of sexual activity. Some of the following suggested questions may be helpful:

> *"Are you having any sexual problems?"*
> *"Are you satisfied with your sexual performance?"* *"Do you think your partner is?"*
>   If not, *"What is unsatisfactory to you (your partner)?"*
> *"Have you had any difficulty achieving orgasm?"*
> *"How frequently does it occur that your partner desires sexual intercourse and you do not?"*
> *"What activities and positions does your sex include?"*
> *"Are there any questions pertaining to your sexual performance that you would like to discuss?"*
> *"Most people experience some disappointment in their sexual function. Can you tell me what disappointments you might have?"*

"Many people experience what others may consider unusual sexual thoughts or wish to perform sexual acts that others consider abnormal. We often are bothered about these thoughts. What has been your experience?"

Domestic violence, rape, child abuse, and *elder abuse* are rampant and have reached staggering proportions. It is, therefore, critically important to ask all patients if they have ever been emotionally, physically, or sexually abused. Much of the violence against women is perpetrated by their intimate partners or in relationships that are commonly protective, such as that of father and daughter. As many as one of every seven women seen in an emergency room has symptoms relating to abuse. Clinicians frequently treat the injuries only symptomatically and often fail to recognize the abuse. According to Federal Bureau of Investigation records, nearly 100,000 cases of domestic violence against women were reported in 1990. It is recognized, however, that such violence is vastly underreported; the actual number of cases is probably double the number reported. According to the *Washington Post,* from 1981 to 1991 the rate of rape in the United States increased fourfold compared with the overall crime rate. It has been estimated that 60–80% of all college women have been sexually assaulted by dates or friends.

Although many women who are victims of abuse do not volunteer any information, they will often discuss the incident(s) if asked simple, direct questions in a nonjudgmental way and in a confidential setting. Begin with the following: "Since domestic violence is so common, I've begun to ask about it routinely. At any time, has your partner hit, kicked, or otherwise hurt or frightened you?" If the patient answers in the affirmative, encourage her to talk about it. You might ask, "What would you like to do about it?" Always listen nonjudgmentally to encourage the woman to continue talking about the episode(s). Showing support is very important. A statement such as "You are not alone" or "Help is available for you" shows empathy. It is critical to assess the danger to the patient as quickly as possible before she leaves the medical facility. If the patient is in imminent danger, determine if she can stay with friends or family. A shelter for battered women may be an alternative. Finally, provide her with the telephone number of the local domestic violence hotline. If the patient answers "No" to the introductory query, be aware of any injury to the head, neck, torso, breasts, abdomen, or genitalia. Any of these injuries must have a plausible explanation. If not, it is appropriate to ask further questions; make sure the partner is not present. You might say, "It looks like you've been hurt. Can you tell me how it happened?" Another approach could be, "Sometimes when people feel the way you do, it's because they may have been abused. Is this happening to you?" Even if a woman is in an abusive setting and she fails to acknowledge it once you have provided an opportunity, allow her to return to discuss it at a later date. Serious injury and homicide often result once a woman attempts to leave her abusive partner. Let her make the decision. You have indicated to her your support.

In 1986 more than 1.5 million children nationwide were reported as abused, an increase of 74% since 1980. Reports of childhood sexual abuse have tripled since 1980, with now more than 350,000 cases per year. A history of childhood sexual abuse is nearly always associated with enduring physical and psychological sequelae. There are many somatic disorders that may result after abuse. These include eczema, sleep disorders, sexual dysfunction, substance abuse, eating disorders, headaches, "mystery" pain, depression, asthma, and a wide variety of phobias. Health-care providers have an ethical and legal responsibility to report all cases of suspected child abuse and to protect the child from further abuse. Any injury without an adequate explanation should raise the concern about either nonaccidental injury or neglect. Injuries to the skin are seen in 90% of abused children. See Figure 22–18. Multiple injuries in various stages of healing almost always indicate repeated beatings.

Male rape is also on the rise. According to the District of Columbia Rape Crisis Center, one of every seven males in the United States will be raped before the age of 18 years. Most male rape victims are raped by other men, in the sense that they are forced to submit to anal intercourse, masturbation of the offender, oral sex, or other sex act. Information about male rape is scarce because male victims, like their female counterparts, feel humiliation and shame and are reluctant to report it. Many males believe that if they have been raped by another male, it implies the victim has homosexual habits.

The *reproductive and gynecologic history* obtains information about a woman's age at menarche, regularity of menstrual flow, and duration of periods. In addition, the number of pregnancies, number of deliveries, number of abortions (spontaneous or induced), and complications of pregnancies are included in this part of the history. It is also vital to determine whether the woman was exposed to diethylstilbestrol (DES) through her mother's use during pregnancy. This is particularly important in any woman born before 1975. Other important questions are further discussed in Chapter 17, Female Genitalia.

In the reproductive history for a man, it is important to inquire about sexual interest, function, satisfaction, and any sexual problem(s). Has the man been unable to procreate? If so, is he aware of the reason(s)? Other questions for men are discussed in Chapter 16, Male Genitalia and Hernias.

Review of Systems

The *review of systems* summarizes in terms of body systems all the many symptoms that may have been overlooked in the history of the present illness or in the medical history. By reviewing in an orderly manner the list of possible symptoms, the interviewer can specifically check each system and uncover additional symptoms of "unrelated" illnesses not yet discussed. The review of systems is best organized from the head down to the extremities. Patients are told that they are going to be asked whether they have ever had a particular symptom and that they should answer just "yes" or "no." If they answer in the affirmative, further direct questioning is appropriate. The interviewer need not repeat questions that were previously answered, unless clarification of the data is necessary.

Table 1–1 is the review of systems that should be asked of all patients. The questions should be asked of the patient in a way in which he or she will understand them. For example, a question regarding paroxysmal nocturnal dyspnea should be asked in this manner:

"Do you ever awaken in the middle of the night with sudden shortness of breath or sudden difficulty in breathing?"

Each of the organ- and system-specific chapters that follow discusses a review of specific symptoms that further elaborates on the symptoms related to the specific organ or system. Hints about specific questioning and pathophysiologic features of the symptoms are also provided in each chapter.

Not infrequently, a patient may answer all the questions in the affirmative. If the interviewer detects that this is occurring, it may be useful to ask a question about a physiologically impossible condition. If when asked "Do your stools glow in the dark?" the patient answers in the affirmative, the interviewer should not continue with the review of systems. The interviewer can state in the written history or in the verbal presentation that "the patient has a positive review of systems."

Because the goal of the medical history is to acquire as much information about each illness as possible, other specific questions related to that particular patient may be indicated. Look at the patient shown in Figure 1–1. If you were to see such a patient, you may wish to try to determine when the facial changes occurred. In such a case, it is important to ask the man whether he has noticed a change in his hat size and when he first noticed it.

Look at Figure 1–2, in which the right hand of the same patient is compared with the right hand of a normal individual. Asking about a change in glove size is also useful with this particular patient. It would also be appropriate to inquire whether there has been a change in shoe size as well.

A useful bit of information may be an old photograph of the patient to help determine when the suspected changes occurred. Compare the photograph in Figure 1–3 (of the same patient, taken 20 years earlier) with Figure 1–1. Notice the bulging forehead and the prominent jaw in the later photograph. The patient has acromegaly, a condition of abnormal, excess growth hormone secreted by a pituitary tumor. The changes are insidious throughout many years. The photograph was helpful in determining the change in bone and soft tissue structure.

Table 1-1　Review of Systems

General
Usual state of health
Fever
Chills
Usual weight
Change in weight
Weakness
Fatigue
Sweats
Heat or cold
　intolerance
History of anemia
Bleeding tendencies
Blood transfusions and
　possible reactions
Exposure to radiation

Skin
Rashes
Itching
Hives
Easy bruisability
History of eczema
Dryness
Changes in skin color
Changes in hair
　texture
Changes in nail texture
Changes in nail
　appearance
History of previous
　skin disorders
Lumps
Use of hair dyes

Head
"Dizziness"
Headaches
Pain
Fainting
History of head injury
Stroke

Eyes
Use of eyeglasses
Current vision
Change in vision
Double vision
Excessive tearing
Pain
Recent eye
　examinations
Pain when looking at
　light
Unusual sensations
Redness
Discharge
Infections
History of glaucoma
Cataracts
Injuries

Ears
Hearing impairment
Use of hearing aid
Discharge
"Dizziness"
Pain
Ringing in ears
Infections

Nose
Nosebleeds
Infections
Discharge
Frequency of colds
Nasal obstruction
History of injury
Sinus infections
Hay fever

Mouth and Throat
Condition of teeth
Last dental appointment
Condition of gums
Bleeding gums
Frequent sore throats
Burning of tongue
Hoarseness
Voice changes
Postnasal drip

Neck
Lumps
Goiter
Pain on movement
Tenderness
History of "swollen glands"
Thyroid trouble

Chest
Cough
Pain
Shortness of breath
Sputum production (quantity,
　appearance)
Tuberculosis
Asthma
Pleurisy
Bronchitis
Coughing up blood
Wheezing
Last x-ray
Last test for tuberculosis
History of bacille Calmette-Guérin
　vaccination

Cardiac
Chest pain
High blood pressure
Palpitations
Shortness of breath with exertion
Shortness of breath when lying flat
Sudden shortness of breath while
　sleeping
History of heart attack
Rheumatic fever
Heart murmur
Last electrocardiogram
Other tests for heart function

Vascular
Pain in legs, calves, thighs, or hips
　while walking
Swelling of legs
Varicose veins
Thrombophlebitis
Coolness of extremity
Loss of hair on legs
Discoloration of extremity
Ulcers

Breasts
Lumps
Discharge
Pain
Tenderness
Self-examination

Gastrointestinal
Appetite
Excessive hunger
Excessive thirst
Nausea
Swallowing
Constipation
Diarrhea
Heartburn
Vomiting
Abdominal pain
Change in stool color
Change in stool caliber
Change in stool consistency
Frequency of bowel
　movements
Vomiting blood
Rectal bleeding
Black, tarry stools
Laxative or antacid use
Excessive belching
Food intolerance
Change in abdominal size
Hemorrhoids
Infections
Jaundice
Rectal pain
Previous abdominal x-rays
Hepatitis
Liver disease
Gallbladder disease

Urinary
Frequency
Urgency
Difficulty in starting the stream
Incontinence
Excessive urination
Pain on urination
Burning
Blood in urine
Infections
Stones
Bed-wetting
Flank pain
Awakening at night to urinate
History of retention
Urine color
Urine odor

Male Genitalia
Lesions on penis
Discharge
Impotence
Pain
Scrotal masses
Hernias
Frequency of intercourse
Ability to enjoy sexual relations
Fertility problems
Prostate problems
History of venereal disease and
　treatment

Female Genitalia
Lesions on external genitalia
Itching
Discharge
Last Pap smear and result
Pain on intercourse
Frequency of intercourse
Birth control methods
Ability to enjoy sexual
　relations
Fertility problems
Hernias
History of venereal disease
　and treatment
History of diethylstilbestrol
　exposure
Age at menarche
Interval between periods
Duration of periods
Amount of flow
Date of last period
Bleeding between periods
Number of pregnancies
Abortions
Term deliveries
Complications of pregnancies
Description(s) of labor
Number of living children
Menstrual pain
Age at menopause
Menopausal symptoms
Postmenopausal bleeding

Musculoskeletal
Weakness
Paralysis
Muscle stiffness
Limitation of movement
Joint pain
Joint stiffness
Arthritis
Gout
Back problems
Muscle cramps
Deformities

Neurologic
Fainting
"Dizziness"
"Blackouts"
Paralysis
Strokes
"Numbness"
Tingling
Burning
Tremors
Loss of memory
Psychiatric disorders
Mood changes
Nervousness
Speech disorders
Unsteadiness of gait
General behavioral change
Loss of consciousness
Hallucinations
Disorientation

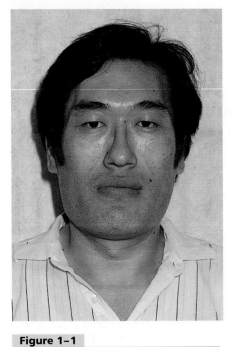

Figure 1–1

Acromegaly: facial characteristics.

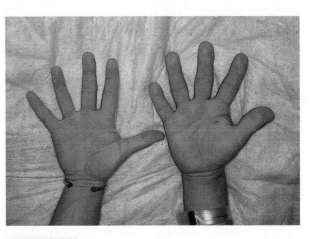

Figure 1–2

Acromegaly: characteristics of hands. Note the hand with stubby fingers of the patient on the right compared with the fingers of a normal hand on the left.

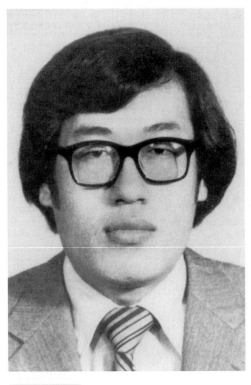

Figure 1–3

Photograph of the patient shown in Figure 1–1, taken 20 years earlier. Compare the facial features with those shown in Figure 1–1.

Concluding Thoughts

A medical history must be dynamic. Every history is different. All patients are asked the standard questions, but each patient should be evaluated individually. There is no limit to the questions to be asked.

The *written history* is a permanent, legal document of the patient's health history. The information that is recorded must be accurate and objective. On the basis of all the information gleaned from the patient's history, the interviewer carefully summarizes all the data into a readable format. Anything that is written in a patient's record could be presented to a court of law. Only objective data should be included. Opinions or statements about previous care and therapy must be avoided.

By convention, when the review of systems is stated or written, all symptoms that the patient has experienced are indicated first. Symptoms never experienced are indicated afterward. The *pertinent positive symptoms* are symptoms that have possible relevance to the present illness. *Pertinent negative symptoms* are symptoms that are not present but that may often be related to the present illness.

If information in the review of systems has been described previously in the history of present illness, for example, it is correct to indicate under the systems review of that symptom, "see history of present illness."

As you proceed with the interview, you may sense that it is not going well. Is the patient comfortable? Is there a language barrier? Did you say or do something to interfere with the rapport? Is the patient intimidated? Is the patient concerned about confidentiality? Is the patient reluctant to talk in the presence of family members? Is the patient able to express his or her feelings? These are just a few of the common reasons for lack of progression of an interview. If you can alleviate the problems, do so. Perhaps interviewing the patient on another day and using the same approach will be more successful.

The key to success in an interview is the ability to put the patient at ease. To do so, the interviewer must be relaxed. What techniques are available to the interviewer and patient to relax? One useful approach is the visualization of color. For example, if the interviewer were to say, "Close your eyes and visualize the color blue," the patient would feel a definite response in body as well as in mind. If the patient were then to let that image dissolve, take a few breaths, close the eyes again, and visualize the color red, he or she would notice that the response to this color is quite different. Red creates a different state of mind than does blue, green, yellow, and so forth.

Whether this is entirely a result of psychological association or not is irrelevant to this discussion. The point is that because people respond strongly to color, interviewers can influence the state of mind of patients and themselves by suggesting an atmosphere of color that calms, warms, cheers, cools, and so forth, depending on what is called for in the situation. Because color can help a patient to relax, it can have beneficial effects on blood pressure, heart rate, and other bodily functions.

The same is true of the visualization of environments that are pleasant, beautiful, and peaceful. Having the patient take a few moments, with eyes closed, to imagine himself or herself in an environment such as a garden or a quiet pine forest can substantially lessen nervousness and tension. The connection between relaxation and health is becoming more widely understood and accepted. According to recent studies in behavioral medicine, the practice of meditation has a beneficial effect in the treatment of hypertension, some heart problems, depression, and anxiety, among other illnesses.

Many visualization techniques are far from new. In the Tibetan approach to medicine, a system that developed between the 4th and 12th centuries, there is a direct connection between the state of a person's mind and the state of his or her health.

In the next chapter, the patient's responses to the questions are investigated, and the influence of background and age on those responses are observed.

Bibliography

Adler G, Buie DH: The misuses of confrontation with borderline patients. Int J Psychoanal Psychother 1:109, 1972.

Alpert EJ, Cohen S: Educating the Nation's Physicians about Family Violence and Abuse. Acad Med 72, 1997.

Benson H, Klipper MZ: The Relaxation Response. New York, Wing Books, 1975.

Bernstein J: Conversations in public places. J Communication 25:85, 1975.

Billings JA, Stoeckle JD: The Clinical Encounter. Chicago, Year Book Medical, 1989.

Bird B: Talking with Patients. Philadelphia, J.B. Lippincott, 1973.

Brown BL, Strong WJ, Rencher AC: Perceptions of personality from speech: Effects of manipulation of acoustical parameters. Acoust Soc Am J 54:29, 1973.

Buchwald D, Caralis PV, Gany F, et al: The medical interview across cultures. Patient Care 27:141, 1993.

Buckman R: How to Break Bad News: A Guide for Health Care Professionals. Baltimore, The Johns Hopkins University Press, 1992.

Bush B, Shaw S, Cleary P, et al: Screening for alcohol abuse using the CAGE questionnaire. Am J Med 83:231, 1987.

Chafetz ME: No patient deserves to be patronized. Med Insight 2:68, 1970.

Clark WD: The medical interview: Focus on alcohol problems. Hosp Prac 11:59, 1985.

Cohen-Cole SA: The Medical Interview: The Three-Function Approach. St. Louis, Mosby Year Book, 1991.

Coulehan JL, Block MR: The Medical Interview: A Primer for Students of the Art. Philadelphia, F.A. Davis, 1992.

Council on Scientific Affairs, American Medical Association: Violence Against Women: Relevance for Medical Practitioners. JAMA 267:3184, 1992.

Ende J. Rockwell S, Glasgow M: The sexual history in general medicine practice. Arch Intern Med 144:558, 1984.

Ewing JA, Rouse BA: Identifying the hidden alcoholic. Presented at the 29th International Congress on Alcohol and Drug Dependence. Sydney, Australia, Feb 3, 1970.

Faust S, Drickey R: Working with interpreters. J Fam Pract 22:131, 1986.

Francis V, Korsch BM, Morris MJ. Gaps in doctor-patient communication. N Engl J Med 280:535, 1969.

Goldman RH, Peters JM. The occupational and environmental health history. JAMA 246:2831, 1981.

Gregg D: Reassurance. Am J Nurs 55:171, 1955.

Haffner L: Translation is not enough: Interpreting in a medical setting. West J Med 157:255, 1992.

Jewell ME, Jewell GS: How to assess the risk of HIV exposure. Am Fam Physician 40:153, 1989.

Kraytman M: The Complete Patient History. New York, McGraw-Hill, 1991.

Landrigan PJ, Baker DB: The recognition and control of occupational disease. JAMA 266:676, 1991.

Larsen KM, Smith CK: Assessment of nonverbal communication in the patient-doctor relationship. J Fam Pract 12:48, 1981.

Lief HI, Karlen A (eds): Sex Education in Medicine. New York, Spectrum Publications, 1976.

Matthews D, Hingson R: Improving patient compliance: A guide to physicians. Med Clin North Am 61:879, 1977.

Myerscough PR: Talking with Patients: A Basic Clinical Skill. Oxford, England, Oxford University Press, 1992.

Peabody FW: The care of the patient. JAMA 88:877, 1927.

Rosenstock L, Cullen M: Textbook of Clinical Occupational and Environmental Medicine, 2nd ed. Philadelphia, W.B. Saunders Co., 1994.

Roter D, Stewart M (eds): Communication with Medical Patients. Newbury Park, CA, Sage Publications, 1989.

Spiro II: What is empathy and can it be taught? Ann Intern Med 116:843, 1992.

The Physician's Guide to Helping Patients with Alcohol Problems. U.S. Dept. of Health and Human Services. NIH Publication 95-3769, 1995.

CHAPTER 2

The Patient's Responses

It is our duty to remember at all times and anew that medicine is not only a science, but also the art of letting our own individuality interact with the individuality of the patient.

Albert Schweitzer
1875–1965

Responses to Illness

Health is characterized by a state of well-being, enthusiasm, and an energetic pursuit of life's goals. Illness is characterized by feelings of discomfort, helplessness, and a diminished interest in the future. Once patients recognize that they are ill and possibly face their own mortality, a series of emotional reactions occur. These include anxiety, fear, depression, denial, projection, regression, anger, frustration, withdrawal, and an exaggeration of symptoms. These psychological reactions are general and are not specific to any particular physical illness. Patients must learn to cope not only with the symptoms of the illness but also with life as it is altered by the illness.

Anxiety

Anxiety is a state of uneasiness in which the patient has a sense of impending danger. It is the fundamental response to stress of any kind, such as separation, injury, social disapproval, or decreased self-esteem. Anxiety and fear are common reactions to the stress of illness. The terms *anxiety* and *fear* are often used interchangeably. There are, however, two important differences. First, fear tends to be specific and is triggered by a specific event or object. In contrast, anxiety tends to be more diffuse, often occurring without a specific trigger. Second, fear is more acute and tends to come on rapidly, whereas anxiety develops more slowly and takes longer to resolve. The feelings of loss of control, guilt, and frustration contribute to the patient's emotional reaction. Illness makes patients feel helpless. Recognizing the body's mortality leads patients to an intense feeling of anxiety. In addition to the emotional reaction, fear can be manifested physiologically by restlessness, gastrointestinal problems, or headaches. Other common symptoms of anxiety include difficulty in falling asleep, nightmares, frequency of urination, palpitations, fatigue, vague aches and pains, paresthesias, and shortness of breath. Not uncommonly, patients may feel that they are "falling apart."

The young man who has been stricken with a heart attack feels helpless. As he lies in his intensive care unit bed, he begins to recognize how mortal he really is. The patient believes that he must be dependent on everyone and everything: the nurse, the doctor, the intravenous line, even the monitor. His anxiety, based on helplessness, is a normal response to his illness. His sudden illness and the threat of possible death oppose his belief that he is indestructible.

A 72 year old man who has lived alone for years since his wife died is admitted to a hospital for a transurethral prostatectomy. He is anxious that he may become dependent upon his children. He may be more threatened by his fear of dependency than by the illness itself.

The hospitalized patient who is brought to the radiology department for a routine chest x-ray and is forced to wait for 2 hours for a transporter to bring her back to her room suffers anxiety. She is angry to have been left waiting and perhaps missed some visitors. But she says nothing. Her anxiety is based on the fear of expressing anger to the nurses and staff members on the floor. She believes that if she were to express her anger, the hospital personnel might interfere with her medical care.

Some hospitalized patients cannot accept the love and care expressed by family or friends. This inability to accept tenderness is a common source of anxiety. Such patients feel threatened by these affectionate acts because they serve to reinforce their dependency.

There is anxiety in all patients admitted to a hospital. The patients must put their most important commodity, their lives, into the hands of a group of strangers who may or may not be competent to assume responsibility for the patients' survival. This is the fear of strangers.

It is most important for the interviewer to identify the causes or roots of a patient's fear or anxiety as well as to acknowledge the existence of the patient's feelings without expressing judgment. Whenever possible, the interviewer should provide some information to allay the patient's fear or anxiety.

Depression

Depression is a term used to describe a chronic state of lowering of mood. Some patients have a predilection for depression, but depression is a common state, occurring in more than 20% of all patients with major illnesses, particularly cancer.

Depression is a psychological reaction to the loss of health, a loved one, or one's own self-esteem. Certain degrees of depression probably accompany every chronic illness. There are many types of depression: reactive, neurotic, manic, melancholic, and agitated, to name only a few. In general, patients with depression have pessimistic tones in speech and a downcast facial expression. They may express feelings of futility and self-accusation. They respond to questions with brief answers. Their speech is slow; their volume is low; their pitch is monotonous. Typically, the speech pattern tends to put the interviewer to sleep. Depressed patients feel inadequate, worthless, and defeated. They also suffer profound feelings of guilt. A remark such as *"You look sad"* allows these patients to talk about their depression. Crying allows relief of severe depressive feelings and permits patients to continue their story. Although crying may be brought on by patients' concern for their own illness, crying usually occurs when patients think of an illness or death of a loved one or of a potential loss. They often have much hostility and resentment and suffer from rejection and loneliness. Self-accusative and self-depreciative delusions can occur in severely depressed patients. When these delusions are present, such feelings of worthlessness are so overwhelming that patients may believe that suicide is the only way out.

A 23 year old law student is engulfed with anxiety when he learns that he has acquired immune deficiency syndrome (AIDS). When his friends and family learn of the illness, he is immediately excluded from all relationships. He has violent feelings of guilt. His depression is worsened when he learns that his university has asked him to leave his studies. He is found later hanged in his parents' attic. His only way of coping with his illness was through suicide.

Depression may be the most common reaction to illness as well as the most frequently overlooked. The most important diagnostic symptoms of depression are the following:

- Markedly diminished interest or pleasure in almost all activities
- Insomnia
- Change in appetite and/or weight
- Fatigue or loss of energy
- Agitation
- Feelings of guilt or worthlessness
- Decreased ability to think or concentrate
- Thoughts of death or suicide

Do not ignore any talk of suicide. Get the assistance of someone experienced in the field.

Denial

Denial is acting and thinking as if a part of reality were not true. Denial is one of the most common psychological mechanisms of defense and is seen in both patients and health-care providers. Denial is often an emotional response to inner tension and prevents a painful conflict from producing overt anxiety. It is actually a form of self-deception. Denial is often seen in patients with terminal illnesses or with chronic, incurable diseases. In general, the more acute the illness, the greater is the patient's acceptance; the more insidious, the greater the denial.

A patient dying slowly from cancer can observe his weight decreasing and the side effects of his medications. His frequent visits to the hospital for chemotherapy or radiotherapy confirm the severity of his illness; yet, in spite of all this, he will continue to deny his illness. He will make plans for the future and talk about when he will be cured. Denial is the psychological mechanism that keeps this patient going. The interviewer should not confront his denial despite its apparent absurdity. Telling such a patient to "face the facts" is cruel. Breaking down denial in such a patient only serves to add to the dying patient's misery. However, the patient's family must understand and accept the poor prognosis.

Denial can sometimes obstruct proper medical care. A woman presents to a breast clinic with an orange-sized mass in her breast. The mass has already started to ulcerate, with a resultant foul-smelling infection. When asked how long she has had the mass, she responds that she noticed it just yesterday. It is often best to interview a reliable informant when the patient with denial is recognized.

Projection

Projection is another common defense mechanism by which people unconsciously reject an unacceptable emotional feature in themselves and "project" it onto someone else. It is the major mechanism involved in the development of paranoid feelings. For example, hostile patients may say to interviewers, "Why are you being so hostile to me?" In reality, such patients are projecting *their* hostility onto the interviewers.

Patients commonly project their anxieties onto doctors. Patients who use projection are constantly watching a doctor's face for subtle signs of their own fears. For example, a 42 year old woman with a strong family history of death from breast cancer has intense fears of developing cancer. During the inspection portion of the physical examination, the patient may be watching the physician's face for information. If the physician frowns or makes some type of negative gesture, the patient may interpret this as "He sees something wrong!" The physician may have made this expression thinking about the amount of work still to be done that day or what type of medication to prescribe for another patient. The patient has projected her anxiety onto the physician. The physician must be aware of these silent "conversations."

In some instances, projection may have a constructive value, saving the patient from being overwhelmed by the illness.

Regression

Regression is a common defense mechanism by which the patient with extreme anxiety attempts unconsciously to return to earlier, more desirable stages of development. During these periods, the individual enjoyed full gratification and freedom from anxiety. Regressed patients become dependent on others and free themselves from the complex problems that have created their anxiety.

For example, consider a middle-aged married man who has recently been told that he has inoperable lung cancer that has already spread to his bones. He is stricken with grief and intense anxiety. There are so many unanswered questions. How long will he live? Will his last months be plagued with unremitting pain? How will his wife be able to raise their young son by herself? How will she manage financially without his income? By regression, the patient can flee this anxiety by becoming child-like and dependent. The patient becomes withdrawn, shy, and often rebellious; he now requires more affection.

A teenager learns that the cause of his 6 month history of weakness and bleeding gums has been diagnosed as acute leukemia. He learns that he will spend what little time he has left in the hospital undergoing chemotherapy. His reaction to his anxiety may be regression. He now needs his parents at his bedside around the clock. He becomes more desirous of his parents' love and kisses. His redevelopment of enuresis, or bed-wetting, is part of his psychological reaction to his illness.

A 25 year old woman with inflammatory bowel disease has had many admissions to hospitals for exacerbations of her disease. She fears the future and the possibility that a cancer may have already started to develop. She is engulfed by a feeling of terror and apprehension. She fears that some day she may require a colostomy and that she will be deprived of one of her most important functions: bowel control. She acts inappropriately, has temper tantrums, and is indecisive. Her dependency on her parents is a manifestation of regression.

Responses to the Interviewer

Much of the enjoyment of medical practice comes from talking with patients. Each patient brings a challenge to the interviewer. Just as there are no two identical interviews, there are no two people who would interview the same patient in the same manner. This section describes a few characteristically troubling patient "types" and indicates some strategies for how the interview may be modified in each case.

Many of these difficult patients can arouse intensely negative feelings in the interviewer; as such, these patients have been collectively called "the hateful patient." The interviewer should recognize these feelings and deal with them directly so that they will not interfere with the interaction. The interviewer must recognize early in the interaction the general characteristics of these patient types so that he or she can facilitate the interview appropriately.

A variety of pejorative labels have unfortunately been given to many of these patient types. The labels serve only to reduce the interviewer's stress through the use of humor. This humor is demeaning to patients as well as often not allowing patients to have proper medical care.

The Silent Patient

Some patients have a lifelong history of shyness. Some of these individuals lack self-confidence. They are very concerned about their self-image and do not want to say or do the wrong thing. These patients are easily embarrassed. Other individuals become hostile or silent as fear of illness develops. The silent patient frequently is seriously depressed. This may be primary to an illness or a secondary response to it. These patients commonly have many of the other signs of depression, as seen in their attitude, facial expressions, and posture. The use of open-ended questions with these patients is generally of little value. Carefully directed questioning may yield some of the answers.

The Overtalkative Patient

The overtalkative patient presents a challenge to the novice interviewer. These patients dominate the interview; the interviewer can hardly get a word in. Every question gets a long answer. Even the answers to "yes-no" questions seem endless. There is usually an aggressive quality to this patient's communications. Every answer is overdetailed. A courteous interruption followed by another direct question will focus on the subject of the interview. The use of open-ended questions, facilitations, or silence is to be avoided, as these techniques encourage such a patient to continue speaking. If all else fails, the interviewer should try to relax and accept the problem.

The Seductive Patient

One of the most difficult types of patients for the novice to interview and examine is the seductive patient. In many ways, the seductive patient is more difficult than a hostile patient. Many of these patients are hysterics who have fantasies of developing an intimate relationship with their physician. These patients are often attractive and are flashy in the way they dress, walk, and talk. They commonly offer inappropriate compliments to the interviewer to gain his or her attention. The patients are frequently emotionally labile. Not uncommonly, these patients expose themselves physically early in the interview. The interviewer may elect to cover the patient, but usually this is unsuccessful. Coping with one's own feelings when one finds oneself attracted to such a patient is difficult. The feeling of attraction is a natural one, and the interviewer must accept it. However, the interviewer must always maintain a strictly professional demeanor. Empathy and reassurance must be kept to a minimum, as these supportive techniques stimulate further fantasies in the patient. The interviewer must always maintain professional distance. It may be necessary to say, "Thank you for your nice compliments, but in order for me to help you, we must keep our relationship strictly professional. I hope you understand." If necessary, the interviewer should get the advice of someone he or she trusts.

The Angry Patient

Angry, obnoxious, or hostile patients are common. Some are demeaning or sarcastic, whereas others are demanding, aggressive, and blatantly hostile. Some patients may remain silent during most of the interview. At other times, they may make inappropriate remarks that are condescending to the novice or even to the experienced clinician. The interviewer may feel resentment, anger, threatened authority, impatience, or frustration. Reciprocal hostility and a power struggle can develop.

The interviewer must realize that these reactions are the patient's responses to *illness* and not necessarily a response to the interviewer. These reactions may be deep-rooted in the patient's past. Every interviewer should be aware that the same emotions, such as rage, envy, or fear, are present in both the patient and the interviewer. A patient may express feelings toward the interviewer, who must act in a detached, professional way and not feel offended or become defensive.

Students of the health-care professions have always been taught that they must like their patients in order to treat them appropriately. Ambivalence in the interviewer can be a problem. Health-care providers must treat patients medically correctly and with respect, but they in fact do not have to like the patient. Because of illness, patients may have feelings of loss of control, threatened authority, and fear. Their anger is the mechanism by which they can handle their fears. Once interviewers gain this insight and become aware of their own feelings, they can better treat such patients. Interviewers must accept and restrain their own negative feelings toward the patients so that their professional judgment will not be distorted. Interviewers' awareness of their own anxieties and feelings will aid in a more productive interview. Conscious expression of one's own feelings in a frank and noninsulting manner will facilitate the interviewing process. Regulation and control of the interviewer's feelings is the goal.

Confrontation may be a useful technique for interviewing such patients. By saying, "You sound very angry," the interviewer allows patients to vent some of their fears. Another confrontational approach is to say, "You're obviously angry about something. Tell me what you think is wrong." Maintain equanimity and avoid becoming defensive. If at the beginning of the interview the patient is angry, try to calm the patient. Proceed slowly with questioning, avoid interpretations, and ask questions that are confined to the history of the present illness.

The Paranoid Patient

The paranoid patient constantly asks, "Why are you asking me that? Do I have _____?" When the interviewer asks the many questions in the review of systems, the patient responds, "Who told you about that?" Paranoid patients think there is some devious plan and that people are constantly talking about them. The patients' suspiciousness can sometimes be handled by the interviewer saying, "These are routine questions that I ask all my patients." Reassurance tends to be threatening to these patients and should not be used because it tends to produce more paranoia. The patients' delusion is beyond reason. The interviewer should therefore complete the questioning and not try to convince such patients about their false ideations. Avoidance of any anger in the interviewer is of paramount importance.

The Insatiable Patient

Insatiable patients are never satisfied. They have many questions, and despite adequate explanations, they feel that the interviewer has not answered all their questions. They tend to be very sensitive, anxious individuals. These patients are best handled with a firm, noncondescending approach. A definite closing statement is helpful, such as, "We have reached the end of our time for today, but I will be back." Alternatively, the interviewer could say, "We have reached the end of our time for today. I will refer your concerns to Dr. _____."

The Ingratiating Patient

The ingratiating patient attempts to please the interviewer. Such patients believe that everything they answer must satisfy the interviewer. They think that if they answer a question to the disapproval of the interviewer, the interviewer will abandon them. Intense feelings of rejection are present in this type of patient. The interviewer must recognize that anxiety is the cause of the patient's behavior and should try not to respond to that behavior. The interviewer should recognize the patient's tendency of trying to please and should stress to the patient how important it is to be accurate.

The Aggressive Patient

The aggressive patient often has a personality disorder. Such patients are easily irritated and often fly into a rage when dealing with the normal stresses of daily life. They are domineering and try to control the interview. However, if allowed to have their way, they may be quite pleasant. Frequently, aggressive patients have intense dependency needs that they cannot consciously handle. These patients mask the primary problem by becoming aggressive and hostile to disguise their anxiety and feelings of inadequacy and inferiority. Aggressive patients are difficult to interview. One must try carefully to stay away from areas provoking anxiety early in the interview. Once a rapport is established, the interviewer may attempt to delve into the deeper areas. In general, aggressive patients refuse any type of psychotherapy.

The Help-Rejecting Patient

Help-rejecting patients are generally not hostile. They describe having been seen by many "expert" physicians for help and are smug in telling interviewers that no one can find out what's wrong with them. They return again and again to the doctors' offices, indicating that the physicians' suggestions "didn't work." Commonly, when a symptom appears relieved, another suddenly appears in its place. These patients use their symptoms to enhance their relationship with their doctors. Such patients are often very depressed, although they deny it. They believe that they have made many self-sacrifices and have had countless disappointments, which they attribute to their "illness." The best approach to these individuals is strong emotional support and gentle reasoning. Despite the need for psychiatric help, these patients generally refuse to accept it.

The Demanding Patient

The demanding patient makes demands of everyone: the physician, the nurse, the student, the aide. These patients use intimidation and guilt to force others to take care of them. They view themselves as being neglected and abused. They may have outbursts of anger toward physicians, who may fear for their own reputations. A power struggle may result.

The Compulsive Patient

Compulsive patients are concerned about every last detail of their lives. These patients pride themselves on their ability to solve all problems, but when their health deteriorates, they lose their composure because they cannot deal with ambiguity or uncertainty. They deny their feelings of anger and anxiety, and projection is a common reaction to their illness. In dealing with the compulsive patient, the interviewer must provide very detailed and specific information to the patient in a straightforward manner. The patient should be allowed as much control as possible, and all the possibilities discussed should be explained clearly.

The Dependent Patient

The dependent patient finds life difficult without the help of others. These other persons provide the necessary support, both emotional and physical. If this support is removed, the patient feels hurt and deserted and demands even more help. When dependent persons become ill, they imagine that their illness will lead to loss of their support groups. Thus, dependent patients need to be cared for most closely. Sometimes, however, these patients can take advantage of a compassionate health-care provider by demanding enormous amounts of time. Be as direct as possible when informing such patients of the appropriate limits without leaving them rejected. The interviewer might say, "You've given me a lot to think about. I do have to leave now. Please don't feel I'm rejecting you. I'll be back later to discuss some of your other problems."

The Masochistic Patient

The masochistic, or self-defeating, patient goes through life suffering. Although these patients need to continue to suffer mentally, they do not seek physical abuse or pain. The masochistic patient is dedicated to a life of self-sacrifice. In contrast to other types of patients, this type adapts well to illness and, in fact, may feel threatened by recovery. This is why such patients frustrate physicians. The goal for these patients is to be able to function despite their problems. Do not promise cures because this creates more problems for the patient and the health-care provider.

The Borderline Patient

Borderline patients are defined as individuals with a personality disorder who have an instability in their personal relationships, engage in impulsive behavior, and have unstable moods. Intense, fluctuating emotions of love and hate are typical of borderline patients. They need emotional support because they are constantly threatened by people and circumstances. It is often very difficult to develop a good doctor-patient relationship with borderline patients because the swings of affect are rapid. Borderline patients are always afraid, but this fear may be masked by outbreaks of anger. These patients are best handled with reassuring words.

Influence of Background and Age on Patient Response

Although disease is universal, patients respond to their illnesses differently. A particular question asked of different patients will be answered in a style that is governed by the patient's ethnic background, emotions, customs, age, medical history, social history, and family history. These factors determine the way in which a patient perceives and responds to a question. This section illustrates the importance of understanding a patient's background as an aid to better communication. The important influence of ethnic and cultural background on the patient response is discussed at length in Chapter 3, Caring for Patients in a Culturally Diverse Society.

The Child Who Is Ill

Children tend always to be "on guard." Ill children are especially vulnerable and wary. First of all, they are taken from their "friendly" home environment. Second, doctors, nurses, and students are constantly staring at them with a wide variety of facial expressions. Many older children believe that the physician has some sort of "magical eye" that can see through them and know everything about them. All of this adds up to a frightening experience for youngsters. Frequently, tests that may cause discomfort may have to be performed by those "people in white." The health-care providers become a symbol of danger and pain.

When the physicians, nurses, or technicians take the youngster for a test, the child experiences his or her greatest fear: separation from parents. This separation produces intense fear and anxiety, manifested by wailing, irritability, and aggressive behavior. The child's fear stems from concern that he or she will not see his or her parents again. This fear may actually be subconscious. Health-care providers should explain to the child, if old enough, that they know why the child is crying and should assure the child that he or she will see his or her parents soon. Parents should be urged to talk to their children, informing them that the doctor is going to help them. The parents should be careful *not* to indicate that the doctor will *not* hurt the child, because if the child has pain as a result of a test, the child-parent relationship may be jeopardized.

The parent should be encouraged to stay with the child in the hospital as long as possible and even sleep in the child's room at night, if permitted. Studies have shown that when parents are permitted to stay with their children, the recovery is quicker and there is less emotional trauma. An important part of caring for children is talking to the parents. If the parents understand the situation, they can do much to help the doctor-child relationship.

Disabled children, like disabled adults, are extremely apprehensive of the atmosphere in the hospital. It reminds them of previous experiences. The interviewer must take time to play with the child while talking to the parent or the person accompanying the child. Complimenting the youngster with statements such as "How pretty you are" or "What a nice outfit you're wearing" seems to foster good will. These children crave love, affection, and attention. The parent has to be reassured that the staff members are reliable and caring. This will give the parent peace of mind. If a child wishes to keep a favorite toy or blanket, there should be no restrictions. Separation from home and family is a terrible experience for any child, but even more so for the disabled one, who functions better in familiar surroundings.

The Aged Patient

The aged patient requires a lot of attention. Depression is prevalent among the elderly. Aged patients must frequently cope with the loss of loved ones and other important persons in their environment. They are also stressed by changes in their own self-images and the way they are perceived by others. A deterioration in bodily function also contributes to depression in aged patients.

A patient's depression may be so severe that he or she may consider suicide a reasonable alternative to living with a severe chronic illness or living alone after the death of a spouse. Among this bereaved population, more deaths from suicide occur within the first 4 years following the spouse's death than from all other causes (McMahon and Puch, 1965).

The interviewer must never assume that older patients' complaints are natural for their age. People do not die of old age; they die of illnesses. Most of these patients are alert and capable of independent living. The ones who are unable to care for themselves are usually accompanied by a family member or an attendant. The interviewer must obtain as much information as possible from these sources. The interviewer should also refrain from using patronizing mannerisms that belittle the individual. A friendly, respectful approach will reassure the patient. Aged patients should be advised about everything that will be done to them. This makes patients confident that there will be no unpleasant surprises. Because of advanced age, such patients may be afraid of dying. Those who are afraid should be reassured that everything possible will be done to make them better. Many people survive an illness because of their desire to live and therefore fight to stay alive. Overzealous reassurance is not appropriate for all aged patients; many regard death as a reasonable outcome.

The Widowed Patient

Many widowed patients come to the hospital alone, with the thought that because their spouses are gone, nobody cares about them. They may be suffering from depression as a result of loneliness. The interviewer should inquire gently whether there are any children, relatives, or friends who can be contacted or will come to visit. These patients may be at odds with their children and may prefer that they not know that the patient has entered a hospital. In other cases the family may live far away. The patients do not want their family to worry, so they do not tell the family. In these cases, it is advisable for the physician to alert the social worker to the particular situation. Volunteers visiting the patient as well as members of the clergy can bring soothing counsel. A warm handshake and reassurance are effective ways of putting this patient in a relaxed state of mind. Many widowed patients are quite active. The clinician should not presume that all widowed individuals are isolated.

The Post-traumatic Stress Disorder Patient

Although the effects of natural calamities and their aftermaths have been recognized since the times of ancient Greece, it is only since 1980 that the American Psychiatric

Association included post-traumatic stress disorder (PTSD) in its handbook of psychiatric disorders, *Diagnostic and Statistical Manual of Mental Disorders (DSM-III)*. One of the first descriptions of PTSD was made by the Greek historian Herodotus. In 490 BC he described, during the Battle of Marathon, an Athenian soldier who suffered no injury from war but became permanently blind after witnessing the death of a fellow soldier. Health-care providers are only beginning to recognize the enormous toll that trauma can take in personal suffering and functional impairment. PTSD may also impact future generations through effects on parental (or guardian) behavior and competence.

For many years PTSD was considered only a wartime affliction. It has been estimated that 25–30% of veterans of the Vietnam War are affected with PTSD. These patients have a variety of symptoms, including nightmares, sleep disturbances, avoidance reactions, guilt, intrusive memories, and dissociative flashbacks. In addition, as much as 9–10% of the U.S. population may have some form of PTSD. Studies have shown that PTSD develops in 2% of those exposed to any type of accident, 30% of those exposed to a community disaster, 25% of those who have experienced traumatic bereavement, 65% of those experiencing nonsexual assault; 85% of battered women in shelters; and 50–90% of those who were raped. Of all psychiatric disorders, PTSD poses one of the greatest challenges to the health-care provider due to its complexity and variability of signs and symptoms.

In 1987, the *DSM-III-R* defined PTSD as including those traumatic events that were "outside the range of usual human experience and that would be markedly distressing to almost anyone." PTSD is a normal reaction to an abnormal amount of stress. Although trauma is usually considered as an injury to a body part, it may be even more devastating to the psyche. Wounding of emotions, spirit, the will to live, dignity, and the sense of security can be traumatic. Some traumatic events may go on for months or years, whereas others may occur in a few seconds and have the same lasting effects as longer events. In minutes, a person's sense of self and sense of the world as a secure place can be shattered.

One problem with the *DSM-III-R* description is that it fails to recognize the importance of the subjective appraisal of the event; this includes the ethnocultural aspects of PTSD. The new *DSM-IV* now lists PTSD as the only diagnosis that identifies the origin of symptoms from external events rather than from within the individual. All of the following *DSM-IV* criteria must be met to make a diagnosis of PTSD:

1. Experience of a traumatic event
2. Re-experience of the trauma
3. Evidence of numbing or other avoidance behavior
4. Exhibition of signs of hyperarousal
5. Evidence of symptoms for at least 1 month
6. Experience of difficulties at home, work, or in other important areas of life as a result of the symptoms

Life is filled with many crises, such as losing a parent or being robbed. Although these events can be stressful, they are not considered "traumatic." A *traumatic event* is defined as an unusual occurrence that is not part of normal human experience that evokes extreme helplessness, fear, and despair. Examples of traumatic events include a natural catastrophe, such as a tornado, hurricane, volcano, earthquake, fire, landslide, or flood; a human catastrophe, such as war, concentration camps, refugee camps, sexual assault, physical assault, or other forms of victimization; witnessing a death, rape, torture, or beating; a suicide of a family member or close friend; and any exposure to danger of one's own safety and life.

Re-experiencing the trauma can take many forms, including dreams, flashbacks, or situations that remind the person of the traumatic event. While dreaming, the person may shout, shake, or thrash about the bed. Although the person may awake suddenly, he or she may not remember the nightmare, but the intense feeling may persist for long periods.

Psychic or emotional numbing is a form of self-protection against unbearable emotional pain. After the event, the individual may experience periods of feeling emotionally dead or numb. That person may have great difficulty in expressing tenderness or loving feelings. *Avoidance behavior* is another important aspect of PTSD. People with PTSD often feel alienated and apart from others. They may lose interest in activities that once gave them pleasure. Others are unable to remember certain aspects of the traumatic event.

Hyperarousal symptoms include difficulty in falling or staying asleep, irritability, outbursts of anger, difficulty in concentration, overprotectiveness of oneself or others, and an exaggerated startle response. People who were abused in a bed commonly experience insomnia. People with an exaggerated startle response may jump at loud noises or if someone touches them on the back.

Duration of symptoms is variable, but according to the official criteria for PTSD, the symptoms must endure at least 1 month.

The last criterion relates to the *impact of the psychic trauma on one's lifestyle.* Survivors of human catastrophes, in general, suffer longer than survivors of natural catastrophes. In addition, the devastating effects of emotional trauma may be influenced by exposure of the individual to one or more traumatic events. Rape is traumatic, but multiple rapes are even more traumatic. Do the person's symptoms interfere with his or her ability to work, study, socialize, or maintain healthy familial relationships?

There are many recognized trauma-related disorders. These include brief reactive psychosis, multiple personality disorder, dissociative fugue, dissociative amnesia, conversion disorder, depersonalization disorder, dream anxiety disorder, somatization disorder, borderline personality disorder, and antisocial personality disorder. Many other trauma-related disorders have been postulated. These disorders and the trauma that may precede them are indicated as follows:

Brief reactive psychosis: any event(s) that would be stressful to anyone
Multiple personality disorder: abuse or other childhood emotional trauma
Dissociative fugue: severe psychological stress such as marital quarrels, military conflict, natural disaster, or personal rejection
Dissociative amnesia: severe psychological stress such as the tragic death of a loved one, abandonment, or a threat of personal injury
Conversion disorder: extreme psychological stress such as warfare or a recent, tragic death of a loved one
Depersonalization disorder: severe stress such as military combat or an automobile accident
Dream anxiety disorder: any major life stress, depression, substance abuse, or substance withdrawal
Somatization disorder: early childhood abuse
Borderline personality disorder: early childhood trauma
Antisocial personality disorder: early childhood abuse

Learned helplessness syndrome is a condition that is frequently seen in trauma survivors, commonly women and children, prisoners of war, concentration camp survivors, refugee camp survivors, or other tortured survivors. The name developed from animal experiments by Seligman (1975). Animals subjected to electric shocks and unable to escape despite their attempts would sink into listlessness and despair. Later, they were reshocked, but although trained to press a lever to stop the shocks, the animals made no effort to do so. The animals had learned to be helpless. It has been postulated that there is an adrenal neurotransmitter problem in animals and humans exposed to severe, repeated traumatic events that may serve as the biological basis for the hyperarousal and numbing phases of PTSD.

Although almost any symptom can result from PTSD, some of the more common ones are as follows:

- Eating disorders
- Anger or rage
- Self-condemnation
- Self-mutilation
- Depression
- Self-hatred
- Suicidal thoughts
- Homicidal thoughts
- Headaches
- Backaches
- Chronic gastrointestinal problems

■ Worsening or activation of chronic medical problems (e.g., diabetes, hypertension)
■ Drug abuse
■ Overworking
■ Self-isolation

An example of a person with PTSD is the Holocaust survivor. Holocaust survivors have complex problems that have affected their lives for more than 50 years. They are *survivors*; therefore, they never stopped fighting for survival. They are especially frightened of becoming sick because, in the past, to survive meant to be in good health; the alternative was to face doom. These patients are afraid of losing control of their lives as well as losing their dignity.

Holocaust-survivor patients may have many psychosomatic complaints commonly related to the gastrointestinal tract. Chest pain, often relieved by belching, may be related to frequent air swallowing. These patients experience vivid dreams and nightmares. They are suspicious and do not trust people readily because they suffered so much in the past. The interviewer must be especially kind and understanding. The majority of the survivors of the Nazi concentration camps are now 74–75 years of age and older, and many suffer from PTSD. Many suffer from severe depression, panic attacks, and anxiety. The interviewer must be careful when asking about family history and background. Most survivors lost entire families; many lost their first spouse and children. The psychological wounds are deep, and anything can trigger an outpouring of grief. It is frequently difficult to find out anything about the family history because the patient's parents and grandparents might have been killed at early ages. These patients should be reassured that they will be treated gently and competently. They, like all PTSD patients, must be assured of security. Feeling safe is the highest priority in their lives.

The Sick Physician

Perhaps the most difficult of all patients to care for is the sick physician. The anxiety of sick physicians should not be underestimated. The expression "A little knowledge is a dangerous thing" applies to the sick physician. Every medical or nursing student goes through the "student syndrome," which is the suspicion that he or she has been stricken with the disease about which he or she is learning. Imagine the anxiety that occurs when the physician *is* stricken. In addition to anxiety about health, there is the new role identification of being the patient. Physicians feel helpless and have great difficulty divorcing themselves from the role of physician. They constantly ask what the electrocardiogram shows and for the results of blood tests. They try to suggest additional tests or even disagree with the tests that have been ordered. The novice interviewer should provide ample time for the sick physician to express fears and anxieties. With the interviewer's support, sick physicians eventually recognize and accept their new role as patient.

Influence of Disease on Patient Response

Just as background and age govern a patient's response, so do the patient's present illness and past medical illnesses. This section illustrates the influence of disease on the type of response.

The Disabled Patient

Disabled patients may come to the hospital with great apprehension and mistrust. They are usually familiar with the shortcomings of hospitals because they have probably been hospitalized for painful tests or surgery. They may be burdened with an inferiority complex and may feel unattractive. The interviewer must take all this into consideration and assure patients that everything will be done to make them comfortable. The interviewer must sort out the emotional problems of disabled persons from the physical ones that brought them to the hospital. A friendly smile or a few kind words can help make these patients cooperate, thereby securing a better doctor-patient relationship.

Many disabled people have developed their own routines that work for them. They often do not want medical personnel to impose their way of doing something if the patient's way works.

Patients with a hearing impairment need to be treated differently than other disabled patients. Sit directly in front of these patients to allow them to benefit from lip reading. Make sure that the lighting in the room is correct so that your face is well illuminated. It is important to speak slowly with appropriate gestures and expressions to punctuate the question. Ask these patients if it is necessary for you to raise your voice. If they wear a hearing aid, raising your voice may not be necessary. If all else fails, the use of written questions can be helpful.

Another special type of disabled patient is the visually impaired patient. Because the patient with limited or no vision has no reference for you in the room, it is useful for you to occasionally touch the patient on the arm or shoulder. This can be done instead of the more standard nonverbal facilitations, which are of no value in this patient.

The severely mentally retarded patient must be accompanied by a family member or guardian in order to provide a proper history.

The Cancer Patient

The cancer patient has five major concerns: loss of control, pain, alienation, mutilation, and mortality. Loss of control makes this patient feel helpless. The knowledge of something growing uncontrolled within a patient's body creates frustration, fear, and anger. Suffering with pain is one of the most feared aspects of cancer. The feeling of alienation stems from the reactions of people around the patient.

Fears of mutilation are common among cancer patients. The fear of being perceived as lacking "wholeness" contributes to depression and anxiety. The young woman with breast cancer who requires a mastectomy fears that she will be rejected as no longer being a complete woman. Supportive family members are the key in reassuring this patient that they will love her just as before her surgery. A diagnosis of cancer makes a patient aware of mortality and leads to intense fear of unremitting pain.

Family members and friends often express grief before death occurs. Resentment and anger may be directed toward the cancer patient. Physicians often harbor feelings of inadequacy about these patients and have difficulty speaking with them. The patients are thus rejected by their own physician. The physician is afraid that the patient may ask some questions, perhaps about death, that the physician cannot handle. The physician must recognize his or her emotional and behavioral reaction and be realistic about the limitations of medical science.

The interviewer should allow the patient to vent anxieties and promote dialogue. Listening to the patient aids the doctor-patient relationship.

The AIDS Patient

Patients with AIDS are fearful for their lives and of being stigmatized as a member of an undesirable group. They are aware that their chance of survival is slim. The fear and misunderstanding common in high-risk groups result in delayed medical treatment. Denial is the important factor in most of these patients. The patient has an intense fear of physicians, nurses, students, and paramedical personnel, who may have strong emotions related to this disease and its risk groups. The patient's fear is paralleled by the anxiety of the hospital workers who have to treat an individual with this deadly disease. Their fear of contracting the disease, even by casual contact, is formidable. These fears are also present among the patient's friends and family, who often banish the patient from all activities. The patient may have been fired from a job because the employer is afraid of catching the disease. There is an unsympathetic rejection of AIDS patients. They suffer emotional turmoil, which contributes to intense anxiety, hostility, and depression. They may have to die alone.

The interviewer should be as supportive as possible without giving false reassurances. Most patients with AIDS recognize their prognosis. They should be given as many facts as appropriate, and the staff members tending to them must be educated concerning the disease.

The Dysphasic Patient

The dysphasic patient has an impairment of speech and cannot arrange words correctly. Dysphasia is usually caused by a cerebral lesion, such as a stroke. The degree of dysphasia can vary enormously, almost to complete aphasia. Although patients may appear relatively unresponsive, they may be totally aware of all conversation. Therefore, all discussions conducted in the presence of such patients must be made with the assumption that the patients can understand. Before the interview, the interviewer may give patients a pen and paper to determine whether they can respond by writing. "Yes" and "No" answers may be given by a nod of the head.

The Psychotic Patient

Psychotic patients have an impairment of their reality-testing abilities. They have a gross inability to communicate effectively. They may also suffer from hallucinations, delusions, or feelings of persecution. Psychotic patients cannot deal with their fear. They are constantly struggling with the ever-changing demands of their environment. It is most important that the interviewer recognize the psychotic patient early and to remain as calm as possible. If the patient has had violent episodes, have assistance standing by.

In general, interviewing psychotic patients presents a difficult task for the inexperienced interviewer. Some of these patients tend to be inarticulate and preoccupied with fantasies, whereas others are reasonably lucid. The symptoms and signs of their psychosis are not clearly evident at first assessment. There are several clues to the existence of a psychosis. Pay particular attention to the speech pattern and its organization. Is there a jumble of ideas? Psychotic patients are easily distracted, and the interviewer must constantly remind them of the subject. These patients fail to complete any train of thought and cannot follow any idea to completion. They can have bizarre impressions about their bodies. They may complain that they have noticed that one arm has recently shortened or that their external genitalia have suddenly shrunk or enlarged. In addition, they may have evidence of an inappropriate affect. The patient may laugh while telling about the death of a friend or relation.

A special type of psychotic personality disorder is found in patients with *Münchausen's syndrome.* Such patients are the classic hospital malingerers. They are pathologic liars and travel from clinician to clinician, from hospital to hospital. They complain of a wide variety of symptoms and, in fact, *create* signs of illness to seek an advantage. Their histories are well rehearsed, and they have a masochistic perpetuation of self-injury. For example, the Münchausen patient may actually prick the skin under a fingernail so it will not be obvious, drop some blood into the urine, and call the clinician, stating that there is blood in the urine. These patients frequently seek out painful diagnostic and therapeutic procedures. At times, they may even undergo surgical procedures.

The Demented and Delirious Patient

Demented patients have lost previously acquired intellectual function, most typically memory. Delirious patients have a disorder of consciousness that does not allow them to interact correctly with the surroundings. Delirious patients frequently become more confused when taken out of their normal environment, especially at night. The term *sundowning* is used in such circumstances. Fear is common in both types of patients. In interviewing these patients, try to be sensitive to their emotions as best as possible, and above all try to allay their fears. Be particularly aware of questions possibly threatening to the patient.

Patients with an organic mental syndrome present a special problem. At times these patients seem lucid; at other times they are disoriented with regard to person, place, or time. If the patient is able to answer some of the questions, record the answers. The same questions should be asked again later to determine whether the patient will respond similarly. These patients have defects in attention span, memory, and abstract thought. Be alert to inconsistent and slow, hesitant responses. Occasionally, patients may interject some humor to try to cover up for their difficulty in memory. A careful mental status examination will indicate the problem. It may be useful to remind the patient of your name and tell him or her that you will ask for the name in a few minutes. Frequently, such patients have forgotten it. Furthermore, the history these patients give may not be reliable.

The Acutely Ill Patient

The acutely ill patient demands prompt attention. In these situations, a concise history and physical examination are in order. A careful history of the present and past illnesses must be taken expeditiously so that the diagnosis may be made and treatment begun. It may be appropriate in this setting to interview the patient while doing the physical examination. Time is of the essence. However, patients who are acutely ill may respond to questions more slowly than normal because of pain, nausea, or vomiting. Be considerate of their problems and allow them time to answer questions. After a patient has been stabilized, there will be time to go back and take a more complete history.

The Surgical Patient

Patients faced with a surgical procedure may be scared despite a calm appearance. They may feel helpless and out of control. The fear of anesthesia, disfigurement, disability, or death is always present. The fear of not awakening from the anesthesia can be devastating. When they awaken, will they find that their body is no longer "whole"? Did the surgeon find something that was not expected? These patients fear the unknown. A question about the surgeon's ability is an expression of the patient's anxiety. Often, patients have tests and are told they are normal "except" for a small area: they will need surgery to "check it out." This lack of communication by the surgeon adds to the patient's anxiety. A surgeon's schedule is frequently erratic. Surgery may be delayed or postponed, which adds to the surgical patient's anxiety and anger. Many possible communication difficulties exist. The best way to avoid the unnecessary anxiety-provoking situations is to maintain open communication among the patient, the physician, and the patient's family. In the postoperative period, the patient's relief of having lived through surgery may be displayed in a variety of ways. The patient may be apathetic and show a general lack of interest or may be moody, irritable, aggressive, angry, or tearful. Subconsciously patients may wish to harm the surgeon for "cutting" into their bodies, whereas consciously they want to thank the surgeon. This dichotomy may be the root of the anger so commonly seen in postoperative patients. In other patients, depression may be seen as a result of the loss of part of the body. The best example of this is the "phantom limb." Patients who have undergone an amputation of a leg frequently claim sensation in their lost limb. Some of this may be physiologic, but certainly some of the phantom leg pain is related to depression. The caring interviewer should allow the patient time to release these tensions and feelings of loss.

The Alcoholic Patient

Alcoholic patients have a physiologic and/or psychological dependence on alcohol. Most of the time, interviewers conduct the sessions when the patient is not inebriated. Excessive drinking is often an attempt to deaden feelings of guilt and failure. The more patients drink, the more they are abandoned by their family and friends. They feel castigated and alone. They are left to their only "friend:" alcohol. They are often ready to talk, and their account of their drinking habits may be interesting. Alcoholics generally have a low opinion of themselves. They may even be upset about their persistent drinking habits. Their hatred of themselves may be a manifestation of a self-destructive wish. Alcoholic patients may also have fears about sexual inadequacy or homosexuality. It is not easy to open up such topics, because these patients are likely to respond explosively. The sensitive interviewer should approach these issues in a manner that is neither condescending nor moralistic.

The Psychosomatic Patient

Just as physical illness can produce psychological problems, so can psychological problems create physical ailments. The intimate interaction of the mind and body is clearly demonstrated in the psychosomatic disorder.

Psychosomatic patients express emotional discomfort and distress in the form of bodily symptoms. They may be totally unaware of the psychological stress in their lives or the relationship of stress to the symptoms.

There are many ways of dealing with psychosomatic patients. First, identify the disorder: do not miss the possible diagnosis of an affective or anxiety disorder. Treatment of somatization is directed toward teaching the patient to cope with the psychological problems. The physician should be aware that somatization operates unconsciously; the patient really is suffering. Above all, *never* tell the patient that his or her problem is "in your head." Anxiety, fear, and depression are the main psychological problems associated with psychosomatic illness. The list of associated, common symptoms and illnesses is long and includes chest pain, headaches, peptic ulcer disease, ulcerative colitis, irritable bowel syndrome, nausea, vomiting, anorexia nervosa, urticaria, tachycardia, hypertension, asthma, migraine, muscle tension syndromes, obesity, rashes, and dizziness. Answers to an open-ended question such as "What's been happening in your life?" often provide insight into the problems.

Finally, the interviewer should legitimize patients' suffering by telling them that their suffering is "real." The interviewer must help patients recognize the way in which stress can create physical suffering. Giving patients the freedom to discuss hopes and fears is often more beneficial than a written prescription for medications.

The Dying Patient

Few patients are as conscious of taking up a physician's time as those who have less time remaining. Dying patients may initially have many questions, but as time goes by, they ask less and less of their caretakers.

Many health-care providers have a dread of death that is so intense that they behave irrationally. They avoid patients who are dying or those with incurable diseases. The emotional needs of the dying patients may be largely ignored. Many patients have a greater fear of dying than of death itself. The fear of living as a chronically ill patient can be almost as intolerable as (and often more so than) the fear of death.

Dying patients suffer from the pain, nausea, or vomiting caused by the disease or treatment. They may be rejected by their families, hospital staff members, or even their own physicians. Many patients have strong feelings of anger, guilt, resentment, and frustration. "Why me?" "It should have been diagnosed earlier." They may envy healthy individuals. They may deny their imminent death; this is the first stage of dying. Not uncommonly, a dying patient will be interviewed and not tell the interviewer about the illness. Even when asked specifically about the disease, the patient will deny any knowledge of having a fatal disease. This mechanism of denial allows the patient to cope with life as it is. Each person faces death differently. Some can deal with it head-on; others cannot. Some approach it with fear and tears, whereas others grow to accept it as an inevitable event. Given sufficient time and the necessary understanding, most dying patients can arrive at the final stage of dying: acceptance. This stage is characterized by apathy and social withdrawal. Counselors specifically trained in the grieving process are often helpful to the patient, family, and health-care providers.

The dying patient needs to speak to someone. The clinician should be alert for subtle clues that the patient wishes to discuss the topic of death. For example, if a patient remarks that his "wife is well provided for," it is correct to pursue this point by making an interpretive statement such as, "I sense that you are very worried about your illness." Although the conversation that ensues might be emotionally draining for the interviewer, it is incumbent upon the interviewer to allow the dying patient to speak. Sometimes the most appropriate response to an expression of grief is a thoughtful period of silence.

Bibliography

Adelman RD, Greene MG, Charon R: Issues in physician–elderly patient interaction. Ageing Soc 11:127, 1991.

Adler G: The physician and the hypochondriacal patient. N Engl J Med 304:1394, 1981.

Cassem NH, Hackett TP: Psychological aspects of myocardial infarction. Med Clin North Am 61: 711, 1977.

Cousins N: Anatomy of an illness (as perceived by the patient). N Engl J Med 295:1458, 1976.

Davidson JRT, Foa EB (eds): Posttraumatic Stress Disorder: DSM-IV and Beyond. Washington, DC, American Psychiatric Press, Inc., 1993.

Dombro RH: The surgically ill child and his family. Surg Clin North Am 50:759, 1970.

Gorlin R, Zucker HD: Physician's reactions to patients: A key to teaching humanistic medicine. N Engl J Med 308:1057, 1983.

Groves JE: Taking care of the hateful patient. N Engl J Med 298:883, 1978.

Hahn SR, Feiner JS. Bellin EH: The doctor-patient-family relationship: A compensatory alliance. Ann Intern Med 109:884, 1988.

Helman CG: Culture, Health and Illness. London, Wright, 1990.

Kornfield DS: Psychiatric problems of an intensive care unit. Med Clin North Am 55:1353, 1971.

Kraut AM: Healers and strangers: Immigrant attitudes toward the physicians in America—A relationship in historical perspective. JAMA 263:1807, 1990.

Kübler-Ross E: On Death and Dying. New York, Macmillan, 1969.

Lipsett DR: Medical and psychological characteristics of "crocks." J Psychiatry Med 1:15, 1970.

Lock M: The relationship between culture and health or illness. In Christie-Seely J (ed): Working with the Family in Primary Care. New York, Praeger, 1984.

McMahon B. Puch G: Suicide in the widowed. Am J Epidemiol 81:23, 1965.

Matsakis A: I Can't Get Over It: A Handbook for Trauma Survivors, 2nd ed. Oakland, CA, New Harbinger Publications, Inc., 1996.

Mezzich JE, Kleinman A, Fabrega H Jr, et al (eds): Culture and Psychiatric Diagnosis: A DSM-IV Perspective. Washington, DC, American Psychiatric Press, Inc., 1996.

Pynoos RS (ed): Posttraumatic Stress Disorder: A Clinical Review. Lutherville, MD, The Sidran Press, 1994.

Rainwater L: The lower class: Health, illness, and medical institutions. In Millon T (ed): Medical Behavioral Science. Philadelphia, W.B. Saunders, 1975.

Reichel W: Care of the elderly. In Taylor RB (ed): Family Medicine: Principles and Practice. New York, Springer-Verlag, 1983.

Sansone RA, Sansone LA: Borderline personality disorder: Office diagnosis and management. Am Fam Physician 44:194, 1991.

Seligman M: Helplessness: On Depression Development and Death. San Francisco, W.H. Freeman, 1975.

Senescu RA: The development of emotional complications in the patient with cancer. J Chron Dis 16:813, 1963.

Smith RC: Somatization disorder: Defining its role in clinical medicine. J Gen Intern Med 6:168, 1991.

Stern M, Pascale L, Ackerman A: Life adjustment postmyocardial infarction. Arch Intern Med 137: 1680, 1977.

Tseng WS: The nature of somatic complaints among psychiatric patients. The Chinese case. Compar Psychiatry 16:237, 1975.

US Department of Commerce, Bureau of the Census, 1990 Census, Washington, DC, US Government Printing Office, 1990.

Waxman HS: The patient as physician. Ann Int Med 126:656, 1997.

Williams JGL, Jones JR, Workman MC, et al: The psychological control of preoperative anxiety. Psychophysiology 12:50, 1975.

CHAPTER 3

Caring for Patients in a Culturally Diverse Society

What the scalpel is to the surgeon, words are to the clinician . . . the conversation between doctor and patient is the heart of the practice of medicine.

Philip A. Tumulty, M.D.
1912–1989

The cultural aspects of physical diagnosis and medicine have become increasingly important. By the middle of the 21st century, the majority of the population of the United States will no longer be white (Hodgkinson, 1992). It is imperative for all members of the health-care professions to focus on the diversity of cultural beliefs and practices that exists within U.S. society. Every health-care provider must understand the dimensions and complexities of caring for individuals of culturally diverse backgrounds. Equally important is the provider's knowledge of the cultural and socioeconomic factors that affect the patient's access to and use of health-care resources. When treating recent immigrants, it is necessary to be aware that their attitudes toward illness and treatment may be very different from those of the indigenous population. Second-generation immigrants may have yet a different appreciation.

The United States is home to one of the most ethnically and culturally heterogeneous populations in the world. There are more than 100 ethnic groups and 400 tribes of Native Americans in the United States, each with specific practices and beliefs. This chapter provides a sampling of cultural diversity and is intended to sensitize the health-care provider to the importance of understanding the impact of cultural diversity on health-care delivery. This chapter is not comprehensive because not all groups are represented; no culture was omitted purposely. The chapter is divided into three main sections: a discussion of some general considerations in delivery of health care in a multicultural society; selected cross-cultural perspectives; and a review of traditional Chinese medicine.

Studies have shown that the frequency of use of unconventional therapy in the United States is far greater than previously reported (Eisenberg et al, 1993). Unconventional medicine consists of relaxation techniques, imagery, massage, spiritual healing, herbal medicine, acupuncture, folk remedies, and prayer, to name a few. An estimated one in three persons in the U.S. adult population used these and other alternate healing methods in 1990. The number of visits to providers of this health care was greater than the number of visits to all primary care medical doctors nationwide. The money spent for these visits amounted to approximately $13.7 billion, $10.3 billion of which was paid out-of-pocket. This figure is comparable to the $12.8 billion spent out-of-pocket annually for all hospitalizations in the United States. One of the reasons for patients seeking alternate therapies may be due to failures in the doctor-patient relationship. Health-care providers often fail to discuss the use of alternate therapies because they lack adequate knowledge in this area. This lack of communication may prove to be detrimental to the patient, because the use of some forms of unconventional medicine, if unsupervised, may be dangerous to the patient.

Health care should be considered in the context of the consumer, not solely that of the provider. The examples of health-care practices in this chapter illustrate *traditional* cultural differences. It should not be misinterpreted that all patients of a certain group have these beliefs. Many patients who are now second- or third-generation Americans may not follow or believe in these practices but may know of them from parents or grandparents.

The names used to identify various groups change with time. Within a cultural group, there are variations as to how its members identify themselves and what name they prefer. The names of cultural groups often grow out of ethnic and ideologic movements.

Stereotyping the patient by race, lifestyle, cultural or religious backgrounds, economic status, or level of education can be detrimental to establishing a solid doctor-patient relationship. The following is not intended to stereotype or label any particular group, but rather to teach about how to recognize common cultural characteristics and to better understand the needs of patients. The health-care provider must recognize that there is also great intra-group variability. Such knowledge of race, culture, and religion can be used to help understand a patient's expressed attitudes and behavior.

General Considerations

According to the 1990 census, there are 248,709,873 people in the United States, an increase of more than 22 million since the 1980 census. This number includes 199,686,070 (80.2%) whites; 29,986,060 (12.1%) African-Americans; 7,273,662 (3%) Asians/Pacific Islanders; and 1,959,234 (0.8%) Native Americans (American Indian, Inuit and Inupiat, and Aleut). There are 22,354,059 people (9%) of Hispanic American origin who comprise a multiculturally diverse group. The members of the Asian/Pacific Island community have their origins in China, Hawaii, the Philippines, Japan, Korea, Cambodia, Laos, Thailand, Malaysia, and Vietnam. The actual numbers are probably several million higher, given that many people are uncounted because of their undocumented status (i.e., no immigration papers) and inadequate census counts.

The results of the 1990 census with regard to European ancestry were as follows: 23.3% German; 15.6% Irish; 13.1% English; 5.9% Italian; 4.1% French; 3.8% Polish; 2.5% Dutch; 2.3% Scottish-Irish; 2.2% Scottish; 1.9% Swedish; 1.6% Norwegian; and 0.4% Spanish.

As regards people of Latino origin, 62.6% are from Mexico; 11.4%, Puerto Rico; 6.0%, Central America; 4.9%, Cuba; 4.8%, Spain; 4.7%, South America; and 2.4%, Dominican Republic. The United States now ranks sixth in terms of the numbers of Latinos residing within its borders.

There have been significant changes in the U.S. population in the past few decades: the white majority is shrinking and aging, whereas the proportion of African-Americans, Asian Americans, and Native Americans is young and growing. It has been projected that by the year 2010 there will be a decrease in white youth by 3.8 million and an increase in nonwhite youth by 44 million (Hodgkinson, 1992).

Language can be a significant barrier to good health care. According to the 1990 census, there are more than 14 million people in the United States who have "limited English proficiency."* More than 5% of the population of California, New York, Texas, New Mexico, and Hawaii have limited English-language skills (ASTHO, 1992).

Race, Culture, and Ethnicity

Race, as defined by *Merriam Webster's Collegiate Dictionary,* 10th edition, is a "class or kind of people unified by a community of interests, habits, or inherited physical characteristics." The term *culture* has a broad meaning. It refers to the unifying beliefs of any group of people of similar religion, values, attitudes, ritual practices, family structure, language, and/or mode of social organization. Culture provides values that are shared by members of a specific society or a social group within a society. Culture socializes its members on how to perceive the world, how to behave in the world, and how to experience the world emotionally. Elements such as language, social or familial roles, beliefs about the universe, the nature of good and evil, appropriate dress, eating and hygienic habits, manners, and food represent cultural values and notions. Culture pervades all lives and shapes all human identity. All personal experiences and norms are perceived through the culture from which they emerge. Culture shapes human perception of reality and influences societal forms of conduct. Different cultures reinforce different behaviors; what is acceptable in one culture may be considered deviant in another.

Cultural values, in part, determine how a person will behave as a patient—the types of treatment accepted and follow-up permitted—and who will make the deci-

---

* "Limited English proficiency" is a term used by the United States Department of Health and Human Services to define the portion of the population that is non–English speaking or limited–English speaking.

sions. From a U.S. medical point of view, it is the clinician and the patient who make the decisions, but due to influence from a patient's family, the picture can be very different. In some traditional cultures, the family takes this over for the patient. Authority figures such as parents or grandparents often take precedence. For example, in the case of Gypsy patients, the primary decision-maker may not even be a relative. Among Orthodox Jewish patients, a medical decision may be made only after consultation with their rabbi. Among the Amish, the entire community may play a role in decision-making.

Ethnicity is a cultural group's sense of identification associated with the group's common social and cultural heritage. The *Harvard Encyclopedia of American Ethnic Groups* defines ethnicity as "a common geographical origin, language, religious faith, and cultural ties (e.g., shared traditions, values, symbols, literature, music, and food preferences)." It is often used as a polite word for race.

Disease, Illness, and Health

The terms *disease* and *illness* are often used interchangeably. Medical sociologists and cultural anthropologists, however, make a distinction. The word *disease* refers to a disorder in which there is a change from normal in the body's structure or function, involving one or more organs of the body. *Illness* is the subjective distress felt by the patient and by those close to the patient, rather than the actual state of ill health. The patient's culture often determines how the patient interprets, explains, responds to, and deals with a disease. It also influences when a patient will seek health-care decisions and from whom. Some cultures try to "normalize" their symptoms, maintaining that symptoms are not abnormal for a person of that age group. They might say that they have experienced the symptoms before and that therefore the symptoms are normal for them. Other cultures dictate immediate care even if symptoms are minimal. Some cultures teach that to be ill is a punishment or curse, whereas others may emphasize that to be ill is to be weak, irresponsible, or unmasculine. For many people in the United States, the clinician is only one of many health-care providers, and often not the first. Patients are likely to consult a healer from their own tradition before seeking consultation from a Western-trained clinician. Two patients from different cultures may respond differently to the same disease or symptoms. Thus, treating illness, rather than treating disease, requires the health-care provider to have not only a broad understanding of medicine but also an understanding of the patient's cultural background.

Health, as defined in *The Random House Dictionary of the English Language,* is "the general condition of the body or mind with reference to soundness and vigor." It is often defined more abstractly as the "absence of disease." In some cultures, health is viewed as the freedom from evil. Other cultures regard health as day and illness as night. By extrapolation, health becomes daylight and clean, and illness becomes darkness and dirty. These depictions form the basis of the beliefs of many cultures, which are discussed later in this chapter.

Culture and Health

It is critical for any health-care provider to have an appreciation of cross-cultural family values, language, norms, religion, and political ideology. An estimated 80–90% of all self-recognized episodes of illness are managed exclusively outside a formal health-care system. Traditional healers, mediums, self-help groups, and religious practitioners provide a substantial proportion of this health care.

Within the United States, there are many culturally distinct groups. Even within these groups, there are many variables such as educational achievement, socioeconomic class, generational status, and political relationship between the country of origin and the United States. All these factors figure into establishing the dynamic reality of an ethnic group. Patients, newly arrived or native born, who are in a low socioeconomic bracket appear to be a strong predictor of whether ethnicity will influence their behavior. The following are other predictors of behavioral ethnicity:

- Emigration from rural areas
- Frequent return to the native area
- Lack of formal education

- Immigration to the United States at an older age
- A major difference in dress or diet

Newly arrived immigrants often experience prejudice; the toll to their psyche may be a heavy one. Cultural change is not limited merely to immigration. Moving around within the same country or changing professions may easily result in *culture shock*. The new culture may be viewed as unempathetic, cruel, and critical. The newcomer frequently experiences frustration, irritability, fatigue, loss of flexibility, and an inability to communicate feelings to others. Distrust, paranoid tendencies, depression, anxiety, and physical and psychosomatic illnesses may develop. It is therefore necessary to include a patient's and family's immigrational and migrational history in the evaluation of the patient. The family is the carrier of ethnic traits and identity.

Cross-cultural marriages can offer the best and worst of both worlds. The reconciliation of different norms and traditions may provide an enriching experience, but a clash of different cultural traits may lead to strained relations of spouses and families.

The influence of ethnicity and culture on health and health-belief practices has long been recognized as a result of the presence of racially related diseases and syndromes as well as societal predispositions to illness. It is very important to inquire about patients' perceptions of their symptoms and illness. To better understand the cultural influences on a patients' medical problem, Lipkin et al have suggested several questions for eliciting patients' explanations for their symptoms or health-belief practices. These include the following:

- *"What do you call your problem?"*
- *"What causes your problem?"*
- *"Why do you think it started when it did?"*
- *"How does it work—what is going on in your body?"*
- *"What kind of treatment do you think would be best for this problem?"*
- *"How has this problem affected your life?"*
- *"What frightens or concerns you most about this problem and treatment?"*

Genetic Diseases

The simultaneous manifestation of two or more forms or alleles of a gene in a population is a genetic polymorphism. Certain genetic polymorphic states, such as blood groups, are well associated with disease. As early as 1953, an association of blood group A with gastric carcinoma was recognized. The causal relationship of hemoglobin S to sickle cell anemia is well known. Thalassemia comprises more than 50 genetic disorders characterized by ineffective erythropoiesis that leads to severe anemia, fever, hyperuricemia, and skeletal deformities. The association of these disorders with patients of Mediterranean background has been established. The human leukocyte antigen gene complex and the many diseases associated with it continue to receive attention. Table 3–1 summarizes some specific diseases based on geographic distribution and ethnic populations.

Traditional Medical Beliefs

People interpret traditional medical beliefs about the body's shape and size, inner structure, and functions in terms of their cultural background. To illustrate various cultural beliefs about body functions, consider that patients often ascribe their symptoms to blood that is "too thin," "too thick," "too little," or "too slow." Blood can be used as an index of an emotional state (blushing); a personality type ("cold-blooded" or "hot-blooded"); a kinship ("blood is thicker than water"); a diet ("thin blood"); or a social relationship ("bad blood between people"). "Bad blood" is also frequently used to refer to syphilis.

As another example of the cultural beliefs about blood, consider menstruation. A study in 1977 by Snow and Johnson evaluated the views of inner city women in a public clinic in Michigan. Many of the 40 women interviewed felt that menstruation was a method of ridding the body of impurities that could cause illness or poison the body. Many of these women believed that, when the uterus was "open" during menstrual flow, they were vulnerable to disease. They also felt that it was only at this time when a woman could become pregnant. At all other times in the menstrual cycle, the

Table 3–1   Geographic and Ethnic Distributions of Specific Diseases

Specific Disease	Highest Incidence
Cancer of the skin	Eastern Australia
Cancer of the cheek	Southern India
	New Guinea
Cancer of the nasopharynx	Southeast Asia
	Kenya
Cancer of the esophagus	Northern France (Brittany)
	South Africa
	Eastern Rhodesia
	Western Kenya
	East of the Caspian Sea
Cancer of the stomach	Japan
	Korea
	Eastern Finland
	Mountain region of Colombia
	Eastern Zaire
	Southwest Uganda
Cancer of the colon	North America
	Western Europe
Cancer of the liver	Subsaharan Africa
Burkitt's lymphoma	Africa (100° north and south of equator)
Appendicitis	North America
	South America
	Europe
Diverticular disease	North America
	Western Europe
	Australia
	New Zealand
Hemorrhoids	North America
	South America
	Europe
Cholelithiasis	Southwestern United States
	Sweden
Stenosing duodenal ulcer	Southern India
	Eastern Zaire
Ischemic heart disease	North America
	South America
	Europe
	Finland
Hypertension	Japan
	Taiwan
Venous thrombosis	North America
	South America
	Europe
Varicose veins	North America
Diabetes	North America
	South America
	Europe
Urinary bladder stones	Rural Thailand
Multiple sclerosis	Northern United States
	Northern Europe
Rosacea	Great Britain, especially Scotland
Vogt-Koyanagi-Harada syndrome	Japan
	Italy
Takayasu's disease	Japan
Lactase deficiency	Greece
	The Jewish People
	African-Americans
	Thailand
	Eskimos
	Japan
Choroideremia	Northern Finland
Abetalipoproteinemia	Ashkenazic Jews
Glycosphingolipidoses	Ashkenazic Jews
Gaucher's disease	
Niemann-Pick disease	
Tay-Sachs disease	
Familial Mediterranean fever	Sephardic Jews
	Armenians

uterus was "closed," and pregnancy was impossible. Another common fear among the women was that of impeded menstrual flow. They feared that stoppage might cause a backup of poison and hence a stroke, cancer, or sterility. This fear may be a reason why the women avoid the use of certain methods of contraception, such as intrauterine devices and diaphragms.

Another belief about menstruation was studied by Skultans (1970) in two groups of women from a small mining village in South Wales. One group of women felt that menstruation was a process by which the body "cleansed" itself; the longer the period or greater the blood loss, the better. These women regarded menstruation as normal and essential to a healthy life. On the other hand, another group of women from the same mining town viewed menstruation as damaging to their overall health; they feared that the blood loss was threatening to their health and welcomed the thought of menopause.

Finally, Ngubane (1977) described the beliefs of South African Zulu women about menstruation. They felt that menstruating women had a "contagious pollution" that was deleterious to other living creatures and to the natural world. A man's virility would be reduced if he had sexual relations with a menstruating woman. Crops would be ruined and cattle would die if menstrual blood came in contact with them. In some of these African communities, menstruating women are isolated from the community because of their "dangerous pollution."

Although food is a source of nutrition, it plays many roles and is deeply embedded in almost all aspects of everyday life. Some foods eaten in one society are forbidden in others. Each culture has its own rules of food preparation: how it is served and how it should be eaten. Every culture defines foods that are edible and those that are not. In France, frogs' legs and snails are delicacies, whereas in the nearby United Kingdom they are rarely eaten. Some foods are considered sacred and others are prohibited. Food abstentions occur during the Jewish fast of Yom Kippur and the Muslim fast of Ramadan. In Hinduism, orthodox Hindus are forbidden to kill or eat any animal, especially the cow. However, milk or milk products may be consumed because they do not require the death of the animal. Orthodox followers of Islam and Judaism are prohibited from eating pork products. Only the meat from mammals that chew their cud and that have cloven hoofs is edible, provided that the animal was slaughtered ritually—*halal* (Islam) or *kosher* (Jewish). Among Orthodox Jews, meat and milk products are never eaten together. In Sikhism, pork is allowed but never beef. The Rastafarians are generally vegetarians, and alcohol is strictly forbidden.

Some cultural groups in the Islamic world, the Indian subcontinent, Latin America, and China believe in the *"hot-cold theory" of disease*. This belief, which is intuitive and common throughout Latin America, states that the body is regulated by hot and cold "humors." The belief stems from Hippocratic humoral theories brought to this hemisphere in the 16th and 17th centuries by the Spanish and Portuguese. Health is the balance of these hot and cold body fluids. Illness is defined by a humoral imbalance of these forces. All mental states, illnesses, and natural and supernatural forces are grouped into hot and cold categories. Foods, herbs, and medications are also classified as hot or cold and serve to restore the body to its natural balance. Although it may seem that the system is based on temperature, the thermal state in which the foods or medications are taken is not important. Certain types of herb tea, served hot, are considered cold, whereas cold beer, due to its alcoholic content, is considered hot. In the hot-cold theory of disease, conditions that are hot, such as ulcer disease, constipation, pregnancy, diarrhea, and rashes, should be balanced and treated with cold foods, such as coconut, avocado, sugar cane, and lima beans. Menstruating or postpartum women who believe in the hot-cold theory may avoid certain "cold" vegetables and fruits because these fruits are liable to clot their "hot" menstrual blood, impeding its flow, causing it to flow backward into the body and cause nervousness or insanity. Cold illnesses, such as arthritis or joint pains, are treated with hot therapy, such as aspirin, iron tablets, penicillin, chili peppers, chocolate, evaporated milk, onions, garlic, or cinnamon.

As another example, consider the following. A patient may be on diuretic therapy and require potassium supplementation. The physician may advise the patient to eat foods high in potassium, such as oranges or bananas. If the patient gets an upper respiratory infection, which is a cold disease, he or she may stop eating these fruits, which are classified as cold, because eating will only worsen the imbalance. This belief should be recognized because it contributes significantly to a patient's noncompliance with therapy. Problems can arise when a physician prescribes a "hot" medication for a "hot" disease or a "cold" medication for a "cold" disease. The hot-cold theory is even more complex in that the assignment of the "hot" or "cold" qualities varies from culture to culture, It is often difficult for the health-care provider to remember the various hot-cold combinations. If there are Latino patients with these beliefs, ask Latino colleagues on the medical team or the patient and family directly. Inquiring respectfully about the patient's culture can be effective in enhancing doctor-patient relationships. To achieve maximum therapeutic benefits for patients who believe in the hot-cold theory of disease, the health-care provider is advised to work within its framework, if possible, in prescribing medicines and diet. Try to consult medical colleagues, nurses, and social workers who share the patient's background.

Belief in *witchcraft* as a cause of illness is widespread. In the Latino population, terms such as *mal puesto, mal de ojo, mal artificial, brujería, hechicería,* and *enfermedad endañada* are used to describe the "illness of damage"; someone has done something to cause injury, illness, or death. *Mal de ojo,* or evil eye, is believed to result from excessive respect or love from another person, especially toward newborn children. A recurring theme in witchcraft belief is that animals are present in the body and are introduced by magical means. Almost always, the offending animal is a reptile, insect, or amphibian. These animals have been dried and pulverized, sprinkled onto food, and reconstituted in the body of the victim. Symptoms are often described as animals crawling over the body or wriggling throughout the intestines. The belief is that this is as magical expression of friends, relatives, or strangers wishing bad luck to come to an individual. A *hex* is an evil spell, a misfortune, or a case of bad luck that a person can impose on another. The use of magical oils, incenses, religious items, and candles may be used to repel the evil. In the Latino community, a *botánica,* or religious artifact shop, sells many of these items. The shopkeeper serves as a consultant on health and related issues. Figures 3–1 and 3–2 were taken in the Otto Chicas Rendon Botánica on 116th Street in New York City. Often, the entrance to a botánica, as shown in Figure 3–1, shows predominant Roman Catholic imagery. Candles, flowers, plants, and bowls of coconut and molasses frequently surround the Christian statues. Notice the influence of Christianity as well as the African and Arabic cultures in the idols shown in Figure 3–2. As of mid-1997, there were more than 500 botánicas listed in the business telephone books in the United States, with more than 40 in Manhattan in New York City. There are probably many more that are not listed.

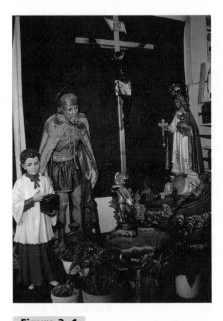

Figure 3–1

Entrance to Otto Chicas Rendon Botánica on 116th Street, New York City.

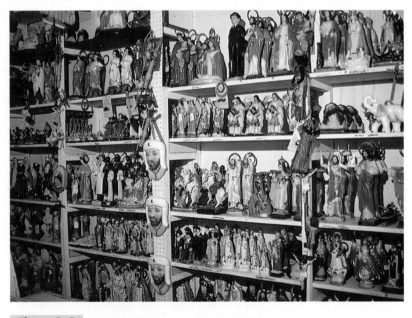

Figure 3–2

Idols in a botánica.

Very often, patients who believe they are victims of witchcraft will not seek medical attention from a clinician. Certain members of their community may be consulted to chant special prayers and incantations to cure the illness. At other times, they may require exorcism or some other dramatic therapy to drive the illness out of the body. Other common "cures" include turpentine, kerosene, mothballs, and carbon tetrachloride.

Culture and Response to Pain

The sociocultural variations in physical pain expression are important to recognize (Todd et al, 1993). Pain is an important form of biofeedback and is essential, as a warning signal, for survival. The experience of physical pain, however, has three components: (1) a person's sensation of pain, (2) a person's tolerance for pain, and (3) a person's expression of pain. Health-care providers must rely on the pain sufferer to describe the symptom of pain, the sum of these three components. Of the three, the last is culturally mediated. Some studies have indicated that there may be cultural variations in the tolerance for pain as well. In some cultures, the complaints of pain are rewarded with increased attention and comforting behavior.

Individuals of Latino background or from the Middle East or Mediterranean areas commonly voice their pain with great emotion. Some believe that they must openly express their pain; if they do not, they may aggravate their illness. In contrast, Southeast Asian, Japanese, and Native American patients believe that emotional control is extremely important. Their cultures encourage stoicism; these people rarely openly express or even indicate the presence of pain, unless it is extremely severe. In many instances, the ability to withstand great pain is a sign of "manhood," "reliability," and "moral uprightness."

The anthropologist Zborowski studied pain in four groups of male patients in a veterans' hospital (Zborowski, 1952). Third-generation Americans generally expressed pain with little emotional behavior and became withdrawn from their friends. Italian and Jewish men were very expressive and preferred to be with others while in pain. Irish men endured pain as a "private" event and neither sought any medication for it nor wanted to socialize with others. These generalizations about cultural responses to pain must be used cautiously and not become the basis of stereotyping.

It is also important for the health-care provider to recognize that many patients from Southeast Asian and Native American cultures frequently express their illness through altered states of consciousness such as trances and hallucinations. The clinician who is unaware of this type of presentation may incorrectly diagnose it as some form of psychosis.

Ethnicity and Pharmacotherapy

Over the past few years, it has become recognized that there are ethnic differences in the response to pharmacologic agents. For example, in psychopharmacology, new research has begun to provide insight concerning the biological mechanisms that underlie this differential response. Data have been accumulated about the ethnic differences in drug metabolism as well as the plasma proteins that bind psychotropic agents. Several ethnic differences in drug metabolism appear to be related to different genetic forms in the cytochrome P-450 enzyme system, which is the main pathway of human drug metabolism. It has been demonstrated that a high percentage of Asians and African-Americans have an enzyme form that metabolizes drugs at a much slower rate; individuals with this form may develop potentially toxic blood levels of drugs after administration of standard doses of certain psychotropic agents. Some Chinese herbs, such as ginseng and muscone, have been shown to have potent stimulating effects on cytochrome enzymes; other herbs substantially inhibit the activities of these enzymes. It is therefore important to determine the serum levels of drugs in a patient in whom an atypical response had developed. Other studies have shown that Asian and Latino patients with schizophrenia require lower doses of neuroleptics, such as chlorpromazine, than do white patients. Asian patients are also more likely to exhibit the extrapyramidal side effects of the neuroleptics than are white patients.

Cross-Cultural Differences in Morbidity and Mortality Rates

It is important to be aware of the considerable cultural diversity in patterns of morbidity and mortality rates in the United States. Some patterns may be purely genetic, as in Tay-Sachs disease among persons of Eastern European Jewish (Ashkenazic) descent or sickle cell anemia among African-Americans. The pattern of health for African-Americans, who are considered the largest ethnic minority in the United States, is very different from that of their white counterparts. The average life expectancy for African-Americans is 69.6 years compared with 75.9 years for whites. Part of this may be related to a higher infant mortality rate among African-Americans. The incidence of hypertension and the consequences of it are much greater in African-Americans than in whites. African-American men die from cerebral vascular accidents at almost twice the rate of white men. In addition, death from coronary artery disease in African-American women is more common than in white women. Diabetes is 35% more common among African-Americans than among the white population. Many African-Americans, like other groups, have had negative experiences with the Western medical system. The perception of a judgmental or impersonal attitude in a white health-care provider may contribute to a fear or distrust of the traditional health-care system. This lack of trust frequently results in the African-American patient seeking alternative medical treatment.

Latinos (Mexican-Americans, Puerto Ricans, and Cuban-Americans) are the fastest growing minority in the United States. Many are at increased risk of alcoholism, cirrhosis, hypertension, specific cancers, and tuberculosis (HHS, 1992). Latinos have a higher than average incidence of diabetes and cancers of the gallbladder, liver, pancreas, cervix, and stomach. Cervical and stomach cancer occur more than twice as often in Latinos as among non-Latino whites. There is also an increased incidence of acute promyelocytic leukemia in Latinos. Within the Latino group, the Puerto Ricans have the poorest health. This may be related to the fact that many older patients do not trust conventional medicine or health-care providers. In addition, migrant people are often forced to live in areas of crowding and poor sanitation. Language may also be a barrier.

The rate of tuberculosis among Chinese-Americans is higher than in the general population. In fact, the incidence of tuberculosis is more than 40 times higher among Southeast Asians than among the non-Asian population. Both first- and second-generation Chinese-Americans have a greater incidence of coronary artery disease than Asian Chinese, presumably because of a difference in diet and stress in the United States. The Japanese and Koreans have the highest incidence of gastric cancer, presumably related to diet and their high consumption of salt. The incidence of liver cancer is more than 12 times higher among the Chinese, Japanese, and Koreans than within the non-Asian population. Hepatitis B is also more common in Southeast Asians.

Native Americans have one of the highest morbidity and mortality rates; their death rate is 30% higher than that of the general population in the United States. This may be linked to the fact that Native Americans are one of the most disadvantaged ethnic groups in the United States. They have a high incidence of fetal alcohol syndrome and fetal alcohol effects. In addition, the incidence of congenital adrenal hyperplasia is greater in Native Americans than in the white population.

Traditional Healing Systems

Traditional, or folk, healers still play a large role in medicine in industrialized societies. Each culture has its own healers: spiritual healers, mediums, herbalists, shamans, fire doctors, medicine men, astrologists, occult healers, bone setters, lay midwives, and leg lengtheners, to name a few. Meditation, prayer, massage, exercise, relaxation techniques, acupuncture, acupressure, hypnosis, imagery, therapeutic touch, martial arts, and herbs are important therapeutic modalities of many of these healers. Spiritual healing is widespread. Christian Science healing, started in 1879 in Boston, teaches that those who follow Jesus must follow him in healing, which is done through the mind.

The Latino groups call their traditional healers by different names, such as the Mexican-American *curanderos(as)* and *parteras,* Puerto Rican *espiritistas,* and Cuban *santeros*. The Haitian voodoo healers, Inuit and African shamans,* Hawaiian *kahunas*, and Navaho singers are also important folk healers for their ethnic groups. It is critical for the health-care provider to respect those patients who follow these practices and to encourage them to express their need for these providers without shame or fear. Discuss with the patients how to combine the help of these providers and medical therapy.

In addition to the natural healing traditions, there are many magicoreligious traditions. As stated previously, religion plays a major role in one's perception of illness. The "evil eye" is one of the oldest and most widespread of all superstitions. The nature of the evil eye is defined differently by different groups, but it is generally accepted that an evil eye causes a sudden injury or illness that may be prevented or cured by rituals or symbols. The afflicted person may or may not know the source of the evil eye. There are several traditional practices used in the protection of health; they include wearing objects, such as charms, that protect the wearer. Figure 3–3 was taken in a *botánica* and shows eye bead charms that are worn on a string or chain around the neck, wrist, or waist to protect an individual. The blue eye bead is commonly worn by Greeks to ward off the evil eye. The *mal occhio* is worn by people of Italian descent; the *mano milagroso* by Mexicans; the *mano negro* by Puerto Rican babies; the Hand of God by Israelis; the *ayn* by the Arabic cultures; the Thunderbird by Hopi Indians; knotted hair or fragments of the Koran by people of South Asia; and red ribbons by Eastern European Jews. The Chinese wear jade to protect them from disease. When the green or red jade object discolors or turns brownish, it is replaced because the person has been exposed to an evil eye or other disease. Figure 3–4 shows several jade bracelets and charms. This photograph was taken in a Chinese jewelry shop in San Francisco's Chinatown.

Various traditional cultures use food substances to protect health. Many people eat raw garlic or onions or wear them around their neck to prevent disease. Members of Greek, Italian, or Native American ethnic groups hang onion and garlic in their homes to protect themselves. Chicken soup, a Jewish remedy, has long been thought to protect health and speed recovery. *Nervo forza* is a Guatemalan vitamin tonic commonly used in Central America. Traditional Chinese eat "1000-year-old" eggs to prevent illness. The most famous of all Chinese herbs is *ginseng (Panax schinseng)*, which is derived from the root of a plant resembling a human figure. Figure 3–5 shows a typical ginseng root. Ginseng has been revered for thousands of years as a general

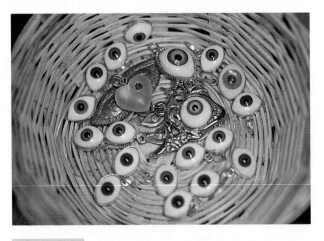

Figure 3–3

Eye beads to protect from the "evil eye."

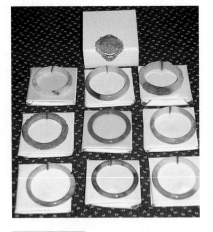

Figure 3–4

Jade bracelets and charms.

---

* The shaman is a medicine man or priest. He cures illness, directs communal sacrifices, and escorts the souls of the dead to the other world. He accomplishes these tasks by his power to leave his body at will during a trance-like state. A person becomes a shaman by inheriting the shamanistic profession or by election by a supernatural agency. Most self-made shamans are regarded as weaker than those who inherit the profession. The shaman who is born to his role is said to have more bones or teeth than others.

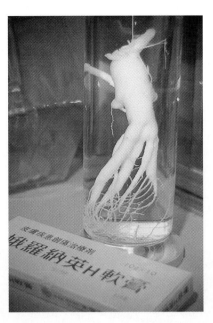

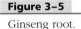
Figure 3–5

Ginseng root.

panacea. Known as an "adaptogen," ginseng has many medicinal purposes; it naturally "adapts" the vital functions of the human system to compensate for adverse conditions such as stress, malnutrition, and the deterioration associated with aging. Ginseng is a slightly bitter root that is used to promote secretion of bodily fluids, and it is recommended for more than 25 medical problems. It is commonly used for anemia, indigestion, impotence, depression, to replenish energy, and to improve sleep. By "building the blood" and stimulating vital organ energies, it is intended to balance the *yin* and *yang* throughout the body. Ginseng must be prepared in earthenware and not in metal because the metal will destroy its healing properties. Ginseng is contraindicated in patients with excess heat. Figure 3–6 shows a bowl of ginseng roots and other ginseng preparations.

Finally, there are many religious objects that are worn to protect individuals from disease. The Virgin of Guadalupe is the patron saint of Mexico. It is believed that she will protect people and their homes from the evil eye. Her image is pictured on medallions. Baptism and the mikva (or ritual bath) are religious practices that cleanse

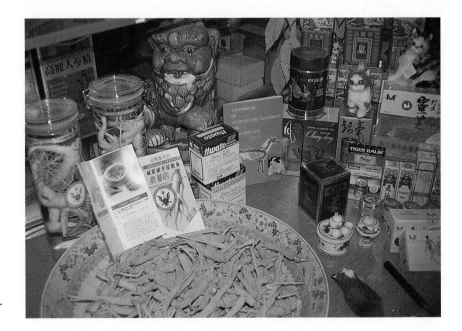

Figure 3–6

Bowl of ginseng roots.

the body and soul. In the Roman Catholic tradition, there are many saints who are concerned with specific illnesses. People may wear medals with the name and the image of the saint on them to prevent the development of a problem. Figure 3–7 shows holy cards with the pictures of saints. These are used to cure and protect individuals from disease. *Gris-gris* are symbols of voodoo; they may take a variety of forms and be used either to protect or harm a person.

Many traditional Asian medical practices are becoming more recognized in the United States. These include acupuncture, acupressure *(shiatsu),* and herbal medicines. They are discussed later in this chapter.

In addition to traditional healers, chiropractic medicine, osteopathic medicine, homeopathy, naturopathy, hydrotherapy, and aromatherapy are other important alternative medical systems. It is beyond the scope of this book to discuss them. The reader is directed to the references at the end of this chapter.

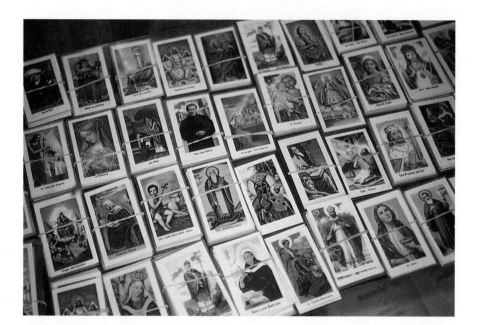

Figure 3–7

Holy cards.

Specific Cross-Cultural Perspectives

In this section, some cross-cultural perspectives, including some common beliefs regarding health and illness, are examined. This section also discusses some strategies that can be applied to improving care of patients. The intention is to sensitize the reader to the vast differences among the major ethnic groups in the United States. It is beyond the scope of this book to include all ethnic groups; the reader is again referred to the bibliography at the end of this chapter.

African-Americans

African-Americans constitute a heterogeneous ethnic group, and therefore it is impossible to make generalizations because there is no prototypical black patient. African-Americans live in all areas in the United States and are represented in every socioeconomic group, with a disproportionate number living in poverty. Any patient in a low socioeconomic bracket is concerned with maintaining dignity and autonomy, and this should never be compromised in the eyes of the clinician. In addition, a respectful attitude can greatly assist in attaining any patient's confidence and trust. This is especially true for many African-American patients as well as patients of other groups who are poor and fear that they will not be treated respectfully. Addressing the patient by the appropriate title, such as Dr., Ms., Mr., or Mrs., is important.

In many inner city populations, lack of access to quality health care has particular deleterious consequences affecting many African-Americans. One alarming result is that many preventable diseases often progress to life-threatening stages. Some diseases are highly prevalent among African-Americans: for example, diabetes mellitus and hypertension. Consequently, when examining an African-American patient regardless of socioeconomic status, the clinician should screen for these diseases and educate both the patient and the patient's family. Because of media stereotyping, African-Americans may react negatively to a general screening for human immunodeficiency virus or substance abuse. Clinicians need to approach this with sensitivity and reserve this testing for the segment of the African-American community that is at risk.

Traditionally, in Africa illness has been attributed to several causes, primarily to demons and evil spirits. Beliefs regarding the role of spirits in causing disease may persist.

Dietary patterns are particularly important to investigate in the African-American patient. Certain ethnic foods, such as rice, plantain, yams, and okra, have deep cultural roots and should not be eliminated from the diet, if possible. Other ethnic foods, such as collards and turnips that are often heavily seasoned with salt and cured meat, may pose a health problem. Without the salt, these foods are wholesome parts of a diet. The eating of Argo starch has an historical basis. Slaves ate clay and dirt, having been taught that these were rich in iron and other minerals. Some African-Americans even today consume Argo starch as a substitute for clay and a source of minerals.

As culture defines health and illness, it also defines acceptable health care and treatment practices. All cultures offer home remedies as part of self-care. For some African-Americans, the following is a partial list of home remedies:

- Poultices to fight infection
- Herbal teas
- Hot lemon tea with honey for colds
- Hot toddies for colds and congestion
- Raw onions placed on the feet in cases of fever
- Placing the white membrane from a raw egg over a boil to bring it to a head
- Hot camphorated oil and mustard plaster on the chest for chest congestion
- Garlic placed on an ill person or in the person's room to remove evil spirits

Latinos

The fastest-growing minority groups in the United States are the Spanish-speaking peoples from various parts of the Western hemisphere: Puerto Rico; Cuba; the Dominican Republic, Mexico, and other Central American countries; and South America. The Latinos residing in the United States are one of the youngest of the ethnic groups, the median age being 25.5 years as of the 1990 census. Demographers predict that, given the Latinos' young age, their high fertility rate, and their migratory patterns, by 2010 the Latinos will become the largest ethnic group in the United States, accounting for 42% of the population (Spencer, 1986). Although bonded by a common language and grouped together by their Spanish surnames, the Latino group has great heterogeneity and diversity in their many different traditions. Although Spanish has no dialects, many words may carry different meanings for various Latino groups, depending on their community of origin. The prevention of illness is a common practice frequently accomplished with praying, keeping relics in the home, and wearing religious amulets or medals. Figure 3–8 shows some religious amulets; Figure 3–9 shows a variety of rosaries and good-luck beads hanging in the foreground and magical oils and elixirs in the background. These photographs were taken in a *botánica* in New York City.

The Latinos, as other traditional groups, are known for having a close-knit family unit, *la familia*. Latino families have strong ties and have maintained many of the qualities of the extended family system. They may have a great fear of being hospitalized, thus being separated from their families. Those who speak only Spanish are concerned that they will not be able to communicate with the medical personnel when help is necessary. They have a sense of obligation toward each other and are expected to be responsible to all members of the family. It is not uncommon for a 90 year old patient who speaks no English to be accompanied to the hospital by his or her children, grandchildren, great-grandchildren, and even great-great-grandchildren. Deci-

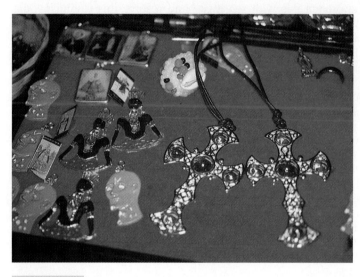

Figure 3–8

Religious amulets.

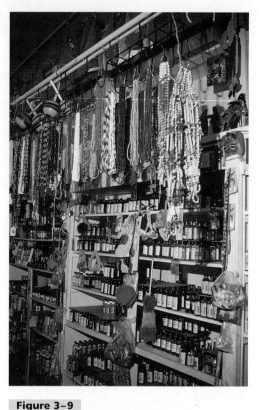

Figure 3–9

Beads, rosaries, and magic oils.

sion-making is likewise a family matter. Never pressure the patient into making a decision. Allow the patient time to discuss an issue with his or her family.

It is common for first- and second-generation Latino U.S. residents, as do many other immigrant groups, to face health-care institutions with a certain amount of distrust. When caring for a Latino patient, it is imperative that the clinician take the family into account. Some Latinos (more often the elderly, recent immigrants, the less educated) still believe in *curanderos(as), espiritistas,* or *santeros,* who are the holistic, family folk practitioners and spiritual counselors. These spiritualists believe that illness is caused by an intentional act of God, supernatural forces, or the ill will of others, and they emphasize healing through religious or medical ceremonies, potions, and amulets. They use a variety of *yerbas* (herbs, especially teas), charms, massages, and magical rituals. *Limpias,* or cleansing, is performed by passing an unbroken egg or selected herbs tied together over the body of the ill person. These healers do not advertise but are well-known throughout their individual communities and play an important role in Latino health care. A *yerberia* or *botánica* is a traditional community resource for purchasing traditional remedies and charms. Figure 3–10 shows containers with dried exotic herbs and teas. Again, notice the Christian and Arabic influences.

Patients are often fearful of discussing these health-care practices with clinicians. For this reason, when they feel trusting enough to do so, it is important that the health-care provider receive this information in a way so that the patient does not feel disrespected. Try to work with the belief. Because many herb remedies are pharmacologically active, it may be necessary to ask the patient not to consume them simultaneously with pharmaceuticals. There is usually a close, personal relationship between the patient and the healer. By using medical knowledge and adapting it to the patient's beliefs, the clinician can gain the patient's confidence and enhance cooperation.

Candles play an important role in traditional healing. The votive candles are for specific deities or saints or for specific requests, such as money, love, health, and success. The candles are lit, and prayers are recited. Figure 3–11 shows some of the candles for sale in a *botánica.*

Two important values in the Latino culture are *respeto* and *dignidad. Respeto* is demonstrated to a Latino patient when the health-care provider dresses in the tradi-

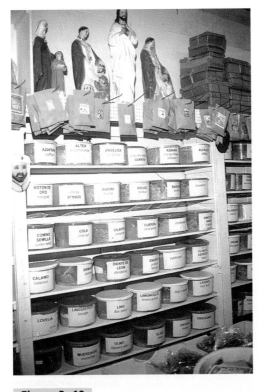

Figure 3-10

Dried exotic herbs and teas in a botánica.

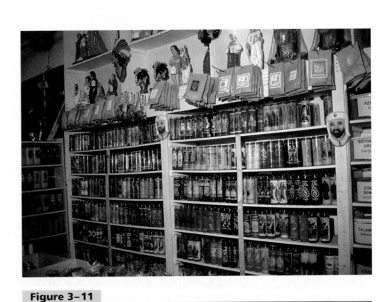

Figure 3-11

Votive candles.

tional garb of the profession expected by the Latino patient and communicates an interest in his or her life and health. Latinos also enjoy a brief social conversation before a discussion of their illness. This helps to develop a sense of *confianza,* or trust.

The belief in *Santería* originated more than 400 years ago in Cuba out of traditions of the African Yoruba people from Nigeria and Benin. These people were transported to Cuba to work as slaves on sugar plantations. From Cuba, this religious cult spread to the neighboring islands and to the United States; it arrived in New York in the late 1940s. Santería blends elements of West African beliefs with Roman Catholicism. Once only a ghetto religion, Santería has a growing following of middle-class professionals, including whites, African-Americans, Latinos, and Asian Americans. The followers believe in one Supreme Being but also in African divinities known as *orishas,* each of which represents a human characteristic, such as power, and an aspect of nature, such as thunder. Each of these deities is worshiped in the image of a Catholic saint. There are several orishas related to health problems: the orisha Chango is linked to Saint Barbara,* who is the god of thunder, lightning, and violent death; orisha Bacoso, with Saint Christopher (infections); orisha Ifa, with Saint Anthony (fertility). Statues of saints or deities are commonly purchased for the home.

Figures 3-2 and 3-12 show some religious statues sold in a New York City *botánica.* The believers pray to these idols to intervene with God to improve their lives and obtain blessings. Many of these idols are used for prayers for health. Notice the African elements blended with Catholicism in the idols. The seated figure with the red tie is Maximón, a Guatemalan believed to have powers for producing health, tranquility, protection, happiness, wealth, and improved sexual performance. The standing figure in the black suit to the right is the Venezuelan physician, Dr. José Gregorio Hernandez Cisnero. He was known for his health-related miracles, and patients pray to him for health. The figure in the reddish-pink and gold robe with the crown is the

---

* St. Barbara's father was struck by lightning as he beheaded her for her faith.

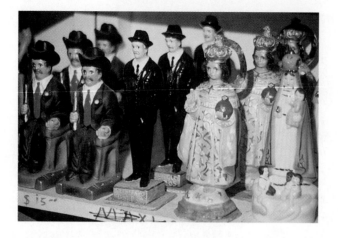

Figure 3–12

Religious Santería statues.

famous statue of Baby Jesus of Prague (also, Atacha), known in Spanish as *El Niñito Jesus de Prague* (also, *Atacha*). Figure 3–13 shows the orisha Chango.

There is a very structured hierarchy in the practice of *Santería.* In charge is the *babalow;* next is the *presidente,* the head medium; and the third practitioner is the *santero.* The *santero,* an important, respected member of the Latino community, is said to possess the magical power of the orishas, known as *ache.* Ritual devotions involving African rhythms and dancing; offerings of food and animal sacrifice; divination with shells, bones, and eggs; trance-like states; and other rites are thought to reveal the sources of problems and to help in their resolution. During the ritual, the *santero* dresses in white robes with beaded necklaces and bracelets. Santería can be practiced in homes, parks, storefronts, or basements.

La partera or *la comadrona* is the traditional midwife or traditional birth attendant of the Latino culture. These women are described as warm, caring, and cooperative. Their role is to give advice to pregnant women, to treat pregnant women for illnesses with herbs and massages, and to be in attendance during labor and delivery. The women offer both emotional and instrumental support during and after childbirth. Most of the *parteras* have birthing rooms in their homes.

There are several traditional, or *culture-bound,* illnesses of the Latinos. A culture-bound illness is one that is culturally defined. It may or may not have an equivalent from a Western medical perspective. Emotional trauma and strong emotions are recognized throughout Latin America as causes of illness. Conditions such as *mal de ojo, empacho, ataque de nervios, susto, male aire,* and *caida de mollera* are examples of Latino "culture-bound" syndromes.

Mal de ojo,* or evil eye, is the result of dangerous imbalances in social relationships; illness is blamed on the "strong glance" of an envious person. Fever, sleepless-

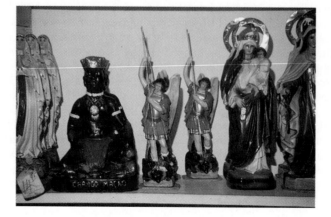

Figure 3–13

The orisha Chango on the left.

* Also used by some groups to refer to actual eye disease.

ness, and headaches are common symptoms. *Empacho,* or upset stomach, occurs when a Latino patient is psychologically stressed during or immediately after eating. The main symptom is a feeling of a "ball in the stomach" associated with abdominal pain. *Ataque de nervios* is manifested by a sudden outburst of shouting or swearing, accompanied by a variety of symptoms including dyspnea, chest tightness, memory loss, trembling, sense of heat, palpitations, dizziness, and paresthesias; it may be accompanied by, or due to, hyperventilation. It is often seen when the patient is confronted with stressful life events, such as an accident, an acute severe illness, a funeral, or a death. During the episode, the person may fall to the ground with convulsions or lay motionless. An *ataque de nervios* may progress to *susto,* which is a prolonged condition that a patient experiences after having been exposed to a traumatic event. The patient is depressed, lacks interest in living, is introverted, and has a disruption of eating and hygienic habits. *Susto,* a nonkinetic fugue state, is a common stress reaction and may be described in part as a state of disorientation and confusion. Ritual prayers and herbal remedies are the common treatment. *Mal aire,* or bad air, is said to cause pain, facial twitching, and paralysis in children. Mothers are concerned that their young children will develop *mal aire* when exposed to cold air. It is therefore important to keep Latino children covered during an examination. *Caida de mollera,* or fallen fontanelle, affects infants; the fontanelle is displaced from its normal position at the top of the head. Diarrhea and restlessness are associated symptoms. It is important to reiterate that beliefs in folk healing cannot be generalized to all Latinos. These traditional beliefs vary from generation to generation and depend largely on the extent of assimilation into the mainstream culture.

Asian Americans

Asian-American patients place much emphasis on obligation, authority, and honor. Those who have disgraced their families consequently suffer guilt. This guilt can be transformed into psychosomatic disease, which is common in this culture. Asian-American patients rarely complain of pain. They may suffer with it, but their complaints are few. If the health-care provider suspects that a patient is having pain, it is fitting to ask if pain is present. In general, after being asked, the patient will acknowledge the pain. Older-generation Chinese individuals tend not to display emotions openly to strangers. Neither do they usually accept comfortably any type of comforting physical contact, such as touching a shoulder or hand, as a form of empathy. Unlike the Chinese or Japanese, in the Korean culture, touching is common among men and women. In fact, it is far more common than in Western cultures.

Titles are important in communicating with the Japanese patient, as with other groups. The family name is usually written first. Bowing is very common and indicates respect; it is used when greeting and leaving. Avoiding eye contact, particularly in the older Japanese patient, demonstrates respect. Another aspect of dealing with Japanese or Korean patients relates to the "yes-no" question and the infrequent use of the word "no." Most older Japanese and Koreans feel that to answer "No" puts an individual on the defensive. Therefore, they may answer "Yes," meaning that they understand, not necessarily answering in the affirmative to the question. Nodding the head generally indicates attentiveness of the Japanese patient and not necessarily agreement. With some Japanese patients, as in other cultures, giggling is often a sign of embarrassment. Interviewers require patience and may need to proceed more slowly when questioning the Asian patient about intimate information, such as sexual behavior (Nilchaikowit et al, 1993). It is generally best to avoid humor when interviewing a Japanese patient, especially an older patient.

Many Asian Americans believe in traditional medicine and distrust Western medicine. The "hot-cold" theory of disease is still accepted by some Asian Americans. Another example of the balancing of internal forces is seen in the Chinese belief in *yin* and *yang.* Everything in the world consists of both *yin* and *yang* forces.

The key to good health is the balance between *yin* and *yang;* Chinese herbs and acupuncture help restore this balance. A common problem among Chinese patients is related to medication. According to traditional Chinese medicine, one dose of an herbal remedy will usually "cure" an illness. Prescriptions of Western medications require multiple doses for longer periods. Chinese patients may have difficulty in complying with this schedule. It is the clinician's responsibility to explain carefully this difference in "medical" therapy.

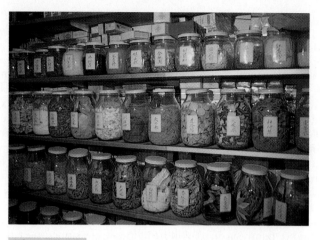

Figure 3–14

Medicinal Chinese herbs.

Figure 3–14 was taken in a traditional herbal pharmacy in San Francisco; it shows jars containing medicinal Chinese herbs. Deer antlers, mercury, turtle shells, bull testicles, snake meat, seahorses, and rhinoceros horns are other popular Chinese cures. The interviewer must respect the patient's belief and, by attempting to understand it, will be equipped to provide better care.

Many Chinese and Vietnamese, like others, have a fear of being admitted to a Western hospital (D'Avanzo, 1992). This anxiety stems from the language barrier, inability to find a translator, fear of isolation from the family, different practices, and even food. Many Southeast Asians are lactose-intolerant. Explain in detail the plan of treatment to the patient and the family members. If an interpreter is needed, make sure that the interpreter speaks the same dialect.

Like other traditional cultures, Asian Americans have several important culture-bound syndromes: *hwa-byung, taijin kyofusho, hsieh-ping, amok, wagamama, shink-eishitsu,* and *koro. Hwa-byung* is a common, multiple somatic and psychological disorder, seen usually in married Korean women. Epigastric pain is the presenting symptom; fear that the pain will lead to death, insomnia, dyspnea, palpitations, and muscle aches are associated symptoms. It often appears that anger is the precipitating cause. *Taijin kyofusho* is a syndrome of Japanese patients in which the patients complain that their body parts or functions are offensive to others. *Hsieh-ping* is a trance-like state in which Chinese patients believe themselves to be possessed by a dead relative or friend whom they have offended. *Amok,* which afflicts Malay men, is a sudden spree of violent attacks on people, animals, and objects. *Wagamama* is seen in Japanese patients and presents with apathetic childish behavior with emotional outbursts. *Shink-eishitsu* is a form of severe anxiety and obsessional neurosis seen in young Japanese patients. *Koro,* a name of Malay origin, is a delusional condition seen in Southeast Asian and Chinese male patients; the patient suddenly grasps his penis, fearing that it will retract into his abdomen and ultimately cause his death. Family members are frequently called upon to hold the penis. This disorder may continue for several days. The condition may be linked to another associated belief called "semen anxiety," in which the patient feels that he has a deficiency of semen, which is believed to be a fatal condition.

Asian Indians

Asian Indians are people from India, Pakistan, Nepal, Bangladesh, and Sri Lanka. Although most Asian Indians speak English well, avoid using idioms that may produce confusion. The most common religious groups among Asian Indians are Hindus, Muslims, and Sikhs. The Hindus believe that life is a circle, continuous without a beginning or end. There is also a strong belief in astrology. The Hindu family is a very strong unit, and health-care decisions are commonly made by the senior members of the family. The cow is considered sacred; eating beef or veal, therefore, is strongly prohibited.

Muslims follow the teachings of Mohammed and Islam. The main principles of Islam are generosity, fairness, respect, cleanliness, and honesty. Smoking and the consumption of alcohol, pork, or lard is strictly prohibited. Sex education, autopsies, and cremation are also commonly forbidden. Older Muslim patients may have a fatalistic attitude, which can interfere with compliance with medical therapy. Muslim women wear a veil over their head when in the presence of males outside the family and prefer women health-care providers. In some cases, if a patient's husband is present, a male physician may be allowed to examine the patient.

Sikhism started in the 15th century in northern India. The Sikhs believe in a single God and in reincarnation. Baptized Sikhs do not cut their hair and do not smoke or drink alcohol; many are vegetarians. A traditional Sikh greeting, similar to that of other Asian Indians, is with the palms of the hands pressed together in front of the chest. Women generally do not shake hands, and eye contact may be considered disrespectful.

The Asian-Indian population relies heavily on a wide-ranging pharmacopeia. Remedies can come from almost any natural substance. *Ayurvedic medicine* is the ancient Indian medical system; it teaches that imbalance in the body humors results in illness. Treatment is to restore the balance. Although Western medicine is recognized in India, it is estimated that there are nearly 4000 people for every Western-taught physician (Sharma et al, 1991).

It is important for the clinician to recognize that taste and food are important parts of Asian-Indian beliefs. Each taste is believed to have special properties: sweet increases phlegm and appeases hunger and thirst; acid increases salivation and improves digestion; salt purifies the blood; pungent food provokes the appetite; bitter food stimulates the appetite and clears the complexion. The study of medicines is more important than the study of illness; the traditional healer deals with symptoms and usually ignores the disease.

Native Americans

Native Americans constitute a heterogeneous group that comprises over 400 federally recognized nations. American Indians, Aleuts, and Inuits (and Inupiats)* are the largest groups of Native Americans. The traditional belief about health is that it reflects living in total harmony with nature and having the ability to survive under dire circumstances. People must treat their bodies with respect. Many Native Americans believe that there is a reason for every illness; illness is the price paid for something bad that had occurred or will occur. Several tribes associate illness with evil spirits. Illness may also result from breaking a taboo or the attack of a ghost or witch.

The traditional healer is the medicine man or woman. Often, the medicine man or woman uses meditation and crystal balls. Occasionally, the medicine man or woman uses the root of jimsonweed to produce a trance to enable him or her to better treat the patient. The cause of illness is diagnosed by three types of divination: motion of the hand, star gazing, and listening. Chanting is a major part of the process. Many Native Americans also believe in witchcraft. Herbal remedies and an act of purification are major steps to curing illness.

Two important problems of Native Americans are alcohol abuse and domestic violence (Aday, 1993). Alcohol abuse is a critical health-care problem that is widespread and is immeasurably costly to the Native American community. In the older, traditional Native American home, alcohol abuse was not common. Currently, domestic violence is a major problem, and it is frequently related to alcohol abuse. The rate of suicide is also high among this population. In addition, there is a higher proportion of postnatal deaths among Native Americans, presumably because the women have inadequate prenatal care.

---

* The Eskimo people are identified by place of residence. The Eastern Eskimos live from eastern Greenland to northern Alaska. The Western Eskimos live to the west of Alaska: Bering Sea, St. Lawrence Island, and northern Pacific. The term *Eskimo* is now thought to be unflattering. Speakers of the Eastern Eskimo language call themselves *Inuit,* based on the *Inuit* language they speak. Although the term *Inuit* has been used to describe all Eskimos, it is appropriate only for those speaking the eastern language. In Alaska, the Eskimo people call themselves *Inupiat,* based on the Inupiat dialect of the Inuit language. The Western Eskimos are now referred to as *Yupik,* based on the language they speak.

The Jewish People

Approximately 7 million Jewish people live in the United States. There are two large groups: the *Ashkenazim,* whose origins can be traced to Eastern or Northern Europe, and the *Sephardim,* whose origins are from the Mediterranean countries or the Iberian peninsula. The majority of the Jews in the United States follow the Ashkenazi traditions. The Ashkenazi are linked linguistically through Yiddish, and the Sephardi are linked by Ladino, Spanish, Portuguese, French, or Arabic.

In the United States, there are three main divisions of the Jewish people, based on adherence to traditional practices and interpretation of Jewish law: Orthodox, Conservative, and Reform. Although most Orthodox Jews dress indistinguishably from others, some individuals observe Jewish law by covering their heads with a skullcap called a *yarmulke* or *kippah*. Many married Orthodox women cover their heads with hats, wigs, or kerchiefs. Because of tradition, men and women are commonly separated in social situations. Another division of Jewish people is the *Hasidim*. This group broke off from mainstream Judaism in the 17th century in order to serve God without the necessity for immersion in religious study that was the standard in the Eastern European Jewish community at that time. Hasidim usually wear 17th century–type black robes or suits with black hats. The men twirl their hair into ringlets at the sides of their face. Hasidim are generally passionate in their worship and adhere strictly to the biblical laws. These laws include restrictions regarding permissible foods (laws of Kashrut or *Kosher**) and forbidden foods (pork products or shellfish).

The Sabbath is a strictly observed day of rest. When scheduling appointments, be aware of the Sabbath and do not schedule tests or clinic visits from Friday afternoon until after Saturday evening. Many religious Jews do not use anything electrical on the Sabbath. Therefore, when visiting a religious Jewish person in the hospital, you may find that the rooms are dark because they are not allowed to turn on the lights; you may, however, turn them on. Despite the many rules of Orthodox Judaism, health always comes first. Even on fasting days, pills may be taken.

Many Jewish holidays are not marked on calendars. Ask the patient about them when scheduling tests to determine if holidays will present a problem with appointments. Many Jewish people may want to consult their rabbi before having a certain test performed or taking some form of medication. This should not be misconstrued as a mistrust of the health-care provider; it is often culturally mediated.

Jewish tradition is rich with mystical beliefs, but there is great respect for conventional medicine and health-care providers. There are several genetic conditions that exist more frequently in the Jewish population. These include Tay-Sachs disease, Gaucher's disease, Bloom's syndrome, ataxia-telangiectasia, Creutzfeldt-Jacob disease, familial Mediterranean fever, Glanzmann's thrombasthenia, pemphigus vulgaris, polycythemia vera, and Niemann-Pick Disease.

When an Orthodox Jew dies, the body is never left alone from the time of death until burial; Orthodox friends and family will pray around the body. The body is not embalmed, and the burial is usually within 24 hours. One exception to this rule would be if the death occurred on a Friday evening (the Sabbath); the burial would then be on Sunday. There is no belief in an afterlife. Autopsies are usually not allowed, unless approved by the family's rabbi.

The primary group targeted for annihilation in World War II were the Jewish people. Because of these experiences, Jewish patients, especially the older, immigrant generation, may manifest greater discomfort, fear, and anxiety when confined in a hospital and when decisions are made about them. For more information, refer to the section on post-traumatic stress disorder in Chapter 2.

Krishna Consciousness Group

An important, small, originally Indian group in the United States is the Krishna Consciousness Group. Its members believe in four rules of conduct: (1) no eating of meat, fish, or eggs; (2) no illicit sex; (3) no intoxicants; and (4) no gambling. They believe

---

* The rules of the *kosher* diet mandate the exclusion of shellfish and pork products. In addition, only fish with scales and fins and only certain types of meat from animals with a cloven hoof and that chew the cud can be eaten.

that the body is ruled by passion and the soul by serenity. The Krishna lifestyle is strictly regulated, and illness should never interfere with these activities. Followers seek medical assistance only when they are extremely ill.

Romanies

The tradition of the Romanies, or Gypsies, poses important health-care problems. According to the Gypsy culture, the sources of all disease are demons, the evil eye, breaking taboos, and the fear of disease itself. Several Romany treatments involve transferring disease symbolically to another person or object. In general, Gypsies turn to organized health-care only during times of crisis. They do not hesitate to come to the hospital for serious illness; often, the extended family or entire tribe may accompany the patient. Preventive medicine and follow-up care is rarely used. Romany women are extremely reluctant to expose themselves to male health-care providers.

In order to protect their anonymity, Gypsies are reluctant to identify themselves as Gypsies, often use assumed names, and may not provide truthful answers to non-Gypsies. Once a trusting relationship with a health-care provider has been established, however, many Gypsies will feel more inclined to rely on that individual.

Traditional Chinese Medicine

There are many traditional medical practices. Of particular note are the Chinese, Ayurvedic, and Greek systems of healing. Due to the limitations of space in this chapter, one traditional system of healing, Chinese medicine, which has influenced so many other systems, is considered.

There are almost 10 million people who constitute the Asian and Pacific Islander group, which represents the third largest majority group in the United States. The Chinese approach to healing is a rich and complex tradition. It emphasizes the importance of promoting balance and harmony in body, mind, and spirit and became the foundation for many other traditional medical systems. Chinese medicine has its origins over 2500 years ago and is still in use to treat millions of people in China and throughout the world. As a result, to the Chinese healers, allopathic medicine is new and experimental.

Chinese medicine is based on the idea that the human system is a microcosmic mirror of the macrocosmic universe. No one thing can exist without the existence of the others. Each person is subject to the same laws that govern the stars, the planets, the trees, and the land. *Tao,* sometimes translated as "the infinite origin," is the single unified source from which all life and the entire universe originated; it is the way to ultimate reality. To follow the laws of nature is to be blessed with good health, long life, and good fortune. Since nature is the most enduring manifestation of *Tao,* much of the traditional terminology of Chinese medicine is derived from natural phenomena, such as fire and water, wind and heat, and dryness and dampness. When the elements in the human body remain in balance, "fair weather" is said to prevail in the body, and the human is well both physically and mentally.

Tao created two opposing forces, *yin* and *yang,* which are the opposites that combine to create everything in the world. *Yin* is a force of darkness and is associated with such qualities as femininity, cold, rest, passivity, emptiness, inwardness, and negative energy. *Yang* is a force of brightness and is associated with masculinity, heat, stimulation, activity, excitement, vigor, fullness, outwardness, and positive energy. Table 3–2 lists the aspects of *yin* and *yang* polarity.

Chinese medicine recognizes five *yin* internal organs (heart, lungs, spleen, liver, and kidneys) and six *yang* internal organs (gallbladder, stomach, small intestine, colon, urinary bladder, and "triple burner"). "Triple burner" is the English translation for this organ, the anatomy of which is not known. It is believed that it is required for water regulation. The function of the *yin* organs is to produce, transform, and regulate the five essential substances listed in the next paragraph. The function of the *yang* organs is to receive, break down, and absorb that part of the food that is transformed into the fundamental substances and excrete the unused portion. Chinese medicine recognizes the following categories of illness:

- *Yin* excess due to *yang* deficiency
- *Yang* excess due to *yin* deficiency

Table 3–2   **Aspects of *Yin* and *Yang* Polarity**

Aspect	Yin	Yang
Cosmic bodies	Earth	Sun
	Moon	
Energy condition	Passive	Aggressive
	Mentally active	Physically active
	Asleep	Awake
	Weak	Strong
	Empty	Full
	Deficient	Excessive
	Cold	Hot
Time of day	Night	Day
Season	Fall	Spring
	Winter	Summer
Magnetic pole	Negative	Positive
Temperature	Cold	Hot
Speed	Slow	Fast
Body location	Interior	Upper torso
	Lower torso	Upper extremities
	Lower extremities	Head
	Feet	Left side
	Right side	Front
	Back	
	Exterior	
Gender	Female	Male
Numbers	Even	Odd
Distance	Near	Far
Relative moisture	Very moist, saturated	Dry
Light	Dark	Light
Acid/base	Alkaline	Acid
Speed	Slow	Fast
Metabolism	Anabolism	Catabolism
Psychic type	Contemplative	Active
	Introverted	Extroverted
	Gentle	Robust

- *Yang* deficiency due to *yin* excess
- *Yin* deficiency due to *yang* excess

There are five essential substances from which life emerges and in which harmony and disharmony exist: *Qi, Shen, Jing, Xue,* and *Jin-Ye. Qi* (anglicized as chee) is the vital life force that pulses throughout everything in the universe. The idea of *Qi* is fundamental to Chinese medical thinking, and no English word can capture its true meaning. In the body *Qi* has five major functions: it is the source of all movement in the body; it protects the body; it is the source of harmonious transformation in the body; it holds the organs in their proper places; and it warms the body. There are five main types of *Qi:* organ, meridian, nutritive, protective, and ancestral (chest).

Meridians are a unique part of Chinese medical theory; they are the channels through which *Qi* flows among the organs, adjusting and harmonizing their activities. The meridians, which are not blood vessels, are 20–50 millimicrons in diameter and link together all the fundamental substances and organs. They are bilateral and exist beneath the surface of the skin. The places at which the branches reach the skin surface are designated as acupuncture sites. Each meridian has an entry and exit point; energy enters through the entry point and flows through to the exit point. There are twelve primary meridians of the body, each running vertically, bringing *Qi* and the other four essential substances to specific parts of the body. No part of the body is without *Qi;* a blockage causes an imbalance in the flow of the life force.

Shen is the fluid, unique to human life, that is responsible for the spirit, consciousness, emotions, and thoughts. It is associated with the force of human personality. *Jing* is the fluid that is the basis of reproduction and development. *Xue* (sch-whey) moves in the same channels as *Qi* and is similar to blood but is produced by food, refined in the spleen, and transported to the lungs where nutritive *Qi* turns it into *Xue*. *Jin-Ye* is all fluids other than *Xue*. It includes sweat, urine, saliva, mucus, bile, and gastric juice. These five essential substances are the basics for the Chinese traditional medical system.

There are two main concepts in traditional Chinese medicine. The first is that the occurrence of disease represents a failure in preventive health care. The second is that health is a responsibility shared equally by the patient and doctor. A Chinese proverb states, "The superior physician teaches his patients how to stay healthy." In traditional Chinese medicine, the doctors treat the patient as a whole system rather than dealing with separate parts, as is common in Western medicine. An important belief is that the mind is engaged to control and guide energy to heal and repair the body. Chinese medicine is a system of preserving health and curing disease that treats the mind, body, and spirit as a whole.

Whereas the Western clinician starts with a symptom and tries to search for the cause of a specific disease, the Chinese clinician directs his or her attention to the whole patient and forms a "pattern of disharmony." This pattern describes the situation of "imbalance" in the patient's body. The Chinese clinician does not ask "Which *A* is causing *B*?" but "What is the relationship between *A* and *B*?" The patterns of disharmony provide the framework for therapy. In Chinese medicine, a person does not catch the flu; a person develops a disharmony. If a patient requires an antibiotic, herbs or acupuncture may be used to dispel the disharmony. Regardless of the ailment, the mind, body, and spirit must be treated as a whole. Healing is achieved by rebalancing *yin* and *yang* and restoring harmony in the whole person.

The traditional Chinese clinician inspects a patient in four stages: looking, listening or smelling, asking, and touching. Inspection of the tongue and palpation of the pulse are the two most important examinations. The tongue is believed to be the clearest indicator of the nature of the disharmony. The Chinese recognize more than 100 different conditions of internal energy imbalance, based on the color and texture of the tongue "fur." The condition of the five major organ-energy systems is evaluated according to their corresponding areas on the tongue. These systems are the kidneys, liver, spleen, lungs, and heart.

In traditional Chinese medicine, pulse diagnosis is evaluated at the radial artery near the wrist. It is believed that disharmonies of the body leave a specific impression on the pulse. There are at least 28 specific types of pulse abnormalities. The pulse is evaluated by placing subtle pressure by the three middle fingers on three points on the radial pulse. When the pulse is strong and regular, the person is considered to be in good health. The Chinese clinician can evaluate six organs on each wrist.

The dominant form of therapy in traditional Chinese medicine is acupuncture. Acupuncture is a therapy used for prevention and treatment of disease and for maintenance of health by manipulating the flow of *Qi* and *Xue* through the body channels. Although most Western clinicians have heard of acupuncture, few understand it. The Chinese have used acupuncture for more than 6000 years to stimulate or awaken the natural power within the body. It is estimated that there are 9 to 12 million treatments a year in the United States. Acupuncture involves the use of nine fine needles, each with a specific purpose. There are as many as 2000 specific points, each 3 mm in diameter, along the meridian lines on the skin into which these needles can be inserted. Most acupuncturists use only 150 of these points. The Chinese have different names for each acupuncture point. Figure 3–15 shows a male model on which the meridians and acupuncture sites are indicated. The needles act as antennae to direct *Qi* to organs of the body. At other times, the needles may drain *Qi* when it is excessive.

Ear acupuncture, known as auriculotherapy, is practiced by traditional Chinese acupuncturists for the diagnosis and therapy of organ system disharmony. Figure 3–16 shows the acupuncture sites of the ear. Auriculotherapy is based on the concept that there are specific parts of the ear that can be related to specific parts of the body. Knowledge of the locations is useful for surgical anaesthesia of most of the areas of the body because it will avoid needles being placed near the surgical field.

Moxibustion is a specific form of acupuncture utilizing burning herbs to stimulate specific acupuncture sites. If a disease fails to respond to traditional acupuncture, moxibustion is used. Moxa leaves *(Artemisia chinensis)* are either rolled into a cigar-

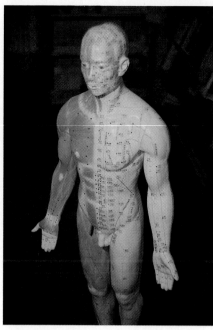

Figure 3–15

Meridians and acupuncture sites on male model.

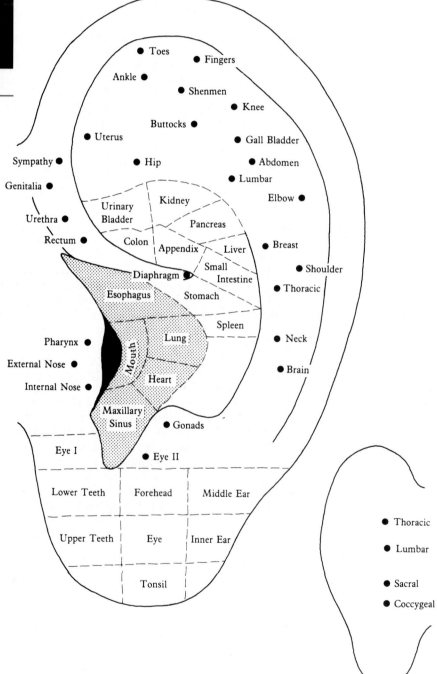

Figure 3–16

Acupuncture sites of the ear.

66

shaped stick or pulverized and made into a cone. The moxa stick is lit, and the glowing end is held over the vital spot to be treated; the cone is placed on the skin over the acupuncture site and ignited, letting it burn slowly toward the skin. Moxibustion is used for conditions in which there is an excess of *yin* and is contraindicated for heat and excess *yang* disharmonies.

The Chinese have used iron balls for health since the Ming Dynasty, dating to 1368–1644. Originally solid, the balls currently are hollow with a sounding plate within them. Each pair has one that produces a high tone and the other a low tone. The iron balls are believed to enhance the user's health and well-being. By moving the iron balls with the fingers, various acupuncture points on the hand are stimulated, resulting in increased circulation of vital energy and blood to the internal organs. Those who use these balls believe that, with daily use, the brain can be kept in good health with improved memory, fatigue will be relieved, and life will be prolonged.

Another major concept in traditional Chinese medicine is the *five element theory,* also known as the *five phases (Wu Xing).* This theory attempts to classify phenomena in terms of five quintessential processes represented by wood, fire, earth, metal, and water. Each phase has qualities and functions that describe the various processes in the body and their interactions with the environment. The phases are as follows:

- *Wood*—proper and straight; characterizes the liver, gallbladder, anger, sour taste, and windy weather
- *Fire*—ascending and blooming; characterizes the heart, small intestine, joy, bitter taste, and hot weather
- *Earth*—solid and quiet; characterizes the spleen, stomach, melancholy, sweet taste, and damp weather
- *Metal*—firm and strong; characterizes the lung, colon, grief, pungent taste, and dry weather
- *Water*—inward and clear; characterizes the kidney, urinary bladder, fear, salty taste, and cold weather

Traditional Chinese healers use this theory to diagnose and treat illness. Often plotted on a circle, the five phases show a unity in the world and in the body. There are many corresponding conditions to the five phases. Table 3–3 lists some of the medically relevant associations.

Acupressure and massage are also important aspects of the traditional Chinese healing arts. Acupressure, or *dian hsueh,* is the forerunner to the Japanese technique called *shiatsu.* Acupressure is the technique of transferring energy from the therapist's body directly into the patient's system by pressing thumb and hands into the patient's vital areas. Acupressure involves the application of deep pressure to the same points along the channels used in acupuncture. Once a point is located, rotating pressure is applied for 10–15 seconds, released, and then repeated as often as the therapist feels necessary. Massage *(tui na),* in contrast, focuses primarily on the muscle masses, ear, abdomen, foot, and spine. Massage offers the energy of acupuncture, the serenity of meditation, and spiritual refreshment. *Tui na* stimulates circulation and energy within the body, activates and drains the lymph, tones the muscles, and enhances nerve function.

Tui na therapy is accompanied by cupping, a technique called *ba guan. Ba guan* uses glass or bamboo cups containing small amounts of alcohol. The cups are applied to the areas of disease and are ignited, creating a vacuum inside. The underlying tissue swells up and the vacuum pressure draws out heat, damp, or wind energies. This technique has been adapted by many other ethnic groups.

Table 3–3   Five Phases Correspondences

	Wood	Fire	Earth	Metal	Water
Taste	Sour	Bitter	Sweet	Pungent	Salty
***Yin* organ**	Liver	Heart	Spleen	Lungs	Kidney
***Yang* organ**	Gallbladder	Small intestine	Stomach	Colon	Urinary bladder
Orifice	Eyes	Tongue	Mouth	Nose	Ears
Tissue	Tendons	Blood vessels	Flesh	Skin	Bones

Chinese herbal therapy encompasses eight methods: sweating, vomiting, purging, harmonizing, warming, removing, supplementing, and reducing. There are 5767 herbal remedies known in traditional Chinese medicine, less than 10% of which are commonly used currently. The majority are derived from plants. Through clinical experience, Chinese medicine recognizes that each herbal remedy has an affinity for a particular meridian or organ. If an illness is due to heat, cooling with herbal therapy is used; if due to a deficiency, with drugs that restore. In a manual of Chinese herbal remedies, each herb is listed as to the part used (P), the taste and nature (T&N), the meridian or organ affected (M), the actions (Act), the amount and form of use (A&F), and the cautions and contraindications (C&C). As an example:*

Acorus gramineus (Japanese sweet flag)

Shichangpu

P: Root stalk
T&N: Acrid; slightly warm
M: Heart, liver, spleen
Act: To open ostia and conduits, to eliminate sputum, to regulate *Qi,* to mobilize blood, to disperse Wind, to excrete Dampness
A&F: 3–6 g (fresh 9–24 g) as decoction, pill, or powder
C&C: Waning *yin* with waxing *yang*, restlessness with diaphoresis, cough, vomiting of blood, spontaneous semen emission

Figure 3–17 was taken in a traditional Chinese herbal pharmacy. Note the prescription written in Chinese, which is necessary to purchase these herbal medications.

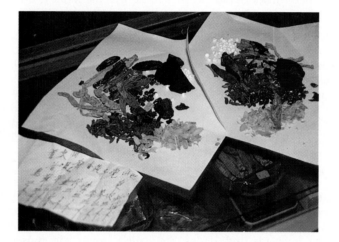

Figure 3–17

Prescription with herbal medications.

Conclusion

Health-care professionals cannot be expected to know everything about each culture but rather to know it is important to keep in mind cultural considerations in the treatment process and the doctor-patient relationship. Alternative medicine has long played a key role in the health care of people in the United States. Most health-care providers have failed to recognize the magnitude of these forms of healing. Many of the therapies are not based on any sound medical knowledge. Some have been derived from ethnic and folk traditions, semireligious cults, metaphysical movements, and health-care groups who rebel against technology and the perceived impersonaliza-

---

*Adapted from *A Manual of Chinese Herbal Medicine: Principles & Practice for Easy Reference* by Warner J-W. Fan, M.D., Shambhala Publications, Inc., 1996.

tion of 20th century medical care. This chapter has introduced the health-care provider to the richness of several of these alternative therapies. Ideally, the clinician can be better prepared to deal with patients who use alternative medicine and with the challenges of caring for patients in a multicultural society.

Bibliography

Aday LA: At Risk in America—The Health and Health Care Needs of Vulnerable Populations in the United States. San Francisco, Jossey-Bass, 1993.

Adler NE, Boyce WT, Chesney MA, et al: Socioeconomic inequities in health: No easy solution. JAMA 269:3140, 1993.

Association of State and Territorial Health Officials: ASTHO bilingual health initiative: Report and recommendations. Washington, DC, Office of Minority Health, 1992.

Blackhall LJ, Murphy ST, Frank G, et al: Ethnicity and attitudes toward patient autonomy. JAMA 274:820, 1995.

Brooks T: Pitfalls in communication with Hispanic and African-American patients: Do translators help or harm? J Natl Med Assn 84:941, 1992.

Buchwald D, Caralis PV, Gany F, et al: Caring for patients in a multicultural society. Patient Care 15:105, 1994.

Carrese JA, Rhodes LA: Western bioethics on the Navajo reservation: Benefit or harm? JAMA 274:826, 1995.

Chang ST: The Complete Book of Acupuncture. Berkeley, Celestial Arts, 1976.

Cohen MR, Doner K: The Chinese Way to Healing: Many Paths to Wholeness. New York, Perigee, 1996.

D'Avanzo CE: Barriers to health care of Vietnamese refugees. J Prof Nurs 8:245, 1992.

Eisenberg DM: Advising patients who seek alternative medical therapies. Ann Intern Med 127:61, 1997.

Eisenberg DM, Kessler RC, Foster C, et al: Unconventional medicine in the United States: Prevalence, costs, and patterns of use. N Engl J Med 328:246, 1993.

Fan WJW: A Manual of Chinese Herbal Medicine: Principles and Practice for Easy Reference. Boston, Shambhala Publications, Inc., 1996.

Freund PES, McGuire MB: Health, Illness, and the Social Body: A Critical Sociology, 2nd ed. Englewood Cliffs, NJ, Prentice Hall, 1995.

Goston L: Informed consent, cultural sensitivity, and respect for persons. JAMA 274:844, 1995.

Haffner L: Translation is not enough. West J Med 157:255, 1992.

Hannay DR: Lecture Notes on Medical Sociology. Oxford, Blackwell Scientific Publications, 1988.

Hartog J, Hartog EA: Cultural aspects of health and illness behavior in hospitals. West J Med 139:106, 1983.

Helman CG: Culture, Health and Illness, 2nd ed. London, Wright, 1990.

Herrera J, Lawson W (eds): Cross-Cultural Issues in Psychopharmacology. Mt Sinai J Med 63, 1996.

Hodgkinson HL: A Demographic Look at Tomorrow. Washington, DC, Institute for Educational Leadership, 1992.

Hsu H, Peacher WG (eds): Chinese Herb Medicine and Therapy. New Canaan, CT, Keats Publishing, Inc., 1982.

Kaptchuk TJ: The Web That Has No Weaver: Understanding Chinese Medicine. Chicago, Congdon & Weed, Inc., 1983.

Lipkin M, Putnam SM, Lazare A (eds): The Medical Interview: Clinical Care, Education, and Research. New York, Springer-Verlag, 1995.

McIvor RJ: Making the most of interpreters. Brit J Psych 165:268, 1994.

Mezzich JE, Kleinman A, Fabrega H Jr, et al (eds): Culture and Psychiatric Disorder: A DSM-IV Perspective. Washington, DC, American Psychiatric Press, Inc., 1996.

Mollina CW, Aguirre-Molina M (eds): Latino Health in the U.S.: A Growing Challenge. Washington, DC, American Public Health Association, 1994.

Monte T: World Medicine: The East-West Guide to Healing Your Body. New York, G.P. Putnam's Sons, 1993.

Murray RH, Rubel AJ: Physicians and healers: Unwitting partners in health care. N Engl J Med 326:61, 1992.

Ngubane H: Body and Mind in Zulu Medicine. London, Academic Press, 1977.

Nilchaikowit T, Jill JM, Holland JC: The effects of culture on illness behavior and medical care: Asian and American differences. Gen Hosp Psychiatry 15:41, 1993.

O'Connor BB: Healing Traditions. Philadelphia, University of Pennsylvania Press, 1995.

Penny CA: Interpretation for Inuit patients essential element of health care in eastern Arctic. Can Med Assoc J 150:1860, 1994.

Polednak AP: Racial and Ethnic Differences in Disease. New York, Oxford University Press, 1989.

Ramakrishna J, Weiss MG: Health, illness, and immigration: East Indians in the United States. West J Med 157:265, 1992.

Reid D: The Shambhala Guide to Traditional Chinese Medicine. Boston, Shambhala Publications, Inc., 1996.

Sharma HM, Triguna BD, Chopra D: Maharishi Ayur-Veda: Modern insights into ancient medicine. JAMA 265:2633, 1991.

Sisty-LePeau N: Oral healthcare and cultural barriers. J Dent Hyg 67:156, 1993.

Skultans V: The symbolic significance of menstruation and the menopause. MAN 5:639, 1970.

Snow LF: Folk medical beliefs and their implications for care of patients: A review based on studies among Black Americans. Ann Intern Med 81:82, 1974.

Snow LF, Johnson SM: Modern-day menstrual folklore. JAMA 237:2736, 1977.

Spector RE: Cultural Diversity in Health and Illness, 4th ed. Stamford, CT, Appleton & Lange, 1996.

Spencer G: Projections of the Hispanic population: 1983 to 2080. Current Population Reports. Series P-25, no. 995, Washington, DC, US Bureau of the Census, 1986.

Todd KH, Samaroo N, Hoffman JR: Ethnicity as a risk factor for inadequate emergency department analgesia. JAMA 269:1537, 1993.

Trill MD, Holland J: Cross-cultural differences in the care of patients with cancer: A review. Gen Hosp Psychiatry 15:21, 1993.

Tumulty P: What is a clinician and what does he do? N Engl J Med 283:20, 1970.

U.S. Bureau of the Census: Statistical Abstract of the US 1990 Census, 113th ed. Washington, DC, U.S. Bureau of the Census, 1993.

U.S. Dept. of Health and Human Services: Healthy people 2000: National health promotion and disease prevention objectives—Special population objectives. Washington, DC, U.S. Dept. of Health and Human Services, 1989.

U.S. Dept. of Health and Human Services: Healthy people 2000: National health promotion and disease prevention objectives—Full report with commentary. Boston, 1992.

Watt IS, Howel D, Lo L: The health care experience and health behavior of the Chinese: A survey based in Hull. J Public Health Med 15:129, 1993.

Wensel LO (ed): Acupuncture in Medical Practice. Reston, VA, Reston Publishing Company, Inc., 1980.

Woloshin S, Bickell NA, Schwartz LM, et al: Language barriers in medicine in the United States. JAMA 273:724, 1995.

Zborowski M: Cultural components in response to pain. J Soc Issues 8:16, 1952.

Zborowski M: People in Pain. San Francisco, Jossey-Bass, 1969.

CHAPTER 4

Putting the History Together

The doctor may also learn more about the illness from the way the patient tells the story than from the story itself.

James B. Herrick
1861–1954

In the first two chapters, the interviewer's questions and the patient's responses were discussed. In this chapter, these materials are put together to shape a mock interview.

In the ensuing interview, note the way in which the interviewer allows the patient to speak and how the various techniques are incorporated.

The footnotes refer to the type of technique used or to some other important aspects of the interview.

Interview of Mr. John Doe

Mr. John Doe, the patient, is lying comfortably in a four-bedded room in Mount Hope Hospital. He is a white man, is slightly obese, and is in his mid-40s. Mr. Doe is watching television. The interviewer enters the room, wearing a white coat.

Interviewer *(smiling, extending hand for a firm handshake)*

Good morning, Mr. Doe. I'm Susan Smith, a second year medical student. I've been asked to interview and examine you today.

Patient *(smiling, appearing friendly)*

Dr. James, my resident, told me you'd be coming to see me.

Interviewer *(draws curtain around bed; pulls up a chair at the patient's bedside and sits down; legs crossed, arms in lap)*

Would you mind if we turn off the TV?

Patient *(turns off television)*

Not at all.

Interviewer How are you today?

Patient OK. No pain for the past 2 days.

Interviewer What was the problem that brought you to the hospital, Mr. Doe?*

Patient I've been having terrible chest pain for the past 6 months. . . .

(pause)

I guess I should start at the beginning. . . . About 4 years ago, I started having this strange sensation in my chest. It wasn't pain exactly . . . it was a dull aching discomfort. I didn't pay any attention to it. I guess I should have. . . . Well, anyway, I was able to go to work, play tennis, and have fun. Occasionally when I had an argument at work, I would get this sensation.

(looking sad)

---

* Inquiring about the chief complaint by using an open-ended question.

My wife never knew anything about it. I never told her. No one knew. I didn't want to upset them. Then all of a sudden on July 15, 1996, it happened.

(silence)

Interviewer	It happened?*
Patient	Yeah. I had my first heart attack.† I was playing tennis when I got this awful pain. I never had anything like that before. I was just getting ready to serve when this pain hit me. All I could do was lie down on the court. My partner ran over to me, and all I remember was that pain. . . . I woke up in Kings Hospital.

(pause)

They told me I lost consciousness and was taken to the hospital by ambulance. I remember that, when I came to in the hospital, I still had the pain. I was there for 2 weeks. |
Interviewer	How did you feel when you left the hospital?
Patient	I really felt fine. No more chest pain. My doctor there had given me some pills and said I would be fine.‡
Interviewer	Then what happened?§
Patient	I went back to work after about 3 weeks. I really felt great!

(smiles) |
Interviewer	What type of work do you do?
Patient	I'm a lawyer.
Interviewer	You mentioned that this was your *first* heart attack. Have you had others?
Patient	Unfortunately . . .

(looking down)

yes. |
| **Interviewer** | Tell me about it.‖

(leaning forward¶) |
| **Patient** | Six months later, I had my second attack.

(pause) |
| **Interviewer** | What were you doing? |
| **Patient** | Playing tennis.

(silence)

This time I don't remember anything . . . not even the pain. I remember being on the court and waking up in the intensive care unit of Kings Hospital. They said I had a massive heart attack and had some irregularity of my pulse that made me faint. But I left the hospital in 3 weeks feeling much better. I went back to work after 3 weeks at home. |
| **Interviewer** | Did you have any tests while you were in the hospital? |
| **Patient** | No . . .

(pause, hand over mouth)

the doctor just gave me some pills to strengthen my heart and for the irregularity. |

---

* This is an example of reflection.
† The patient is now telling the history of the present illness.
‡ Possibly false reassurance from the physician, or the patient heard what he wanted to hear.
§ Continues obtaining information with another open-ended question about the present illness.
‖ An example of verbal facilitation.
¶ An example of nonverbal facilitation.

	(silence)
Interviewer	*(silence, then after 10 seconds)*
	Your silence makes me think that you want to tell me something.*
Patient	I should have listened to him.
	(pause, shaking head)
Interviewer	To whom?
Patient	My doctor suggested after my first heart attack that I should have cardiac catheterization. I told him that I was fine . . . I didn't need it. . . . Even after my second attack, I didn't listen to him.
	(pause)
	I hope it's not too late.
Interviewer	Too late?
Patient	Yeah. That's why I'm here. I'm going to have the cardiac catheterization tomorrow. Emily finally convinced me to have it.
	(pause)
	I've really not been able to do anything for the past 6 months.
	(pause, looking down)
	I had to give up my work at the office. Sure, they still call me for advice, but it's not the same.
	(pause, almost tearful)
	The commuting by car just got to me.
	(pause)
	My son and his friends yelling around the house.
	(longer pause)
	I just can't take it anymore.
Interviewer	What did your doctor tell you about the test?†
Patient	The doctor told me if I have some blockage, he'll operate or fix it with a balloon. Will I be normal again?
Interviewer	*(pause)*
	After the study your doctor will be in the best position to answer that question.‡
	(pause)
	Tell me about the pain you've been having.
Patient	It seems I have the pain all the time. I can hardly walk up the stairs at home without getting the pain.
Interviewer	What's the pain like now?
Patient	It's an awful tightness, like a vise . . .
	(closes fist over chest§)
	right here.

---

* An example of confrontation.
† Inquiring about the patient's understanding of the test.
‡ The interviewer does not want to give false reassurances. Therefore, she chooses not to answer the question directly. Notice how the interviewer gets the narrative back on course.
§ This example of body language has been termed Levine's sign. It is discussed in Chapter 12, The Heart.

Interviewer	When you get the pain, do you feel it anywhere else?
Patient	Yeah. It goes straight to my back and my left arm. . . . The arm feels so heavy.
Interviewer	Are there any other times when you get the pain?
Patient	It seems I get it with the slightest effort or emotion.
Interviewer	Do you get the pain during sexual intercourse?
Patient	I had to stop even that 6 months ago. I'd get the pain just when I'm about to come . . . and . . . and . . . I'd have to stop.
Interviewer	Have you had any difficulty breathing?
Patient	When I get the pain, I get short of breath.
Interviewer	Do you ever get short of breath without the pain?
Patient	I find I just can't walk far any more without getting winded.
Interviewer	How many level blocks can you walk now without getting short of breath?
Patient	About one block.
Interviewer	How much could you walk 6 months ago?
Patient	I guess about two to three blocks.
Interviewer	Since your heart attack, have you had any skipped beats or fluttering of your heart?
Patient	No, never.
Interviewer	Has anyone ever told you that your cholesterol or fats in your blood were high?*
Patient	No.
Interviewer	Have you ever smoked?
Patient	I stopped after my first heart attack.
Interviewer	How much did you smoke?
Patient	About two packs a day.
Interviewer	For how long?
Patient	Oh . . . since I was about 18.
Interviewer	May I ask your age?†
Patient	I'm 42.
Interviewer	Have you ever had high blood pressure?
Patient	Yep. . . . My doctor gave me some medications for it but . . . but . . . I never refilled the pills after they ran out. . . . I felt fine.
Interviewer	Do you know how high your pressure was?‡
Patient	Not really.
Interviewer	Do you have diabetes?
Patient	Thank goodness, I don't. . . . My father does, though. . . . He's been pretty sick lately. . . . He's got some sort of a problem with his eyes. The doctor said that it's from his diabetes. He's going to see a specialist in a couple of weeks. . . . He's had a lot of problems. He broke his hip a few years ago when he was walking our dog. Some big guy came pulling a cart out of the supermarket and knocked my father over. He was hospitalized for several weeks since he really couldn't take care of himself. His hip is fine now. He would. . . .

---

*The interviewer is now starting to ascertain whether the patient has any risk factors for coronary artery disease.

†Notice that the interviewer has just now decided to ask the patient's age.

‡Notice that the interviewer ignores the statement that the patient didn't take his medications. Questioning the patient "Why not?" would only put the patient on the defensive.

Interviewer	*(interrupting)*
	I'm glad his hip is well healed. Is there anyone else in your family who has diabetes?*
Patient	No.
Interviewer	Anyone who's had a heart attack?
Patient	I think my mother's father died of a heart attack.
Interviewer	How old was he?
Patient	About 75.
Interviewer	What about your mother?†
Patient	She died when she was age 64 . . . right after my first heart attack. She had stomach cancer. She really suffered. . . . I guess it's a blessing.
Interviewer	Do you have any brothers or sisters?
Patient	My sister is 37 and she's fine. . . .
Interviewer	Any other siblings?
Patient	My brother is 45. . . . He had a heart attack when he was 40.‡
Interviewer	Do you have any children?
Patient	One boy who's 10.
Interviewer	How's your son's health?
Patient	No problem, except he's a little overweight.
Interviewer	Are you married?§
Patient	To a great gal. Emily's the one who convinced me to have the test.‖
Interviewer	Does anyone in your family have high blood pressure?
Patient	No.
Interviewer	Asthma?
Patient	No.
Interviewer	Tuberculosis?
Patient	No.
Interviewer	Birth defects or congenital diseases?
Patient	Not that I know of.
Interviewer	Have you ever been hospitalized here at Mount Hope Hospital?
Patient	No.¶
Interviewer	Have you ever been hospitalized at any time other than for your heart attacks?
Patient	I had my appendix taken out when I was 15.
Interviewer	Do you remember the surgeon's name and the hospital?

---

* Notice that the patient was beginning to ramble. The interviewer politely interrupted and redirected the interview. She is now inquiring about the family history.

† Notice that the interviewer does not assume anything about the mother's well-being or health. Because the patient approached the family's health history, the interviewer is now directing her questions to that history.

‡ Notice that the patient did not mention his brother when first asked about other family members with heart attacks or when asked about other brothers or sisters. The patient did not even acknowledge his brother's cardiac problem.

§ Notice that the interviewer does not assume that Mr. Doe is married *now*, even though he referred to his wife at the beginning of the interview and has acknowledged "Emily." "Emily" may *not* be his wife.

‖ In this case, "Emily" *is* the patient's wife. It is extremely important for the patient to identify family members. Never make an assumption that another person with the patient or described in the history is related to the patient.

¶ Had the patient answered in the affirmative, the interviewer would have asked when, and the patient's record would have been reviewed later.

Patient	I think it was a Dr. Meyers at Booth Hospital. We were living in Rochester.
Interviewer	Any other operations?
Patient	No.
Interviewer	Have you ever been hospitalized for any other reason?*
Patient	No, what do you mean?
Interviewer	Just a routine question. Do you have any allergies?
Patient	No.
Interviewer	How was your health as a child?
Patient	I guess OK. I had the usual sore throats and earaches that most kids get.
Interviewer	Did anyone ever tell you you had rheumatic fever?†
Patient	No.
Interviewer	Did you have any of these illnesses:‡ chickenpox? . . . measles? . . . diphtheria? . . . polio? . . . mumps? . . . whooping cough?
Patient	*(shakes head "no")*
Interviewer	Do you take any medications?
Patient	Just Inderal and Isordil.
Interviewer	Do you know the dosages?
Patient	I take Inderal LA 120 mg once daily and Isordil 20 mg four times a day.
Interviewer	Do you think the medications help you?
Patient	I guess so. I think I feel better with them.
Interviewer	Any other medications?
Patient	*(pause)* Nitroglycerin . . . when I get the pain.
Interviewer	How long does the nitroglycerin take to work?
Patient	Real quickly.
Interviewer	How long is that?
Patient	About 4 to 5 minutes.
Interviewer	Do you take any other medications . . . *(pause)* cold medicine? . . . vitamins? . . . anything else?
Patient	*(thinking)* I take Chlor-Trimeton when I get a cold . . . but that's about it.
Interviewer	Have you ever had any other health problems?
Patient	No.
Interviewer	Any problems with your liver? . . . kidneys? . . . stomach? . . . lungs?§
Patient	*(shakes head "no")*

---

* The interviewer is specifically asking about nonmedical hospitalizations, e.g., for psychiatric reasons. This type of question is not offensive. If the patient has had such admissions to hospitals, he can generally describe them at this time. If not, as in this case, watch how the interview progresses. (Notice how the interviewer continues directly with the next question.)

† This question can follow nicely after the history of sore throats.

‡ The interviewer slowly asks about each illness, after which she pauses for the patient to respond.

§ Because this patient has demonstrated so much denial, the interviewer wishes to ask specifically about diseases of the major organs. Each question is asked slowly, and the interviewer pauses after each question, waiting for a response.

Interviewer	How's your appetite?
Patient	Pretty good. I haven't been real hungry lately.
Interviewer	Starting with breakfast yesterday, what did you eat?
Patient	Toast, coffee, and juice for breakfast . . .
	(pause)
	a ham sandwich with a Tab for lunch . . .
	(pause)
	oh yeah, blueberry pie for dessert . . .
	(pause)
	and . . . uh . . . steak with a baked potato and salad for dinner.
Interviewer	Any snacks between meals?
Patient	I had a cupcake with milk before I went to bed.
Interviewer	Do you eat fish?
Patient	Sometimes.
Interviewer	How often?*
Patient	Maybe . . .
	(pause)
	once every 2 weeks. I enjoy shrimp, but I know it's not good for me.†
Interviewer	Have you had any weight change recently?
Patient	I lost about 10 pounds in the past 3 months . . .
	(pause)
	but I wanted to. . . .
Interviewer	Were you on a diet?
Patient	No . . . not exactly. . . . I just haven't been too hungry lately.
Interviewer	How well do you sleep?‡
Patient	Like a baby . . .
	(pause)
	although I've been getting up pretty early recently.
Interviewer	Mmmm?
Patient	Yeah . . . recently I go right to sleep . . . but seem to get up about 3 in the morning . . . and can't go back to sleep. . . .
	(pause)
	I guess I've got a lot on my mind. . . .
	(pause, looking down, hand to mouth)
Interviewer	You seem depressed.§
Patient	*(pause)*
	I guess I am. . . . What's going to happen to me? . . . I really want to live. . . .

---

* The interviewer is not satisfied with qualitative statements. She pursues each question to quantify as best as possible.

† Despite the fact that he knows that shrimp is not as healthy as fish, he still eats it. This is further denial of his illness.

‡ The interviewer has now picked up some other somatic element of depression and will now pursue it.

§ An example of an interpretation.

(beginning to cry)

I've been so stupid . . .

(pause)

My kid's only 10. . . . He's a great kid. . . . He needs me. . . . What's the test gonna show? . . . I hope I can have the surgery or the balloon to get relief from this pain.*

Interviewer   *(silent, handing a box of tissues to the patient)*†

Patient   *(sobbing, trying to control his emotions)*

I'm sorry . . . I can't help it . . .

(wiping his tears)

I guess we'll have to wait till tomorrow.

Interviewer   I just have a few more questions for you. Do you drink alcohol?

Patient   *(shaking head "no")*

Just socially . . . one drink . . . maybe after work, sometimes.

Interviewer   Do you ever feel that you have a need for a drink as the day goes on?

Patient   Yeah . . . I sure do!

Interviewer   Have you ever felt the need to cut down on your drinking?

Patient   No.

Interviewer   Have people annoyed you by criticizing your drinking?

Patient   Never . . . but my wife doesn't like me drinking.

Interviewer   Have you ever felt bad or guilty about your drinking?

Patient   Yeah. . . . Once about 10 years ago my friend's father made some wine. . . . We got really drunk . . . it was terrible . . . but never again!

Interviewer   Do you drink in the morning?

Patient   Never.

Interviewer   Do you ever drive while intoxicated?

Patient   No! That's suicide.

Interviewer   Do you drink coffee or tea?

Patient   About three cups of coffee a day at work. I have tea only when I'm sick with a cold.

Interviewer   Have you ever used street drugs?

Patient   I've tried pot a couple of times . . . never did anything to me. . . . Nothing else.

Interviewer   What's your usual day like?‡

Patient   Before I stopped working at the office, I got up about 5:30, dressed, and was at my desk in the office by 7:30. I usually left the office about 7 and got home by 8:15. We'd have dinner, and I'd be in bed by 11:30, after the news.

Interviewer   Sounds like you have a pretty busy day.

Patient   Yeah . . . I enjoy my work . . . or at least I used to.

Interviewer   How long have you been working with your present office?

---

*The interviewer could have elected to ask the patient his reactions if surgery cannot be performed. How will he face life? Is there a possibility of suicide? The interviewer chose not to create further anxiety at this time.

†An example of empathetic support. The interviewer cannot answer the patient's questions, but she allows the patient to express his emotions. She is, in essence, saying, "I'm with you."

‡Interviewer is inquiring about the patient's lifestyle and psychosocial history.

Patient	I started right after law school. I guess I've been there . . . about . . . 17 years. I'm one of the senior partners.
	(pause)
	I was just promoted. . . . A lot of good that will do now.
Interviewer	I now have several questions that I would like to ask you. You can answer just "yes" or "no" to each.*
	(pause)
	Have you had any recent fevers?
Patient	No.
Interviewer	Chills?
Patient	No.
Interviewer	Sweats?
Patient	No.
Interviewer	Rashes?
Patient	No.
Interviewer	Changes in your hair or nails?
Patient	No.
Interviewer	Headaches?
Patient	Rarely, about once every 2 to 3 months.
Interviewer	For how long have you been having headaches?
Patient	Years . . . I guess about 20 to 25 years.
Interviewer	Can you describe them to me?
Patient	That's hard. They're right here.
	(pointing to the center of his forehead)
	They last about 1 to 2 hours.
Interviewer	What relieves them?
Patient	Usually, aspirin.
Interviewer	Have you noticed a change in the pattern or severity of your headaches?
Patient	No.
Interviewer	Have you had any head injuries?
Patient	Never.
Interviewer	Have you ever fainted?
Patient	No.
Interviewer	Do you have any problems with. . . .†
	(the interviewer completes the review of systems and then asks)
	Is there anything else you would like to tell me that I haven't asked about?
Patient	No . . . you've certainly been very thorough.

---

* The interviewer will now begin asking the *review of systems*. She will ask about each symptom. If the patient answers in the affirmative, further questioning is appropriate.

† The interviewer continues through the entire review of systems, asking further questions when necessary.

Interviewer	I'd like to summarize your history briefly to make sure I have the details correct before I proceed with your physical examination. This is your first time here at Mount Hope Hospital. You had your first heart attack on July 15, 1996, while playing tennis. You were hospitalized in Kings Hospital for 2 weeks. Your second heart attack was 6 months later. You were again hospitalized in Kings Hospital. Your medications since then have been Inderal LA 120 mg once daily and isosorbide dinitrate (Isordil) 20 mg, four times a day. Because of a worsening of your chest pain and an increase in your shortness of breath in the past 6 months, you're now being admitted for cardiac catheterization. Is that correct, Mr. Doe?
Patient	Exactly!
Interviewer	Do you have any questions for me before I begin your physical examination?
Patient	No . . . I can't think of any.
Interviewer	*(The interviewer stands up, sets up the equipment on the night table, and goes to the sink to wash her hands. The physical examination then commences.)*
Interviewer	*(concluding the physical examination)*
	I want to thank you for your time.
Patient	Well . . . what do you think? Will I make it?
Interviewer	*(opening curtain around patient's bed)*
	I'm now going to meet with my preceptor. Afterwards, we'll be back.*

Written History of Mr. John Doe

The preceding interview has revealed much about this 42 year old lawyer. Superficially, he is a patient with coronary artery disease. Just as important as his physical illness is his emotional reaction to it. As the interview progressed, the interviewer recognized that the patient is scared and anxious. What will happen "after tomorrow"? Will he be a candidate for balloon angioplasty? Can it be performed? Is he a good candidate for bypass surgery? Will he live? The anxiety from these questions has resulted in his depression, which must be dealt with as well.

The written history is a summary of the information obtained during the interview. It is usually written after the interview and the physical examination have been completed. The following is an example of the written history of Mr. Doe, based on the preceding interview.

Chief Complaint. "Chest pain for the past 6 months."

History of Present Illness. This is the first Mount Hope admission for Mr. John Doe, a 42 year old lawyer with coronary artery disease. His history dates back to approximately 4 years before admission, when he started to experience a vague discomfort in his chest. He describes it as "a dull ache," provoked by emotional upsets at work. He suffered his first heart attack on July 15, 1996, while playing tennis. He was hospitalized for 3 weeks in Kings Hospital. After 3 weeks at home, he returned to work. Six months later, he suffered his second heart attack, again while playing tennis. He was again hospitalized at Kings Hospital and was told that he had "irregularity" of his heart. He was started on some medications for this irregularity. The patient denies any palpitations since then.

Over the past 6 months, the patient has had increasing chest pain with radiation down his left arm despite Inderal LA 120 mg daily and isosorbide dinitrate (Isordil) 20 mg qid.† The patient's chest pain is produced by exercise, emotion, and sexual intercourse. The patient takes nitroglycerin as needed, with relief within 5 minutes. One block dyspnea on exertion is also present. This has worsened in the past 6 months, before which he could walk two to three blocks. The patient's risk factors for coronary artery disease include a

---

* By indicating to the patient that the interviewer and her preceptor will be back, the patient is less likely to press the interviewer for her opinion at this time. The interviewer should never provide an answer at this point. False reassurances can be dangerous.

† Four times a day.

history of untreated hypertension, a 40 pack-year history of smoking (2 packs per day for 20 years), and a brother with a myocardial infarction at the age of 40 years. The patient's brother is now 45 years of age. The patient denies any history of diabetes or hyperlipidemia. At his physician's and wife's request, he has entered the hospital for elective cardiac catheterization. The patient has a significant denial of his illness and a secondary depression.* Although cardiac catheterization was suggested after the patient's first heart attack, he refused to accept it until this admission.

Past Medical History. The patient was hospitalized at age 15 years for an appendectomy in Booth Hospital in Rochester, New York. The surgery was performed by a Dr. Meyers. The only other hospitalizations were for the patient's two heart attacks, as indicated previously. The patient is predominantly a red meat eater with little fish in his diet. Recently, presumably owing to depression, there has been a loss of appetite with a 10 pound weight loss. The patient admits to a sleeping problem. He falls asleep normally but awakens early and cannot go back to sleep. His only medications are indicated in the history of present illness. There is no history of renal, hepatic, pulmonary, or gastrointestinal disease. There is no history of allergy.

Family History. The patient's father is 75 years of age and has a history of diabetes. He apparently has some ocular problem (cataracts or retinopathy). The patient's mother died at age 64 years from stomach cancer. The patient's older brother, as mentioned previously, is 45 years of age and has coronary artery disease. The patient has a younger sister who is 37 years of age and is well. There is no history of congenital disease. The patient is married and has a 10 year old son, who is well.

Psychosocial History. The patient is a "type A" personality. He admits to having a need to drink alcohol occasionally after work. He drinks coffee about three times a day. He has used only marijuana on rare occasions, and he denies the use of other street drugs.

Review of Systems. There is a 20–25 year history of headaches without any recent change in their pattern or severity. The patient denies any head injury. There is. . . .† There is no history of claudication.‡ The remainder of the review of systems is noncontributory.§

Bibliography

Bird B: Talking with Patients. Philadelphia, J.B. Lippincott, 1973.
Cassell EJ: Talking with Patients: Clinical Technique. Cambridge, MA, MIT Press, 1985.
Cassell EJ: Talking with Patients: The Theory of Doctor-Patient Communication. Cambridge, MA, MIT Press, 1985.
Enelow AJ, Swisher SN: Interviewing and Patient Care. New York, Oxford University Press, 1979.
Feinstein AR: Clinical Judgment. Baltimore, Williams & Wilkins, 1967.
Morgan WL Jr, Engel GL: The Clinical Approach to the Patient. Philadelphia, W.B. Saunders, 1969.

---

* Notice that the history of the present illness summarizes all the information related to the present illness chronologically, regardless of when the information was obtained during the interview.

† The review of systems would then indicate any of the other symptoms that may be present.

‡ Notice that the positive symptoms are indicated first. The important, or pertinent, negatives are then listed. A pertinent negative in this patient is the lack of claudication. Coronary artery disease is often associated with peripheral vascular disease. The absence of a major symptom of peripheral vascular disease, claudication, makes claudication in this patient a pertinent negative. Chapter 13, The Peripheral Vascular System, has a further discussion on pertinent positives and negatives.

§ This statement indicates that none of the other symptoms is either present or contributes to the patient's present illness.

The Science of the Physical Examination

CHAPTER 5

The Physical Examination

Don't touch the patient—state first what you see; cultivate your powers of observation.

Sir William Osler
1849–1919

The Basic Procedures

In the previous chapters, the general rules for mastering the art of taking the history have been discussed. The specific skills necessary to perform a proper physical examination are discussed in this chapter. The four principles of physical examination are the following:

1. Inspection
2. Palpation
3. Percussion
4. Auscultation

To achieve competence in these procedures, the student must, in the words of Sir William Osler, "teach the eye to see, the finger to feel, and the ear to hear." The ability to coordinate all this sensory input is learned with time and practice.

Even though examiners will not use all these techniques for every organ system, they should think of these four skills before moving on to the next area to be evaluated.

Inspection

Inspection can provide an enormous amount of information. Proper technique requires more than just a glance. Examiners must train themselves to look at the body using a systematic approach. All too often, the novice examiner will rush to use the ophthalmoscope, stethoscope, or otoscope before the naked eyes have been used for inspection.

An example of what is meant by "teaching the eye to see" can be demonstrated in the following illustration. Read the sentence in the box. Then count the number of "F's" in the sentence.

> Finished files are the result of years of scientific study combined with the experience of years.

How many did you count? The answer is in a footnote at the end of this chapter. This example clearly shows that eyes have to be trained to see.*

While taking the history, the examiner should observe certain aspects of the patient:

- General appearance
- State of nutrition
- Body habitus
- Symmetry
- Posture and gait
- Speech

---

*This test has been circulated widely in the medical community. The original writer is unknown.

The *general appearance* includes the state of consciousness and personal grooming. Does the patient look well or sick? Is he comfortable in bed, or does he appear in distress? Is he alert, or is he groggy? Does he look acutely or chronically ill? The answer to this last question is sometimes difficult to determine from inspection. There are some useful signs to aid the examiner. Poor nutrition, sunken eyes, temporal wasting, and loose skin are associated with chronic disease. Does the patient appear clean? Although the patient is ill, she does not have to appear unkempt. Is her hair combed? Does she bite her nails? The answers to these questions may provide useful information about the patient's self-esteem and mental status.

Inspection will provide an evaluation of the *state of nutrition*. Does the patient appear thin and frail? Is the patient obese? Most individuals with chronic disease are *not* overweight. These patients are cachectic. Long-standing ailments such as cancer, hyperthyroidism, or heart disease can result in a markedly wasted-looking individual.

The *body habitus* is useful to observe because certain disease states are more common in different body builds. The asthenic, or ectomorphic, patient is thin, has poor muscle development and small bone structure, and appears malnourished. The sthenic, or mesomorphic, patient is the athletic type with excellent development of the muscles and a large bone structure. The hypersthenic, or endomorphic, patient is the short, round individual with good muscle development, but frequently has a weight problem.

Because the body is a *symmetric* structure, any asymmetry should be noted. Many systemic diseases provide clues that can be uncovered on inspection. With an obvious unilateral supraclavicular swelling or a less obvious unilateral miotic pupil, each clue serves to aid the examiner in reaching a final diagnosis. The left supraclavicular swelling in a 61 year old man may represent an enlarged supraclavicular lymph node and could be the only sign of gastric carcinoma. The miotic pupil in a 43 year old woman may be a manifestation of interruption of the cervical sympathetic chain by a tumor of the apex of the lung. The recent onset of a left-sided varicocele in a 46 year old man could be related to a left hypernephroma.

The patient is usually in bed when introduced to the examiner. If the patient were walking about, the examiner could use this time to observe the patient's *posture* and *gait*. The ability of a person to walk normally involves the coordination of the nervous and musculoskeletal systems. Does the patient drag a foot? Is there a shuffling gait? Does the patient limp? Are the steps normal?

The examiner can learn much about the patient from the *speech patterns*. Is the speech slurred? Does the patient use words appropriately? Is the patient hoarse? Is there an unusual high- or low-pitched voice?

Is the patient oriented to person, place, and time? This can easily be evaluated by asking the patient, "Who are you?"; "Where are you?"; "What is the date, season, or month?"; and "What is the name of the President of the United States?" These questions certainly do not have to be asked at the beginning, but they should be asked at some time during the interview and examination. These questions provide an insight into the mental status of the patient. The mental status examination is discussed further in Chapter 19, The Nervous System.

The examiner must be able to recognize the cardinal signs of inflammation: swelling, heat, redness, pain, and disturbance of function. Swelling results from edema or congestion in local tissues. Heat is the sensation resulting from an increased blood supply to the involved area. Redness is a manifestation of the increased blood supply. Pain often results from the swelling that exerts an increased pressure on the nerve fibers. Because of the pain and swelling, a disturbance of function may occur.

Palpation

Palpation is the use of the tactile sense to determine the characteristics of an organ system. For example, an abnormal impulse may be felt in the right chest that could be related to an ascending aortic aneurysm. A pulsatile mass in the abdomen might be an abdominal aneurysm. An acutely tender mass in the right upper quadrant of the abdomen that descends with inspiration is probably an inflamed gallbladder.

Percussion

Percussion relates to the tactile sensation and sound produced when a sharp blow is struck to an area being examined. This provides valuable information about the structure of the underlying organ or tissue. The difference in the sensation in comparison with normal may be related to fluid in an otherwise nonfluid-containing area. Collapse of a lung will change the percussion note, as will a solid mass in the abdomen. Percussion that produces a dull note in the midline of the lower abdomen in a man probably represents a distended urinary bladder.

Auscultation

Auscultation involves listening to sounds produced by internal organs. This technique furnishes information about an organ's pathophysiology. The examiner is urged to learn as much as possible from the other techniques before using the stethoscope. This instrument should corroborate the signs that were suggested by the other techniques. Auscultation should not be used alone to examine the heart, chest, and abdomen. This technique should be used together with inspection, percussion, and palpation. Listening for carotid, ophthalmic, or renal bruits can provide lifesaving information. The absence of normal bowel sounds could indicate a surgical emergency.

Preparation for the Examination

The physical examination generally begins after taking the history has been completed. The examiner should have a portable case designed to contain all equipment, which should include the items listed in Table 5–1.

The examiner should place the equipment on the patient's night table or bedstand. By presenting all the "tools," the examiner will be less likely to forget to perform a specific examination. It is preferable to use daylight for illumination, because skin color changes may be masked by artificial light. The patient's curtains should be drawn at the start of the interview.

Before you examine the patient, wash your hands, preferably while the patient is watching. Washing with soap and water is an effective way to reduce the transmission of disease.

The patient should be wearing a gown that opens at the front or back. Pajamas are also acceptable. It is most important for you to consider the comfort of the patient. You should allow the patient the use of pillows if requested. There are few relationships in which individuals will expose themselves to a stranger after only a brief contact.

Table 5–1   Equipment for Physical Examination

Required	Optional	Available in Most Patient Care Areas
Stethoscope	Nasal illuminator†	Sphygmomanometer
Oto-ophthalmoscope	Nasal speculum	Tongue blades
Penlight	Tuning fork:	Applicator sticks
Reflex hammer	512 Hz	Gauze pads
Tuning fork: 128 Hz		Gloves
Safety pins or a box of straight pins*		Lubricant gel
Tape measure		Guaiac card for occult blood
Pocket visual acuity card		Vaginal speculum

* A new pin should be used in examining each patient as a precaution against transmission of the AIDS and hepatitis viruses.
† Attachment for the otoscope handle.

It is important that you become facile in each organ system examination. Incorporate the individual evaluations into the complete examination with the least amount of movement of the patient. Regardless of age, patients tire quickly when asked to "sit up," "lie down," "turn on your left side," "sit up," "lie down," and so on. You should perform as much of the examination as possible with the patient in one position. It is also important that the patient never be asked to sit up in bed without support for any extended period of time.

By convention, the examiner stands to the *right* of the patient as the patient lies in bed. The examiner uses the right hand for most maneuvers of the examination. It has been a common experience that even left-handed individuals will learn to perform the examination from the right side using their right hand. Each of the following organ system chapters discusses the placement of hands.

Although it will be necessary for the patient to disrobe completely, the examination should be carried out by exposing only the areas that are being examined at that time, without undue exposure of other areas. When examining a woman's breast, for example, it is necessary to check for any asymmetry by inspecting both breasts at the same time. After inspection has been completed, the physician may use the patient's gown to cover the breast not being examined. The examination of the abdomen may be done discreetly by placing a towel or the bedsheet over the genitalia. Examination of the heart with the patient in the supine position may be performed with the right breast covered. This caring for the patient's privacy will go a long way in establishing a good doctor-patient relationship.

While performing the physical examination, the examiner should continue speaking to the patient. The examiner may wish to pursue various parts of the history as well as to tell the patient what is being done. The examiner should always refrain from comments such as "That's good" or "That's normal" or "That's fine" in reference to any part of the examination. Although this is initially reassuring to the patient, if the examiner fails to make such a statement during another part of the examination, the patient will automatically assume that there is something wrong or abnormal.

The chapters that follow discuss the individual organ system examinations. After they have been presented, Chapter 20, Putting the Examination Together, summarizes a method of putting all the individual evaluations together into one smoothly continuous examination.

Precautions to Take During the Examination

The student and clinician are frequently exposed to patients with hepatitis or acquired immunodeficiency syndrome (AIDS). The fear many clinicians have about this disease frequently interferes with the development of a good doctor-patient relationship. Once clearly defined procedures are implemented to ensure the safety of health-care workers, this fear can be better handled.

Several precautionary guidelines have been established by the Centers for Disease Control and Prevention (1986) and the Occupational Safety and Health Administration (OSHA) Bloodborne Pathogens Standard (1991). These guidelines should be followed routinely by all health-care workers whenever there is a possibility of exposure to potentially infectious materials such as blood or other body fluids.

1. The use of gloves should provide adequate protection when performing the physical examination or when handling blood-soiled or body fluid–soiled sheets or clothing.
2. Gloves should be worn when examining any individual with exudative lesions or weeping dermatitis.
3. When a procedure is performed, the use of fluid-resistant gowns, masks, and eye covers is indicated if splattering or aerosolization of body fluid is anticipated.
4. Hands or other contaminated skin surfaces should be washed thoroughly and immediately if accidentally soiled with blood or other body fluids.
5. All sharp items, such as needles, scalpel blades, and other pointed items, must be handled with extraordinary care to prevent injuries.
6. To prevent needlestick injuries, needles should *not* be recapped. They should be disposed in clearly marked puncture-resistant containers.

7. If mouth-to-mouth contact is necessary, mouthpieces, resuscitation bags, or other ventilatory devices should be used.
8. Blood and other body fluid specimens should be handled with gloves.
9. Areas that have been soiled with blood or other body fluids should be cleaned and decontaminated with an appropriate disinfectant.
10. All reusable items should be processed with current recommendations. The level of disinfection and/or sterilization is based on the specific tissues that the item had contacted.
11. If a sharp injury or exposure to blood or body fluid occurs, the area should be cleansed immediately, and if mucous membranes are exposed, they should be irrigated thoroughly with water. The incident should be reported, and the exposed person referred promptly for management and counseling.
12. All health-care providers who have direct contact with patients should complete the hepatitis B vaccine series. In certain populations, testing for immunity prior to the vaccine may be indicated.

A patient may be in isolation or on special precautions, which indicates that he or she is suffering from a contagious disease, such as tuberculosis or varicella-zoster infection, or is colonized with a multiresistant organism. Consult the institutional infection control manual for guidelines regarding restrictions on entry into the patient's room and protective attire.

The Goal of the Physical Examination

The goal of the physical examination is to obtain valid information concerning the health of the patient. The examiner must be able to identify, analyze, and synthesize the accumulated information into a comprehensive assessment.

The validity of a physical finding depends on many factors. Clinical experience and reliability of the examination techniques are most important. False-positive or false-negative results reduce the precision of the techniques. Variance can occur when techniques are performed by different examiners, with different equipment, on different patients. The concepts of validity and precision are discussed further in Chapter 25, Clinical Decision-Making.

Unconscious bias is an important concept to understand. It is well known that unconscious bias in an examiner can influence the evaluation of the physical finding. For example, in patients with rapid atrial fibrillation, the ventricular rate is irregular and varies from 150 to 200 beats per minute. The radial pulse rate is significantly less, owing to a pulse deficit (explained in Chapter 12, The Heart). If examiners record the apical heart rate first, they will find that the rate varies from 150 to 200 beats per minute. If they then check the radial pulse, they will detect a faster pulse rate than if they had measured the radial pulse first. The first observation, therefore, biases the second observation. Alternately, if examiners determine the radial pulse first and the heart rate second, the apical heart rate will be slower, but the chance of bias is lower because observer error is less at the apex (Chalmers, 1981).

It is important to review the concepts of *sensitivity* and *specificity*. Sensitivity is the frequency of a positive test or technique in individuals with a disease or condition. Specificity is the frequency of a negative test or technique in individuals without a disease or condition. Sensitivity and specificity refer to properties of the test or technique, whereas the health-care provider is interested in properties or characteristics of the patient, which are given by the predictive values. The *positive predictive value* is the frequency of disease in patients with a positive test. The *negative predictive value* is the frequency of nondisease in patients with a negative test. The question, "What is the possibility that a woman with a stony hard breast mass has cancer?" addresses the positive predictive value. Predictive value depends on the prevalence of disease in the respective population as well as the sensitivity and specificity of the test. A positive test in an individual from a population with a low prevalence of disease will still yield a low positive predictive value.

For example, eliciting the presence of shifting dullness is a highly sensitive technique for detecting ascites. Thus, an examiner who does not detect shifting dullness in the abdomen of a patient can be reasonably sure that this negative finding rules out ascites. In contrast, the finding of microaneurysms in the macular area of the retina is a highly specific finding for diabetes. For example, an examiner who finds microaneurysms at the macula can be reasonably confident that this finding rules in diabetes, because normal individuals without diabetes do not have macular microaneurysms. That is, the finding of microaneurysms at the macula has a high degree of specificity. Unfortunately, a technique is rarely both very sensitive and very specific. Several techniques must be applied together to be able to make an appropriate assessment.

In summary:

1. A technique or test with high sensitivity can be confidently used to rule out disease for a patient with a negative finding.
2. A technique or test with high specificity can be confidently used to rule in disease for a patient with a positive finding.

These concepts are more clearly discussed in Chapter 25, Diagnostic Reasoning in Physical Diagnosis.

Useful Vocabulary

The vocabulary of medicine is difficult and broad. Memorization of a term is less useful than trying to determine the meaning by understanding its etymology, or roots. The spelling of terms will also be easier.

Listed here are some general roots that are important to understand. At the end of the following chapters, there is a section on specific roots and terminology for that area of the body. The following list should not be memorized at this time. It should be used in conjunction with the roots listed in the subsequent chapters.

Prefix/Root	Pertaining To	Example	Definition
ab-	away from	*ab*duction	Away from the body
ad-	toward	*ad*duction	Toward the body
aden-	gland	*aden*opathy	Glandular disease
an-	without	*an*osmia	Without the sense of smell
aniso-	unequal	*aniso*coria	Unequal pupils
asthen-	weak	*asthen*opia	Eye fatigue
contra-	against; opposite	*contra*lateral	Pertaining to the opposite side
diplo-	double	*diplo*pia	Double vision
duc-	lead	ab*duc*tion	Turning outward
dys-	bad; ill	*dys*uria	Painful urination
eso-	in	*eso*tropia	Eye deviated inward
eu-	good; advantageous	*eu*pnea	Easy breathing
exo-	out	*exo*tropia	Eye deviated outward
hemi-	half	*hemi*plegia	Paralysis of one side of the body
hydro-	water	*hydro*philic	Readily absorbing water
hyper-	beyond	*hyper*emia	Excess of blood
hypno-	sleep	*hypno*tic	Inducing sleep
idio-	separate; distinct	*idio*pathic	Of unknown causation
infra-	below	*infra*hyoid	Below the hyoid gland
intra-	within	*intra*cranial	Within the skull
ipsi-	self	*ipsi*lateral	Situated on the same side
iso-	equal	*iso*tonic	Equal tension
leuko-	white	*leuko*cyte	White cell
lith-	stone	*lith*otomy	Incision of an organ to remove a stone
macro-	large	*macro*cephaly	Abnormally large head
neo-	new	*neo*plasm	Abnormal new growth
pedia-	child	*pedia*trics	Branch of medicine treating diseases of children
peri-	around	*peri*cardium	Sac around heart
poly-	many	*poly*cystic	Many cysts
presby-	old	*presby*opia	Impairment of vision due to advancing years
retro-	situated behind	*retro*bulbar	Behind the eye
soma-	body	*soma*tic	Pertaining to the body
sten-	narrowed	*sten*osis	Narrowed
trans-	through	*trans*urethral	Through the urethra

Suffix/Root	Pertaining To	Example	Definition
-dynia	pain	cephalo*dynia*	Headache
-ectomy	removal of	append*ectomy*	Removal of the appendix
-gnosis	recognition	stereo*gnosis*	Recognizing an object by touch
-gram	something written	myelo*gram*	X-ray film of the spinal cord
-ism	state; condition	gigant*ism*	State of abnormal overgrowth
-itis	inflammation of	col*itis*	Inflammation of the colon
-kinesia	movement	brady*kinesia*	Abnormal slow movement
-lysis	dissolution	hemo*lysis*	Liberation of hemoglobin into solution
-malacia	softening	osteo*malacia*	Softening of bones
-megal-	enlargement	cardio*megaly*	Cardiac enlargement
-mycosis	fungus	blasto*mycosis*	A specific fungal infection
-oid	resembling	human*oid*	Resembling a human
-ologist	specialist in study of	cardi*ologist*	A specialist in heart disease
-oma	tumor; growth	fibr*oma*	A tumor of fibrous tissue
-orrhaphy	suture; repair	herni*orrhaphy*	Repair of a hernia
-osis	diseased state	endometri*osis*	Disease state of abnormally located uterine tissue
-pathy	disease	uro*pathy*	Disease of the urinary tract
-phobia	fear; pain	photo*phobia*	Abnormal intolerance of light
-plasty	repair	valvulo*plasty*	Surgical repair of a valve
-plegia	paralysis	hemi*plegia*	Paralysis of one half of the body
-ptosis	drooping	blepharo*ptosis*	Drooping eyelids
-rrhagia	hemorrhage	oto*rrhagia*	Hemorrhage from the ear
-rrhexis	rupture	gastro*rrhexis*	Rupture of stomach
-scope	instrument for examining	ophthalmo*scope*	Tool for examination of the eye
-spasmos	spasm	blepharo*spasm*	Twitching of the eyelids
-stom-	opening	ileo*stomy*	Surgical creation of an opening into the ileum
-tome	cut	micro*tome*	An instrument for cutting thin slices

The preceding list represents the more common prefixes, roots, and suffixes. Each chapter will further enhance your knowledge with more organ-specific roots.

Bibliography

Centers for Disease Control (CDC): Recommendations for preventing transmission of infection with human T-lymphotrophic virus type III lymphadenopathy-associated virus during invasive procedures. MMWR 35:221, 1986.

Chalmers TC: The clinical trial. Milbank Mem Fund Q 59:324, 1981.

U.S. Department of Labor, Occupational Safety and Health Administration 29 CFR Part 1910.1030: Occupational Exposure to Bloodborne Pathogens, 1991.

Answer to Puzzle: There are six "F's" in the sentence in the box. Go back and count them. Most individuals count only three. Include the "F's" in the three "ofs".

CHAPTER 6

The Skin

What is the hardest of all? That which you hold the most simple; seeing with your own eyes what is spread out before you.

Johann Wolfgang von Goethe
1749–1832

General Considerations

The skin, which is the largest organ of the body, is one of the best indicators of general health. Even the untrained person is capable of detecting changes in skin color and texture. The trained examiner can detect these changes and at the same time evaluate more subtle cutaneous signs of systemic disease.

Diseases of the skin are common. Approximately one third of the population in the United States has a disorder of the skin that warrants medical attention. Nearly 8% of all adult outpatient visits are related to dermatologic problems. Skin cancer is the most common malignancy; more than 400,000 new cases are diagnosed annually. Although most of these patients are treated and cured, skin cancer still causes over 5000 deaths a year.

The incidence of malignant melanoma is rising at a faster rate than that of any other tumor. This year, 35,000 new cases diagnosed and 7000 deaths from this tumor are predicted. The incidence of melanoma has increased 7% per year during the last decade, and it is estimated that by the year 2000, the rate of development of melanoma during a lifetime will be 1 in 75. The reasons for this are unclear, but excessive sun exposure is a major factor.

Early detection and treatment of malignant melanoma, as with most cancers, offers the best chance of a cure. Among patients with a superficial melanoma (less than 0.76 mm in depth), the survival rate is more than 99%, whereas among those with a larger lesion (greater than 3.64 mm in depth), the 5 year survival rate is only 42%. The external nature of melanoma gives the examiner an opportunity to detect these small, curable lesions.

The most important function of the skin is to protect the body from the environment. The skin has evolved in humans to be a relatively impermeable surface layer that prevents the loss of water, protects against external hazards, and insulates against thermal changes. It is also actively involved in the production of vitamin D. The skin appears to have the lowest water permeability of any naturally produced membrane. Its barrier to invasion retards potentially noxious agents from entering the body and causing internal damage. This barrier protects against many physical stresses and prohibits the invasion of microorganisms. By observing patients with extensive skin problems, such as burns, the importance of this organ can be appreciated.

Structure and Physiology

The three tissue layers of the skin are the

- Epidermis
- Dermis
- Subcutaneous tissue

These layers are depicted in Figure 6–1.

The *epidermis* is the thin, outermost layer of the skin. It is composed of several layers of keratocytes, or keratin-producing cells. Keratin is an insoluble protein that provides the skin with its protective properties. The stratum corneum is the outermost

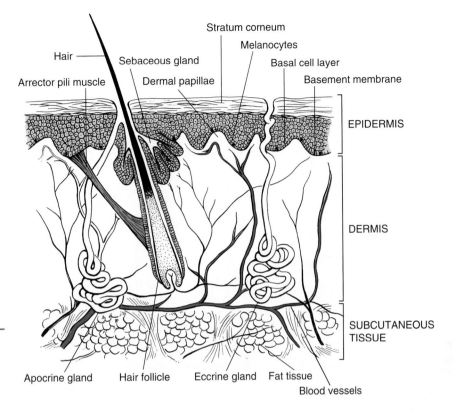

Hair

Sebaceous gland

Stratum corneum

Melanocytes

Basal cell layer

Basement membrane

Arrector pili muscle

Dermal papillae

EPIDERMIS

DERMIS

SUBCUTANEOUS
TISSUE

Apocrine gland   Hair follicle   Eccrine gland   Fat tissue

Blood vessels

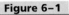

Figure 6–1

Cross section through the skin, showing the structures in the epidermis, and subcutaneous tissues.

layer and serves as a major physical barrier. The stratum corneum is composed of keratinized cells, which appear as dry, flattened, anuclear, and adherent flakes.

The *basal cell layer* is the deepest layer of the epidermis. The basal cell layer forms a single row of rapidly proliferating cells that slowly migrate upward, keratinize, and are ultimately shed from the stratum corneum. The process of maturation, keratinization, and shedding takes approximately 4 weeks. The cells of the basal layer are intermingled with melanocytes, which produce melanin. The number of melanocytes is approximately equal in all people. The difference in skin color is related to the amount and type of melanin produced as well as to its dispersion in the skin.

Beneath the epidermis is the *dermis,* which is the dense connective tissue stroma forming the bulk of the skin. The dermis is bound to the overlying epidermis by fingerlike projections that project upward into the corresponding recesses of the epidermis. In the dermis, blood vessels branch and form a rich capillary bed in the dermal papillae. The deeper layers of the dermis also contain the hair follicles with their associated muscles and cutaneous glands. The dermis is supplied with sensory and autonomic nerve fibers. The sensory nerves end either as free endings or as special end-organs that mediate pressure, touch, and temperature. The autonomic nerves supply the arrector pili muscles, blood vessels, and sweat glands.

The third layer of the skin is the *subcutaneous tissue,* which is composed largely of fatty connective tissue. This highly variable adipose layer is a thermal regulator as well as a protection for the more superficial skin layers from bone prominences.

The sweat glands, hair follicles, and nails are termed *skin appendages.* The evaporation of water from the skin by the sweat glands provides a thermoregulatory mechanism for heat loss. Figure 6–2 illustrates the types of sweat glands.

Within the skin, there are 2 to 3 million small, coiled *eccrine glands.* The eccrine glands are distributed over the body surface and are particularly profuse on the forehead, axillae, palms, and soles. They are absent in the nail beds and in some mucosal surfaces. These glands are capable of producing over 6 liters of watery sweat in 1 day. The eccrine glands are controlled by the sympathetic nervous system.

The *apocrine glands* are larger than the eccrine glands. The apocrine glands are found in close association with hair follicles but tend to be much more limited in distribution than the eccrine glands. The apocrine glands occur mostly in the axillae, the areolae, the pubis, and the perineum. They reach maturity only at puberty secreting

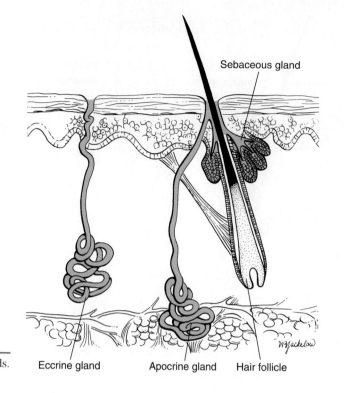

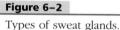
Figure 6–2

Types of sweat glands.

a milky, sticky substance. Apocrine glands are adrenergic mediated and appear to be stimulated by stress.

The *sebaceous glands* are also found surrounding hair follicles. The sebaceous glands are distributed over the entire body; the largest glands are found on the face and upper back. They are absent on the palms and soles. The secretory product, sebum, is discharged directly into the lumen of the hair follicle, where it lubricates the hair shaft and spreads to the skin surface. Sebum consists of sebaceous cells and lipids. The production of sebum depends on gland size, which is directly influenced by androgen secretion.

Nails are derived by keratinization of cells from the nail matrix, which is located at the proximal end of the nail plate. The nail plate consists of the nail root embedded in the posterior nail fold, a fixed middle portion, and a distal free edge. The whitish nail matrix of proliferating epithelial cells grows in a semilunar pattern. It extends outward past the posterior nail fold and is called the *lunula*. The structural relationships of the nail are shown in Figure 6–3.

Hair is a dead, keratinized structure that grows out of the hair follicle. Its lower end, called the *hair matrix,* consists of actively proliferating epithelial cells. Hair is

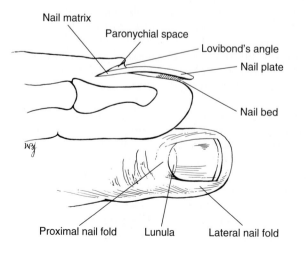

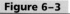
Figure 6–3

Structural relations of the nail: cross section and from above.

present over the entire body surface except on the palms, soles, lips, eyelids, glans penis, and labia minora. The arrector pili muscles attach to the follicle below the opening of the sebaceous gland. Contraction of this muscle erects the hair and causes "goose bumps." The structure of a hair follicle is shown in Figure 6–4.

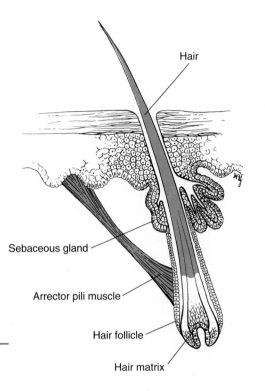

Hair

Sebaceous gland

Arrector pili muscle

Hair follicle

Hair matrix

Figure 6–4

The hair follicle and its surrounding structures.

Review of Specific Symptoms

The main symptoms of disease of the skin, hair, and nails are the following:

- Rash or skin lesion
- Changes in skin color
- Itching (pruritus)
- Changes in hair
- Changes in nails

Rash or Skin Lesion

There are some important points to clarify when interviewing a patient about a new rash or skin lesion. The specific time of onset and location of the rash or skin lesion are critical. A careful description of the first lesions and any changes is vital. The patient with a rash or skin lesion should be asked the following questions:

"Was the rash initially flat? raised? blistered?"
"Did the rash change in character with time?"
"Have there been new areas involved since the rash began?"
"Does the rash itch or burn?"
"Is the lesion tender or numb?"
"What makes the rash better? worse?"
"Was the rash initiated by sunlight?"
"Is the rash aggravated by sunlight?"
"What kind of treatment have you tried?"
"Do you have any joint pains? fever? fatigue?"
"Does anyone near you have a similar rash?"

"Have you traveled recently?" If so, *"To where?"*
"Have you had any contact with anyone who has had a similar rash?"
"Is there a history of allergy?" If so, *"What are your symptoms?"*
"Do you have any chronic disease?"

Note whether the patient has used any medications that may have changed the nature of the skin disorder.

Inquire whether the patient uses any prescription medications or any over-the-counter drugs. Ask specifically about aspirin and aspirin-containing products. Patients can suddenly develop a reaction to medications that they have taken for many years. Do not ignore a long-standing prescription. Has the patient had any recent injections or taken any new medications? Does the patient use "recreational" drugs? Ask the patient about the use of soaps, deodorants, cosmetics, and colognes. Has the patient changed any of these items recently?

A family history of similar skin disorders should be noted. The effect of heat, cold, and sunlight on the skin problem is important. Can any contributing factor be brought to bear, such as occupation, specific food allergies, alcohol, or menses? Is there a history of gardening or household repair work? Has there been any contact with animals recently? The interviewer should also remember to inquire about psychogenic factors that may contribute to a skin disorder.

Determine the patient's occupation, if it is not already known. Ascertain avocational and recreational activities. The information is important even if the patient has been exposed to chemicals or similar agents for years. Manufacturers frequently change the basic constituents without notifying the consumer. It may also take years for a patient to become sensitized to a substance.

Changes in Skin Color

Patients may complain of a *generalized* change in skin color as the first manifestation of an illness. Cyanosis and jaundice are examples of this type of problem. Determine whether the patient is aware of any chronic disease that may be responsible for these changes. *Localized* skin color changes may be related to aging or to neoplastic changes. Certain medications can also be responsible for skin color changes. The examiner should inquire whether the patient is taking or has recently taken any medications.

Pruritus

Pruritus, or itching, may be a symptom of a generalized skin disorder or an internal illness. Ask the following questions of any patient with pruritus:

"When did you first notice the itching?"
"Did the itching begin suddenly?"
"Is the itching associated with any rash or lesion on your body?"
"Are you taking any medications?"
"Has there been any change in the sweating or dryness of your skin?"
"Have you been told that you have a chronic illness?"
"Have you traveled recently?" If so, *"To where?"*

Diffuse pruritus is seen in biliary cirrhosis and in cancer, especially lymphoma. Pruritus in association with a diffuse rash may be dermatitis herpetiformis. Determine whether the pruritus has been associated with a change in perspiration or dryness of the skin, because either of these conditions may be the cause of the pruritus.

Changes in Hair

The interviewer should inquire whether there has been a loss of hair or an increase in hair. Ascertain any changes in distribution or texture. The interviewer should ask the following questions:

"When did you first notice the changes?"
"Did the change occur suddenly?"
"Is the hair loss symmetric?"

"Has the change been associated with itching? fever? recent stress?"
"Are you aware of any exposure to any toxins? commercial hair compounds?"
"Have you changed your diet?"
"What medications are you taking?"

Changes in diet and medications are frequently responsible for changes in hair patterns. Hypothyroidism is frequently associated with loss of the lateral third of the eyebrows. Vascular disease in the legs often causes hair loss on the legs. Alternately, ovarian and adrenal tumors can cause an increase in body hair.

Changes in Nails

Changes in nails may be splitting, discoloration, ridging, thickening, or separation from the nail bed. Ask the patient the following questions:

"When did you first notice the nail changes?"
"Have you had any acute illness recently?"
"Do you have any chronic illness?"
"Have you been taking any medications?"
"Have you been exposed to chemicals at work or at home?"

Fungal disease will cause thickening of the nail. Acute illnesses are associated with lines and ridges in the nail bed and nail. Medications and chemicals are notorious for causing nail changes.

General Suggestions

All patients should be asked whether there have been any changes in moles, birthmarks, or spots on the body. Determine any color changes, irregular growth, pain, scaling, or bleeding. Any recent growth of a flat, pigmented lesion is relevant information.

Ask all patients whether there are any red, scaly, or crusted areas of skin that do not heal. Has the patient ever had skin cancer? If the patient has had skin cancer, further questioning regarding the body location, treatment, and description is appropriate.

Impact of Skin Disease on the Patient

Diseases of the skin play a profound role in the way the affected patient interacts socially. If located on visible skin surfaces, long-standing skin diseases may actually interfere with the emotional and psychological development of the individual. The attitude of a person toward self and others may be markedly affected. Loss of self-esteem is common. The adult with a skin disorder often faces limitation of sexual activity. This disruption of intimacy increases the patient's hostility and anxiety. Skin is a sensitive marker of an individual's emotions. It is known that blushing can reflect embarrassment, sweating can indicate anxiety, and pallor or "goose bump" skin may be associated with fear.

Patients with rashes have always evoked feelings of revulsion. Rashes have been associated with impurity and evil. Even today, friends and family may reject the individual with a skin disease. Patients with skin that is red, oozing, discolored, or peeling are rejected not only by family members but also perhaps even by their physicians. At other times, skin lesions cause others to stare at the patient, causing further discomfort. Some skin disorders may be associated with such extreme physical or emotional pain that marked depression may result and occasionally lead to suicide.

Skin diseases are often treated palliatively. Because numerous skin disorders have no cure, many patients go through life helpless and frustrated, as do their physicians.

The role of anxiety as a natural stressor in producing rashes is frequently observed. Stress tends to worsen certain skin disorders, such as eczema. This creates a vicious cycle, because the rash then exacerbates the anxiety. Rashes are common symptoms and signs of psychosomatic disorders.

Clinicians should discuss these anxieties with the patient in an attempt to break the cycle. The interviewer who tries to elicit the patient's feelings about the disease will allow the patient to "open up." The fears and fantasies can then be discussed. The examiner should also be comfortable in touching the patient for reassurance. This tends to improve the doctor-patient relationship, as the patient will have a lesser sense of isolation.

Physical Examination

> The only equipment necessary for the examination of the skin is a penlight.

The examination of the skin consists of

- Inspection
- Palpation

The examination of the skin is dependent on inspection, but palpation of a skin lesion must also be performed. Although most skin lesions are not contagious, it is prudent to wear gloves to evaluate any skin lesion. This is especially true due to the prevalence of skin disease associated with the human immunodeficiency virus (HIV). Palpation of a lesion helps define its characteristics: texture, consistency, fluid, edema in the adjacent area, tenderness, and blanching.

The patient and the examiner must be comfortable during the examination of the skin. The lighting should be adjusted to produce the optimal illumination. Natural light is preferable. Even in the absence of complaints related to the skin, a careful examination of the skin must be performed on all patients because the skin may provide subtle clues of an underlying systemic illness. Examination of the skin may be performed as a separate system approach, or preferably the skin should be examined when the other parts of the body are evaluated.

General Principles

The examiner should be suspicious of any lesion that the patient describes as having increased in size or changed in color. The development of any new growth warrants attention.

When examining the skin, the initial evaluation is made to determine the general aspects of the skin. Evaluate the *color, moisture, turgor,* and *texture* of the skin.

Note any *color* changes, such as cyanosis, jaundice, or pigmentary abnormalities.

Red vascular lesions may be either extravasated blood into the skin, known as petechiae or purpura, or angiomas, which are malformed elements of the vascular tree. When pressure is applied by a glass slide over an angioma, it will blanch. This is a useful test to differentiate an angioma from petechiae, which will not change when pressure from a glass slide is applied.

During the physical examination, inspect all pigmented lesions and be aware of the **ABCD** warning signs associated with malignant melanoma:

Asymmetry of shape
Border irregularity
Color variation
Diameter larger than 6 mm

Asymmetry means that half the lesion appears different from the other half. *Border irregularity* describes a scalloped or poorly circumscribed contour. The *color variation* may show shades of tan and brown, black, and sometimes white, red, or blue. A *diameter* larger than 6 mm, which is the size of a pencil eraser, is considered a danger sign for melanoma.

Remember the axiom in dermatology: "There are more errors made by not looking than by not knowing."

Excessive *moisture* may be seen in normal individuals, or it may be associated with fevers, emotions, neoplastic diseases, or hyperthyroidism. Dryness is a normal aging change, but it may also be seen in myxedema, nephritis, and certain drug-induced states. Look for excoriations, which might indicate the presence of pruritus as a clue to an underlying systemic illness.

When palpating the skin, evaluate its *turgor* and *texture*. Tissue turgor provides a mechanism for estimating the patient's general state of hydration. If the skin over the forehead is pulled up and released, it should promptly reassume its normal contour. In a patient with decreased hydration, the skin will show a delayed response.

It is often difficult for the inexperienced examiner to evaluate the texture of the skin because texture is a qualitative parameter. Softness has occasionally been likened to the texture of skin over a baby's abdomen. "Soft" textured skin is seen in secondary hypothyroidism, hypopituitarism, and eunuchoid states. "Hard" textured skin is associated with scleroderma, myxedema, and amyloidosis. "Velvety" skin is associated with Ehlers-Danlos syndrome.

Examination with Patient Seated

When the patient is seeded, examine the hair and the skin on the hands and upper extremities.

Inspect the Hair

The hair and scalp are evaluated for any lesions. Is alopecia or hirsutism present? Pay attention to the pattern of distribution and texture of hair over the body. In certain diseases, such as hypothyroidism, the hair becomes sparse and coarse. In contrast, patients with hyperthyroidism have hair that is very fine in texture. Loss of hair occurs in many conditions: anemia; heavy metal poisoning; hypopituitarism; and some nutritional disease states, such as pellagra. Increased hair patterns are seen in Cushing's disease; Stein-Leventhal syndrome; and several neoplastic conditions, such as tumors of the adrenals and gonads.

Inspect the Nail Beds

Evaluation of the nails can provide important clues about diseases. The nails may be affected in many systemic and dermatologic conditions. Nail-bed changes are usually not pathognomonic for a specific disease. Disorders stemming from renal, hematopoietic, or hepatic conditions may be evident from the nails. Inspect the nails for shape, size, color, brittleness, hemorrhages under the nail transverse lines or grooves in the nail or nail bed, and an increased white area of the nail bed. Figure 6–5 illustrates some typical nail changes associated with medical diseases.

Beau's lines are transverse grooves parallel to the lunula, often associated with significant infections or renal or hepatic diseases. This abnormality is caused by diseases that cause the nail to grow slowly or even cease to grow for short intervals. The point of arrested growth is seen as a transverse groove in the nail. Beau's lines may

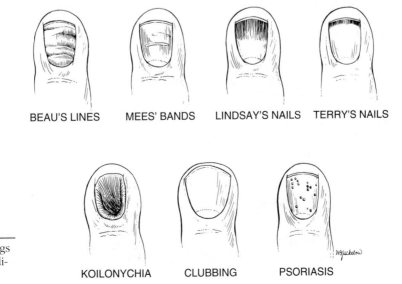

BEAU'S LINES   MEES' BANDS   LINDSAY'S NAILS   TERRY'S NAILS

KOILONYCHIA   CLUBBING   PSORIASIS

Figure 6–5

Common nail findings associated with medical diseases.

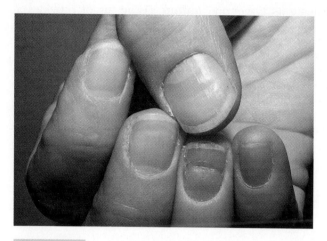

Figure 6–6

Beau's lines.

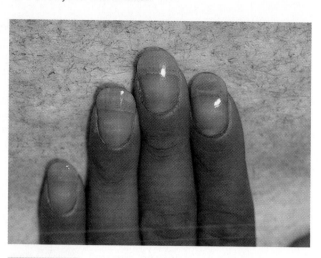

Figure 6–7

Mees' bands.

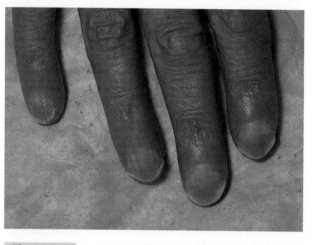

Figure 6–8

Lindsay's nails.

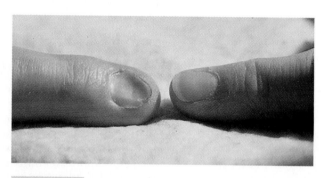

Figure 6–9

Koilonychia.

also result from coronary occlusion, surgical procedures, and anti-cancer agents. Figure 6–6 shows a patient's fingers with Beau's lines on the nails. Notice that all of the nails are involved. Occasionally, a white transverse line or band, instead of a groove, will result from poisoning or an acute systemic illness. These lines, called *Mees' bands,* are historically associated with chronic arsenic poisoning. These lines or bands are also parallel to the lunula. By measuring the width of the line and approximating nail growth at 1 mm per week, it may be possible to determine the duration of the antecedent acute illness. Figure 6–7 shows the fingernails of a patient who was ill with pneumonia 6 weeks earlier.

Lindsay's nails are also called "half-and-half nails." The proximal portion of the nail bed is whitish, whereas the distal part is red or pink. Chronic renal disease and azotemia are associated with this type of nail abnormality. Figure 6–8 shows Lindsay's nails secondary to hypoalbuminemia. *Terry's nails* are white nail beds to within 1–2 mm of the distal border of the nail. These nail findings are most commonly associated with cirrhosis and hypoalbuminemia.

Is *koilonychia* present? Koilonychia, or spoon nail, is a dystrophic state in which the nail plate thins and a cup-like depression develops. Spoon nails are most commonly associated with iron deficiency anemia but may be seen in association with thinning of the nail plate from any cause, including local irritants. Figure 6–9 shows a normal fingernail compared with a nail showing koilonychia secondary to iron deficiency anemia.

Inspect the Nails for Clubbing

The angle between the normal nail base and finger is about 160°, and the nail bed is firm. The angle is referred to as *Lovibond's angle*. When clubbing develops, this angle straightens out to greater than 180°, and the nail bed, when palpated, becomes spongy or floating. As clubbing progresses, the base of the nail becomes swollen, and Lovibond's angle greatly exceeds 180°. A fusiform enlargement of the distal digit may also occur. In Figure 6–10, a normal finger is compared with a clubbed finger.

To examine for clubbing, the patient's finger is placed on the pulp of the examiner's thumbs, and the base of the nail bed is palpated by the examiner's index fingers. Figure 6–11 illustrates the technique for assessing whether early clubbing is present.

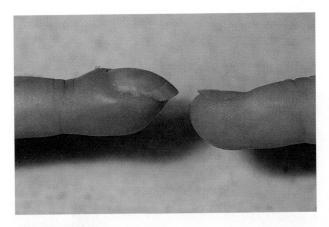

Figure 6–10

Late clubbing.

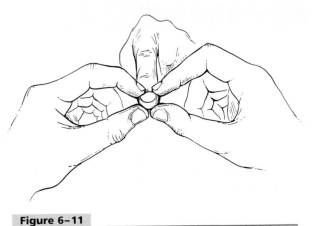

Figure 6–11

Technique for assessing whether clubbing is present.

Clubbing of the nails is associated with congenital cyanotic heart disease, cystic fibrosis, and acquired pulmonary disease. The most common acquired pulmonary cause is bronchogenic carcinoma. In a patient with chronic obstructive pulmonary disease who manifests clubbing, other causes, including bronchiectasis or bronchogenic carcinoma, should be sought. The initial manifestation of clubbing is a softening of the tissue over the proximal nail fold.

Inspect the Nails for Pitting

Pitting of the nails is commonly associated with psoriasis and psoriatic arthropathy. Involvement of the nail bed and nail matrix by psoriasis causes the nail plate to be thickened and pitted. Nail involvement occurs in about 80% of all patients with psoriasis. Multiple pits in the nail are produced by discrete psoriatic lesions in the nail matrix. Minor degrees of pitting are also seen in persons with no other skin complaints. A

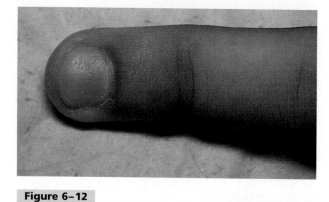

Figure 6–12

Psoriasis: nail pitting.

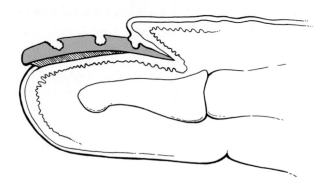

Figure 6–13

Cross section of nail pitting.

Figure 6–14

Psoriatic nail lesions.

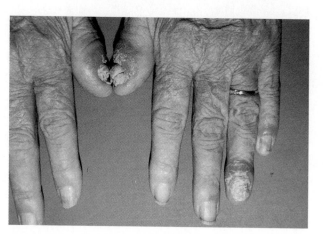

patient with psoriatic nail pitting is shown in Figure 6–12. Figure 6–13 illustrates a cross-section of pitting. Figure 6–14 shows another patient with psoriatic nail lesions. Notice the characteristically dystrophic nail changes due to subungual hyperkeratosis.

Inspect the Skin of the Face and Neck

Evaluate the eyelids, forehead, ears, nose, and lips carefully. Evaluate the mucous membranes of the mouth and nose for ulceration, bleeding, or telangiectasis. Is the skin at the nasolabial fold and mouth normal?

Inspect the Skin over the Back

Examine the skin of the patient's back. Are any lesions present?

Examination with Patient Lying

Inspect the Skin of the Chest, Abdomen, and Lower Extremities

Ask the patient to lie down in order to complete the examination of the skin. Inspect the skin of the chest and abdomen. Particular attention should be paid to the skin of the inguinal and genital area. Inspect the pubic hair. Elevate the scrotum. Inspect the perineal area. The pretibial areas are evaluated for the presence of ulcerations or waxy deposits.

The feet and soles are carefully examined for any skin changes. The toes should be spread in order to evaluate the webs between them thoroughly.

The patient is asked to roll onto the left side so that the skin on the back, gluteal, and perianal areas may be examined.

Description of Lesions

If a skin lesion is found, it should be classified as a *primary* or *secondary* lesion, and a description of its shape and its distribution should be given. Primary lesions arise from normal skin. They result from anatomic changes in the epidermis, dermis, or subcutaneous tissue. The primary lesion is the most characteristic lesion of the skin disorder. Secondary lesions result from changes in the primary lesion. They develop during the course of the cutaneous disease.

The first step in identifying a skin disorder is to characterize the appearance of the primary lesion. In the description of the skin lesion, note whether the lesion is flat or raised and whether it is solid or contains fluid. A penlight is often useful to determine whether the lesion is slightly elevated. If a penlight is directed to one side of a lesion, a shadow will form according to the height of the lesion.

The location of the lesion on the body is important. Therefore, the distribution of the eruption is crucial in making a diagnosis. It may be rewarding to inspect a patient's clothing when contact dermatitis or pediculosis (infestation with lice) is suspected. Occasionally, occupational exposure may leave traces of contamination with oils or other materials that may be visible on the clothing and help in the assessment.

The three specific criteria for a dermatologic diagnosis are based on *morphology, configuration,* and *distribution,* morphology being the most important. The purpose of the following section is to acquaint the reader with the morphology of the primary and secondary lesions and the vocabulary associated with them.

Primary and Secondary Lesions

To facilitate reading, the primary lesions are listed with respect to being flat or elevated and solid or fluid-filled (Figs. 6–15 to 6–18). There is no "standard" size of a primary lesion. The dimensions indicated are only approximate. The secondary lesions are grouped according to their occurrence below or above the plane of the skin (Figs. 6–19 and 6–20). Other important lesions are shown and described in Figure 6–21.

Primary Skin Lesions	Nonpalpable, flat	
Lesion	**Characteristics**	**Examples**
Macule	Smaller than 1 cm	Freckles, moles
Patch	Greater than 1 cm	Vitiligo, café au lait spots

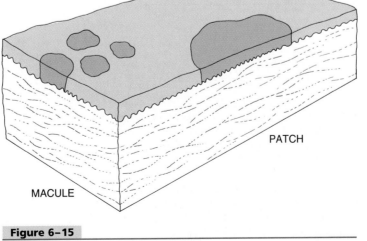

PATCH

MACULE

Figure 6–15

Primary Skin Lesions	Palpable, solid mass	
Lesion	**Characteristics**	**Examples**
Papule	Smaller than 1 cm	Nevus, wart
Nodule	1–2 cm	Erythema nodosum
Tumor	Greater than 2 cm	Neoplasms
Plaque	Flat, elevated, superficial papule with surface area greater than height	Psoriasis, seborrheic keratosis
Wheal	Superficial area of cutaneous edema	Hives, insect bite

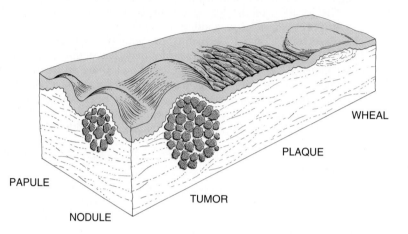

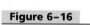
Figure 6–16

Primary Skin Lesions	Palpable, fluid filled	
Lesion	**Characteristics**	**Examples**
Vesicle	Smaller than 1 cm; filled with serous fluid	Blister, herpes simplex
Bulla	Greater than 1 cm; filled with serous fluid	Blister, pemphigus vulgaris
Pustule	Similar to vesicle; filled with pus	Acne, impetigo

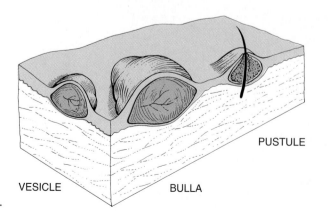

Figure 6–17

Special Primary Skin Lesions

Lesion	Characteristics	Examples
Comedo	Plugged opening of sebaceous gland	Blackhead
Burrow	Smaller than 10 mm, raised tunnel	Scabies
Cyst	Palpable lesion filled with semiliquid material or fluid	Sebaceous cyst
Abscess	A specific type of primary lesion with localized accumulation of purulent material in the dermis or subcutis. Generally, the accumulation is so deep that the pus is not visible from the skin's surface.	
Furuncle	A specific type of primary lesion that is a necrotizing form of inflammation of a hair follicle	
Carbuncle	A coalescence of several furuncles	
Milia	Tiny, keratin-filled cysts representing an accumulation of keratin in the distal portion of the sweat gland	

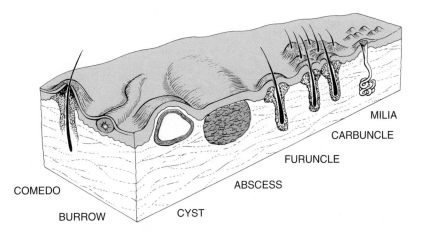

Figure 6–18

Secondary Skin Lesions Below the Skin Plane

Lesion	Characteristics	Examples
Erosion	Loss of part or all of the epidermis; surface is moist	Rupture of a vesicle
Ulcer	Loss of epidermis and dermis; may bleed	Stasis ulcer, chancre
Fissure	Linear crack from epidermis into dermis	Cheilitis, athlete's foot
Excoriation	A superficial linear, or "dugout," traumatized area, usually self-induced	Abrasion, scratch mark
Atrophy	Thinning of skin with loss of skin markings	Striae
Sclerosis	Diffuse or circumscribed hardening of skin	

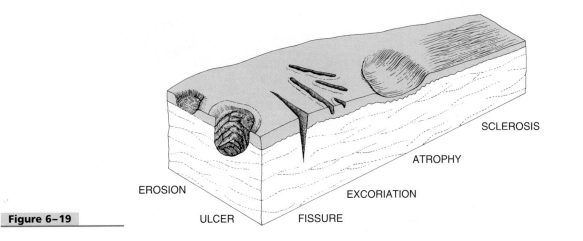

Figure 6–19

Secondary Skin Lesions Above the Skin Plane

Lesion	Characteristics	Examples
Scaling	Heaped-up keratinized cells; exfoliated epidermis	Dandruff, psoriasis
Crusting	Dried residue of pus, serum, or blood	Scabs, impetigo

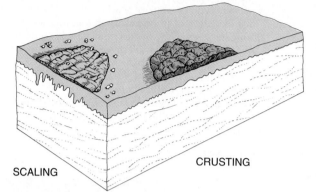

Figure 6–20

Vascular Skin Lesions

Lesion	Characteristics	Examples
Erythema	Pink or red blanchable discoloration of the skin secondary to dilatation of blood vessels	
Petechiae	Reddish-purple; nonblanching; smaller than 0.5 cm	Intravascular defects
Purpura	Reddish-purple; nonblanching; greater than 0.5 cm	Intravascular defects
Ecchymosis	Reddish-purple; nonblanching; variable size	Trauma, vasculitis
Telangiectasia	Fine, irregular dilated blood vessels	Dilatation of capillaries
Spider angioma	Central red body with radiating spider-like arms that blanch with pressure to the central area	Liver disease, estrogens

Miscellaneous Skin Lesions

Lesion	Characteristics	Examples
Scar	Replacement of destroyed dermis by fibrous tissue; may be atrophic or hyperplastic	Healed wound
Keloid	Elevated, enlarging scar growing beyond boundaries of wound	Burn scars
Lichenification	Roughening and thickening of epidermis; accentuated skin markings	Atopic dermatitis

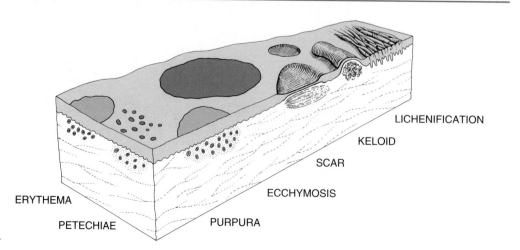

Figure 6–21

Configuration of Skin Lesions

It is not essential for the examiner to make a definitive diagnosis of all skin disease. A careful description of the lesion, the pattern of distribution, and the arrangement of the lesion will often lead the examiner to a group of related disease states with similar presenting dermatologic signs (e.g., confluent macular rashes, bullous diseases, grouped vesicles, papular rashes on an erythematous base). For example, grouped urticarial lesions with a central depression suggest insect bites. Listed in Figure 6–22 are the terms used to describe the configurations of lesions.

Descriptive Dermatologic Terms

Lesion	Characteristics	Examples
Annular	Ring shaped	Ringworm
Arcuate	Partial rings	Syphilis
Bizarre	Irregular or geographic pattern *not* related to any underlying anatomic structure	Factitial dermatitis
Circinate	Circular	
Confluent	Lesions run together	Childhood exanthems
Discoid	Disc shaped without central clearing	Lupus erythematosus
Discrete	Lesions remain separate	
Eczematoid	An inflammation with a tendency to vesiculate and crust	Eczema
Generalized	Widespread	
Grouped	Lesions clustered together	Herpes simplex
Iris	Circle within a circle; a bull's-eye lesion	Erythema multiforme (iris)
Keratotic	Horny thickening	Psoriasis
Linear	In lines	Poison ivy dermatitis
Multiform	More than one type of shape or lesion	Erythema multiforme
Papulosquamous	Papules or plaques associated with scaling	Psoriasis
Reticulated	Lace-like network	Oral lichen planus
Serpiginous	Snake-like, creeping	Cutaneous larva migrans
Telangiectatic	Relatively permanent dilatation of the superficial blood vessels	Osler-Weber-Rendu disease
Universal	Entire body involved	Alopecia universalis
Zosteriform*	Linear arrangement along a nerve distribution	Herpes zoster

* Also known as dermatomal.

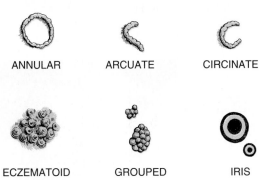

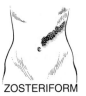

ANNULAR   ARCUATE   CIRCINATE   CONFLUENT   DISCOID

ECZEMATOID   GROUPED   IRIS   KERATOTIC   LINEAR

RETICULATED   SERPIGINOUS   TELANGIECTATIC   ZOSTERIFORM

Figure 6–22

Clinicopathologic Correlations

Skin disorders are frequently perplexing to the examiner. When one sees a rash, the common thought is, "Where do I begin?" All too often, the examiner may become frustrated and not even attempt to make a diagnosis. Dermatologic terms are complicated, and the names of dermatologic disorders may be intimidating. Often the descriptions of skin disorders in textbooks are more confusing than helpful.

There are over 2500 separately named dermatologic diagnoses. In view of the low frequency of most of these diseases, only 10 to 15 common conditions compose about 50% of all dermatologic diagnoses. If the 50 most common conditions were considered, a diagnosis could be rendered for over 95% of all patients.

In approaching a skin lesion, do the following:

- First, identify the primary lesion
- Second, identify its distribution
- Third, identify any associated findings
- Fourth, consider the age of the patient

Skin diseases evolve and their manifestations change. A lesion may evolve from a blister to an erosion, from a vesicle to a pustule, or from a papule to a nodule or tumor.

There are many common skin disorders or lesions with which the examiner should be familiar. Illustrated in the figures in this chapter are examples of some of these conditions; these cross-sectional diagrams illustrate the locations of these abnormalities in the skin and the involvement of the various skin layers in the pathogenesis of the conditions. The text describes the primary lesions.

A *wart* is a common, benign growth caused by an infection of an epidermal cell by a virus. This results in a thickening and vacuolation of the epidermis with scaling and an upward growth of the dermal papilla. Figures 6–23 and 6–24 illustrate a wart.

A *squamous cell carcinoma* is a malignant neoplasm of keratocytes in the epidermis and is locally invasive into the dermis. The tumor results in a scaling, crusting nodule or plaque that can ulcerate and bleed. Squamous cell carcinoma is a potentially dangerous lesion that can infiltrate the surrounding structures and metastasize to lymph nodes and other organs. The causes vary but include ultraviolet radiation, x-rays, polycyclic hydrocarbons (e.g., tar, mineral oils, pitch, and soot), mucosal diseases (e.g., lichen planus and Bowen's disease), scars, chronic skin disorders, genetic diseases (e.g., albinism and xeroderma pigmentosum), and human papillomavirus. Figure 6–25 shows two examples of squamous cell carcinoma of the skin. Notice that the lesion in Figure 6–25*A* is ulcerated with a firm, raised indurated margin. Figure 6–26 shows a squamous cell carcinoma in a surgical scar. Figure 6–27 shows a cross section through a squamous cell carcinoma.

A *basal cell carcinoma* is a malignant neoplasm of the basal cells of the epidermis and is the most common skin malignancy. The epidermis is thickened, and the dermis may be invaded by the malignant basal cells. It may manifest as a lesion with a pearly,

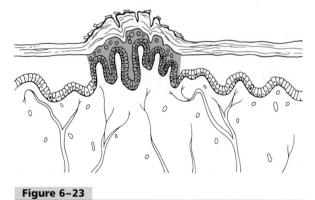

Figure 6–23

Cross section through a wart. Note the thickened epidermis and hyperkeratosis.

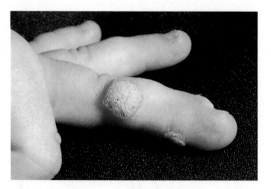

Figure 6–24

Wart.

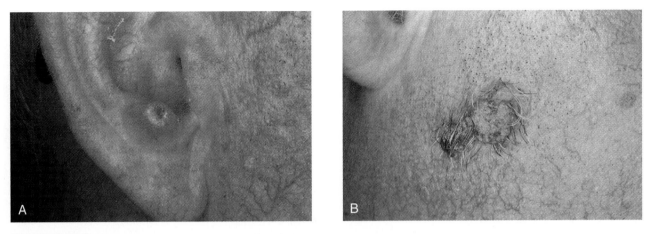

Figure 6–25

Squamous cell carcinoma of the skin.

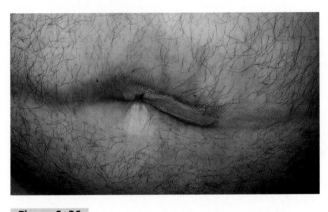

Figure 6–26

Squamous cell carcinoma in scar.

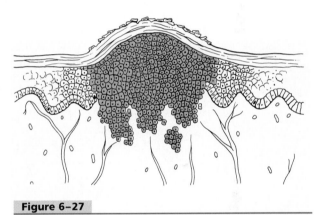

Figure 6–27

Cross section through a squamous cell carcinoma. Note the invasion into the dermis.

rolled, well-defined margin and a central ulcerated depression. Although sunlight is an important etiologic factor, basal cell carcinomas are almost always seen on the face and rarely in other sun-exposed areas. They are slow-growing tumors and rarely metastasize in contrast to squamous cell carcinomas. They are locally invasive, and when located near the eye or nose they may invade the cranial cavity. If ulceration, bleeding, and crusting occur, a *rodent ulcer* is said to be present. Any nonhealing lesion should be carefully evaluated for the possibility of a basal cell carcinoma. Figures 6–28 to 6–30 illustrate the typical features of a basal cell carcinoma.

A *melanoma* is a malignant neoplasm of the melanocytes of the epidermis. If untreated or unrecognized, a melanoma will cause fatal metastases. Most melanomas have a prolonged superficial, or horizontal, growth phase in which there is a progressive lateral expansion. With time, the melanoma enters the vertical, or deep, phase by penetrating into the dermis, and metastatic spread may occur.

Malignant melanomas are the most common malignancy seen by dermatologists. The incidence of malignant melanoma is increasing faster than that of any other form of malignancy. Most melanomas have atypical pigmentation in the epidermis, such as shades of red, white, gray, blue, brown, and black, all in a single lesion. There are four types of malignant melanoma: lentigo maligna melanoma, superficial spreading melanoma, nodular malignant melanoma, and acral-lentiginous malignant melanoma. Figure 6–31 shows the typical features of a lentigo maligna melanoma on the face. The lentigo maligna melanoma is seen frequently in the geriatric population. This type of melanoma has a prolonged horizontal growth phase and appears in areas of sun-

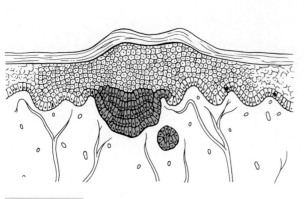

Figure 6–28

Cross section through a basal cell carcinoma.

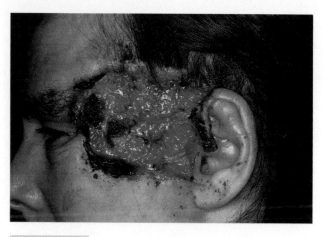

Figure 6–29

Basal cell carcinoma (rodent ulcer).

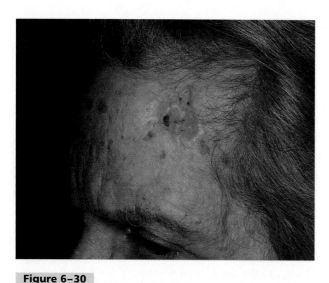

Figure 6–30

Basal cell carcinoma. Notice the rolled, well-defined margin.

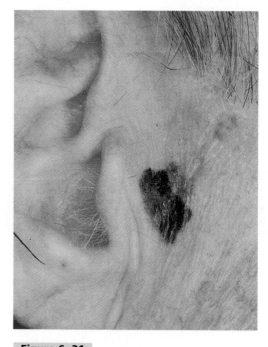

Figure 6–31

Lentigo maligna melanoma.

exposed, sun-damaged skin. The superficial spreading variety, Figure 6–32, is the most common type of melanoma (70% of all melanomas). Typically, an irregularly colored plaque with sharp notches and variegation of pigment is seen. If diagnosed early, the prognosis is excellent, with a 5 year survival of 95%. Figure 6–33 illustrates a cross section through a melanoma. Vertical growth and deep invasion follow the spreading phase of superficial malignant melanomas. Figure 6–34 shows another patient with a superficial spreading melanoma that has developed vertical growth. The nodular melanoma is the second most common type, seen in approximately 15% of cases of melanoma. Unlike the superficial spreading type, these melanomas are usually black, brown, or dark blue and tend to grow rapidly for months.

Melanomas occur in white individuals and have a predilection for the back in men and women and the anterior tibial areas in women. In general, lesions on back, axillae, neck, and scalp (the so-called BANS area) tend to have a worse prognosis than do melanomas on the extremities. A great contrast between the risk of acquiring mela-

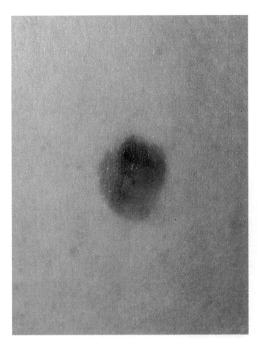

Figure 6–32

Superficial spreading
malignant melanoma.

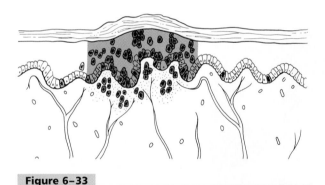

Figure 6–33

Cross section through a melanoma. Note the nests of
melanoma cells in the dermis.

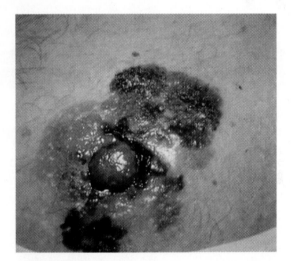

Figure 6–34

Superficial spreading melanoma.

noma and basal or squamous cell carcinoma is that basal and squamous cell carcinomas occur more frequently in individuals who are exposed to constant sunlight, such as sailors and agricultural workers. Melanomas occur more often in rather fair-skinned individuals who are exposed to brief, intense sun exposure such as that acquired during vacations in the southern latitudes.

Fewer than 5% of all melanomas occur in the African-American population. The acral-lentiginous melanoma is the most common form in African-Americans and occurs on the palms, soles, and nail beds. These melanomas have a short superficial growth phase and an early vertical growth phase and, as such, are associated with a poor prognosis. An acral-lentiginous melanoma on the sole of an African-American patient is shown in Figure 6–35.

A *lipoma* is a benign growth of subcutaneous fat and has a rubbery appearance. The epidermis is normal. Frequently, an encapsulated lipoma may grow to a very large size and elevate the overlying dermis and epidermis, as shown in Figure 6–36; a cross section through a lipoma is shown in Figure 6–37. Note that the examiner can easily push into the soft-tissue tumor.

Café au lait spots are patch lesions that are well circumscribed and brownish in color. They may occur as a solitary birthmark in up to 10% of the normal population. The café au lait macule or patch results from an increased number of functionally hyperactive melanocytes. Multiple café au lait patches in a patient may suggest neurofibromatosis. Figure 6–38 shows a patient with neurofibromatosis and a café au lait patch.

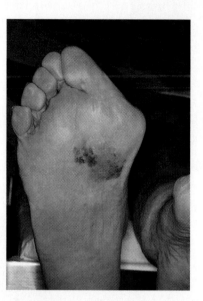

Figure 6–35

Acral-lentiginous melanoma.

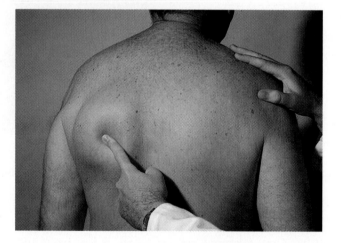

Figure 6–36

Lipoma.

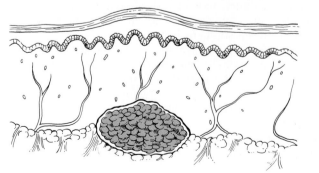

Figure 6–37

Cross section through a lipoma.

A *neurofibroma* is a tumor produced by a focal proliferation of neural tissue in the dermis. The epidermis is normal. Neurofibromas may appear as papules or nodules. Cutaneous neurofibromas are soft in consistency. Neurofibromatosis is a disorder in which multiple neurofibromas are present, sometimes as many as several hundred. Although the tumors are benign, the occurrence of these space-occupying lesions may produce severe disfigurement and/or neurologic disease. Other dermatologic features of neurofibromatosis include multiple café au lait patches and axillary freckling. Figure 6–39 shows several neurofibromas in a patient with neurofibromatosis; a cross-sectional view is shown in Figure 6–40. Figure 6–41 shows axillary freckling in a patient with neurofibromatosis.

Contact dermatitis is an inflammatory reaction of the skin that is precipitated by contact with an irritant or allergen, such as detergents, acids, alkali, plants, medicines,

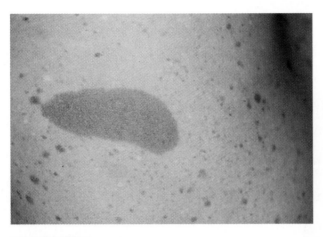

Figure 6–38

Café au lait spot in a patient with neurofibromatosis.

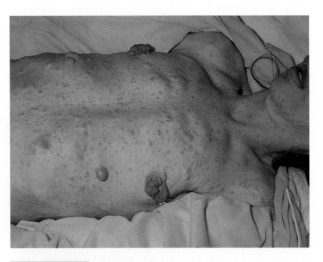

Figure 6–39

Neurofibromatosis.

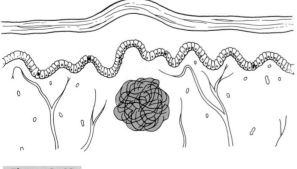

Figure 6–40

Cross section through a neurofibroma. Note that the tumor is a well-delimited mass of loosely packed neural elements.

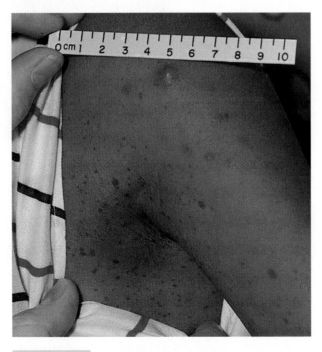

Figure 6–41

Neurofibromatosis: axillary freckling.

and solvents. Vesicles in the epidermis and perivascular inflammation result. Figure 6–42 shows a patient with contact dermatitis to poison ivy; the area is shown in cross section in Figure 6–43. Note the characteristic linear distribution of papules, vesicles, and bullae on this patient's calf where the leaves of the plant touched the leg. The distribution of the bullous lesions together with their location is strongly suggestive of the diagnosis, which was confirmed by biopsy.

Psoriasis is one of the most common noninfectious skin disorders. It is frequently inherited, often chronic, and may also affect the joints and nails. The rash is characterized by well-defined, slightly raised, hyperkeratotic (scaling) plaques. Scratching the lesion will reveal small bleeding points, which is a specific sign of the disease. The lesions are frequently symmetric and can be extremely itchy. The stratum corneum thickens, and erythematous plaques with silvery scales result. Within the dermis, there is capillary proliferation with perivascular inflammation. The lesions are characteristically located on the elbows, knees, scalp, and intergluteal cleft. Figure 6–44 shows the typical, symmetric lesions on the knees of this patient. Figure 6–45 shows the classic scaling lesions at the intergluteal cleft of another patient. Figure 6–46 illustrates a cross section through an area of psoriasis (see also Fig. 6–13). Figure 6–47 shows a patient with psoriasis of the scalp. The lesions commonly extend beyond the hair-bearing areas onto the adjacent skin. Surprisingly, this lesion rarely results in hair loss.

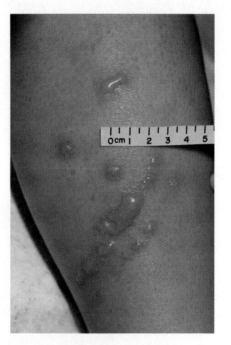

Figure 6–42

Poison ivy reaction.

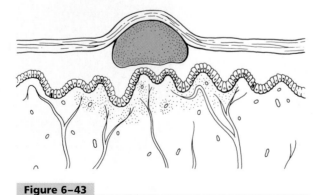

Figure 6–43

Cross section through an area of contact dermatitis. Note the perivascular inflammation in the dermis as well as the vesicles and bullae in the epidermis.

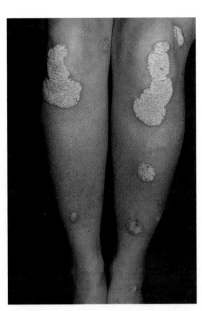

Figure 6-44

Psoriatic lesions on the knees.

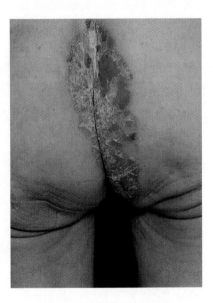

Figure 6-45

Psoriasis of the inter-gluteal cleft.

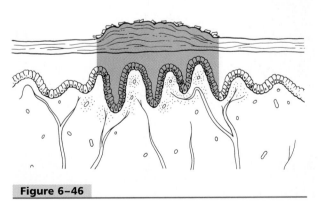

Figure 6-46

Cross section through an area of psoriasis. Note the area of hyperkeratosis.

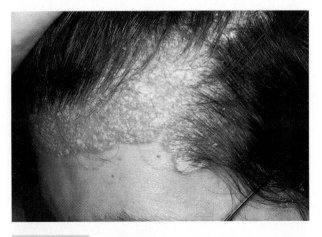

Figure 6-47

Psoriasis of the scalp.

Tinea corporis is "ringworm" infection. Fungal infections of the skin produce a scaling, erythematous patch, often with a reddened, raised, serpiginous border. The term *tinea* indicates the fungal cause, whereas the second word denotes the area of the body involved: *tinea corporis,* body; *tinea pedis,* foot; *tinea faciale,* face; *tinea cruris,* groin; *tinea capitis,* head. In all cases, the epidermis is thickened, with the stratum corneum infiltrated with fungal hyphae. The underlying dermis shows mild inflammation. Figures 6–48 and 6–49 show the classic annular lesion of tinea corporis with its raised erythematous border and central clearing. Figure 6–50 shows a patient with tinea cruris. This common pruritic lesion is seen commonly in young men; it is unusual in women. It spreads outward from the groin, down the thigh, leaving postinflammatory pigmentation. The advancing border is well defined, red, scaly, and slightly raised. If untreated, the eruption can spread onto the lower abdomen, as shown, and the buttocks.

Pityriasis rosea is a common, acute, self-limiting inflammatory disease of unknown cause. Papulosquamous plaques appear over the trunk. The generalized eruption is preceded by a "herald patch," which is a single lesion resembling tinea corporis. In several days, the generalized eruption appears. Although patients may complain of mild itching, they feel quite well. Slight hyperkeratosis of the epidermis with moderate dermal perivascular infiltration occurs. Figure 6–51 shows a herald patch and the characteristic lesions of pityriasis rosea; see Figure 6–52 for a cross-sectional view. Notice the delicate scale at the border of the annular lesion. Secondary syphilis may manifest with a similar eruption. It is therefore important to order a serologic test for syphilis in any individual with pityriasis rosea.

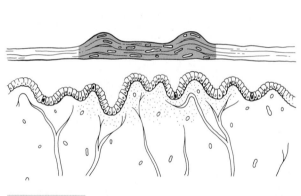

Figure 6–48

Cross section through an area of tinea corporis. Note the thickened stratum corneum, which is infiltrated by the fungus.

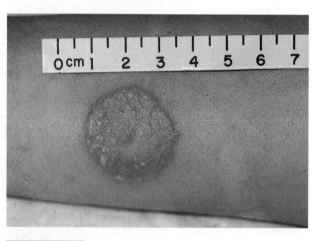

Figure 6–49

Tinea corporis.

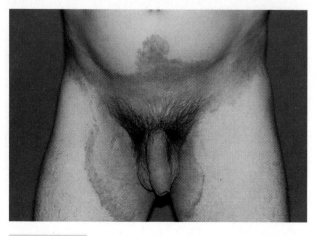

Figure 6–50

Tinea cruris.

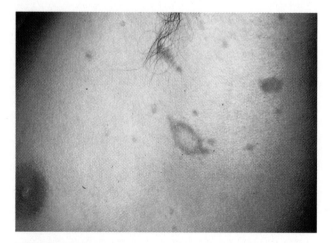

Figure 6–51

Pityriasis rosea. Note the herald patch.

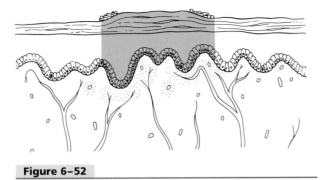

Figure 6–52

Cross section through a lesion of pityriasis rosea.

Herpes zoster, or shingles, is an intraepidermal vesicular eruption occurring in a dermatomal distribution. Bullae and multinucleated giant cells are present in the epidermis, with perivascular inflammation of the dermis. The condition is caused by activation of the zoster-varicella virus. Groups of vesicles and bullae on erythematous bases are present along the distribution of peripheral nerves. Severe pain often precedes the eruption. The distribution may occur along the spinal or cranial nerves. Figure 6–53 shows herpes zoster along the T3 distribution; see Figure 6–54 for a cross section. Figure 6–55 shows a close-up of the typical vesicles on an erythematous base in a dermatomal distribution.

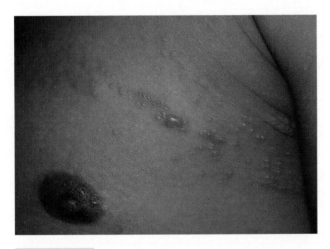

Figure 6–53

Herpes zoster in T3 distribution.

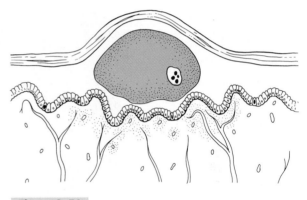

Figure 6–54

Cross section through one of the vesicles in herpes zoster. Note the large epidermal bullae with the classic multinuclear cells.

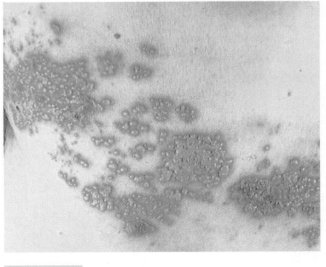

Figure 6–55

Herpes zoster vesicles.

Herpesvirus infections are frequently encountered in patients with HIV infection; approximately 25–50% of patients develop some form of herpetic disease during the course of their illness. Herpesvirus infections are thought to be predictive of future progression from HIV infection to acquired immunodeficiency syndrome (AIDS); this association with progression is 23% at 2 years and up to 73% at 6 years. When CD4+ counts fall below 100 cells/mm³, the likelihood of a herpesvirus infection approaches 95%. Herpes zoster infections may be severe and fulminant in immunocompromised patients such as in the patient shown in Figure 8–15.

Acne is a pustular disease affecting the hair follicles and sebaceous glands. In this condition, pustules, papules, and comedones are the primary lesions. There are collections of intradermal as well as intrafollicular neutrophils. Within the dermis, the hair follicle is occluded by a collection of keratin, sebum, and inflammatory cells. The hair follicle often ruptures into the dermis as a result of increasing pressure, leading to further dermal inflammation (Figs. 6–56 and 6–57).

Tinea versicolor is a common superficial fungal skin infection of young adults. Pregnancy, warm climate, corticosteroids, and debilitation seem to be predisposing factors. The lesion consists of very fine, scaly patches that coalesce as they enlarge.

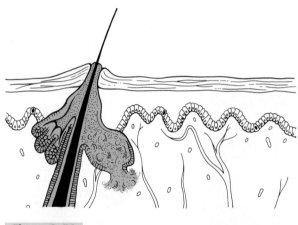

Figure 6–56

Cross section through an area of acne. Note the rupturing of the sebaceous gland in the dermis as a result of a plugged hair follicle, which results in dermal inflammation.

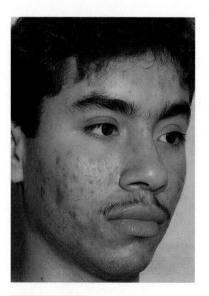

Figure 6–57

Acne.

The hypopigmented lesions are frequently seen on seborrheic areas of the body; neck, upper trunk, upper arms, and groin. The lesions are usually asymptomatic but may be mildly pruritic. Figure 6–58 shows the back of a patient with the classic hypopigmented patches of tinea versicolor.

A *ganglion cyst* is a chronic, painless lesion on the dorsum of the wrist or ankle. It contains fluid from leakage of synovial fluid through the tendon sheath of capsule of the joint. This fluid eventually becomes encapsulated, and a cyst results. Figure 6–59 shows a ganglion in the typical location.

A *spider angioma* is a red lesion, usually less than 2 cm in diameter, with a central arteriole, often raised, surrounded by erythema and radiating legs. If pressure is exerted on the central body, blanching of the spider's legs occurs. These benign lesions are commonly seen on the face, neck, arms, and upper trunk; they are rarely seen on the lower extremities. Although seen in normal individuals, spider angiomas are found more commonly in pregnant women and in patients with liver disease or vitamin B deficiency. These angiomas frequently become more evident during various times of a woman's menstrual cycle. Figure 6–60 shows a young woman with a spider angioma on her face.

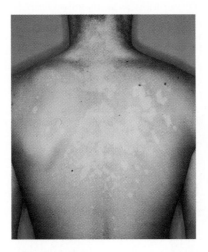

Figure 6–58

Tinea versicolor.

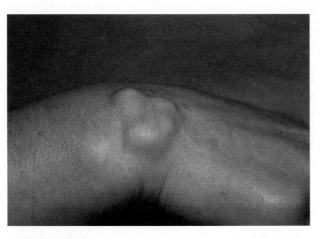

Figure 6–59

Ganglion.

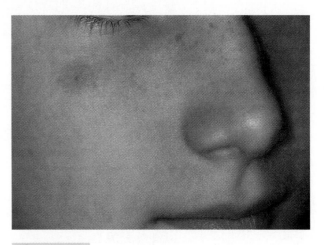

Figure 6–60

Spider angioma.

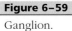

Vitiligo consists of patches of lightened skin resulting from decreased melanin pigmentation. Vitiligo is essentially a large macule that is totally depigmented. The epidermis shows a complete absence of pigment, whereas the dermis is normal. Vitiligo can occur in any area, but it is commonly found on the neck, knees, elbows, and back of the hands. Figure 6–61 shows a woman with extensive vitiligo of her face and neck; a cross section is shown in Figure 6–62.

Urticaria is a common condition. The primary lesion is the wheal, or hive. In urticaria, the epidermis is normal. The dermis shows papillary edema. Inflammatory cells may be found surrounding dilated blood vessels. Itching is a common complaint. There are several mechanisms for the development of urticaria, which include both immunologic and nonimmunologic causes. Regardless of the cause, the common factor is the release of substances, such as histamine, that change the vascular permeability and produce dermal edema. Figure 6–63 shows urticaria, and Figure 6–64 depicts the cross section.

Erythema multiforme is an immunologic reaction in the skin triggered by infection or drugs. As the name implies, the condition includes a variety of lesions: papules, bullae, plaques, and "target lesions." Target lesions are the diagnostic lesions and have three zones of color. A central, tense bulla, or dark area, is surrounded by a zone of relative pallor that is rimmed by a thin area of erythema. Typically, target lesions are seen on the palms and soles. The epidermis is usually normal. In the dermis, there is a subepidermal separation with inflammatory cells in the papillary dermis. Penicillin and sulfonamides are the drugs most commonly implicated as the cause of this condition. The most severe form of erythema multiforme involves the mucous membranes and is called Stevens-Johnson syndrome. The classic skin lesions of erythema multiforme are shown in Figure 6–65; see Figure 6–66 for a cross-sectional view.

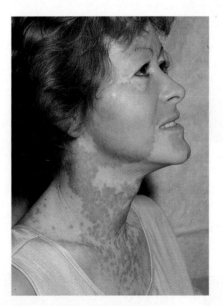

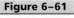
Figure 6–61

Vitiligo.

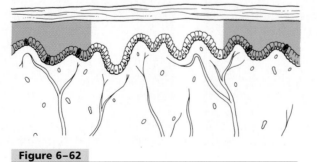

Figure 6–62

Cross section through an area of vitiligo. Note the absence of melanocytes and skin pigment.

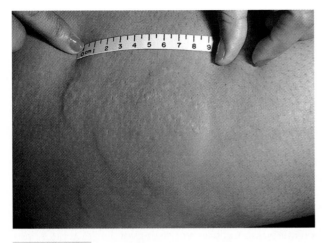

Figure 6–63

Urticaria.

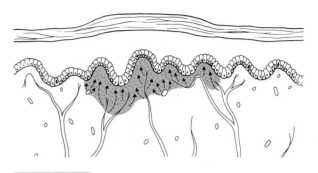

Figure 6–64

Cross section through an area of urticaria.

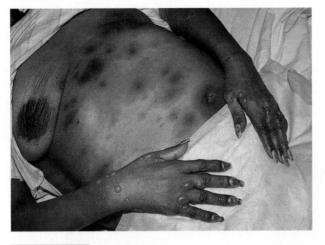

Figure 6–65

Erythema multiforme.

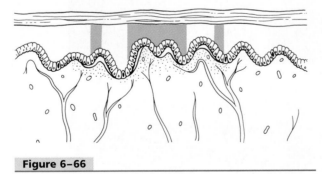

Figure 6–66

Cross section through an area of erythema multiforme.
Note the separation of the epidermis from the dermis.

Scabies is a common, intensely pruritic skin disorder caused by a mite, *Sarcoptes scabiei* var. *hominis.* The female mite burrows into the stratum corneum of the skin and lays her eggs. A month or longer may pass before the symptom of generalized pruritus develops. The diagnostic physical sign is the burrow, which is a serpiginous, palpable track about 1 cm in length that may end in a papule, nodule, or tiny vesicle.

The adult female mite is present in the burrow. The extremely pruritic rash of scabies has a predilection for the web spaces of the fingers and toes as well as the groin. The buttocks is also frequently involved as are the genitals of men and the nipples of women. A generalized papular or urticarial eruption may ensue after localized scabies infection. The presence of papules on the genitalia in a patient with intense pruritus is very suspicious of scabies. Outbreaks of scabies are common in population groups in which HIV is prevalent. Figure 6–67 shows the hands of a patient with scabies. Notice the classic eruption between the fingers. Figure 16–11 shows another patient with scabies; the papular rash in the groin and on the penis is clearly seen.

Norwegian scabies is a rare, highly infectious form of scabies that was once seen in immunosuppressed patients and patients with psychiatric illness; currently, this form of scabies is seen frequently in patients with AIDS. It is characterized by very thick, white hyperkeratotic scales containing thousands of mites. The dorsal aspects of the hands, the feet, and the extensor surfaces of the elbows and knees are commonly involved. Figure 6–68 shows the hand of a patient with Norwegian scabies.

Pyoderma gangrenosum is a cutaneous condition consisting of large, tender, necrotic ulcers having a violaceous, overhanging edge with a purulent base. The lesions are most frequently seen on the face, lower legs, and abdomen. Although most often associated with inflammatory bowel disease, this condition is also seen in association with various blood dyscrasias (especially multiple myeloma), chronic active hepatitis, rheumatoid arthritis, systemic lupus erythematosus, and acute leukemias. Approximately 10% of all patients with ulcerative colitis, however, have cutaneous manifestations, especially pyoderma gangrenosum. The skin lesions of pyoderma gangrenosum are closely linked to the bowel disease; exacerbations of bowel symptoms are associated with extension of existing lesions or development of new ones. Removal of the diseased bowel often leads to improvement in the cutaneous manifestations. See Figure 14–5, which shows a patient with an exacerbation of ulcerative colitis and pyoderma gangrenosum of the shin.

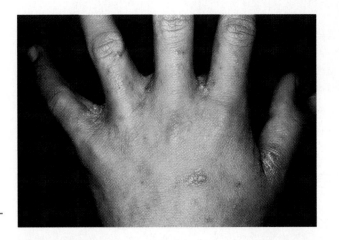

Figure 6–67

Scabies.

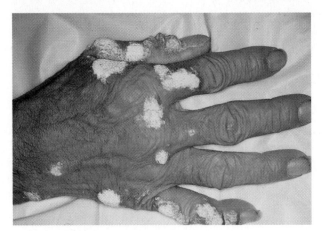

Figure 6–68

Norweigan scabies.

Insect bites are common and should always be considered when a patient complains of a pruritic rash. Papules, vesicles, and wheals amid excoriations suggest the diagnosis. Papules in a linear arrangement on an arm or face suggest bedbug bites. These insects, which live in crevices in furniture, shun the light and feed at night on exposed areas of the body. They bite and then walk only to bite again. Figure 6–69 shows the linear papules on the arm of a patient who was bitten by bedbugs. Flea bites were the cause of the pruritic eruption on the feet of the patient shown in Figure 6–70. Notice the excoriations. The lower legs and feet are common sites for flea bites.

Kaposi's sarcoma (KS) is a neoplasm characterized by dark blue-purple macules, papules, nodules, and plaques. The classic form of the disease is a rare slow-growing neoplasm occurring mostly on the lower extremities, especially the ankles and soles, of elderly men of Mediterranean or Jewish eastern European descent. The male-to-female ratio is 10–15:1, and the majority of patients are from 60 to 80 years of age. Figure 6–71 shows a large reddish-colored plaque, which was slow-growing, on the sole of the foot of a 60 year old man of eastern European origin. Currently, KS is the most frequent neoplasm occurring in AIDS patients. Approximately 35% of AIDS patients are affected, as opposed to about 5% of patients whose infection was acquired from intravenous drug use. Overall, 24% of all AIDS patients develop this rapidly progressive form of the disease, also known as the epidemic HIV-associated form. The widely disseminated lesions are present on the legs, trunk, arms, neck, and head. They start as light-colored papules or nodules and coalesce into larger, darker lesions. Unlike the classic form, the epidemic HIV-associated form is commonly associated with visceral

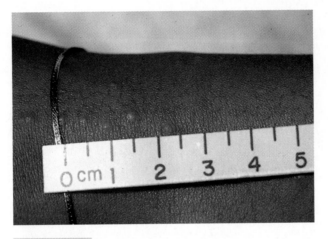

Figure 6–69

Bedbug bites.

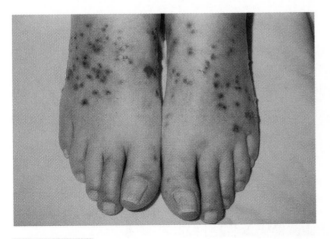

Figure 6–70

Flea bites.

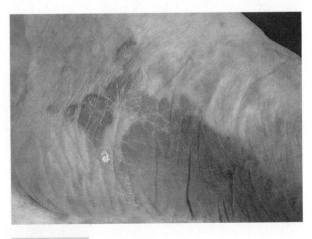

Figure 6–71

Classic Kaposi's sarcoma.

involvement, frequent oral lesions, and lymphadenopathy. The average length of patient survival from the onset of the disease is 18 months. The skin lesions of epidemic HIV-associated Kaposi's sarcoma are shown in Figures 6–72. Figure 6–72*A* shows a patient with the typical lesions on the arm and chest; Figure 6–72*B* shows the widely

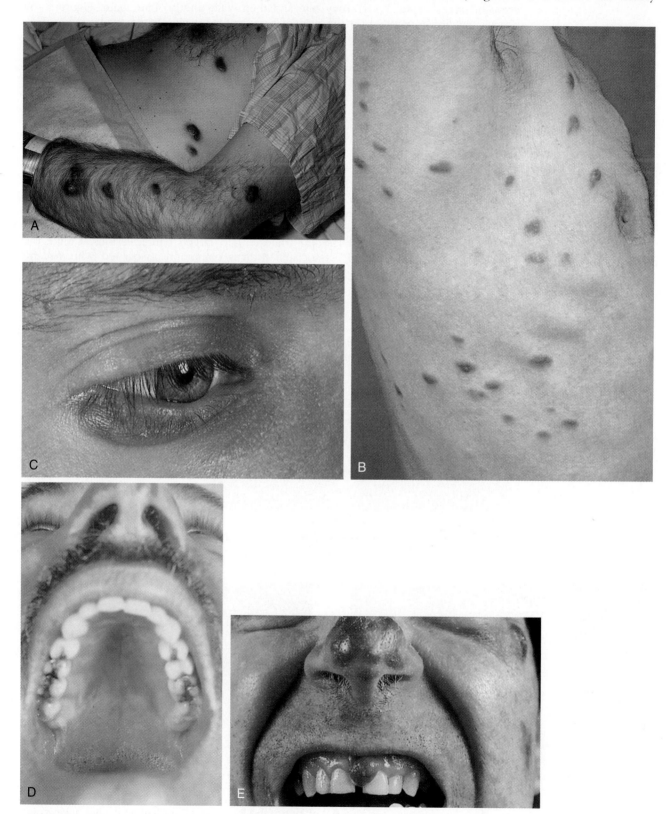

Figure 6–72

Kaposi's sarcoma. *A* and *B*, Plaque lesions. *C*, Violaceous lesion affecting the lateral lower eyelid. *D*, Confluent plaque of Kaposi's sarcoma on the hard palate. *E*, Nodular lesion of Kaposi's sarcoma on the gingiva and the nose.

disseminated plaque lesions varying in color from dark red to violet; Figure 6–72*C* shows a violaceous lesion on the lateral aspect of the lower lid; Figure 6–72*D* shows a large confluent plaque of KS on the hard palate of another patient; Figure 6–72*E* shows a purplish-red, nodular lesion of KS on the gingiva and an infiltrative, violaceous tumor lesion of the nose. Figure 6–73 demonstrates the rapidity of the growth of epidemic KS. Figure 6–73*A* shows the back of a 36 year old homosexual male who presented with only a few macular lesions of KS on his back; a follow-up photograph, taken only 6 months later, shows the widely disseminated, purplish plaques of KS (Fig. 6–73*B*).

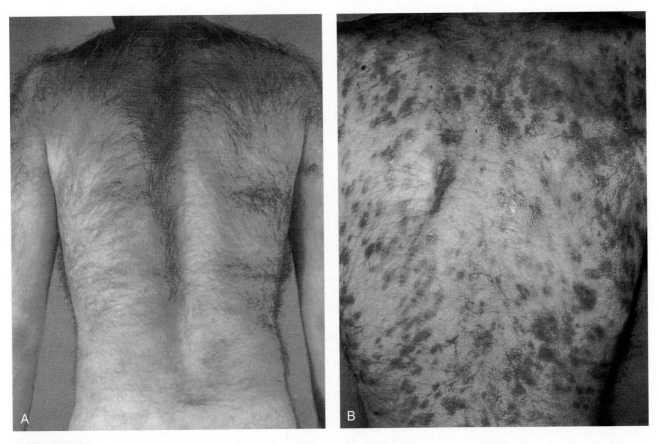

Figure 6–73

A, Early lesions of Kaposi's sarcoma on the back. *B,* Follow-up photograph, 6 months later, showing rapid development of purplish plaques of Kaposi's sarcoma.

Scleroderma, also known as *progressive systemic sclerosis,* is an important rheumatic disease characterized by hardening of the skin. Vascular changes occur with visceral involvement and involve the microvessels and small arteries. The onset of the disease is often heralded by the development of Raynaud's phenomenon, which is discussed in Chapter 13, The Peripheral Vascular System. The cutaneous manifestations of scleroderma involve tightening of the skin, especially on the face and hands. As a result of tendon contractures, flexion of the fingers results. Look at the fingers of the patient with scleroderma shown in Figure 6–74. Notice that the skin is bound tightly and obscures the superficial vasculature. Skin lines are absent. Figure 6–75 shows the face of the same patient. Notice the tightening and wrinkling of the skin around her mouth and the fixed, expressionless countenance as a result of flattening of the nasolabial folds. The patient had great difficulty in opening her mouth. The skin around the mouth has many furrows radiating outward, giving a mouse-like appearance known as "mauskopf."

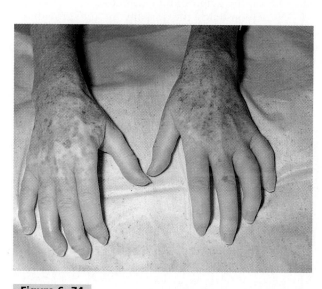

Figure 6–74

Scleroderma: hands.

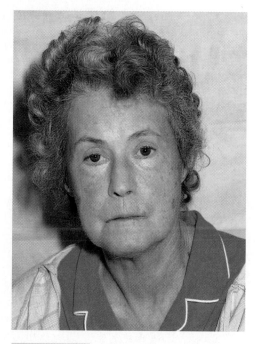

Figure 6–75

Scleroderma: face.

Erythema nodosum is a common reaction associated with streptococcal infections, sarcoidosis, tuberculosis, inflammatory bowel diseases, and fungal diseases. It is infrequently associated with rheumatic disorders. Patients, primarily young women, seek medical attention after the appearance of tender, erythematous nodules on the legs, especially over the anterior tibia. The lesions range in size from 1 to several centimeters in diameter. The lesions then coalesce and spread over the entire leg. The lesions of erythema nodosum begin to regress after 1–2 weeks. As they disappear, they undergo a series of characteristic color changes: bright erythema to shades of purple, yellow, and green. Figure 6–76 shows the early lesions of erythema nodosum in a 33 year old woman in whom sarcoidosis was diagnosed 3 months later.

Lichen planus is a relatively common skin disorder of unknown cause. The primary lesion is a polygonal, shiny, flat-topped papule with a violaceous hue. The pruritic lesions can be seen on any part of the body but have a predilection for the front of the wrists and forearms, the backs of the hands, ankles, shins, genitalia, and lumbar areas. The lesions range in size from 2 mm to more than 1 cm. Figure 6–77 shows a patient with the characteristic rash on the arm. Fine reticulated scales are visible. Oral lesions are seen in 50% of all patients with lichen planus and consist of a

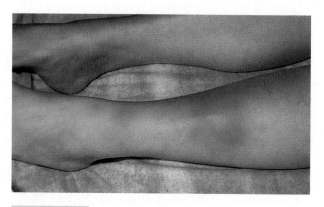

Figure 6–76

Erythema nodosum.

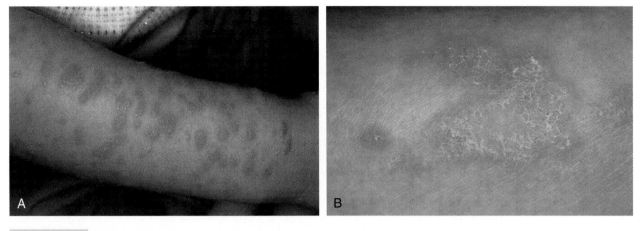

Figure 6-77

Lichen planus. Notice the fine reticulated white scales.

white, lacy network on the buccal mucosa. On occasion, involvement of the mouth may be the only involvement of lichen planus. The patient usually experiences severe pain as the lesions ulcerate. Figure 10–13 shows a patient with lichen planus of the buccal mucosa. Lichen planus may also involve the genitalia. Figure 16–14 shows a patient with lichen planus of the penis. The violaceous rash with the white reticulate pattern can be seen.

Seborrheic dermatitis is a papulosquamous disorder associated with epidermal hyperplasia and scaling. The lesions have a "greasy"-looking scale in a seborrheic distribution: scalp, eyebrows, nasolabial fold, perioral area, midchest, and groin. Seborrheic dermatitis is one of the most common skin conditions associated with HIV infection; it is estimated that 85% of patients infected with HIV have this skin lesion at some time. In some patients, the development of seborrheic dermatitis is the first sign of HIV infection. Figure 6–78 shows a patient with AIDS and the typical greasy scales of seborrheic dermatitis on the face.

Seborrheic warts are common, benign skin tumors, seen in light-skinned individuals; they occur more frequently with advancing age. Also known as *seborrheic keratosis,* seborrheic warts may be solitary or multiple lesions. They occur in any area of the body exposed to ultraviolet light. The lesions are well defined, raised, and have a fissured surface. The lesions result from a failure of keratinocytes to mature normally, which produces an accumulation of immature cells within the epidermis. Sometimes the lesions may be pedunculated. A similar condition known as *dermatosis papulosis nigra* is seen in African-Americans. Figure 6–79 shows the characteristic appearance of a seborrheic wart.

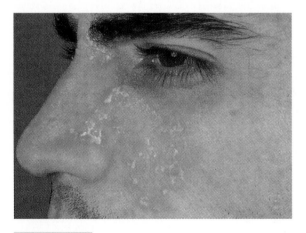

Figure 6-78

Seborrheic dermatitis.

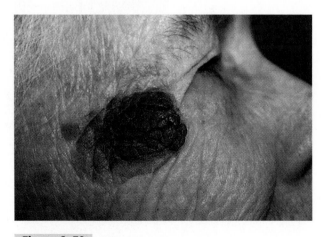

Figure 6-79

Seborrheic keratosis.

A *keloid* is a hyperproliferative response of fibrous tissue to injury, inflammation, or infection. It has a smooth appearance with a shiny surface and is raised and firm to palpation. It is more commonly seen in dark-skinned individuals. The lesion characteristically spreads beyond the site of the initiating factor. Figure 6–80 shows an extensive keloid on the back of this patient.

Nevi are common, localized abnormalities of the skin that may be present at birth or appear within the first few decades of life. Sometimes called "moles," nevi may arise from almost any area of the skin. They are well defined, with a smooth surface and a round shape. Hair may sometimes project from the surface. A *strawberry nevus* is a vascular tumor or hemangioma that occurs shortly after birth and is red and raised. These grow rapidly and are often seen on the face of a child. They may bleed and ulcerate. Fortunately, most strawberry nevi involute by the age of 6 or 7 years of age. Figure 22–7 shows a child with strawberry nevi.

Blistering diseases of the skin are rare but important diseases to recognize. Two disorders, *pemphigus vulgaris* and *bullous pemphigoid,* have been shown to be autoimmune in etiology. Pemphigus vulgaris is a bullous disease of middle age, seen more commonly in Jewish people. The lesions are superficial, flaccid blisters that break easily, leaving the skin denuded and eroded. The broken bullae may crust but do not heal spontaneously. These lesions are nonpruritic and are painful. Figure 6–81 shows a patient with pemphigus vulgaris and the broken bullae. The lesions may be present on any area of the skin, especially the trunk, umbilicus, intertriginous areas, and scalp. The lesions are frequently found in the mucous membranes of the oral cavity, pharynx, and genitalia.

Bullous pemphigoid is a blistering disorder seen more in elderly patients. It is more common than pemphigus vulgaris. There is no racial predilection, and the disease is not as serious as pemphigus. The lesions are intensely pruritic, tense bullae often on an erythematous base and are symmetric on the limbs, inner aspects of the arms, thighs, and trunk. Oral and mucosal lesions are rare compared with those of pemphigus. Figure 6–82 shows a patient with bullous pemphigoid. Notice the tense bullae, which helps to differentiate this disease from pemphigus.

Atopic dermatitis is a common disease associated with other atopic diseases such as asthma and allergic rhinitis. The symptoms of atopic dermatitis often begin at a young age. Infants and young children may have eczematous patches on the face, scalp, and extensor surfaces of the extremities. These patches may erode and ooze. Scaling erythematous plaques often develop. As the child grows older, the atopic dermatitis begins to involve the flexural areas such as the neck, antecubital fossae, and popliteal fossae. The pruritic lesions result in excoriations; thickening and lichenification of the skin with increased skin markings are common. In the adult, oozing,

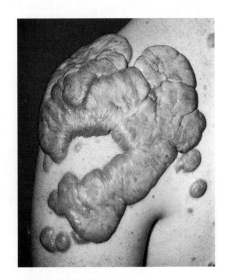

Figure 6–80

Keloid.

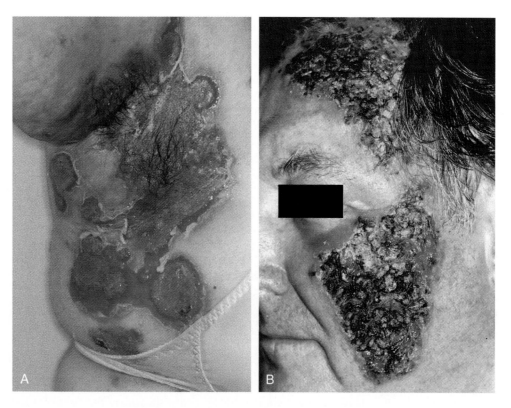

Figure 6–81

Pemphigus vulgaris. *B* shows a vegetative form sometimes called pemphigus vegetans.

weeping, and excoriated plaques may become generalized. Although the pathogenesis of atopic dermatitis is unknown, many patient have elevated levels of serum immunoglobulin E. Figure 6–83 shows a patient with classic lesions of atopic dermatitis in the axilla. Figure 6–84 shows another patient with atopic dermatitis. Notice the oozing lesions and the excoriations.

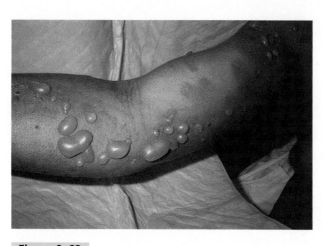

Figure 6–82

Bullous pemphigoid.

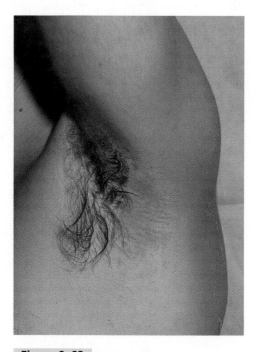

Figure 6–83

Atopic dermatitis.

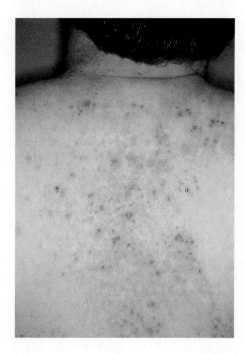

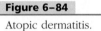

Figure 6–84

Atopic dermatitis.

As indicated in this chapter, there are many cutaneous manifestations of AIDS. Three of these common lesions are shown on the face of a patient with AIDS in Figure 6–85. The umbilicated, white papules on and around the lips, nose, and cheek are lesions of molluscum contagiosum. The verrucous papule on the upper lip is a wart. The violaceous lesions of KS are present on the lips and chin.

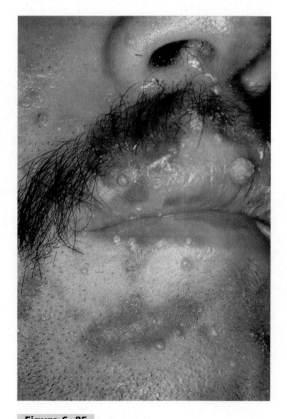

Figure 6–85

Cutaneous manifestations of AIDS.

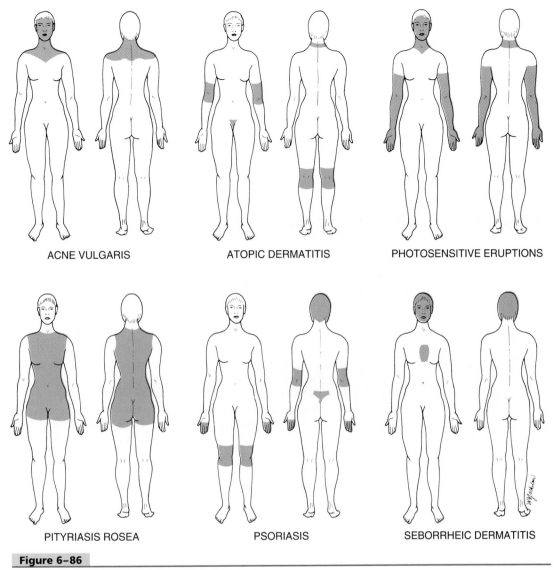

ACNE VULGARIS   ATOPIC DERMATITIS   PHOTOSENSITIVE ERUPTIONS

PITYRIASIS ROSEA   PSORIASIS   SEBORRHEIC DERMATITIS

Figure 6–86

Typical distributions of common skin conditions.

The typical distribution of lesions in six common skin disorders is shown in Figure 6–86.

Table 6–1 describes the differential diagnosis of common maculopapular diseases. Table 6–2 lists the differentiation of some common eczematous disorders and gives some special hints about their causes derived from the history. Table 6–3 provides a differential diagnosis of the vesiculobullous diseases. Table 6–4 classifies some of the common benign tumors by color. Table 6–5 lists some of the common allergens associated with contact dermatitis.

Table 6–1	Common Maculopapular Diseases*				
	Psoriasis	Pityriasis Rosea	Tinea Versicolor	Seborrheic Dermatitis	Lichen Planus
Color	Dull red	Pinkish yellow	Reddish brown	Pinkish yellow	Violaceous
Scale	Abundant	Fine, adherent	Fine	Greasy	Shiny, adherent
Induration	1+†	0	0	1+	1+
Face lesions	Rarely	Rarely	Occasionally	Common	Rarely
Oral lesions	0	0	0	0	2+
Nail lesions	4+	0	0	0	Rarely

* See Figures 6–12, 6–44, 6–45, 6–47, 6–51, 6–58, 6–77, 6–78.
† 0, rarely seen; 1+, occasionally seen; 2+, frequently seen; 4+, nearly always associated.

Table 6–2	Common Eczematous Diseases*			
	Contact Dermatitis	Atopic Dermatitis	Neurodermatitis	Stasis Dermatitis
History	Acute, localized to specific area	History in patient or family member of asthma, hay fever, or eczema	Chronic, in same areas, associated with anxiety	Varicosities, past history of thrombophlebitis or cellulitis
Location	Areas of exposure to allergen	Eyelids, groin, flexural areas	Head, lower legs, arms	Lower legs

* See Figures 6–42, 6–83, 6–84, 13–1.

Table 6–3	Vesiculobullous Diseases*			
	Pemphigus Vulgaris	Dermatitis Herpetiformis	Epidermolysis Bullosa**	Bullous Pemphigoid
Age of patient	40–60 years	Children and adults	Infants and children	60–70 years
Initial site	Oral mucosa	Scalp, trunk	Extremities	Extremities
Lesions	Normal skin at margins	Erythematous base	Bullae produced by trauma	Normal skin at margins
Sites	Mouth, abdomen, scalp, groin	Knees, sacrum, back, elbows	Hands, knees, elbows, mouth, toes	Trunk, extremities
Groupings	0†	4+	1+	0
Weight loss	Marked	None	None	Minimal
Duration	1 or more years	Several years	Normal lifetime	Months to years
Pruritus	0	4+	0	±
Oral pain	4+	0	±	±
Palms/soles involved	No	No	Yes	Yes
Typical lesion	Flaccid bulla	Grouped vesicles	Flaccid vesicles	Tense bulla

* See Figures 6–81 and 6–82.
** Refers to a group of inherited diseases.
† 0, rarely seen, 1+, occasionally seen; 4+, nearly always associated; ±, sometimes present.

Table 6–4	Common Benign Tumors by Color
Color	Benign Tumor
Skin color	Warts (see Fig. 6–24)
	Cysts
	Keloids
	Nevi
Pink or red	Hemangiomas (see Fig. 21–6)
	Keloids
Brown	Seborrheic keratoses (see Fig. 6–79)
	Nevi
	Lentigines
	Dermatofibromas
Tannish yellow	Xanthomata (see Fig. 11–12)
	Xanthelasma (see Fig. 11–15)
	Warts (see Fig. 6–24)
	Keloids
Dark blue or black	Seborrheic keratoses (see Fig. 6–79)
	Hemangiomas
	Blue nevi
	Dermatofibromas

Table 6–5 Allergens Associated with Contact Dermatitis

Location	Possible Allergen
Scalp	Hair dyes
	Shampoos
	Tonics
Eyelids	Eye makeup
	Hair sprays
Neck	Aftershave lotions
	Perfumes
	Soaps
	Washing agents
	Nickel jewelry
Trunk	Clothing
	Washing agents
Axillae	Deodorants
	Soaps
Genitalia	Soaps
	Contraceptives
	Deodorants
	Washing agents
Feet	Shoes
	Sneakers
	Deodorants
	Socks
	Washing agents
Hands	Nickel jewelry
	Soaps
	Dyes
	Plants

Useful Vocabulary

Listed here are the specific roots that are important in order to understand the terminology related to diseases of the skin.

Root	Pertaining to	Example	Definition
kerat(o)-	horny	*kerat*oma	Horny growth
derm(a)-	skin	*derma*titis	Inflammation of the skin
trich(o)-	hair	*trich*oid	Resembling hair
seb(o)-	sebum	*sebo*rrhea	Excess flow of sebum
hidr(o)-	sweat	*hidr*adenitis	Inflammation of sweat glands
onych(o)-	nails	*onycho*mycosis	Disease of the nails caused by fungus

Writing Up the Physical Examination

Listed here are examples of the write-up for the examination of the skin.

- There are oval plaques with well-defined borders and silvery scale symmetrically present on the elbows, knees, scalp, and gluteal cleft. The plaques in the scalp are along the hairline. The scales are large. Examination of the nails reveals pitting of the nail plates. The hair is of normal texture.
- There is an annular lesion 3–4 cm in diameter on the right forearm. Scale is present on the narrow (1–2 mm), raised, erythematous border. The central area is slightly hypopigmented. The hair and nails are unremarkable.
- There is a linear bullous eruption along the lateral aspect of the left leg. The eruption consists of bright red edematous papules and bullae. There are no lesions on the palms or soles or in the mouth.
- A wide variety of lesions are seen on the face, shoulders, and back. The predominant lesions are pustules on an inflammatory base. Many pustules are present, and several have become confluent over

the chin and forehead. Open and closed comedones are present on the face, especially along the nasolabial folds. Inflammatory papules are present on the lower cheeks and chin. Large abscesses and ulcerated cysts are present over the upper shoulder areas. Numerous scars are present over the face and upper back.

- A diffuse erythematous maculopapular rash is present on the trunk. Some excoriations are present over the shoulders and chest. The hair and nails are unremarkable.
- Examination of the skin reveals several types of lesions. The main lesions are small papules in the antecubital and popliteal fossae. The papules in some areas have become confluent, and plaques are present. On the dorsum of the feet, eczema is present with erythema, weeping, crusting, and scaling. Lichenification of the anogenital area, especially the scrotum, is present.
- The skin is slightly cool and dry. Scattered lentigines are present over the trunk. The hair is very fine and soft. There is loss of the lateral one third of the eyebrows. No nail abnormalities are present.

Bibliography

Callen JP, Greer KE, Hood AF, et al: Color Atlas of Dermatology. Philadelphia, W.B. Saunders, 1993.

Ellis RA: Eccrine, sebaceous and apocrine glands. In Zelickson AS (ed): Ultrastructure of Normal and Abnormal Skin. Philadelphia, Lea & Febiger, 1967.

Flowers FP, Krusinski PA: Dermatology in Ambulatory and Emergency Medicine. Chicago, Year Book Medical, 1984.

Friedman-Kien AE, Cockerell CJ: Color Atlas of AIDS, 2nd ed. Philadelphia, W.B. Saunders, 1996.

Habif TP: Clinical Dermatology. St. Louis, C.V. Mosby, 1985.

Lebwohl MG: Atlas of the Skin and Systemic Disease. New York, Churchill Livingstone Inc., 1995.

Lookingbill DP, Marks JG Jr: Principles of Dermatology. Philadelphia, W.B. Saunders, 1986.

Safai B, Johnson KG, Myskowski PL, et al: The natural history of Kaposi's sarcoma in the acquired immunodeficiency syndrome. Ann Intern Med 103:744, 1985.

du Vivier A: Atlas of Clinical Dermatology. Philadelphia, W.B. Saunders, 1986.

CHAPTER 7

The Head and Neck

A lady, aged twenty, became affected with some symptoms which were supposed to be hysterical. . . . After she had been in this nervous state about three months it was observed that her pulse had become singularly rapid. . . . She next complained of weakness on exertion and began to look pale and thin. . . . It was observed that the eyes assumed a singular appearance, for the eyeballs were apparently enlarged. In a few months . . . a tumour, of a horseshoe shape, appeared on the front of the throat and exactly in the situation of the thyroid gland.

Robert James Graves
1796–1853

General Considerations

The appearance of the head and face, their contours and texture, often provides the first insight into the nature of illness. Sunken cheeks, wasting of the temporal muscles, and flushing of the face are important visible clues of systemic illness. Some facial appearances are pathognomonic of disease. The pale, puffy face of nephritis, the startled expression of hyperthyroidism, and the immobile stare of parkinsonism are examples of classic facies.

The appearance of the patient's face may also provide information regarding psychological makeup: is the person happy, sad, angry, or anxious?

Thyroid disease takes many forms. The World Health Organization estimates that over 200 million people in the world have the condition of an enlarged thyroid, known as a *goiter*. The Asians first described the goiter around 1500 BC. Even at that time, they recognized that seaweed in the diet tended to make the goiter smaller. Iodine was not discovered until the 19th century, but it is now believed that these goiters were related to an iodine deficiency that was partially corrected by the iodine that was present in the seaweed.

The ancient Greeks and Romans recognized that when a thin thread tied around the neck of a newly married woman broke, she was pregnant. This was caused by an increase in the size of the thyroid during pregnancy.

In the United States, cancer of the head and neck constitutes about 5% of all malignancies in men and 2% in women. There are more than 28,000 new cases a year. It has been estimated that nearly 90% of these cases are associated with poor dental hygiene, tobacco use, exposure to nickel, and alcohol. Tobacco, whether chewed, smoked, or simply kept in the buccal pouch, predisposes an individual to tumors of the upper aerodigestive tract (Vaughan et al, 1980). Pipe smokers and tobacco chewers are at risk for tumors of the oral cavity, and the Chinese are at risk for nasopharyngeal carcinomas.

Structure and Physiology

The Head

The skull is composed of 22 bones, 14 in the face alone. This bony structure acts as a support and protection for the softer tissues within.

The *facial skeleton* is composed of the *mandible,* the *maxilla,* and the *nasal, palatine, lacrimal,* and *vomer* bones. The unpaired *mandible* forms the lower jaw. The maxilla is an irregular bone and forms the upper jaw on each side. The nasal bones form the bridge of the nose. The other bones are not relevant to this discussion.

The main bones of the *cranial* skeleton include the *frontal, temporal, parietal,* and *occipital* bones. The frontal bones form the forehead. The temporal bones form the anterolateral walls of the brain. The *mastoid* process, which is part of the temporal bone, is particularly important in ear disease and is discussed in a subsequent chapter. The parietal bones form the top and posterolateral portions of the skull. The occipital bones form the posterior portion of the skull. The bones of the face and skull are shown in Figure 7–1.

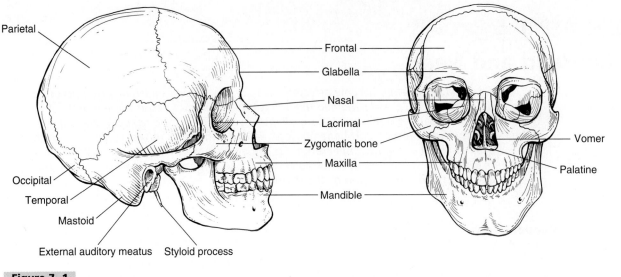

Figure 7–1

Bones of the face and skull.

The principal muscle of the mouth is the *orbicularis oris*. This single muscle surrounds the lips, with numerous other facial muscles inserting into it. The action of the orbicularis oris is to close the lips.

The *orbicularis oculi* muscle surrounds the eye. Its function is to close the eyelids. This muscle and its action are further discussed in Chapter 8, The Eye.

The *platysma* is a thin, superficial muscle of the neck, crossing the outer border of the mandible and extending over the lower anterior portion of the face. The main action of the platysma is to pull the mandible downward and backward, resulting in a mournful facial expression.

The muscles of mastication include the *masseter, pterygoid,* and *temporalis.* These muscles insert on the mandible and effect chewing. The masseter is a strong, thick muscle and is one of the most powerful muscles of the face. The action of the masseter is to close the jaw by elevating and drawing the mandible backward. Tension in the masseter may be felt by clenching the jaw. Although important in the functioning of the jaw, the other muscles of mastication are not clinically relevant to physical diagnosis and are not discussed in this text. The locations of these muscles are shown in Figure 7–2.

The *trigeminal,* or fifth cranial, nerve carries sensory fibers from the face, oral cavity, and teeth and carries efferent motor fibers to the muscles of mastication. The major divisions of this nerve are discussed in subsequent chapters.

The Neck

The neck is divided by the sternocleidomastoid muscle into the anterior, or medial, triangle and the posterior, or lateral, triangle structures. This is illustrated in Figure 7–3.

The *sternocleidomastoid* is a strong muscle that serves to raise the sternum during respiration. The sternocleidomastoid has two heads: the *sternal* head arises from the manubrium sterni, and the *clavicular* head originates on the sternal end of the clavicle. The two heads unite and insert on the lateral aspect of the mastoid process. The sternocleidomastoid is innervated by the *spinal accessory,* or eleventh cranial, nerve.

Anterior to the sternocleidomastoid muscle is the *anterior triangle.* The other boundaries of the anterior triangle are the clavicle inferiorly and the midline anteriorly. The anterior triangle contains the thyroid gland, larynx, pharynx, lymph nodes, submandibular salivary gland, and fat.

The *thyroid gland* envelops the upper trachea and consists of two lobes connected by an isthmus. It is the largest endocrine gland in the body. As seen from the front, the thyroid is butterfly-shaped and wraps around the anterior and lateral portions of the larynx and trachea, shown in Figure 7–4.

The thyroid isthmus lies across the trachea just below the cricoid cartilage of the larynx. The lateral lobes extend along either side of the larynx, reaching the level of

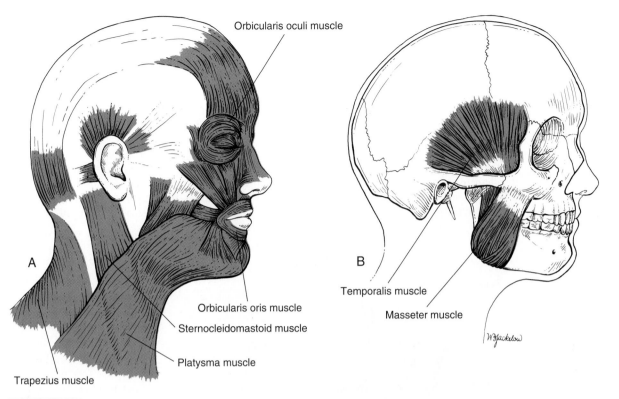

Figure 7–2

Muscles of the face and skull. *A,* The more superficial muscles. *B,* The underlying muscles.

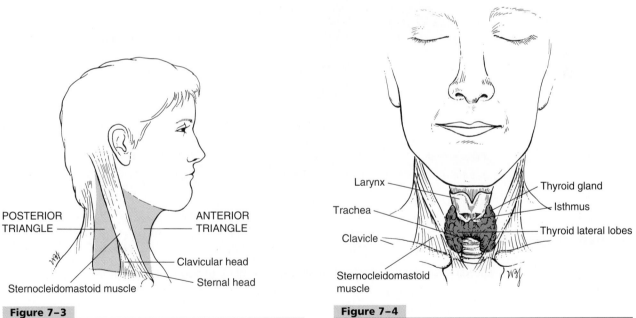

Figure 7–3

The boundaries of the triangles of the neck.

Figure 7–4

The thyroid gland.

the middle of the thyroid cartilage of the larynx. Occasionally, the thyroid gland may extend downward and enlarge within the thorax, producing a substernal goiter. The function of the thyroid gland is to produce thyroid hormone in accordance with the needs of the body.

The pharynx and larynx are discussed in Chapter 10, The Oral Cavity and Pharynx.

The sternocleidomastoid muscle overlies the *carotid sheath*. The carotid sheath lies lateral to the larynx. This sheath contains the common carotid artery, the internal jugular vein, and the vagus nerve.

Posterior to the sternocleidomastoid is the *posterior triangle*. This is bounded by the trapezius muscle posteriorly and by the clavicle inferiorly. The posterior triangle also contains lymph nodes.

It has been estimated that the neck contains more than 75 lymph nodes on each side. The chains of these lymph nodes are named for their location. Starting posteriorly, they are the *occipital, posterior auricular, posterior cervical, superficial* and *deep cervical* (adjacent to the sternocleidomastoid muscle), *tonsillar, submaxillary, submental* (at the tip of the jaw in the midline), *anterior auricular,* and *supraclavicular* (above the clavicle) chains. A knowledge of the lymphatic drainage is important, because the presence of an enlarged lymph node may signal disease in the area draining into it. The main groups of lymph nodes and their drainage areas are shown in Figure 7–5.

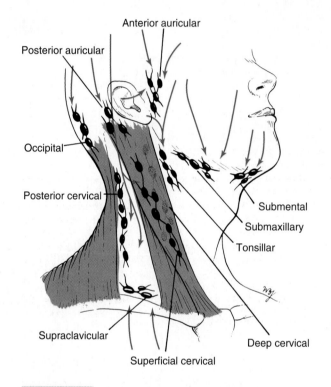

Figure 7–5

Lymph nodes of the neck and their drainage.

Review of Specific Symptoms

The most common symptoms related to the neck include

- Neck mass
- Neck stiffness

Neck Mass

The most common symptom is a lump or swelling in the neck. Once a patient complains of a neck lump, ask the following questions:

"When did you first notice the lump?"
"Does it hurt?"
"Does the lump change in size?"

"Have you had any ear infections? infections in your mouth?"
"Has there been hoarseness associated with the mass?"

If there is associated pain with a mass in the neck, an acute infection is likely. Masses that have been present for only a couple of days are commonly inflammatory, whereas those present for months are more likely to be neoplastic. A mass that has been present for months to years without any change in size will often turn out to be a benign or congenital lesion. Blockage of a salivary gland duct may produce a mass that fluctuates in size while the patient eats.

The *age of the patient* is relevant in the assessment of a neck mass. A lump in the neck of a patient younger than the age of 20 years may be an enlarged tonsillar lymph node or a congenital mass. If the mass is in the midline, it is likely to be a thyroglossal cyst.*

From the ages of 20 to 40 years, thyroid disease is more common, although lymphoma must always be considered. When a patient is older than the age of 40 years, a neck mass must always be considered malignant until proved otherwise.

The *location* of the mass is also important. Midline masses tend to be benign or congenital lesions, such as thyroglossal cysts or dermoid cysts. Lateral masses are frequently neoplastic. Masses located in the lateral upper neck may be metastatic lesions from tumors of the head and neck, whereas masses in the lateral lower neck may be metastatic from tumors of the breast and stomach. One benign lateral neck mass is a branchial cleft cyst, which may manifest as a painless, lateral neck mass near the anterior upper third border of the sternocleidomastoid muscle.

Hoarseness in association with a thyroid nodule suggests vocal cord paralysis by impingement of the recurrent laryngeal nerve by tumor.

Neck Stiffness

Stiffness of the neck is usually caused by spasm of the cervical muscles and is commonly the cause of the tension headache. The sudden occurrence of a stiff neck, fever, and headache should alert suspicion of possible meningeal irritation. Neck pain may be associated with referred pain from the chest. Patients with angina or a myocardial infarction may complain of neck pain.

Impact of Head and Neck Disease on the Patient

The concept of body image is important. The head and neck are the most visible portions of the body. The shape of the eyes, mouth, face, and nose is very important to people. Many dislike their body image and want to change it by cosmetic surgery. Others require cosmetic surgery to repair alterations caused by trauma. Still others suffer from disfiguring head and neck cancer and need to undergo surgical procedures for the removal of these lesions. Many of these procedures themselves are mutilating.

Distortion of the body image, especially on the head and neck, can produce a devastating effect on the patient. The most common reaction to head and neck disease is depression. Many of these patients suffer from feelings of sadness and hopelessness. They look in the mirror hoping someday they will see themselves with a more acceptable body image. Recurrent thoughts of suicide are common. Many of these depressed patients turn to alcohol or other drugs.

Occasionally, patients who have undergone cosmetic surgery are dissatisfied with the results. Many of these patients are trying to escape from feelings of inferiority and social maladjustment. They may have had only minor defects, but these defects are viewed as a major source of interpersonal problems. Cosmetic surgery is a way to change their image in the hope of improving their social maladjustment. Some individuals may even blame the physician for "destroying" their face. Even after further revisions, these patients may never be satisfied. One of the keys to success of cosmetic surgery is the proper selection of patients.

---

*A thyroglossal cyst may arise anywhere along the route of the thyroid gland's descent from the foramen cecum of the tongue to its adult location in the neck. The thyroid gland is a painless, mobile structure that moves on swallowing or with movement of the tongue. See Figure 22–21.

Physical Examination

> No special equipment is needed for the examination of the head and neck.

The examination of the head and neck is performed with the patient seated, facing the examiner. The examination consists of

- Inspection
- Auscultation for carotid bruits (discussed in Chapter 13), The Peripheral Vascular System
- Palpation

Inspection

Inspect the position of the head. Does the patient hold the head erect? Is there any asymmetry of the facial structure? Is the head in proportion to the rest of the body?

Inspect the scalp for lesions. Describe the hair.

Are any masses present? If so, describe their size, consistency, and symmetry. Look at Figure 22–21, which shows a child with a midline *thyroglossal duct cyst*. A thyroglossal duct cyst results from a failure in the obliteration of the embryologic tract along which the thyroid descends from the base of the tongue to the anterior neck, leaving active thyroid tissue along the path. The cyst is smooth, firm, and midline. When the patient is asked to swallow or stick out the tongue, the thyroglossal duct cyst moves upward.

Inspect the eyes for proptosis (a forward displacement, or bulging, of the eyeball). Proptosis may be caused by thyroid dysfunction or by a mass in the orbit.

Inspect the neck for areas of asymmetry. Ask the patient to extend the neck. Inspect the neck for scars, asymmetry, or masses. The normal thyroid is barely visible. Ask the patient to swallow while you observe any upward motion of the thyroid with swallowing. A diffusely enlarged thyroid gland often causes generalized enlargement of the neck. Look at the patient with diffuse thyromegaly shown in Figure 7–6. This patient has Graves' disease with bilateral proptosis.

Is nodularity of the neck seen? A patient with nodular neck masses that are due to a multinodular goiter is shown in Figure 7–7.

Is superficial venous distention present? Venous distention in the neck is important to evaluate, as this finding may be associated with a goiter.

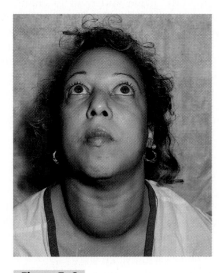

Figure 7–6

Graves' disease.

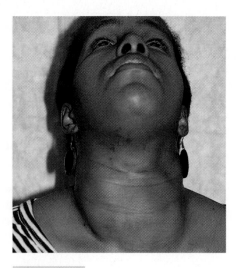

Figure 7–7

Multinodular goiter.

Palpation

Palpate the Head and Neck

Palpation confirms the information obtained by inspection. The head should be slightly flexed and should be cradled in the examiner's hands, as shown in Figure 7–8.

All areas of the cranium should be palpated for tenderness or masses. The pads of the examiner's fingers should roll the underlying skin over the cranium in circular motions to assess its contour and to feel for the presence of lymph nodes or masses. Starting from the occipital region, the examiner's hands are moved into the posterior auricular region, which is superficial to the mastoid process; down into the posterior triangle to feel for the posterior cervical chain; along the sternocleidomastoid muscle to feel for the superficial cervical chain; hooking around the sternocleidomastoid muscle to feel for the deep cervical chain deep to the muscle; into the anterior triangle region; up to the jaw margin to feel for the tonsillar group; along the jaw to feel the submaxillary chain; to the tip of the jaw for the submental nodes; and up to the anterior auricular chain in front of the ear. This sequence of examination is shown in Figure 7–9.

A patient with enlarged posterior auricular and posterior cervical nodes is shown in Figure 7–10.

Any nodes that are felt should be observed for mobility, consistency, and tenderness. Tender lymph nodes are suggestive of inflammation, whereas fixed, firm nodes are consistent with a malignancy.

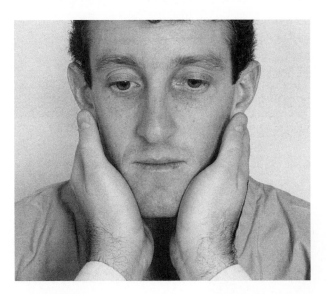

Figure 7–8

Palpation of the head and neck.

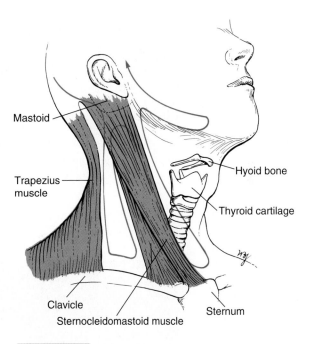

Figure 7–9

Suggested approach for palpation of the lymph nodes of the neck.

Palpate the Thyroid Gland

There are two approaches to palpating the thyroid gland. The anterior approach is carried out with the patient and examiner sitting face to face. By flexing the patient's neck or turning the chin slightly to the right, the examiner can relax the sternocleidomastoid muscle on that side, making the examination easier to perform. The examiner's right hand should displace the larynx to the right, and, during swallowing, the displaced right thyroid lobe is palpated between the examiner's left thumb and index

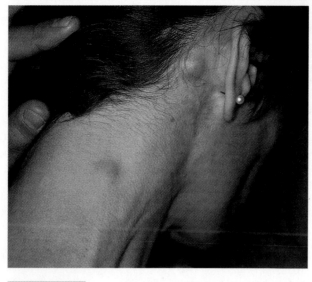

Figure 7–10

Posterior auricular and posterior cervical adenopathy.

fingers. This is demonstrated in Figure 7–11. After the right lobe has been evaluated, the larynx is displaced to the left, and the left lobe is evaluated by reversing the hand positions.

At this point in the examination, the examiner should stand behind the patient to palpate the thyroid by the posterior approach. The posterior approach involves placing the examiner's two hands around the neck of the patient, whose neck is slightly extended. The examiner uses the left hand to push the trachea to the right. The patient is asked to swallow while the examiner's right hand rolls over the thyroid cartilage. As the patient swallows, the examiner's right hand feels for the thyroid gland against the right sternocleidomastoid muscle. The patient is again asked to swallow as the trachea is pushed to the left, and the examiner uses the left hand to feel for the thyroid gland

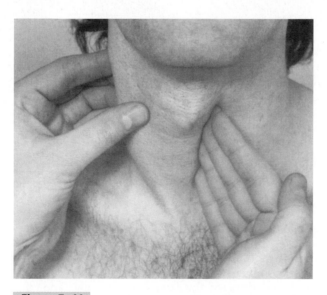

Figure 7–11

Anterior approach for palpation of the thyroid gland.

against the left sternocleidomastoid muscle. Water given to the patient will facilitate swallowing. The posterior approach is shown in Figure 7–12.

Although both the anterior and the posterior approaches of palpation are usually performed, the examiner rarely feels the thyroid gland in its normal state.

The consistency of the gland should be evaluated. The normal thyroid gland has a consistency of muscle tissue. Unusual *hardness* is associated with cancer or scarring. Softness, or sponginess, is often seen with a toxic goiter. *Tenderness* of the thyroid gland is associated with acute infections or with hemorrhage into the gland.

If the thyroid is enlarged, it should also be examined by auscultation. The bell of the stethoscope is placed over the lobes of the thyroid while the examiner listens for the presence of a bruit (a murmur heard when there is increased turbulence in a vessel). The finding of a systolic or a to-and-fro* *thyroid bruit,* particularly if heard over the superior pole, indicates an abnormally large blood flow and is highly suggestive of a *toxic goiter.*

▧ Palpate for Supraclavicular Nodes

The palpation for supraclavicular nodes concludes the examination of the head and neck. The examiner stands behind the patient and places the fingers into the medial supraclavicular fossae, deep to the clavicle and adjacent to the sternocleidomastoid muscles. The patient is instructed to take a deep breath while the examiner presses deeply in and behind the clavicles. Any supraclavicular nodes that are enlarged will be felt as the patient inspires. This technique is shown in Figure 7–13.

The examination of the trachea is discussed in Chapter 11, The Chest. The examination of the carotid arterial and jugular venous pulsations is discussed in Chapter 12, The Heart.

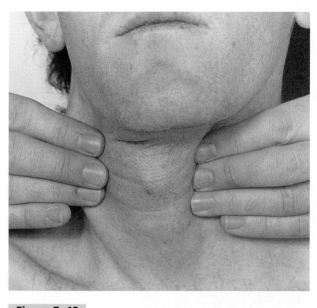

Figure 7–12

Posterior approach for palpation of the thyroid gland.

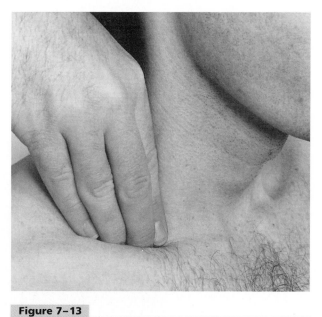

Figure 7–13

Technique for palpation of the supraclavicular lymph nodes.

---

* Refers to two separate murmurs, systolic and diastolic.

Clinicopathologic Correlations

Although iodine deficiency is still a worldwide cause of thyroid enlargement, other important causes of goiter are infection, autoimmune disease, cancer, and isolated nodules. An enlarged thyroid may be associated with *hyper*thyroidism, *hypo*thyroidism, or a *simple* or a *multinodular* goiter of normal function.

As mentioned earlier in this chapter, the thyroid may enlarge into the chest cavity. If the thyroid is large enough, it may impair venous outflow from the head and neck and may even be responsible for airway or vascular compromise. Pemberton's sign is a useful maneuver for detecting latent obstruction in the thoracic inlet. To determine whether the sign is present, the patient is asked to elevate both arms until they touch the sides of the head. If the test is positive, indicating that the Pemberton sign is present, facial suffusion with dilatation of the cervical veins will develop within a few seconds. After 1 to 2 minutes, the face may even become cyanotic. Figure 7–14 shows a patient with a positive Pemberton sign. The patient was a 62 year old man with a known anterior neck mass for 25 years. The upper border of the thyroid was felt on examination, but the lower pole descended below the clavicle and was not palpable.

As indicated in the quote at the beginning of this chapter, hyperthyroidism may manifest with a variety of generalized symptoms and signs. It has been said, "To know thyroid disease is to know medicine" because there are so many generalized effects of thyroid hormone excess. Table 7–1 indicates the variety of clinical symptoms related to thyroid hormone excess.

The nervous, perspiring patient with a stare and bulging eyes offers an unmistakable combination of physical signs associated with hyperthyroidism. The most common type of hyperthyroidism is the diffuse toxic goiter, known as Graves' disease. Graves' disease is viewed as an autoimmune disorder provoked by the elaboration of a thyroid-stimulating immunoglobulin. There are many cutaneous signs of hyperthyroidism, including the following:

- Warm skin
- Erythema
- Hyperhidrosis (increased sweating)
- Alopecia (hair loss)
- Hyperpigmentation
- Nail growth changes

Occasionally Graves' disease manifests with unilateral proptosis, as shown in Figure 7–15. This patient presented with proptosis and was treated for Graves' disease 20 years before this photograph was taken. As is common, the proptosis never disappeared.

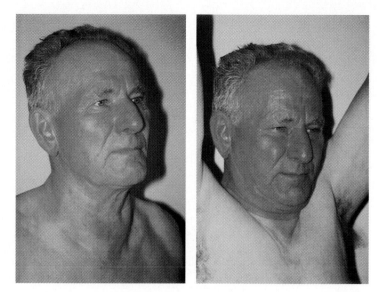

Figure 7–14

The Pemberton sign.

Table 7–1   Symptoms of Hyperthyroidism

Organ System	Symptom
General	Preference for the cold
	Weight loss with good appetite
Eyes	Prominence of eyeballs*
	Puffiness of eyelids
	Double vision
	Decreased motility
Neck	Goiter
Cardiac	Palpitations
	Peripheral edema†
Gastrointestinal	Increased bowel movements
Genitourinary	Polyuria
	Decreased fertility
Neuromuscular	Fatigue
	Weakness
	Tremulousness
Emotional	Nervousness
	Irritability
Dermatologic	Hair thinning
	Increased perspiration
	Change in skin texture
	Change in pigmentation

* Appears to be due to mucopolysaccharide deposition behind the orbit.
† Appears to be due to excessive mucopolysaccharide deposition under the skin, especially in the legs.

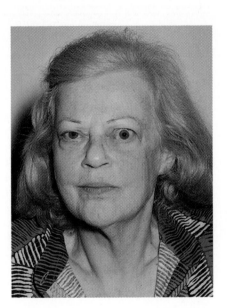

Figure 7–15

Graves' disease.

Sometimes hyperthyroidism is caused by a single hot nodule.* Toxic adenomatous goiter, also known as *Plummer's disease,* accounts for fewer than 10% of all hyperthyroid patients. Hyperthyroidism may be caused by a single, autonomously functioning thyroid adenoma. The adenoma is usually papillary and is unrelated to any autoimmune process. Hyperfunction may also occur in multiple nodules. The distinctive

---

* The terms *hot* and *cold* are descriptions of nodules seen on a thyroid scan and are used to indicate whether a nodule accumulates more or less radioactive iodine than the surrounding thyroid tissue. A hot nodule is functioning thyroid tissue and has a greater uptake than the surrounding tissue. A cold nodule is nonfunctioning and fails to take up the radioactive tracer.

features of hyperthyroidism caused by Graves' and Plummer's diseases are summarized in Table 7–2.

Approximately 5% of the population has a single thyroid nodule larger than 1 cm in diameter. Although most of these nodules are benign and necessitate no therapy, all should be investigated for malignancy. The history and physical examination can provide some clues as to the nature of the lump. Table 7–3 summarizes some of the important characteristics of benign and malignant nodules.

Many symptoms and signs of thyroid disease have been evaluated for their sensitivity and specificity. Most of these findings are specific but are too insensitive to make them useful. Table 7–4 summarizes the operating characteristics of certain findings in the evaluation of a thyroid nodule for malignancy. The most useful signs are a palpable, hard nodule and a fixed mass.

The heavy, puffy-faced, lethargic patient with dry skin, sparse hair, and a hoarse voice provides the classic picture of hypothyroidism. Hypothyroidism develops insidiously. Often the only complaint is a tired or "run down" feeling. The careful interviewer and examiner must be on the alert for any patient, especially older than the age of 60 years, with these symptoms. Patients with hypothyroidism commonly have *hung,* or delayed, reflexes. The measurement of the relaxation time of the Achilles tendon reflex has long been used to follow the effect of treatment in patients with hypothyroidism. However, it is useless as a screening technique because there may be many false-negative or false-positive results.

Table 7–5 lists some of the major symptoms and signs of hypothyroidism.

Table 7–2   Distinctive Features of Graves' Disease and Plummer's Disease

Feature	Graves' Disease (Toxic Diffuse Goiter*)	Plummer's Disease (Toxic Adenomatous Goiter†)
Age of onset	40 years	40 years
Onset	Acute	Insidious
Goiter	Diffuse	Nodular
Signs/symptoms	Clear-cut	Vague
Myopathy (muscle disease)	Present	Absent
Heart involvement	Sinus tachycardia Occasionally atrial fibrillation	Frequently atrial fibrillation Congestive heart failure
Ophthalmopathy	Exophthalmos Vision changes Motility abnormalities Chemosis (conjunctival edema)	Eyelid lag Eyelid retraction

* See Figures 7–6 and 7–15.
† See Figure 7–7.

Table 7–3   Characteristics of Benign and Malignant Thyroid Nodules

Characteristic	Benign Nodule	Malignant Nodule
Age of onset	Adult	Adult
Gender	Female	Male
Patient history	Symptoms present	Previous x-ray treatment to head or neck
Family history	Benign thyroid diseases	None
Speed of enlargement	Slow	Rapid
Change in voice	Absent	Present
Number of nodules	More than one	One
Lymph nodes	Absent	Present
Remainder of thyroid	Abnormal	Normal

Table 7–4   Characteristics of Thyroid Nodules Suspicious for Cancer*

Characteristic	Sensitivity (%)	Specificity (%)
Palpable, hard nodule	42	89
Fixed mass	31	94
Local symptoms	3	97
Dysphagia	10	93
Unilateral adenopathy	5	96
Nodule found on routine examination	50	56
Family history of goiter	17	79

* Data from Kendall and Condon, 1976; and Haff et al, 1976.

Table 7–5   Symptoms and Signs of Hypothyroidism

System	Symptom	Sign
General	Weight gain with regular diet Chilly while others are warm	Obesity
Gastrointestinal	Constipation	Enlarged tongue
Cardiovascular	Fatigue	Hypotension Bradycardia
Nervous	Speech disorders Short attention span Tremor	Hyporeflexia Defective abstract reasoning Spasticity Tremor Depressed affect
Musculoskeletal	Lethargy Thickened, dry skin Hair loss Brittle nails Leg cramps Puffy eyelids Puffy cheeks	Hypotonia Puffy facies
Reproductive	Heavier menses Decreased fertility	

Useful Vocabulary

Listed here are the specific roots that are important in order to understand the terminology related to diseases of the head and neck.

Root	Pertaining to	Example	Definition
capit-	head	*capit*ate	Head-shaped
cephal(o)-	head	*cephalo*metry	Measurement of the head
cleido-	clavicle	*cleido*mastoid	Pertaining to the clavicle and mastoid process
cranio-	skull	*cranio*malacia	Abnormal softening of the skull
occipito-	back portion of the skull	*occipito*parietal	Pertaining to the occipital and parietal bones
odont(o)-	tooth; teeth	*odont*orrhagia	Hemorrhage following tooth extraction
thyro-	thyroid gland	*thyro*megaly	Enlargement of the thyroid gland

Writing Up the Physical Examination

Listed here are examples of the write-up for the examination of the head, neck, and thyroid.

- The head is normocephalic without evidence of trauma. The neck is supple, with full range of motion. No adenopathy is present in the neck. The thyroid is nontender and is not enlarged. No thyroid nodules are felt.
- The head is normocephalic and atraumatic. There is a 2 cm, rubbery, nontender mass in the superficial cervical chain on the left side. The mass is freely mobile and is not fixed to the skin or underlying muscle. Another 4 cm, rubbery, nontender mass is felt in the right supraclavicular fossa. The thyroid is unremarkable.
- There is frontal bossing of the head with prominence of the cheek bones. There is no evidence of trauma. The neck is supple, with no adenopathy present. There is a 2 cm, soft, painless thyroid nodule felt 3 cm from the midline in the upper portion of the right lobe (approximately at 10 o'clock). The nodule is not fixed to the overlying skin or muscles.

Bibliography

Haff RC, Schecter BC, Armstrong RG, et al: Factors increasing the probability of malignancy in thyroid nodules. Am J Surg 131:707, 1976.

Kendall LW, Condon RE: Prediction of malignancy in solitary thyroid nodules. Lancet 1:1019, 1976.

Vaughan CW, Homburger F, Shapshay SM, et al: Carcinogenesis in the upper aerodigestive tract. Otolaryngol Clin North Am 13:403, 1980.

Wallace C, Siminoski K: The Pemberton sign. Ann Intern Med 125:568, 1996.

Werner SC, Ingbar SH (eds): The Thyroid: A Fundamental and Clinical Text. New York, Harper & Row, 1971.

CHAPTER 8

The Eye

*Who would believe that so small a space could contain the images of all the universe?
O mighty process!*

Leonardo da Vinci
1452–1519

Historical Considerations

The eyes are the human windows to the world. Most of the sensory input to the brain is through the eyes. For centuries, the eye has been considered the essence of the person, representing the "I." In mythology and the writings of ancient times, the eye is an organ associated with mystical powers.

The eye has long been associated with mythical gods. In ancient Egypt, the eye was the symbol of the Great Goddess. The Eye of Horus was believed to protect against all evil and to ensure success. The "evil eye" from the myth of Medusa was an expression of envy and greed.

Another interesting association is the subconscious linking of "eyeball" with genitalia. Blindness can symbolize castration, as testicles and eyeballs have the same shape and are important in the development of the sense of identity. This linking goes back to the legend of Oedipus, who pierced his eyeballs when he discovered that he had been married to his mother and had killed his father. This can be thought of as an act of self-castration as well as a means of cutting oneself off from all worldly relationships. Throughout literature, the blinding of an individual was frequently a form of punishment for lust. The age-old notion that masturbation will cause blindness serves to further reinforce this close association of organs.

Structure and Physiology

The external landmarks of the eye are shown in Figure 8–1, and the cross-sectional anatomy of the eye is shown in Figure 8–2.

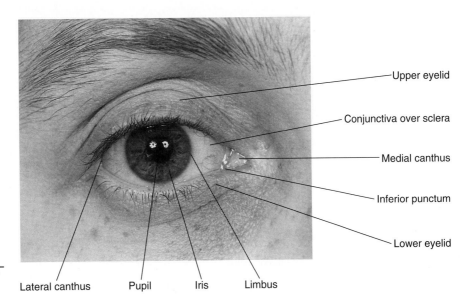

Figure 8–1

External landmarks of the eye.

Upper eyelid

Conjunctiva over sclera

Medial canthus

Inferior punctum

Lower eyelid

Lateral canthus   Pupil   Iris   Limbus

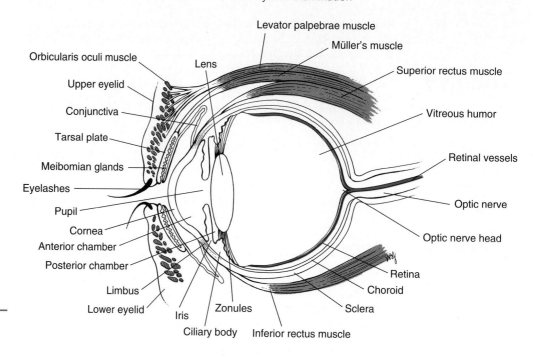

Figure 8–2

Cross-sectional anatomy of the eye.

The *eyelids* and *eyelashes* serve to protect the eyes. The eyelids cover the globe and lubricate its surface. The *meibomian* glands, which are modified sebaceous glands in the eyelids, secrete an oily lubricating substance to retard evaporation. The openings of these glands are at the lid margins.

The *orbicularis oculi* muscle encircles the lids and is responsible for their closure. This muscle is supplied by the facial, or seventh cranial, nerve. The *levator palpebrae* muscle serves to elevate the lids and is innervated by the oculomotor, or third cranial, nerve. Müller's muscle is a small part of the levator muscle, having sympathetic innervation.

The globe has six *extraocular muscles* that control its motion. There are four rectus and two oblique muscles: the medial rectus, the lateral rectus, the superior rectus, the inferior rectus, the superior oblique, and the inferior oblique muscles. These six extraocular muscles are shown in Figure 8–3.

The extraocular muscles work in a parallel, conjugate manner to maintain single, binocular vision. When the head is turned to look left, for example, the *left lateral*

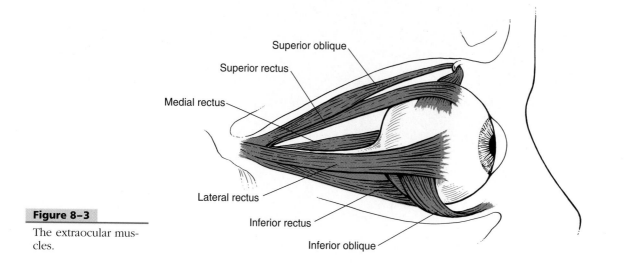

Figure 8–3

The extraocular muscles.

rectus and the *right medial rectus* contract to turn the eyes to the left. The actions and innervations of the extraocular muscles are demonstrated in Table 8–1, and the extraocular movements are illustrated in Figure 8–4.

The *lateral rectus* muscle, which is innervated by the *abd*ucens nerve, *abd*ucts the eye (turns it laterally), as do both oblique muscles.

The *conjunctiva* is a thin, vascular, transparent mucous membrane that lines the lids and the anterior portion of the globe continuously. The *palpebral* portion covers the inner surface of the lids, whereas the *bulbar* portion covers the sclera up to the *limbus,* which is the corneal-scleral junction. The conjunctiva contains many small blood vessels, which when dilated produce a "red" eye. There is little nervous innervation to the conjunctiva.

The *lacrimal apparatus* consists of the lacrimal gland, accessory tear glands, canaliculi, tear sac, and nasolacrimal duct. These are shown in Figure 8–5.

Table 8–1   Actions and Innervations of the Extraocular Muscles*

Muscle	Action	Cranial Nerve Innervation
Medial rectus	Adduction (eye moves nasally)	Oculomotor (III)
Lateral rectus	Abduction (eye moves temporally [away from the nose])	Abducens (VI)
Inferior rectus	Depression (eye moves down) Extorsion (the 12 o'clock position on the cornea rotates temporally) Adduction	Oculomotor (III)
Superior rectus	Elevation (eye moves up) Intorsion (the 12 o'clock position on the cornea rotates nasally) Adduction	Oculomotor (III)
Superior oblique	Intorsion Depression Abduction	Trochlear (IV)
Inferior oblique	Extorsion Elevation Abduction	Oculomotor (III)

* Remember "LR$_6$SO$_4$." This mnemonic states that the lateral rectus (LR) muscle is innervated by the sixth cranial nerve, and the superior oblique (SO) muscle is innervated by the fourth cranial nerve. All the other muscles are innervated by the third cranial nerve.

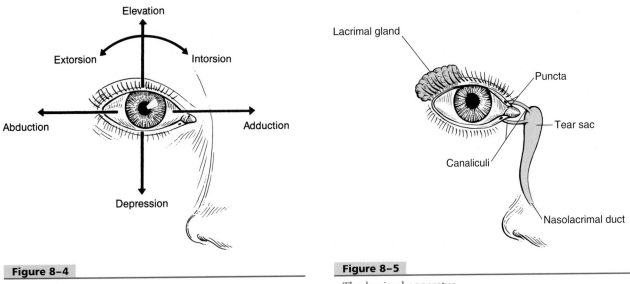

Figure 8–4

Extraocular movements.

Figure 8–5

The lacrimal apparatus.

The *lacrimal gland* produces watery tears and is located above and slightly lateral to the globe. Secretion occurs mostly as reflex tearing or crying. Tears drain through the *puncta* on the lids and into the superior and inferior *canaliculi.* These canaliculi join and enter the *tear sac,* located at the medial *canthus* of the eye. The *nasolacrimal duct* drains the sac to the nose. Of the lacrimal apparatus, only the *puncta* are visible on routine examination.

The *sclera* is the white, fibrous, outer coat of the globe visible just beneath the conjunctiva. The extraocular muscles insert into the sclera.

The *cornea* is a smooth, transparent, avascular tissue that covers the iris and joins with the sclera and conjunctival reflection at the limbus. The cornea functions as a protective window, allowing light to pass into the eye. The cornea is richly innervated by the trigeminal, or fifth cranial, nerve and is therefore exquisitely sensitive to touch.

The *anterior chamber,* or space between the cornea anteriorly and the iris posteriorly, is filled with clear *aqueous humor.* Aqueous humor is produced by the *ciliary body* in the *posterior chamber,* the area behind the iris and in front of the lens. Aqueous humor circulates from the posterior chamber through the pupil into the anterior chamber and is removed through the *canal of Schlemm,* from where it eventually enters the venous system. Pressure within the eye is regulated by this filtration. The *angle* is that formed by the juncture of the cornea and the iris at the lumbus. A section through the eye at this level is shown in Figure 8–6.

The *iris* is the circular, colored portion of the eye. The small, round aperture in the middle of the iris is the *pupil.* The pupil functions much as the aperture of a camera, controlling the amount of light that enters the eye.

When a light is shined on one eye, both pupils constrict consensually. This constriction is the *pupillary light reflex.* In order to understand this reflex, a brief review of the neuroanatomy is in order. Figure 8–7 illustrates the pathways of the pupillary light reflex.

The optic, or second cranial, nerves are composed of 80% *visual* and 20% afferent *pupillary* fibers. The optic nerves leave both retinae and travel a short course to where they join each other. This joining is the *optic chiasm.* At the optic chiasm, the nasal fibers cross and join the uncrossed fibers of the other side, forming the *optic tract.* The *visual* fibers continue in the optic tract to the *lateral geniculate body,* where synapses occur, the axons of which terminate in the primary visual cortex of the occipital lobe. The afferent pupillary fibers bypass the geniculate body and end in the *superior colliculus* and *pretectal* area of the midbrain.

Light impulses to the eye cause the retina to transmit nerve impulses to the optic nerve, the optic tract, the midbrain, and the visual cortex of the occipital lobes. This is the *afferent limb* of the light reflex. In the midbrain, the pupillary fibers diverge and are relayed by crossed fibers to the opposite *Edinger-Westphal* nucleus of the oculomotor, or third cranial, nerve. Some fibers remain on the same side. The third cranial nerve is the *efferent limb,* which goes via the ciliary body to the sphincter muscle of the iris to cause it to contract. The *direct effect* is the constriction of the pupil of the eye upon which the light is shined (the *ipsilateral eye*). The *consensual effect* is the simultaneous constriction of the opposite pupil (the *contralateral eye*).

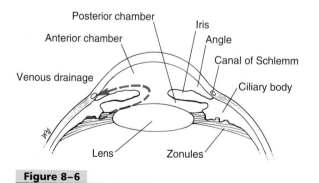

Figure 8–6

Cross section of the normal-angle structures, showing the flow of aqueous humor.

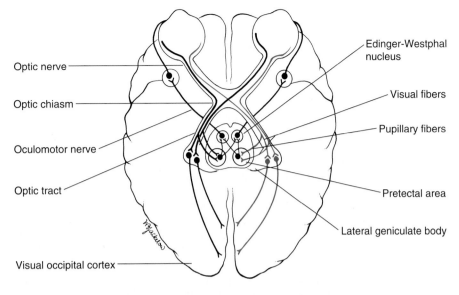
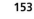

Optic nerve

Optic chiasm

Oculomotor nerve

Optic tract

Edinger-Westphal nucleus

Visual fibers

Pupillary fibers

Pretectal area

Lateral geniculate body

Visual occipital cortex

Figure 8–7

The pupillary light reflex.

The *near reflex* occurs when the subject looks at a near target. The three parts of the near reflex are *accommodation, convergence,* and *pupillary constriction*. Accommodation is defined as the near focusing of the eye, which is effected by increasing the power of the lens by contraction of the ciliary muscle, innervated by the third cranial nerve.

There is also autonomic innervation of the eyes. The iris is supplied by sympathetic and parasympathetic fibers. When the sympathetic fibers are stimulated, pupillary dilatation occurs, as does elevation of the eyelid. Think of the cat stalking its prey, pupils dilated, ready to pounce in the dark. The cat needs all the light it can get. The reflex is purely sympathetic. When the parasympathetic fibers in the oculomotor nerve are stimulated, pupillary constriction occurs.

The *choroid* is the middle, vascular layer of the globe. It acts as a source of nourishment as well as a heat sink, serving to remove the extreme heat produced by the light energy entering the eye.

The *lens* sits directly behind the iris. It is a biconvex, avascular, colorless structure that changes its shape to focus the image upon the retina. The shape is changed by the *ciliary body muscles.*

The *vitreous humor* is the transparent, avascular gel that is located behind the lens and in front of the retina.

The *retina* is the innermost layer, or "camera film," of the eye. Within the retina are several important structures: the optic disc, the retinal vessels, and the macula. Figure 8–8 illustrates the retina.

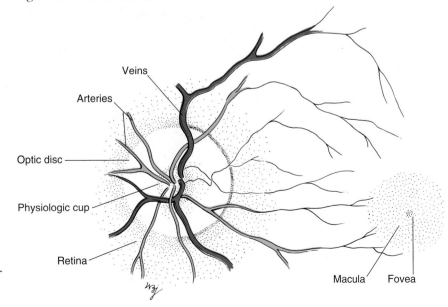

Veins

Arteries

Optic disc

Physiologic cup

Retina

Macula   Fovea

Figure 8–8

The retina of the left eye.

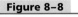

The *optic disc* is located at the nasal aspect of the posterior pole of the retina. This is the head of the optic nerve, from where the nerve fibers of the retina exit the eye. The optic disc is 1.5 mm in diameter and is ovoid. It is lighter than the surrounding retina and appears yellowish-pink. The disc margins are sharp with some normal blurring of the nasal portion. African-American patients may have pigmentation at the margins. The *physiologic cup* is the center of the disc, where the retinal vessels penetrate. This small depression occupies about 30% of the disc diameter.

The *retinal vessels* emerge from the disc and arborize on the retinal surface. The arteries are brighter red and thinner than the veins. An artery-to-vein ratio of 2:3 is normal.

The *macula* is a small, round area, approximately the size of the disc, located 3.5 mm temporal to and 0.5 mm inferior to the disc. The macula is easily seen because it is devoid of retinal vessels. In the center of the macula is the *fovea,* a depressed area composed only of *cones*. Cones provide detailed vision and color perception.

The remaining areas of the retina contain mostly *rods,* which compose the other neurosensory element of the retina. The rods are responsible for motion detection and night vision. It should be remembered that the image on the retina is upside down and reversed left to right. The right world is projected on the left half of the retina. The left world is projected on the right half of the retina. An image in the superior world will strike the inferior part of the retina, and vice versa. This concept is shown in Figure 8–9.

At birth, there is little pigment in the iris, which is why all babies are born with blue eyes. By 6 months, the pigmentation is completed. The lens is more spherical at birth than in later life. Most infants are born hyperopic (farsighted). By 3 months after birth, the medullation process of the optic nerve is completed. As the child grows, hyperopia increases until the age of 8 years and then gradually decreases. After age 8, myopia (nearsightedness) appears to increase.

With advancing age, there is the gradual loss of elasticity of the skin around the eyes. The cornea may show an infiltration of degenerative material around the limbus, which is known as an *arcus senilis*. The lens consistency changes from plastic to rigid, making it progressively more difficult to change its shape in order to focus on near objects. This condition is *presbyopia*. The lens may undergo changes resulting from metabolic disorders that cause its opacification; this condition is called a *cataract.* The vitreous humor may develop condensations, called *floaters.* The retinal arteries may develop *atherosclerosis,* with resultant retinal ischemia or infarction.

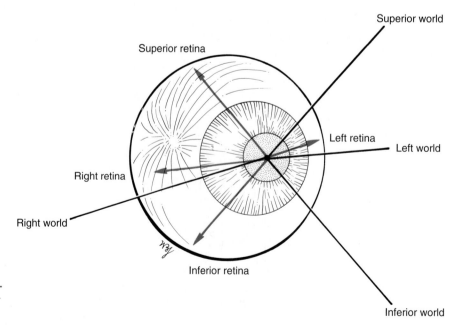

Figure 8–9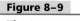

The images on the retina.

Review of Specific Symptoms

The major symptoms of eye disease are the following:

- Loss of vision
- Eye pain
- Diplopia (double vision)
- Tearing or dryness
- Discharge
- Redness

Loss of Vision

When a patient complains of loss of vision, the following two questions must be asked:

"Did the loss of vision occur suddenly?"
"Is the eye painful?"

It is extremely important to ascertain the acuteness of the loss of vision and the presence or absence of pain. Sudden painless loss of vision may result from a retinal vascular occlusion or a retinal detachment. Sudden painful loss of vision occurs in attacks of acute narrow angle glaucoma. Gradual painless loss of vision commonly occurs in chronic simple glaucoma.

Eye Pain

Eye pain may result from a variety of causes. Ask the patient the following questions:

"Can you describe the pain?"
"Did the pain come on suddenly?"
"Does the light bother your eye?"
"Do you have pain when you blink?"
"Do you have the sensation of something in the eye?"
"Do you have headaches?"
"Do you have pain on movement of the eye?"
"Do you have pain over the brow on the same side?"

Pain may be experienced as "burning," "throbbing," "tenderness," or a "drawing sensation." Each of these descriptions may have a range of causes. It is important to determine whether the patient has the sensation of a foreign body in the eye. Pain in the eye while blinking occurs in corneal abrasions and with foreign bodies in the eye. *Photophobia* is eye pain associated with light, as seen in inflammations of the iris and the middle layer of the eye. Inflammations of the conjunctiva, *conjunctivitis,* produce a gritty sensation. Diseases of the cornea are associated with significant pain because the cornea is so richly innervated. Headaches and eye pain are commonly seen in acute narrow-angle glaucoma. Pain on motion of the eye occurs in optic neuritis. Eye pain associated with brow or temporal pain may be an indication of temporal arteritis (see Chapter 23, The Geriatric Patient).

Diplopia

Diplopia, or double vision, is a common complaint. Diplopia results from a faulty alignment of the eyes. Normally, when the eyes fixate on an object, the object is clearly seen despite the fact that the two retinal images are not exactly superimposed. These slightly different images, however, are fused by the brain; it is this fusion that produces *binocular vision,* or the perception of depth. When the eyes are misaligned, the two images fall on different parts of the retinae, only one falling normally on the fovea. The field of vision of the deviated eye is different, so that its image is not projected on its fovea; therefore, this second image will be different and not superimposable. The patient may close one eye to relieve this distressing situation. A compensatory head posture may be used by the patient to relieve the double vision. Elevation or depression of the patient's chin will be used to overcome a vertical deviation. Tilting of the head is often used to counteract the torsional and vertical deviation. Suggested questions for the patient with diplopia are in Chapter 19, The Nervous System.

Tearing or Dryness

Excessive tearing or dryness of the eyes is a common complaint. Abnormal tearing may be caused either by overproduction of tears or by an obstruction of outflow. Dryness results from faulty secretion by the lacrimal or accessory tear glands. A common cause is *Sjögren's syndrome,* which is generalized failure of the secretory glands. This syndrome is associated with a variety of disease states.

Discharge

Discharge from the eye can be watery, mucoid, or purulent. A watery or mucoid discharge is often associated with allergic or viral conditions, whereas a purulent discharge occurs in association with bacterial infections.

Redness

The symptom of the red eye is very common. The interviewer should ask the following questions:

> *"Have you had any injury to the eye?"*
> *"Does anyone else in the family have a red eye?"*
> *"Have you had any recent coughing spells? vomiting?"*
> *"Have you had any associated eye pain?"*
> *"Is there any associated discharge?"*

The eye may appear bloodshot. Redness may result from trauma, infection, allergy, or increased pressure in the eye. Severe coughing spells or recurrent vomiting may cause a patient to have a conjunctival hemorrhage. A family member or friend with viral conjunctivitis may be the source of this patient's red eye. Eye pain and a red eye may indicate acute narrow angle glaucoma. (See Table 8–2 for a summarization of the differential diagnosis for the red eye.)

General Suggestions

It is important to determine the medications that a patient is taking, because many drugs have deleterious effects on the eye. Some antimalarial, antituberculous, antiglaucoma, and anti-inflammatory drugs can cause eye disorders. A thorough family history will reveal familial disease tendencies such as glaucoma, cataracts, retinal degeneration, strabismus, or corneal dystrophies.

There are many specific symptoms related to eye disease. The common visual, nonvisual but painful, and nonvisual and painless symptoms and some possible causes are listed in Tables 8–3, 8–4, and 8–5, respectively.

Impact of Blindness on the Patient

The loss of sight is a terrifying experience. The sighted person lives mostly in a visual and auditory world illuminated by lights and colors. When blindness occurs, the person loses not only the ability to see but also the perceptual center of the world. This center must now be replaced by hearing and touch. Because light is often equated with life, the inability to see light is associated with death. The newly blinded patient must take a new place in society. He or she can no longer read ordinary books, can no longer receive visual stimuli, and is unable to appreciate the world of visual communication. This can result in a reactive depression. The physician must show genuine care for blind patients and try to understand their feelings of discouragement and despair.

The person who is blind from birth or early childhood has little or no conception of the visual world. Having never been able to see, this patient has no frame of reference.

Table 8–2   Differential Diagnosis of Red Eye*

Presentation	Acute Conjunctivitis†	Acute Iritis**	Narrow Angle Glaucoma	Corneal Abrasion
History	Sudden onset Exposure to conjunctivitis	Fairly sudden onset Often recurrent	Rapid onset Sometimes history of previous attack Highest incidence among Jews, Swedes, and the Inuit (Eskimos)	Trauma Pain
Vision	Normal	Impaired if untreated	Rapidly lost if untreated‡	Can be affected if central
Pain	Gritty feeling	Photophobia	Severe	Exquisite
Bilaterality	Frequent	Occasional	Occasional	Usually unilateral
Vomiting	Absent	Absent	Common	Absent
Cornea	Clear (epidemic keratoconjunctivitis has corneal deposits)	Variable	"Steamy" (like looking through a steamy window)	Irregular light reflex
Pupil	Normal, reactive	Sluggishly reactive Sometimes irregular in shape	Partially dilated, oval, nonreactive	Normal, reactive
Iris	Normal	Normal§	Difficult to see, owing to corneal edema	Shadow of corneal defect may be projected on the iris with penlight
Ocular discharge	Mucopurulent or watery	Watery	Watery	Watery or mucopurulent
Systemic effect	None	Few	Many	None
Prognosis	Self-limited	Poor if untreated	Poor if untreated	Good if not infected

* See Figure 8–37.
** See Figure 8–26.
† Can be viral, bacterial, or allergic.
‡ Seeing "rainbow" can be an early symptom during an acute attack.
§ Slit-lamp examination revealing cells in anterior chamber is diagnostic.

Table 8–3   Common Visual Eye Symptoms and Disease States

Visual Symptom	Possible Causes
Loss of vision	Optic neuritis Detached retina Retinal hemorrhage Central retinal vascular occlusion Central nervous system disease
Spots	No pathologic significance*
Flashes	Migraine Retinal detachment Posterior vitreous detachment
Loss of visual field or presence of shadows or curtains	Retinal detachment Retinal hemorrhage
Glare, photophobia	Iritis (inflammation of the iris) Meningitis (inflammation of the meninges)
Distortion of vision	Retinal detachment Macular edema
Difficulty seeing in dim light	Myopia Vitamin A deficiency Retinal degeneration
Colored haloes around lights	Acute narrow angle glaucoma Opacities in lens or cornea
Colored vision changes	Cataracts Drugs (digitalis increases yellow vision)
Double vision	Extraocular muscle paresis or paralysis

* May precede a retinal detachment or may be associated with ingestion of fertility drugs.

Table 8–4   Common Nonvisual, Painful Eye Symptoms and Disease States

Nonvisual, Painful Symptom	Possible Causes
Foreign body sensation	Foreign body Corneal abrasion
Burning	Uncorrected refractive error Conjunctivitis Sjögren's syndrome
Throbbing, aching	Acute iritis (inflammation of the iris) Sinusitis (inflammation of the sinuses)
Tenderness	Eyelid inflammation Conjunctivitis Iritis
Headache	Refractive errors Migraine Sinusitis
Drawing sensation	Uncorrected refractive errors

Table 8–5   Common Nonvisual, Painless Eye Symptoms and Disease States

Nonvisual, Painless Symptom	Possible Causes
Itching	Dry eyes Eye fatigue Allergies
Tearing	Emotional states Hypersecretion of tears Blockage of drainage
Dryness	Sjögren's syndrome Decreased secretion as a result of aging
Sandiness, grittiness	Conjunctivitis
Fullness of eyes	Proptosis (bulging of the eyeball) Aging changes in the lids
Twitching	Fibrillation of orbicularis oculi
Eyelid heaviness	Fatigue Eyelid edema
Dizziness	Refractive error Cerebellar disease Vestibular disease
Excessive blinking	Local irritation Facial tic
Eyelids sticking together	Inflammatory disease of eyelids or conjunctivae

Occasionally, a blind individual recovers sight as a result of a surgical procedure later in life. Many difficulties may arise, owing to the reorganization of the patient's perception. His or her frame of reference has been shifted from touch to sight. Surprisingly, many of these patients become depressed after attaining vision. Facial expressions mean nothing, because only with experience can one understand them. The following quote from a case history illustrates the response of such an individual (Gregory and Wallace, 1963):

> He suffered one of the greatest hardships (blindness) and yet he lived with energy and enthusiasm. When his handicap was apparently swept away, as by a miracle, he lost his peace and self-respect.

Similarly, the patient with normal vision may develop psychosomatic eye problems as a result of anxiety. The loss of vision that can accompany panic disorders should be mentioned. These individuals can have either partial or complete vision loss in one or both eyes. Supportive care of the primary problem usually results in the return of vision.

Physical Examination

> The equipment necessary for the examination of the eye is as follows: an ophthalmoscope, a penlight, a pocket visual acuity card, and a 3 × 5 inch card.

The physical examination of the eye includes the following:

- Visual acuity
- Visual fields
- Ocular movements
- External and internal eye structures
- Ophthalmoscopic examination

Visual Acuity

Visual acuity is expressed as a ratio, such as 20/20. The first number is the distance at which the patient reads the chart. The second number is the distance at which a person with normal vision can read the same line of the chart. The abbreviation OD refers to the right eye; OS refers to the left eye; OU refers to both eyes.*

Using the Standard Snellen Chart

If a standard Snellen eye chart is available, the patient should stand 20 feet from the chart. If the patient wears glasses, he or she should wear them for the examination. The patient is asked to cover one eye with the *palm*† and read the smallest line possible. If the best he or she can see is the 20/200 line, the patient's vision in that eye is 20/200; this means that at 20 feet the patient can see what a person with normal vision can see at 200 feet. If a patient at 20 feet cannot see the 20/200 line, he or she is moved closer until the letters are recognized. If the patient can read these letters at 5 feet, the patient's visual acuity in that eye is 5/200.

Using a Pocket Visual Acuity Card

If the standard Snellen chart is not available, a pocket visual acuity card is helpful. This is viewed at 14 inches. The patient is again asked to read the smallest line possible. If neither eye chart is available, any printed material may be used. The examiner should remember that most patients older than the age of 40 years require reading glasses. Although visual acuity cannot be quantified, whether the patient has any vision can certainly be determined. In such a case, the patient is asked to cover an eye and read the smallest line possible on a given printed page.

Evaluation of Patients with Poor Vision

Patients with poor vision who are unable to read any lines of print should be tested for finger-counting ability. This crude measurement of visual acuity is obtained by holding up fingers in front of one of the patient's eyes with the other eye closed. The patient is then asked how many fingers are seen. If the patient is still unable to see, it is important to evaluate whether he or she has any light perception. This is performed by covering one eye and directing a light at the other eye. The examiner asks the patient whether he or she can see when the light is on and off. *No light perception* (NLP) is the term used when a person cannot perceive light.

Evaluation of Patients Who Cannot Read

For individuals who cannot read, such as young children or the illiterate, the use of the letter "E" in different sizes and directions is helpful. The examiner asks the patient to point in the direction of the letter: up, down, right, left.

Visual Fields

Visual field testing is useful for determining lesions of the visual pathway. Many techniques are used for this purpose. The examiner should learn to perform the

---

* Abbreviations are Latin: OD = *oculus dexter*; OS = *oculus sinister*; OU = *oculus uterque*.
† Always ask a patient to cover the eye with the palm. When fingers are used to cover the eye, a patient may peek between the fingers.

technique known as *confrontation visual field testing*. In this technique, the examiner compares his or her peripheral vision with that of the patient.

■ Assess Fields by Confrontation Testing

The examiner stands or sits 3 feet in front of and at eye level with the patient. The patient is asked to close the right eye while the examiner closes the left eye, each fixating on the other's nose. The examiner holds up fists with the palms facing him or her. The examiner then shows one or two fingers on each hand simultaneously and asks the patient how many fingers he or she sees. The hands are moved from the upper to the lower quadrants, and the examination is repeated. The examination is then repeated, with the other eye of the patient and examiner. The fingers should be seen by both patient and examiner simultaneously. To position the patient to better advantage, the hands are held up slightly closer to the examiner. This provides a wider field for the patient. If the examiner can see the fingers, the patient can see them unless he or she has a field deficit. This technique for examining the patient's right eye is shown in Figure 8–10.

Because lesions along the visual pathway develop insidiously, the patient may not be aware of any changes in visual fields until late in the course of the disease. Confrontation fields, performed by the internist, may provide the first objective evidence that the patient has a lesion involving the visual pathway. An area of depressed vision is called a *scotoma*.

The normal central vision extends approximately 30° in all directions of central fixation. The *blind spot* is the physiologic scotoma located about 15–20° temporal to central fixation, corresponding to the optic nerve head. There are no sensory elements such as the rods or cones that are located on the nerve head.

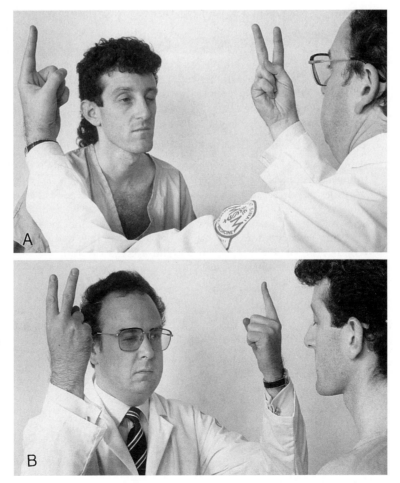

Figure 8–10

Confrontation visual field testing. *A,* View of the patient during examination of the upper fields of the patient's right eye. *B,* Position of the examiner during examination of the upper fields of the patient's right eye.

Visual Field Abnormalities

Pathologic scotomata may be appreciated on visual field testing. Scotomata may result from primary ocular disease, such as glaucoma, or from lesions in the central nervous system, such as tumors. Figure 8–11 illustrates some of the common defects.

Total loss of vision in one eye is a *blind* eye, resulting from a disease of the eye or a lesion of its optic nerve.

Hemianopsia refers to absence of half of a visual field. A defect in both temporal fields is termed *bitemporal hemianopsia*. It results from a lesion involving the optic nerves at the level of the optic chiasm. Pituitary tumors are common causes.

A *homonymous hemianopsia* results from damage to the optic tract, optic radiation, or occipital cortex. The term *homonymous* indicates that the visual loss is in similar fields. A patient with a left homonymous hemianopsia is unable to see the left half of the fields of both eyes. This defect occurs with damage to the right optic tract. Homonymous hemianopsia is the most common form of field loss and occurs frequently in patients with strokes.

A *quadrantanopsia* is a field loss in one quadrant. A patient with a left upper homonymous quadrantanopsia has damage to the right lower optic radiations or the right lower occipital region.

Tunnel vision may occur in advanced glaucoma. However, the visual fields enlarge with increasing testing distance, in contrast to hysteria, in which the field size typically remains the same at all times.

Assess Optokinetic Nystagmus

Occasionally, a patient with psychiatric problems may feign blindness. A useful test to rule out such malingering involves *optokinetic nystagmus* (OKN). OKN is the rapid alternating motion of the eyes that occurs when the eyes try to fixate on a moving

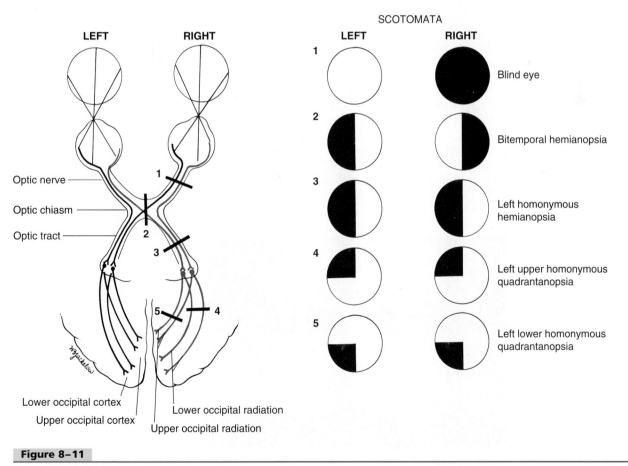

Figure 8–11

Visual field defects.

target. For example, observe the eyes of a person riding a train as it enters the station. The eyes move rapidly back and forth as the person tries to fixate on a station sign. The presence of OKN indicates physiologic continuity of the optic pathways from the retina to the occipital cortex. OKN may be elicited in the examining room by having the patient fixate on the numbers on a tape measure while you rapidly pull out the tape. Because OKN is involuntary, a positive response provides excellent verification that the patient is feigning blindness.

Ocular Movements

Ocular movements are effected by the contraction and relaxation of the extraocular muscles. This results in simultaneous movement of the eyes up or down or from side to side as well as in convergence.

▣ Assess Eye Alignment

Alignment of the eyes is seen by observing the location of reflected light on the cornea. The penlight should be held directly in front of the patient. If the patient is looking straight ahead into the distance, the light reflex should be in the center of each cornea. If the light falls in the corneal center of one eye but is displaced away from the corneal center in the other eye, *deviation* of the eye exists.

The condition of a deviated, or crossed, eye is *strabismus,* or tropia. Strabismus is the nonalignment of the eyes in such a way that the object being observed is not projected simultaneously on the fovea of each eye. *Esotropia* is deviation of an eye nasally; *exotropia* is deviation of an eye temporally; *hypertropia* is deviation upward. An *alternating tropia* is the term used to describe the condition in which either eye deviates. Figure 8–12 shows a patient with a left exotropia.

▣ Perform the Cover Test

The cover test is useful for determining whether the eyes are straight or a deviated eye is present. The patient is instructed to look at a distant target. One eye is covered with a 3 × 5 inch card. The examiner should observe the uncovered eye. If the uncovered eye moves to take up fixation of the distant point, that eye was not straight before the other eye was covered. If the eye did not move, it was straight. The test is then repeated with the other eye.

▣ Evaluate the Diagnostic Positions of Gaze

An important cause of a deviated eye is *paretic* (weak), or paralyzed, extraocular muscle(s). Paralysis of these muscles is detected by examination of the *six diagnostic positions of gaze.* Hold the patient's chin steady with the right hand, and ask the patient to follow the left hand tracing a large "H" in the air. Hold the left index finger about 10 inches from the patient's nose. From the midline, move the finger about a foot to the patient's right and pause; then up about 8 inches and pause, as shown in

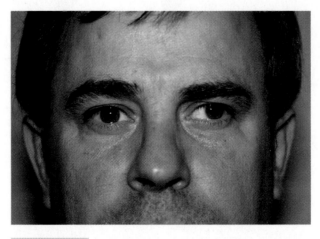

Figure 8–12

Left exotropia.

Figure 8–13; down about 16 inches and pause; and then slowly back to the midline. Cross the midline and repeat the finger movement on the other side. These are the six diagnostic positions of gaze. Observe the movement of both eyes, which should follow the finger smoothly. Look for the parallel movements of the eyes in all directions.

Occasionally when looking to the extreme side, the eyes develop a rhythmic motion called *end-point nystagmus*. There is a quick motion in the direction of gaze, which is followed by a slow return. This test differentiates end-point nystagmus from pathologic nystagmus, in which the quick movement is always in the same direction, regardless of gaze.

If the eye and eyelid do not move together, *lid lag* is present.

The six diagnostic positions of gaze are shown in Figure 8–14, and Table 8–6 summarizes the abnormal ocular motility that is caused by paretic muscles.

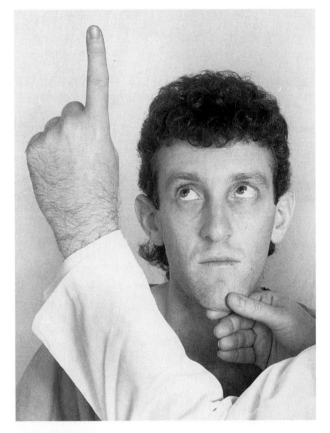

Figure 8–13

Technique for testing ocular motility.

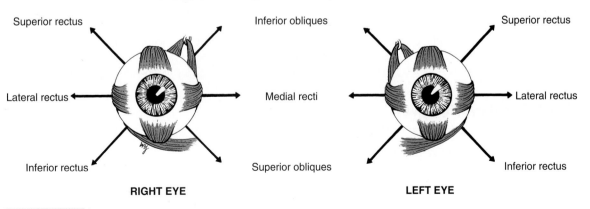

Figure 8–14

Diagnostic positions of gaze. Because the rotational actions of the obliques and vertical recti cannot be assessed, the eye must be moved into the gaze positions to maximize their vertical actions to test their innervations. The oblique muscles are tested in adduction to maximize their vertical action. The vertical recti muscles are tested in abduction, with the superior acting now as a pure elevator and the inferior as a pure depressor.

Table 8–6   Paretic Muscles Causing Abnormal Ocular Motility

Paretic Muscle	Position to Which Eye Will Not Turn
Medial rectus	Nasal
Inferior oblique	Up and nasal
Superior oblique	Down and nasal
Lateral rectus	Temporal
Superior rectus	Up and temporal
Inferior rectus	Down and temporal

The images projected on the retina may be interpreted by the brain in one of three ways: fusion, diplopia, or suppression. Fusion and diplopia have already been discussed. In children, strabismus leads to diplopia, which leads to confusion, then *suppression* of the image, and finally *amblyopia*. Amblyopia is the loss of visual acuity secondary to suppression. Amblyopia is reversible until the retinae are fully developed at about the age of 7 years. Amblyopia is a phenomenon that occurs only in children. An adult who acquires strabismus secondary to a stroke, for example, cannot suppress the deviated eye's image and will have diplopia.

Evaluate the Pupillary Light Reflex

The examiner should ask the patient to look in the distance while he or she shines a bright light in the patient's eye. The light source should come from the side, the nose being used as a barrier to light to the other eye. The examiner should observe the direct and consensual pupillary responses. The examiner then repeats the test on the other eye.

The *swinging light test* is a modification for testing the pupillary light reflex. This test reveals differences in the response to afferent stimuli of the two eyes. The patient fixates on a distant target while the examiner rapidly swings a light from one eye to the other, observing for constriction of the pupils. In some conditions, there is a paradoxical dilatation of the pupil on which the light is shone. This condition, called a *Marcus Gunn pupil,* is associated with an afferent limb defect in the eye being illuminated.

The most extreme example of an eye displaying the Marcus Gunn phenomenon is a blind eye. When light is shined into the blind eye, there is neither a direct nor a consensual response. When the light is moved to the other eye, there is both a direct and a consensual response because both afferent and efferent pathways are normal. When the light is swung back to the blind eye, no impulses are received by the retina (afferent), and the pupil of the blind eye no longer remains constricted; it dilates. There are different degrees of severity of Marcus Gunn pupils, depending on the involvement of the optic nerve.

Evaluate the Near Reflex

The near reflex is tested by having the patient look first at some distant target and then at a target placed about 5 inches away from his or her nose. When the patient focuses on the near target, the eyes should converge, and the pupils should constrict.

External and Internal Eye Structures

The examination of the external eye structures includes the following:

- Eyelids and orbits
- Conjunctiva
- Sclera
- Cornea
- Pupils
- Iris
- Depth of the anterior chamber
- Lens
- Lacrimal apparatus

■ **Inspect the Eyelids and Orbits**

Examine the eyelids for evidence of drooping, infection, erythema, swelling, crusting, tumors, or other abnormalities. In *herpes zoster ophthalmicus* there are rows of vesicles, ulcers, and crusted scabs that are scattered along the course of one or more of the branches of the ophthalmic division of the trigeminal facial nerve. Pain can be excruciating. See Figure 8–15, which shows a patient with acquired immunodeficiency syndrome (AIDS) and herpes zoster ophthalmicus.

Is orbital pigmentation present? Orbital pigmentation, also known as *raccoon eyes,* is an important sign of an orbital fracture. This discoloration is caused by extravasated blood from the fracture of the base of the brain. This is an important sign to recognize, especially in an unconscious patient, when a history may not be attainable. Figure 8–16 shows a patient with an orbital floor fracture. Notice the subconjunctival hemorrhages, which are also frequently present.

Have the patient open and close the eyelids. The motion should be smooth and symmetric.

Inspect the eyelids for *xanthelasma*. Although not specific for hypercholesterolemia, these yellowish plaques are commonly associated with lipid abnormalities and are caused by lipid deposition in the periorbital skin. A patient with xanthelasma is shown in Figure 8–17.

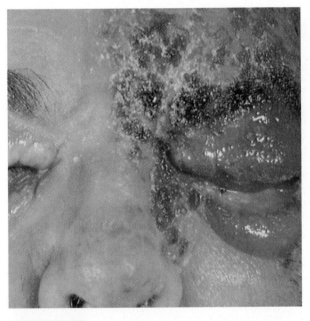

Figure 8–15

Herpes zoster ophthalmicus.

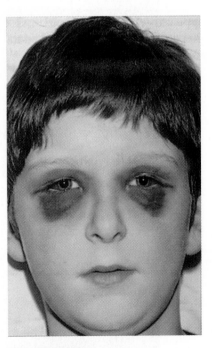

Figure 8–16

Raccoon eyes secondary to an orbital floor fracture.

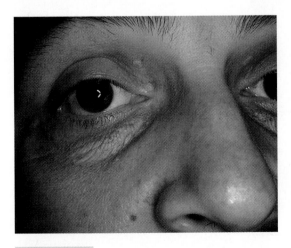

Figure 8–17

Xanthelasma.

A *chalazion* is a chronic granulomatous inflammation of the meibomian gland. It is a localized swelling of the eyelid, generally painless when chronic. Figure 8–18 shows a patient with bilateral chalazions.

A *stye,* or *acute hordeolum,* is a localized abscess in an eyelash follicle and is caused by a staphylococcal infection. It is a painful, red infection that looks like a pimple pointing on the lid margin. *Blepharitis* is a chronic inflammation of the eyelid margins. The most common form is associated with small white scales around the eyelashes, which fall out. This type of blepharitis is often associated with seborrheic dermatitis.

The most common ocular manifestation of AIDS affecting the eyelids is lesions of Kaposi's sarcoma. The initial presentation may be subtle and may be mistaken for blepharitis or a chalazion. Look at Figure 6–72*C*, which shows a patient with AIDS and Kaposi's sarcoma of the eyelid.

When the eye is open, the upper eyelid normally covers only the upper margin of the iris. When the eye is closed, the eyelids should approximate each other completely. The distance between the upper and lower lids is the *palpebral fissure.* Figure 8–19 shows a patient with marked bilateral ptosis and a narrowed palpebral fissure that are due to the muscle-weakening disorder myasthenia gravis.

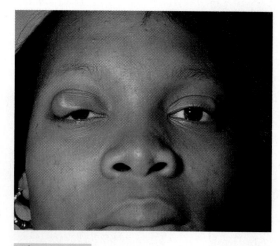

Figure 8–18

Bilateral chalazions.

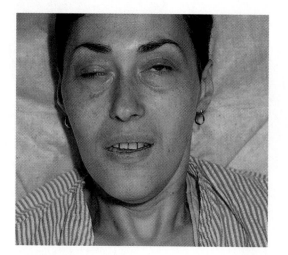

Figure 8–19

Myasthenia gravis.

■ **Inspect the Conjunctiva**

Both conjunctivae should be examined for signs of inflammation (i.e., injection, or dilatation of its blood vessels), pallor, unusual pigmentation, nodes, swelling, and hemorrhage.

The tarsal conjunctiva may be seen by everting the eyelid. Ask the patient to keep the eyes open and look downward. Grasp some of the eyelashes of the upper lid. The eyelid is then pulled away from the globe, and the tip of an applicator stick is pressed against the upper border of the tarsal plate. The tarsal plate is then quickly turned over the applicator stick, using it as a fulcrum. The thumb can now be used for holding the everted lid, and the applicator stick can be removed. After inspection of the tarsal conjunctiva, have the patient look up to return the lid to its normal position.

The normal conjunctiva should be pink. Note the number of blood vessels. Normally, only a small number of vessels are seen. Ask the patient to look up, and pull down on the lower lids. Compare the vascularity in the two eyes. See Figure 8–38.

The conjunctiva is attached to the episclera by loose connections. This potential space can easily be filled with fluids such as blood or serum. *Chemosis* is the presence of fluid in this space. Trauma, allergies, and chronic exposure, as seen in hyperthyroidism and neurologic deficits, are important causes of chemosis. Figure 8–20 shows a patient with chemosis secondary to hay fever.

Two common benign growths on the conjunctiva are the *pinguecula* and *pterygium*. A pinguecula is a whitish-yellow, triangular, nodular growth on the bulbar conjunctiva adjacent to the corneal-scleral junction; it does not cross on to the cornea. A pterygium is a more vascular growth on the bulbar conjunctiva that begins at the medial canthus and extends beyond the corneal-scleral junction to the cornea. This typically triangle-shaped fibrovascular connective tissue may cause astigmatism or even decreased vision if it extends across the pupillary margin. The cause of the pterygium is unknown, but its frequency is higher among people living near the equator. Figure 8–21 shows a patient with a pterygium. Notice its vascularity and position across the limbus.

■ **Inspect the Sclera**

The sclera is examined for nodules, hyperemia, and discoloration. The normal sclera is white. In dark-skinned individuals, the sclera may be slightly muddy in color.

Jaundice, or *icterus,* is a yellowish discoloration of the sclera, skin, and mucous membranes and is caused by retention of bilirubin or its products of metabolism. Jaundice is more easily seen in the sclera of white individuals and may be missed in people of color or in dim light. Carotene may also cause yellowing of the skin but not of the sclera. See Figure 15–5.

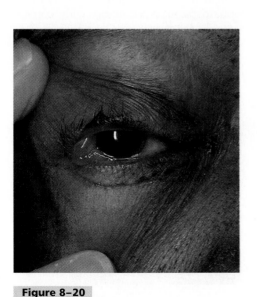

Figure 8–20

Chemosis. Notice the presence of fluid in the subconjunctival space.

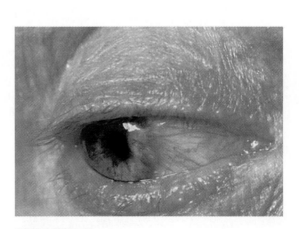

Figure 8–21

Pterygium.

The sclera may appear bluish, normally in infants or pathologically in *osteogenesis imperfecta*. Osteogenesis imperfecta is a group of hereditary disorders with bone fragility. The autosomal dominant form is the most widely recognized form. In this form, the sclerae are very thin and take on a blue hue caused by the uveal pigment shining through the sclera. Individuals with these disorders have bone fractures with little trauma. Deafness is also seen in this form of the disorder. Figure 8–22 shows a patient with osteogenesis imperfecta and blue sclera.

Episcleritis is a benign, usually painless, commonly recurring disorder frequently affecting both eyes of young adults. It is a noninfectious inflammation that is subconjunctival yet superficial to the underlying sclera. The infected area may be either flat and diffuse or localized and nodular (1–4 mm in diameter). Although the cause in most cases is unclear, episcleritis also occurs in patients with inflammatory bowel disease, herpes zoster (7%), collagen vascular disease (5%), gout (3%), syphilis (3%), and rheumatoid arthritis. Figure 8–23 shows a patient with the classic features of episcleritis.

Scleritis is a painful, often bilateral, recurrent, less common disorder than episcleritis that affects the older age groups and occurs in women more often than in men. There is inflammation of the sclera with possible involvement of the cornea, uveal tract (iris, choroid, and ciliary tract), or retina. Scleritis is usually related to a systemic disorder. It occurs much more commonly in patients with connective tissue disorders. The condition may resolve spontaneously.

■ Inspect the Cornea

The cornea should be clear and without cloudiness, ulceration, or opacities.

A whitish ring at the perimeter of the cornea is probably an *arcus senilis*. In patients older than the age of 40 years, this finding is usually a normal aging phenomenon. Although there are many false-positive findings, patients younger than the age of 40 years may have hypercholesterolemia. An arcus senilis is seen in the patient in Figure 8–24.

An abnormal greenish-yellow ring near the limbus, most evident superiorly and inferiorly, is a *Kayser-Fleischer ring*. This ring is a specific and sensitive sign of *Wilson's disease*, which is hepatolenticular degeneration as a result of an inherited disorder of copper metabolism. The Kayser-Fleischer ring is due to deposition of copper in the cornea.

Corneal ulcers are extremely painful lesions due to loss of substance from the cornea by progressive erosion and necrosis of tissue. These ulcers may be caused by a variety of agents, including bacteria, viruses, fungi, and hypersensitivity reactions. *Pneumococcus* is a common bacteria associated with corneal ulceration. *Pseudomonas* infection is less common but is associated with a rapid spread and corneal perforation. Herpes simplex is another common cause of corneal ulceration. Figure 8–25 shows a patient with a corneal ulceration. Marked blepharospasm is common with corneal ulceration.

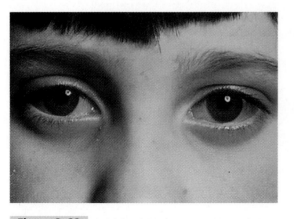

Figure 8–22

Osteogenesis imperfecta and blue sclera.

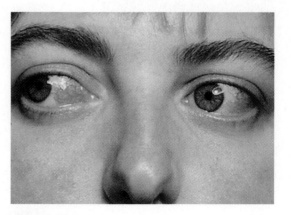

Figure 8–23

Episcleritis.

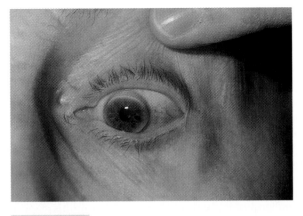

Figure 8-24

Arcus senilis.

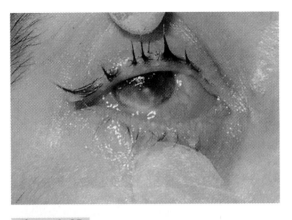

Figure 8-25

Corneal ulceration. Notice the pus in the anterior chamber.

Inspect the Pupils

The pupils should be equal in size, round, and reactive to light and accommodation. In about 5% of normal individuals, pupillary size is not equal; this is called *anisocoria.* Anisocoria may be an indication of neurologic disease. Pupillary enlargement, or *my-driasis,* is associated with ingestion of sympathomimetic agents or with administration of dilating drops. A sluggish, mid-dilated pupil can be seen with acute-angle closure glaucoma. Pupillary constriction, or *miosis,* occurs with ingestion of parasympathomimetic drugs, with inflammation of the iris, and with drug treatment for glaucoma. Many medications can cause anisocoria. It is therefore important to ascertain whether the patient has used any eye drops or has taken any medications.

Pupillary abnormalities are often markers of neurologic disease. A condition known as *Adie's tonic pupil* is a pupil dilated 3-6 mm that constricts little in response to light and accommodation. This pupil is often associated with diminished to absent deep tendon reflexes in the extremities. It occurs more commonly in women 25 to 45 years of age, and the cause is unknown. There are no serious clinical implications. The *Argyll Robertson pupil* is a pupil constricted 1-2 mm that reacts to accommodation but is nonreactive to light. It occurs in association with neurosyphilis. *Horner's syndrome* is sympathetic paralysis of the eye that is due to interruption of the cervical sympathetic chain. In addition to miosis and ptosis, anhidrosis* is also present. Table 8-7 indicates some of the more significant pupillary abnormalities.

Table 8-7   Pupillary Abnormalities

	Adie's Tonic Pupil	Argyll Robertson Pupil	Horner's Syndrome
Laterality	Often unilateral	Bilateral	Unilateral
Reaction to light	Minimally reactive	Nonreactive	Reactive
Accommodation	Sluggishly reactive	Reactive	Reactive
Pupillary size	Mydriatic	Miotic	Miotic
Other signs	Absent or diminished tendon reflexes	Absent knee-jerk reflexes	Slight ptosis† Anhidrosis

† The ptosis is slight, owing to interruption of the sympathetic chain innervating only the Müller's muscle portion of the levator palpebrae. The rest of the levator palpebrae functions normally; thus, ptosis is not severe.

---

* Absence of sweating in this syndrome is related to interruption of the sympathetic chain. The amount of sweating is assessed by examination of the forehead or the axilla of the affected side.

Inspect the Iris

The iris is evaluated for color, nodules, and vascularity. Normally, iris blood vessels cannot be seen with the naked eye or even with slit lamp magnification.

Inflammation of the iris, *iritis* or *iridocyclitis,* is associated with severe pain, photophobia, lacrimation, decreased vision, and circumcorneal congestion. This congestion is due to injection of the deep episcleral vessels (ciliary flush). The dilatation of the iris vessels leads to transudation of protein into the aqueous humor and deposition of inflammatory cells on the corneal endothelium known as keratic precipitates. As a result of this deposition, the iris becomes blurred and loses its distinctive radial appearance and is termed a "muddy iris." There are many causes of iritis, including exogenous infection from perforating injuries; secondary infection from the cornea, sclera, or retina; endogenous infection such as tuberculous, gonorrhea, syphilis, and viral and mycotic infections; and systemic diseases such as rheumatoid arthritis, systemic lupus erythematosis, Reiter's disease, Behçet's syndrome, and relapsing polychondritis. Figure 8–26 show a patient with the classic features of acute iritis.

As a result of the inflammatory reaction of the iris, the iris may adhere to the cornea, forming anterior synechiae; posterior synechiae are adhesions between the iris and lens. Glaucoma is a well-known sequela of iritis and synechiae formation.

Inspect the Depth of the Anterior Chamber

By shining a light obliquely across the eye, a rough estimation of the depth of the chamber can be made. If a crescentic shadow on the far portion of the iris is seen, the anterior chamber may be shallow. *Shallowing* of the anterior chamber refers to the decreased space between the iris and the cornea. The technique for estimating the depth of the anterior chamber is illustrated in Figure 8–27.

The presence of a shallow anterior chamber predisposes an individual to a condition called *narrow-angle glaucoma.* The term *glaucoma* refers to a symptom complex that occurs in a variety of disease states. The characteristic finding in all types of glaucoma is an increased intraocular pressure. This can be measured with the *Schiøtz tonometer,* which is a small, portable instrument used for the quantitative assessment of intraocular pressure. Palpation of the globe to determine intraocular pressure is a technique of low sensitivity. Palpation, if performed incorrectly, may be deleterious, especially in an eye that has been subjected to recent surgery, because a retinal detachment may result. Therefore, palpation of the eye should *not* be performed.

Inspect the Lens

With oblique lighting, inspect the lens. Is the lens clear? Note any opacities that may be visible through the pupil.

The most commonly observed abnormality of the lens is opacification; the most common cause of opacification is aging. Slow, gradual vision loss is the symptom. Other causes include hereditary diseases, such as mongolism and cretinism; ocular diseases, such as high myopia, iritis, and retinal dystrophy; systemic disease, such as diabetes and hypoparathyroidism; medications; and trauma, such as a perforating eye wound.

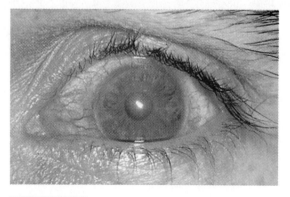

Figure 8–26

Acute iritis.

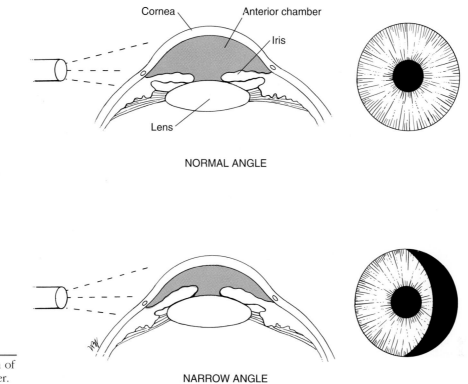

Cornea   Anterior chamber

Iris

Lens

NORMAL ANGLE

NARROW ANGLE

Assessing the depth of
the anterior chamber.

A *cataract* is any opacification of the lens, an opacity that causes reduced visual
acuity, or an opacity that interferes with the patient's everyday life. Figure 8–28 shows
a patient with a cataract of the left eye. Figure 8–29 shows a patient with a dense
nuclear, or central, cataract of the left eye. The red reflex, described in the next section
on ophthalmoscopy, is absent in a patient with a cataractous lens.

▪ Inspect the Lacrimal Apparatus

In general, there is little to be seen of the lacrimal apparatus, with the exception of the
punctum. If tearing, also known as *epiphora,* is present, there may be some obstruction
to flow through the punctum. If excessive moisture is present, check for a blockage of
the nasolacrimal duct by pressing the lacrimal sac gently against the inner orbital rim. If
a blockage is present, material may be expressed through the punctum. Figure 8–30
shows a patient with massive lacrimal gland enlargement as a result of sarcoidosis.

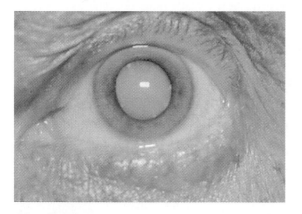

Figure 8–28

Cataract of the left eye.

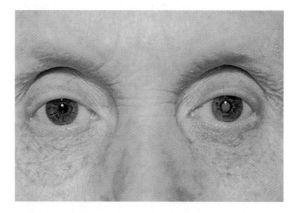

Figure 8–29

Dense nuclear cataract.

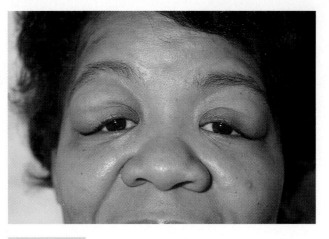

Figure 8–30

Bilateral lacrimal gland enlargement. Notice the classic sigmoid shape of the eyelids.

Ophthalmoscopic Examination

The Ophthalmoscope

Before the examination of the optic fundus is discussed, a few words about the ophthalmoscope are in order. The ophthalmoscope is an instrument with a mirror optical system for viewing the interior anatomy of the eye. There are two dials on the ophthalmoscope: one adjusts the light apertures and filters, and the other changes the lenses to correct for the refractive errors of both the examiner and the patient.

The most important apertures and filters are the *small* aperture, the *large* aperture, and the *red-free* filter. The small aperture is for an undilated pupil; the large aperture is for a dilated pupil; and the red-free filter excludes rays of red light and is designed for visualization of blood vessels and hemorrhages. With this filter, the retina appears gray, the disc appears white, the macula appears yellow, and blood appears black.

Using the Ophthalmoscope

The ophthalmoscope is held in the *right* hand in front of the *right* eye of the examiner in order to examine the *right* eye of the patient. The patient is asked to look straight ahead and fixate on a distant target. If the examiner wears glasses, they should be removed for better visualization of the retina. The ophthalmoscope light is turned on, and the aperture is switched to the small aperture. The examiner should start with the lens diopter* dial set to 0 if he or she does not use glasses. The myopic examiner should start with "minus" lenses, which are indicted by red numbers; the hyperopic examiner needs "plus" lenses, which are indicated by black numbers. The index finger remains on the dial to permit easy focusing.

The ophthalmoscope is placed against the forehead of the examiner while the examiner's left thumb gently elevates the patient's right upper eyelid. The ophthalmoscope and the head of the examiner should function as one unit. The examiner looking through the ophthalmoscope should approach the patient at eye level from about 15 inches away at an angle of about 20° lateral from center, as shown in Figure 8–31. The light should shine on the pupil. A red glow, the *red reflex,* can be seen in the pupil if the path of light is not obstructed by an opaque lens. The examiner should note any opacities in the cornea or lens.

By moving in toward the patient along the same 20° line, the examiner will begin to see the blood vessels of the retina. The examiner should move in close to the

---

* A unit of optical power of a lens to diverge or converge light rays.

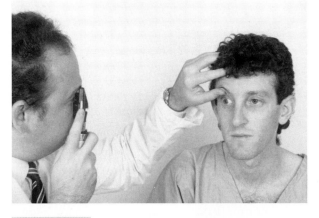

Figure 8–31

Correct position for holding the ophthalmoscope and patient's eye.

patient, bringing the hand holding the ophthalmoscope against the patient's cheek. As contact is made with the patient, the optic disc or vessels will be seen. By rotating the diopter wheel with the index finger, the examiner will bring these structures into sharp focus. Figure 8–32 shows the correct position of the examiner and patient; Figure 8–33 shows a normal optic fundus.

After the right eye is examined, the ophthalmoscope is held in the examiner's *left* hand with the examiner using his or her *left* eye to examine the patient's *left* eye.

Careful assessment of the optic fundus is important for several reasons. The optic fundus is the only area where the blood vessels can be seen *in vivo;* it can provide an excellent idea of the state of the vasculature of other organs. In addition, the optic fundus is frequently involved with manifestations of systemic disease such as AIDS, infectious endocarditis, hypertension, and diabetes; a thorough evaluation of the fundus can provide valuable clues to their diagnosis. Finally, because the eye is an extension

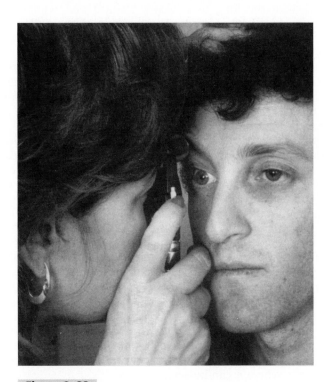

Figure 8–32

Correct position for examining the retina.

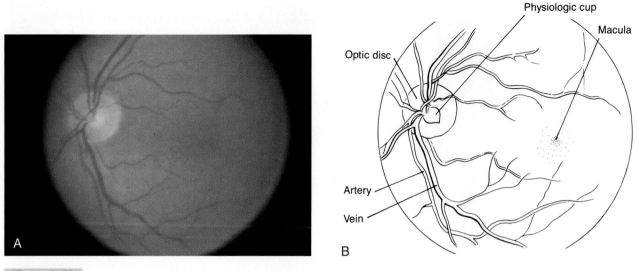

Figure 8-33

A and *B*, Photograph and schematic drawing of landmarks of the retina of the left eye.

of the central nervous system, evaluation of the optic fundus can provide information about many neurologic disorders.

The optic fundus must be assessed methodically, starting at the optic disc, tracing the retinal vessels emerging from it, inspecting the macula, and evaluating the rest of the retina.

Inspect the Optic Disc

The most conspicuous landmark of the retina is the optic disc. The optic disc is the intraocular portion of the optic nerve and is seen with the ophthalmoscope. Its *margins, color,* and *cup-to-disc ratio* should be determined. The disc should be round or slightly oval with the long axis usually vertical and with sharp borders. The nasal border is normally slightly blurred. The disc is pinkish in light-skinned individuals and yellowish-orange in darker-skinned individuals. The relative pallor of the optic disc is caused by the reflection of light from the myelin sheaths of the optic nerve. In the center of the normal optic disc, there is a funnel-shaped depression known as *physiologic cupping.* The cup is the portion of the disc that is central, lighter in color, and penetrated by the retinal vessels. The normal ratio of the cup-to-disc diameter varies from 0.1 to 0.5. The examiner should check the cup-to-disc ratio in both eyes for symmetry.

Myelinated, or *medullated, nerve fibers* is a benign condition seen in 0.3–0.6% of all individuals. In this condition, the nerve fiber layer continues to medullate into the retina beyond the lamina cribrosa. The fibers appear as white patches with feathery borders that radiate from the optic disc and obscure the retinal vessels over which they pass. The condition is present at birth, does not change, and usually causes no visual impairment. Figure 8–34 shows the retina of a patient with medullated nerve fibers.

Inspect the Retinal Vessels

The retinal vessels are evaluated as they arborize over the retina. The central retinal artery enters the globe through the physiologic cup. It divides within the cup and again on the surface, giving rise to four main branches that supply the superior and inferior temporal and nasal quadrants of the optic fundus. The arteries are two thirds to four fifths the size of the veins in diameter and have a prominent *light reflex.* This light reflex is a reflection of the ophthalmoscope's light on the arterial wall and is normally about one quarter the diameter of the column of blood. The veins exhibit spontaneous pulsations in 85% of patients. This can best be demonstrated as the retinal vein enters the optic nerve, where it can be seen on end.

As all the vessels course away from the disc, they appear to narrow. The crossing of the arteries and veins occurs within 2 disc diameters from the disc.

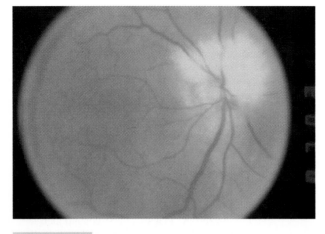

Figure 8–34

Retina with medullated nerve fibers.

The normal vessel wall is invisible, with its thin light reflex. In hypertension, the vessel may have focal or generalized areas of narrowing or spasm, causing the light reflex to be narrowed. With time, the vessel wall becomes thickened and sclerotic, and there is a widening of the light reflex to greater than half of the diameter of the column of blood. The light reflex develops an orange metallic appearance called *copper wiring.* When such an artery crosses over a vein, there appears to be a discontinuity of the venous column as a result of the widened, but invisible, arterial wall. This is termed *arteriovenous nicking.*

Follow the vessels in all four directions: superior temporal, superior nasal, inferior nasal, and inferior temporal. Remember to move your head and the ophthalmoscope as one unit.

Inspect the Macula

When the ophthalmoscope is kept level with the disc and moved temporally about 1.5–2 disc diameters, the macula is seen. This appears as an avascular area with a pinpoint reflective center, the fovea. If the examiner has difficulty in seeing the macula, the patient can be instructed to look directly into the light; the fovea will then be seen. The red-free filter is also helpful in locating the macula.

Describe Any Retinal Lesions

In scanning the fundus, the examiner may detect abnormalities. When a lesion is seen, its color and shape are important in determining its cause. Is it red, black, gray, or whitish? Red lesions are usually hemorrhages. They can be located best by using the green filter of the ophthalmoscope. Linear, or *flame-shaped,* hemorrhages occur in the nerve fiber layer of the retina, whereas round hemorrhages are located in deeper intraretinal layers.

Black lesions that are shaped like bone spicules are associated with retinitis pigmentosa. In this condition, melanin tends to ensheath the retinal vessels. A doughnut-shaped lesion is often found in chronic inactive chorioretinitis. A pigmented, raised, disc-shaped lesion suggests a melanoma. Diffuse spotting of the retina is often a degenerative state. Flat, *gray* lesions are usually benign nevi.

White lesions may appear as soft, cotton-wool areas or may be dense. Soft, cotton-wool spots or exudations are caused by infarctions of the nerve fiber layer of the retina. White lesions are common and are frequently associated with hypertension or diabetes. The differentiation of white lesions of the retina is summarized in Table 8–8.

Difficulties in Using the Ophthalmoscope

Frequently, difficulties arise in the use of the ophthalmoscope. These include the following:

- A small pupil
- Extraneous light

Table 8–8	**Differentiation of Whitish Lesions of the Fundus**			
	Cotton-Wool Spots*	Fatty Exudates†	Drusen‡	Chorioretinitis¶
Etiology§	Hypertension Diabetic retinopathy Acquired immunodeficiency syndrome Lupus erythematosis Dermatomyositis Papilledema	Diabetes mellitus Retinal venous occlusion Hypertensive retinopathy	Can be normal with aging Age-related macular degeneration	Toxoplasmosis Sarcoidosis Cytomegalovirus
Border	Fuzzy	Well defined	Well defined, nonpigmented	Often large with ragged edge, heavily pigmented
Shape	Irregular	Small, irregular	Round, well circumscribed	Very variable
Patterns	Variable	Often clustered in circles or stars	Variable; symmetric in both eyes	Variable
Comments	Caused by an ischemic infarct of the nerve fiber layer of the retina; obscures retinal blood vessels; usually several in number	In deep retinal layer	Often confused with fatty exudates; deep to retinal blood vessels	Acute with white exudate; healed lesion with pigmented scar (toxoplasmosis)

* See Figure 8–39.
† Also known as "edema residues."
‡ Also known as "colloid bodies." See Figure 8–45.
§ The diseases noted do not comprise a complete etiologic list. Only the most common causes are indicated.
¶ See Figures 8–48, 8–49, 8–50, 8–51, and 8–52.

- Improper use of the ophthalmoscope
- Myopia in the patient
- Cataract in the patient

The use of mydriatic drops in order to visualize the retina better is important. Many medical students fear that these drops will precipitate an attack of narrow-angle glaucoma. It is clear from the data that more retinal findings are missed by not dilating the pupils than when the drops precipitate such an attack. Even if the 0.1% of persons who have this reaction should have an attack of glaucoma, they are in the best possible facility for treatment.

The examiner should use one drop of tropicamide 0.5% in each eye. Care should be taken to place the drop on the inside of the lower lid and not on the cornea. The patient should be told that the drop will sting slightly and will cause photophobia in the sunshine. The duration of the mydriatic action depends primarily on the patient's sensitivity to the medication: a more heavily pigmented iris requires more time to achieve mydriasis. The cyclopegic* action lasts for about 6 hours. These drops can be used in patients wearing contact lenses. Atropine should be avoided, because its effect lasts for up to 2 weeks. The large aperture of the ophthalmoscope is used when the eye is dilated. Record in the chart that the patient's eye(s) were dilated and which medications were used.

The room should be darkened as much as possible for the easiest evaluation of the retina. Another common problem is corneal reflection. Often, light is reflected back from the cornea, which makes the examination more difficult. Use of the small aperture or a polarizing filter, which many ophthalmoscopes include, may be helpful.

Patients with myopia provide the most problems for the novice examiner. In myopic eyes, the retinal image is enlarged, making it sometimes difficult to visualize the retina adequately. If the patient is severly myopic, it may be necessary for the patient to wear corrective lenses while being examined.

A cataract does not allow adequate visualization of the retina, especially if the cataract is central.

---

* Producing paralysis of accommodation.

Clinicopathologic Correlations

There are many ophthalmoscopic conditions with which the examiner should be familiar. An image is normally focused directly on the retina. When the image is not focused on the retina, a refractive error is present. Lenses are used to correct refractive errors. The absence of a refractive error is called *emmetropia*. Refractive errors are extremely common. Listed here are the common refractive errors and their causes:

Hyperopia (farsightedness): Light is focused posterior to the retina.
Myopia (nearsightedness): Light is focused anterior to the retina.
Astigmatism: Light is not uniformly focused in all directions. Astigmatism is commonly due to a cornea that is not perfectly spherical.
Presbyopia: Progressive decrease in near vision as a result of a decrease in the eye's ability to accommodate. Presbyopia occurs after age 40 years.

Figure 8–35 illustrates emmetropic, hyperopic, myopic, and astigmatic eyes.

Cataracts are the most common cause of blindness. A cataract is a type of degenerative eye disease. One of the first symptoms that cataract patients experience is a "mistiness" of vision. Patients typically give a history in which vision has become "like looking through a dirty window." As the lenticular opacity increases with time, there is a diminution of visual acuity associated with glare in bright light. This effect is due to pupillary constriction limiting the light rays passing through the lens to the central portion of the lens, where the opacity is often most dense. These patients may wear dark glasses and hold their heads down to avoid excess light.

Narrow-angle glaucoma results from an obstruction to the drainage of aqueous humor at the canal of Schlemm. Patients with narrow-angle glaucoma have periodic attacks of acute elevation of intraocular pressure caused by intermittent obstruction. This is associated with pain, halos, and poor vision. This type of glaucoma commonly occurs in a darkened room, when pupillary dilatation occurs. When the pupil is fully dilated in a person with a narrow angle, the redundant iris folds at its base cause the increased obstruction and decreased drainage.

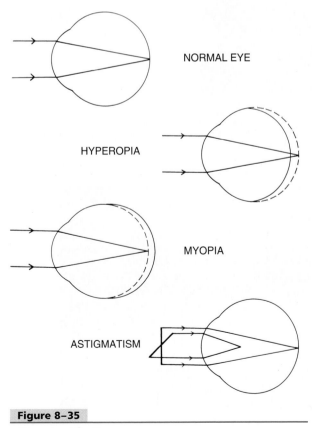

Figure 8–35

Common refractive errors.

Primary open-angle, or chronic simple, glaucoma, in contrast, is associated with an open angle. There are many causes for simple glaucoma, which is a leading cause of slowly progressive blindness. The most important difference diagnostically from narrow-angle glaucoma is that in chronic simple glaucoma, pain is absent. Patients have reduced outflow of aqueous humor through the trabecular meshwork and into the canal of Schlemm, thus resulting in elevated intraocular pressure. As a result, progressive cupping of the optic nerve occurs (i.e., loss of nerve substance), and visual field changes occur. The cup-to-disc ratio increases with loss of symmetry. Peripheral field defects, especially in the nasal aspect, are common early in the disease. As the disease progresses, vision is increasingly impaired. Late in the disease, only a small area on the nasal aspect of the nerve head may remain. Figure 8–36 shows marked glaucomatous cupping of the nerve head with an increased cup-to-disc ratio. Table 8–9 lists the major characteristics of both types of glaucoma.

Acute eye inflammations are common. They may be associated with local or systemic disease. The differential diagnosis of the red eye is important. The presence of pain, visual loss, and irregularities of the pupils are important signs signifying a serious, potentially blinding disorder. Figure 8–37 shows a patient with a red eye. Table 8–2 provides an approach to the diagnosis of the red eye.

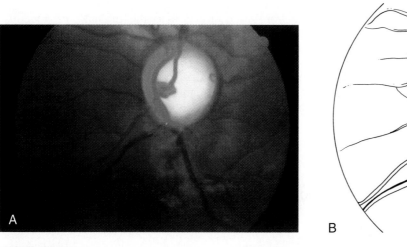
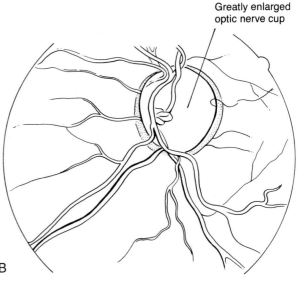

Greatly enlarged optic nerve cup

Figure 8–36

A and *B*, Photograph and labeled schematic showing glaucomatous cupping of the optic nerve head. The cup-to-disc ratio is approximately 85%.

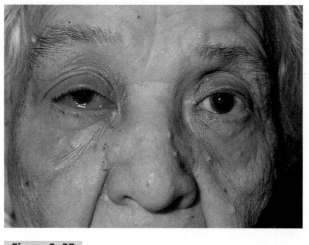

Figure 8–37

Red eye.

Table 8–9   Characteristics of Glaucoma

	Primary Open-Angle Glaucoma	Narrow-Angle Glaucoma
Occurrence	85% of all glaucoma cases	15% of all glaucoma cases
Cause	Unclear*	Closed angle prevents aqueous drainage
Age at onset	Variable	50–85 years
Anterior chamber	Usually normal	Shallow
Chamber angle	Normal	Narrow
Symptoms	Generally none Decreased vision, late	Headache Haloes around lights Sudden onset of severe eye pain Vomiting during attack
Cupping of disc	Progressive if not treated (see Fig. 8–36)	After untreated attack(s)
Visual fields	Peripheral fields involved early Central involvement a very late sign	Involvement is a late sign
Ocular pressure	Progressively higher if not medically controlled	Early: detected with provocative tests only Late: high
Other signs		Fixed, partially dilated pupil Conjunctival injection "Steamy" cornea†
Treatment	Medical Laser surgery	Surgical
Prognosis	Good if recognized early Very dependent on patient compliance	Good

* Thought to be a defect in the trabecular network ultrastructure.
† Like looking through a steamy window.

Diabetes and hypertension are systemic illnesses with retinal manifestations. The retinal findings in a patient with diabetes are shown in Figure 8–38. Diabetic retinopathy is a highly specific vascular complication of type I and type II diabetes mellitus. By 25 years after the onset of diabetes, nearly all patients with type I diabetes and 65% of patients with type II diabetes have some degree of retinopathy. Figure 8–39 shows the retinal changes in a patient with hypertension. Systemic hypertension may be reflected in the retina in terms of irregularities in arteriolar size, tortuosity of the retinal arteries, and changes in the arteriovenous crossings. Progressive changes of hypertension include arteriolar narrowing with increasing areas of retinal ischemia, which is evident by the development of cotton-wool exudates, hemorrhages, retinal edema, and papilledema. As the arterioles thicken their walls as a result of sustained hypertension, they lose their transparency, and noticeable changes are seen at the crossings of the arteries and veins. The vein appears to disappear abruptly on either side of the artery. Some of the arteries develop a burnishing of the red reflex.

Increased pressure in the central nervous system produces a classic picture of papilledema in the retina. Blood dyscrasias are frequently first diagnosed from the examination of the retina.

Occlusive disorders of the retinal circulation are dramatic. A *central retinal artery occlusion* is usually caused by an embolus from the heart or large artery. It results in sudden, painless loss of vision in one eye. The pupillary direct light reflex is lost, and spontaneous venous pulsations are absent. Within minutes, the retina becomes pale with narrowed arteries, and a cherry red spot appears at the macula. This cherry red spot is a result of the fact that in the foveal area the retina is thin, allowing visibility of the underlying choroidal circulation, that is obscured elsewhere by retinal edema. This is a true ocular emergency because if treated within 45 minutes, part of the retina may be saved. Figure 8–40 shows the retina of a patient with a central retinal artery occlusion (CRAO). Notice the pale retina with the cherry red spot at the macula. Figure 8–41 shows the retina of another patient with a CRAO with cilioretinal artery sparing. The cilioretinal arteries are present in 40% of normal individuals. They are derived from

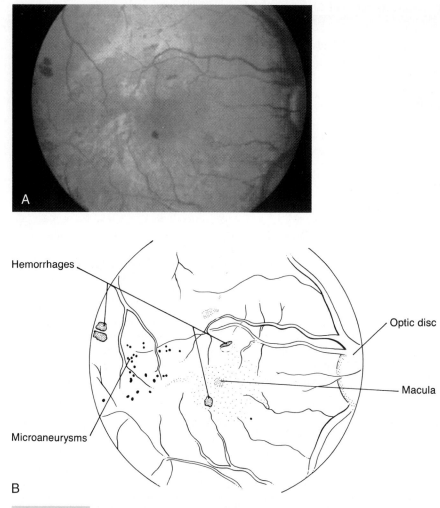

Figure 8–38

A and *B*, Photograph and labeled schematic showing the retinal findings in the right eye in a patient with diabetes. Note the macroaneurysms near the macula.

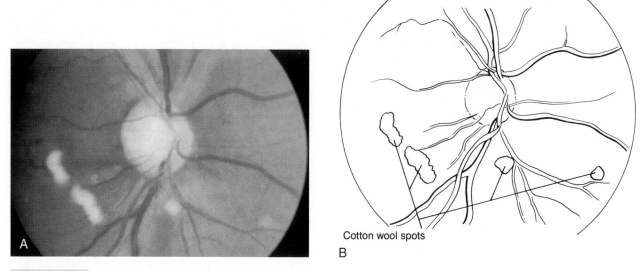

Figure 8–39

A and *B*, Photograph and labeled schematic showing the retinal changes in a patient with long-standing hypertension. Note the cotton-wool spots.

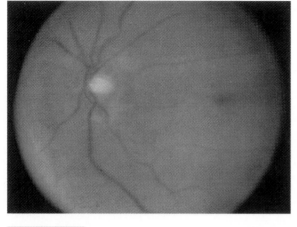

Figure 8–40

Central retinal artery occlusion.

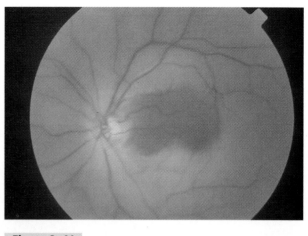

Figure 8–41

Central retinal artery occlusion with cilioretinal artery sparing.

the posterior ciliary circulation and usually emerge from the temporal aspect of the disc to supply a small portion of the retina. Notice the area of spared retina due to perfusion by the cilioretinal artery. Figure 8–42 shows a third patient with a CRAO. Notice that in this example the retina is also pale (ischemic and edematous), but the area of the cherry red spot at the macula is heavily pigmented. This is the finding in dark-skinned individuals with a CRAO.

Venous occlusion is one of the most common retinal vascular disorders. A *central retinal venous occlusion* (CRVO) occurs at the lamina cribosa. The patient experiences painless loss of vision in one eye. The fundus shows venous dilatation and tortuosity, disc edema, flame-shaped hemorrhages in all quadrants, blurred optic disc, cotton-wool spots, and often a large hemorrhage at the macula. The fundus in a CRVO has been described as a "pizza thrown against a wall." The patients are usually from 70 to 80 years of age. The causes of CRVO are many: hypertension, glaucoma, atherosclerosis, diabetes, and hyperviscosity syndromes. Figure 8–43 shows the retina of a hypertensive patient with a central retinal venous occlusion.

The retinal findings of these and other clinical states are summarized in Table 8–10.

Drusen of the optic disc are acellular, calcified hyaline deposits within the substance of the optic nerve that occur secondary to axonal degeneration. The disc

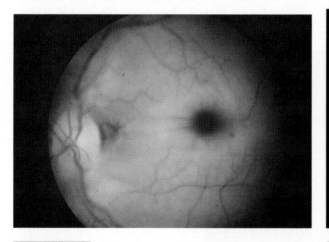

Figure 8–42

Pigmented CRAO.

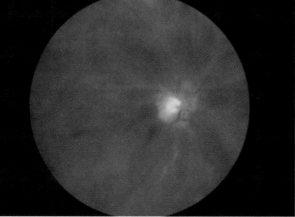

Figure 8–43

Central retinal venous occlusion.

Table 8–10   Retinal Characteristics of Common Diseases

Condition	Primary Findings	Distribution	Secondary Findings
Diabetes (see Figs. 8–38 and 8–54)	Microaneurysms Neovascularization Retinitis proliferans*	Posterior pole	Hard exudates† Deep hemorrhages Retinal venous occlusions Vitreous hemorrhages
Hypertension (see Fig. 8–39)	Arteriolar narrowing "Copper wiring" Flame hemorrhages Arteriovenous nicking	Throughout retina	Hard and soft exudates Retinal venous occlusions Macular stars (see Fig. 8–47)
Papilledema (see Fig. 8–53)	Hyperemia of the disc Venous engorgement Retinal hemorrhages Disc elevation Loss of spontaneous venous pulsations Cotton-wool spots	On or near disc	Hard exudates Optic atrophy, late
Retinal venous occlusion (see Fig. 8–43)	Hemorrhages Neovascularization	Confined to area drained by affected vein	Exudates
Retinal arterial occlusion (see Figs. 8–40 to 8–42)	Pallor of retina Decreased width of artery Embolus possibly visible	Confined to area supplied	Optic atrophy, late
Arteriolar sclerosis	Widening of light reflex "Copper wiring" Arteriovenous nicking	Throughout retina	Decrease in retinal pigment
Blood dyscrasias	Diffuse hemorrhages Venous dilatation, common Roth's spots (hemorrhagic lesions with white centers)		
Sickle cell disease	Sharp cutoff of arterioles Arteriovenous anastomoses Neovascularization in "sea fan" formations (resembling the marine organism with a similar pattern)	Peripheral retina	Vitreous hemorrhages Retinal detachments

* A growth of a light-colored sheet of opaque connective tissue over the inner surface of the retina. Neovascularization of the tissue with tortuous vessels is seen. These vessels bleed easily.

† *Exudate* is the term used for small intraretinal lesions caused by retinal disturbances in a variety of disorders.

margins are irregular or blurred. Drusen are found to be bilateral in 70% of patients, and the condition is transmitted as an irregular dominant trait with incomplete penetrance. Drusen occur almost exclusively in white individuals. Figure 8–44 shows optic disc drusen. Notice the scalloped appearance of the optic nerve border. Because of the irregular disc border, optic disc drusen sometimes can be confused with papilledema. Optic disc drusen should not be confused with *retinal drusen,* an age-related abnor-

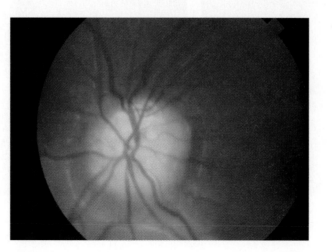

Figure 8–44

Optic disc drusen.

mality, which can be part of the disorder known as *macular degeneration*. These are yellowish-white round spots that may vary in size and are frequently concentrated at the posterior pole. Figure 8–45 shows the retina of a patient with drusen of the retina.

Optic atrophy is reduction in size and substance of the optic nerve caused by loss of axons and myelin sheaths. Optic atrophy may result from a lesion anywhere in the anterior visual pathway between the retina and the lateral geniculate body. The ophthalmoscopic hallmark of optic atrophy is optic disc pallor. The patient may have a loss of visual acuity, narrowed visual fields, deficit in color vision, or an afferent defect. The pallor of the disc is due to the loss of its capillary network and to glial tissue formation. There are two basic types of optic atrophy: "primary," which has disc pallor with a clearly defined margin due to retrobulbar or intracranial disease; and "secondary," which has disc pallor with a blurred disc margin due to optic neuritis or chronic papilledema. Figure 8–46 shows the retina of a patient with optic atrophy.

A *macular star* is an accumulation of edema residues arranged in a stellate pattern around the macula. Macular stars are commonly seen in patients with hypertension, papilledema, papillitis, and CRVO. Figure 8–47 shows the retina of a patient with a macular star, secondary to a viral infection.

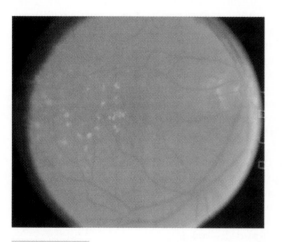

Figure 8–45

Drusen of the retina.

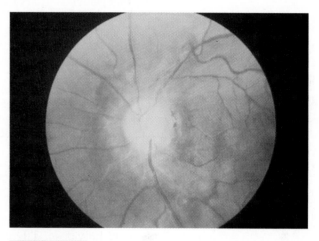

Figure 8–46

Retina with optic atrophy. Notice the marked pallor of the disc.

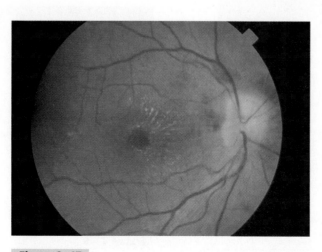

Figure 8–47

Retina with a macular star.

Chorioretinitis is an inflammatory process that originates in the choroidal tissues and subsequently spreads to involve the retina. Most inflammatory changes in the choroid are of endogenous origin, including tuberculosis, syphilis, Q fever, human immunodeficiency virus, herpes zoster, cytomegalovirus, measles, sarcoidosis, histoplasmosis, *Aspergillus, Candida,* cryptococcosis, coccidioidomycosis, toxoplasmosis, *Toxocara,* onchocerciasis, and retinoblastoma. In acute chorioretinitis, there are cloudy vision resulting from vitreous haze, light flashes, and multiple floating spots. Loss of vision may occur if the macula is involved. In chronic chorioretinitis, there is clumping of pigment around the lesions, which look whitish due to the presence of scar tissue and the underlying sclera that is visible because of the destroyed retina and choroid. Toxoplasmosis is usually a congenital condition, transmitted to the fetus from the mother during the first trimester of pregnancy. The early lesions heal once the organisms become encysted; only retinochoroidal scarring is seen on routine ophthalmoscopy. Recurrence may occur with the liberation of the encysted organisms and further retinal damage.

Figure 8–48 shows the retina of the right eye of a patient with AIDS and acute toxoplasmosis chorioretinitis. Notice the multifocal areas of retinal involvement. This patient had similar multifocal lesions in the left eye. The multifocal areas and bilaterality are typical of acute toxoplasmosis retinitis in the AIDS patient. Figure 8–49 shows a retina of a patient with an inactive scar of toxoplasmosis adjacent to an active lesion.

Cytomegalovirus (CMV) chorioretinitis is the most common ocular opportunistic infection in patients with AIDS. Autopsy studies have shown that more than 95% of viral chorioretinitis in patients with AIDS is a result of CMV infection. CMV chorioretinitis is progressive and often preterminal. It appears that the AIDS patient is at greatest risk for CMV retinitis when the CD4+ count is less than $40/mm^3$. Figure 8–50 shows the retina of the left eye of a patient with CMV chorioretinitis. Notice the marked retinal necrosis extending from the optic nerve superiorly and temporally. Figure 8–51 shows the retina of the right eye of another patient with CMV retinitis. There is extensive necrotizing optic neuritis with retinal necrosis and retinal vasculitis. Notice the white sheathing of the retinal vessels (especially superiorly off the disc), which is typical of vasculitis.

Figure 8–52 shows the left retina of a patient with HIV infection. Notice the cotton-wool spots and the extremely large flame-shaped hemorrhage.

Blurring of the disc margins may be the only sign of increased intracranial pressure. This finding, however, does occur with other conditions. Figure 8–53 shows the blurred disc margins of papilledema in a patient with increased intracranial pressure. Table 8–11 provides a differentiation of blurred disc margins.

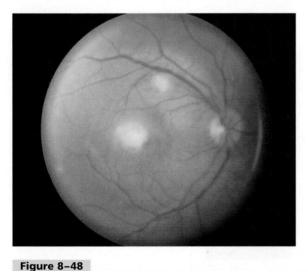

Figure 8–48

Acute toxoplasmosis chorioretinitis in an AIDS patient.

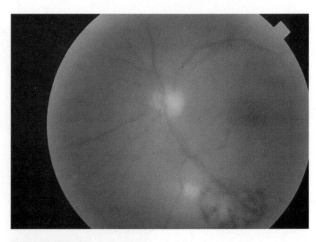

Figure 8–49

Acute and chronic toxoplasmosis chorioretinitis. The large dark lesion is the inactive toxoplasmosis scar.

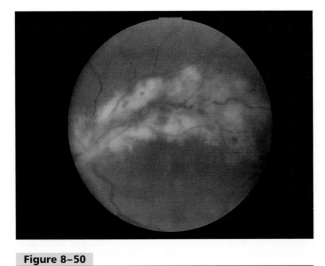

Figure 8–50

CMV chorioretinitis: left retina.

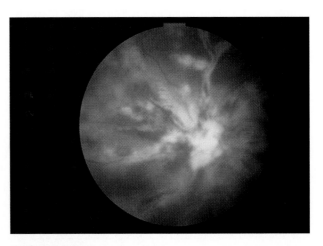

Figure 8–51

CMV chorioretinitis: right retina.

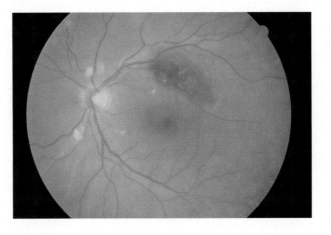

Figure 8–52

HIV chorioretinitis.

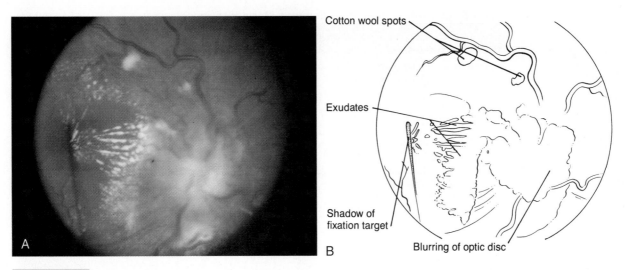

Figure 8–53

A and *B,* Photograph and labeled schematic showing the retinal changes in chronic papilledema. Note the marked blurring of the right optic disc, the cotton-wool spots, and the exudates. The dark line at the macula is a shadow of the target at which the patient was asked to look.

Table 8–11   Differentiation of Blurred Disc Margins

Presentation	Papilledema*	Papillitis†	Drusen‡	Myelinated Nerve Fibers§	Central Retinal Vein Occlusion‖
Visual acuity	Normal	Decreased	Normal	Normal	Decreased
Venous pulsations	Absent	Variable	Present	Present	Generally absent
Pain	Headache	Eye movement pain	No	No	No
Light reaction	Present	Marcus Gunn (see text)	Present	Present	Present
Hemorrhage	Present	Present	Uncommon	No	Marked
Visual fields	Enlarged blind spot	Central scotoma	Enlarged blind spot	Scotomata correspond to areas of myelination	Variable
Laterality	Bilateral	Unilateral	Bilateral	Seldom bilateral	Unilateral

* Edema of the optic disc resulting from increased intracranial pressure. See Figure 8–53.
† Inflammation of the optic disc.
‡ See Figure 8–44.
§ Myelination of the optic nerve ends at the optic disc. When it continues into the retina, white, flame-shaped areas obscure the disc margins. See Figure 8–34.
‖ See Figure 8–43.

Many common diseases display their disorders at the macula of the retina. Table 8–12 provides a differentiation of some of these lesion types. Figure 8–54 shows circinate retinopathy in a diabetic patient.

Abnormalities of gaze are not uncommon. *Ophthalmoplegia* is paralysis of the eye muscles. Lesions causing this paralysis may be acute, chronic, or progressive. Note the patient shown in Figure 8–55. When asked to look straight ahead, the right eye is abducted. Notice the ptosis of the right eyelid. When the patient is asked to look to the far right, both eyes move normally, although the right ptosis is well seen. When the patient is asked to look to the far left, the right eye cannot cross the midline. This patient has an acute oculomotor paralysis secondary to a fungal lesion near the nucleus of the third cranial nerve.

Note the patient shown in Figure 8–56. When the patient is asked to look straight ahead or to the right, both eyes move smoothly in the correct motion. However, when the patient is asked to look to the left, the left eye fails to cross the midline. Diplopia occurred as a result of a left abducens palsy secondary to carcinomatous meningitis.

Table 8–12   Differentiation of Common Macular Lesions

	Macular Degeneration*	Macular Star†	Circinate Retinopathy‡
Appearance	Pigmentary mottling, often with hemorrhage	Whitish exudate that radiates around macula	Broken ring–shaped whitish exudate around macula
Etiology		Hypertension Papilledema Papillitis Central retinal vein occlusion	Diabetes Central retinal vein occlusion

* Often bilateral in the aged.
† See Figure 8–47.
‡ See Figure 8–54.

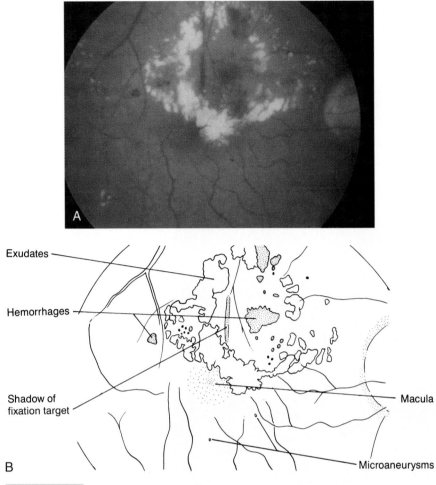

Figure 8-54

A and *B*, Photograph and labeled schematic showing the retinal changes of severe diabetes, called *circinate retinopathy,* which is a ring of exudates around the macula. This is the retina of the right eye.

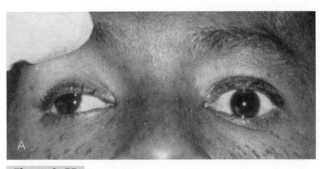

Figure 8-55

Acute right oculomotor nerve paralysis. *A,* When the patient is asked to look straight ahead, the right eye is turned laterally (note the position of the corneal light reflexes). The right palpebral fissure is markedly narrowed, requiring the eyelid to be elevated to visualize the position of the eye. *B,* When the patient is asked to look to the far right, both eyes are able to move in that direction. Note the marked ptosis of the right eyelid. *C,* When the patient is asked to look to the far left, the right eye cannot cross the midline.

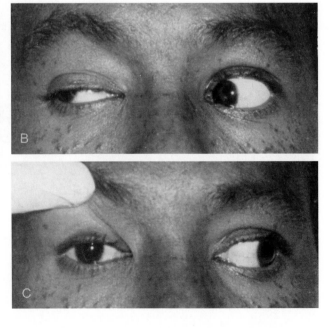

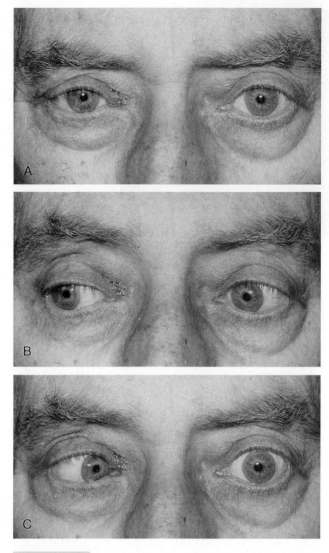

Figure 8–56

Acute left abducens paralysis. *A,* When the patient is asked to look straight ahead, both eyes are straight. *B,* When the patient is asked to look to the right, both eyes turn normally. *C,* When the patient is asked to look to the left, the left eye cannot cross the midline, indicating left abducens palsy.

Useful Vocabulary

Listed here are the specific roots that are important in order to understand the terminology related to diseases of the eye.

Root	Pertaining to	Example	Definition
blepharo-	eyelid	*blepharo*plasty	Surgical repair of eyelid
choroi-	choroid	*choroi*ditis	Inflammation of the choroid
-cor-	pupil	aniso*cor*ia	Unequal pupils
cyclo-	ciliary body	*cyclo*plegia	Paralysis of accommodation
dacryo-	tear	*dacryo*cystitis	Inflammation of the lacrimal sac
-duction	to lead	ab*duction*	Turning outward
irid-	iris	*irid*ectomy	Surgical excision of part of the iris

Root	Pertaining to	Example	Definition
kerato-	cornea	*kerato*pathy	Disease of the cornea
lacri-	tears	*lacri*mal	Pertaining to the tears
nyct-	night	*nyct*alopia	Night blindness
-ocul-	eye	intra*ocul*ar	Within the eye
ophthalm-	eye	*ophthalm*oscope	Instrument for visualizing the retina
-opsia	vision	hemian*opsia*	Blindness in half of the visual field
-phak(os)-	lens	a*phak*ia	Without a lens
photo-	light	*photo*sensitive	Sensitive to light
presby-	old	*presby*opia	Impairment of vision as a result of increasing age
tars-	eyelid structure	*tars*orrhaphy	Surgical suturing of the lid
-trop-	turn	eso*trop*ia	Eye turning inward.

Writing Up the Physical Examination

Listed here are examples of the write-up for the examination of the eye.

- Visual acuity is OD 20/20 and OS 20/30 according to the standard Snellen chart. The visual fields by confrontation are normal. Examination of the external structures of the eyes is normal. The pupils are equal, round, and reactive to light and to accommodation.* The extraocular movements† are normal. On ophthalmoscopic examination, the disc margins are sharp. A normal cup-to-disc ratio is present. The vasculature is normal.

- Visual acuity is OD 20/60 and OS 20/20 according to the pocket visual acuity card. Examination of the eyes reveals marked conjunctival injection on the right with a dilated pupil on the same side. The pupils are round and are reactive to light. Accommodation was not well seen. The visual fields by confrontation field testing are normal. The optic disc margins are sharp, and the vascularity of both retinas appears normal.

- The patient is able to read the newspaper without corrective lenses. The extraocular movements are normal. The left pupil is miotic and is 2 mm smaller than the right pupil. A mild ptosis of the left upper lid is present. Both pupils react to light directly and consensually. Confrontation fields are within normal limits. Funduscopic examination is within normal limits.

- The visual acuity with corrected lenses appears normal. There is a paralysis of abduction of the left eye, accompanied by diplopia on attempted left lateral gaze. The pupils are equal, round, and reactive to light. The optic disc margins are sharp. The vasculature is normal.

- There is decreased visual acuity in both eyes. The patient has difficulty reading 1/4 inch print in the newspaper at about 6 inches with his right eye. There is OS NLP. The examination of the external eye is normal. The extraocular movements are intact. The left optic disc margin is slightly blurred on its nasal aspect. The cup-to-disc ratio is normal. There are multiple, soft, cotton-wool exudates seen bilaterally. A large, flame-shaped hemorrhage is seen in the right eye at the 2 o'clock position. Arteriovenous nicking is present bilaterally.

- The visual acuity is OD 20/40 and OS 20/100 according to the pocket visual acuity card. A bitemporal hemianopsia is present by confrontation field testing. EOMs are normal. Ophthalmoscopic examination reveals blurring of both optic discs with loss of spontaneous venous pulsations. A flame-shaped hemorrhage is present in the right eye 1 disc diameter at the 10 o'clock position.

---

* Often abbreviated as PERRLA.
† Often abbreviated as EOMs.

Bibliography

Albert DM, Jakobiec FA: Atlas of Clinical Ophthalmology. Philadelphia, W.B. Saunders Co., 1996.
Cassirer R: The Philosophy of Symbolic Forms. London, Oxford University Press, 1955.
Chevigny H, Braverman S: The Adjustment of the Blind. New Haven, CT, Yale University Press, 1950.
Diamond BL, Ross A: Emotional adjustments of newly blinded soldiers. Am J Psychiatry 102:367, 1945

Gregory RL, Wallace JG: Recovery from Early Blindness: A Case Study. Monograph 2, Experimental Psychology Society. Cambridge, England, Heffer, 1963.

Havener WH: Synopsis of Ophthalmology. St. Louis, C.V. Mosby, 1984.

Heaton JM: The Eye: Phenomenology and Psychology of Function and Disorder. Philadelphia, J.B. Lippincott, 1968.

Kritzinger EE, Beaumont HM: A Colour Atlas of Optic Disc Abnormalities. London, Wolfe Medical Publications Ltd./Year Book Medical Publishers, Inc. 1987.

Michelson JB, Friedlaender MH: Color Atlas of the Eye in Clinical Medicine. London, Mosby-Wolfe, 1996.

Steinmann WC, Millstein ME, Sinclair SH: Pupillary dilation with tropicamide 1% for fundoscopic screening: A study of duration of action. Ann Intern Med 107:181, 1987.

Zadnik K: The Ocular Examination: Measurements and Findings. Philadelphia, W.B. Saunders Co., 1997.

CHAPTER 9

The Ear and Nose

Yet it was not possible for me to say to people, "Speak louder, shout, for I am deaf."
. . . Alas! how could I declare the weakness of a sense which in me ought to be more
acute than in others—a sense which formerly I possessed in highest perfection, a
perfection such as few in my profession enjoy, or ever have enjoyed.

Ludwig van Beethoven
1770–1827

General Considerations

Most of us are fortunate to hear the sounds of music, noise, and, above all, speech. Sometimes "silence is golden," but silence can be golden only when one can choose not to hear.

Although normal children are born with the apparatus necessary to produce speech, they are not born with speech. The ear and brain integrate and process sound, permitting the child to learn to imitate it. If sound cannot be heard, it cannot be imitated. Sounds will not become words; words will not become sentences; sentences will not become speech; speech will not become language.

Hearing is a perceptual process. To illustrate this concept, consider tinnitus as an example. *Tinnitus,* the name given to a sensation of sound in one or both ears, is a common accompaniment to deafness. When tinnitus is present, there is nearly always some degree of hearing loss. Conversely, when there is no appreciable hearing loss, there is rarely tinnitus. However, children who are born deaf do not complain of tinnitus.

Structure and Physiology

The Ear

The ear can be divided into the following four parts:

- External ear
- Middle ear
- Inner ear
- Nervous innervation

A cross section through the ear is shown in Figure 9–1.

The *external ear* consists of the *pinna* and the *external auditory canal.* The pinna is composed of elastic cartilage and skin. Figure 9–2 illustrates the parts of the pinna.

The external auditory canal is about 1 inch in length. Its outer third is cartilaginous, and its inner two thirds are composed of bone. Within the cartilaginous portion, there are hair follicles, pilosebaceous glands, and *ceruminous,* or wax-producing, glands. Secretions of these ceruminous glands, debris, and desquamated keratin are "earwax." The glands secrete their product around the base of the hairs as shown in Figure 9–3. Figure 9–4 shows earwax in the external ear canal. Earwax color and consistency depend on the type of cerumen secreted, the amount of keratin present, and the presence of debris. The soft, brown form shown here is the most common type. The cartilaginous portion is continuous with the pinna. The canal curves slightly, being directed forward and downward. The innervation to most of the external canal is through the trigeminal, or fifth cranial, nerve. The innermost portion of the canal is innervated by the vagus, or tenth cranial, nerve.*

---

* Occasionally, when the distal external canal is cleaned, coughing may result. This cough reflex is mediated through the vagus nerve.

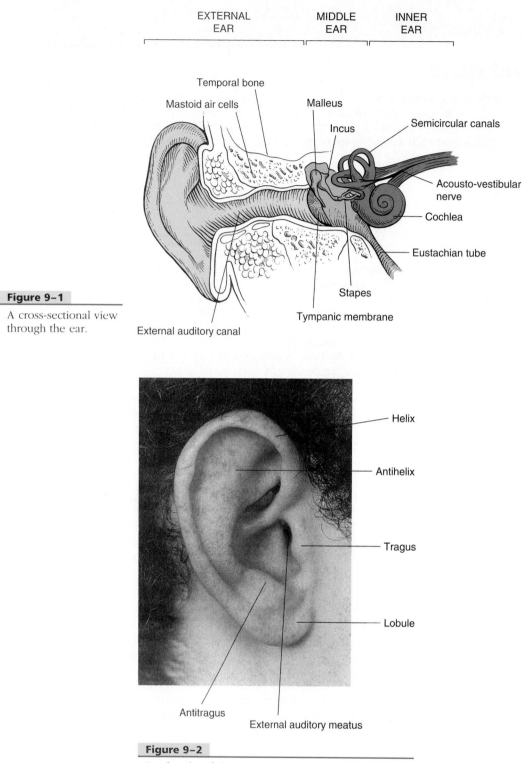

EXTERNAL
EAR

MIDDLE
EAR

INNER
EAR

Temporal bone

Mastoid air cells

Malleus

Incus

Semicircular canals

Acousto-vestibular
nerve

Cochlea

Eustachian tube

Stapes

Tympanic membrane

External auditory canal

Figure 9–1

A cross-sectional view
through the ear.

Helix

Antihelix

Tragus

Lobule

Antitragus

External auditory meatus

Figure 9–2

Landmarks of the pinna.

The *middle ear,* or tympanic cavity, consists of connections to the *mastoid antrum* and to its connecting air cells and, through the *eustachian tube,* to the nasopharynx. The function of the eustachian tube is to provide an air passage from the nasopharynx to the ear to equalize pressure on both sides of the tympanic membrane. The eustachian tube is normally closed but opens during swallowing and yawning.

The *tympanic membrane* forms the lateral boundary of the middle ear. The medial boundary is formed by the *cochlea.* The tympanic membrane is gray, with blood

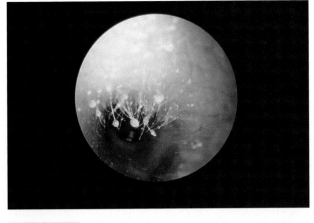

Figure 9-3

Earwax on base of hairs.

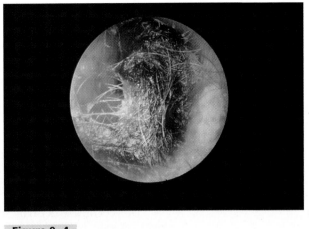

Figure 9-4

Earwax in the external ear canal.

vessels at its periphery. It is composed of two parts: the *pars flaccida* and the *pars tensa*. The pars flaccida is the upper, smaller portion of the tympanic membrane. The pars tensa composes the remainder of the membrane. The handle of the malleus is a prominent landmark and divides the pars tensa into the *anterior* and *posterior folds*. The tympanic membrane is set slightly at an angle to the external canal. The inferior portion is more medial than is the superior portion. Figure 9-5 illustrates the left tympanic membrane.

Sound is conducted from the tympanic membrane to the inner ear by way of three *auditory ossicles:* the *malleus,* the *incus,* and the *stapes.* The malleus is the largest ossicle. At its upper end is the *short process,* which appears as a tiny knob. The *handle* (long process) of the malleus, or *manubrium,* extends downward to its tip, called the *umbo.* The short process and the handle of the malleus attach directly to the tympanic membrane. At the other end of the malleus is its head, which articulates with the incus. The incus then articulates with the head of the stapes, the footplate of which attaches to the *oval window* of the inner ear.

The middle ear also contains two muscles: the *tensor tympani* and the *stapedius.* The tensor tympani muscle attaches to the malleus, and the stapedius muscle attaches to the neck of the stapes. The tensor tympani muscle is innervated by the trigeminal nerve, and the stapedius muscle is innervated by the facial, or seventh cranial, nerve. Both muscles contract in response to high-intensity sound.

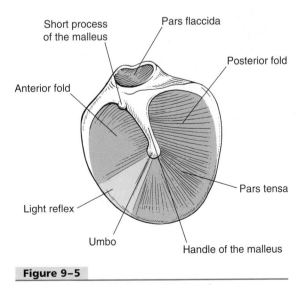

Figure 9-5

Landmarks of the left tympanic membrane.

The facial nerve passes through the middle ear and provides, in addition to the nerve to the stapedius muscle, the *chorda tympani* nerve. The chorda tympani travels through the middle ear between the incus and the malleus and exits near the temporo-mandibular joint. It carries taste sensation from the anterior two thirds of the tongue.

The *inner ear* is the end-organ for hearing and equilibrium. It is situated in the petrous portion of the temporal bone and consists of the three *semicircular canals,* the *vestibule,* and the *cochlea.* Each of these structures is made up of three parts: the *osseous labyrinth,* the *membranous labyrinth,* and the *space between.* The osseous labyrinth is the outer bone casing. The inner membranous labyrinth is within the osseous labyrinth and contains a fluid called *endolymph* and the sensory structures. The space between these two labyrinths is filled with another fluid, called *perilymph.* A cross section through this area is shown in Figure 9–6.

The three semicircular canals are directed posteriorly, superiorly, and horizontally. Each canal has a dilated end, the *ampulla,* which is the sensory end-organ for balance.

The cochlea is a snail shell–shaped structure composed of two and three-quarter turns. Within its membranous labyrinth is the end-organ for hearing. The *acoustic,* or eight cranial, nerve consists of two parts: the *vestibular* and the *cochlear* divisions. These connect to the semicircular canals and cochlea, respectively. They join and pass through the internal auditory meatus to the brain stem.

Sound waves stimulate the afferent fibers either by *bone conduction* or by *air conduction.* Bone conduction is directly through the bones of the skull. Air conduction is through the external auditory canal, tympanic membrane, and ossicles to the oval window. Most hearing is mediated by air conduction.

Sound waves set up vibrations that enter the external canal and are transmitted to the ossicles, which vibrate. This vibration causes an inward motion of the footplate of the stapes and deforms the oval window. Waves are created in the perilymphatic fluid of the labyrinth. These fluid motion changes are transmitted in a wave-like fashion to the endolymphatic fluid, which causes distortion of the *hair cells* of the *organ of Corti.* These hair cells convert the mechanical force into an electrochemical signal that is propagated down the acoustic nerve and is ultimately interpreted as sound. It has been estimated that there are more than 30,000 of these afferent hair fibers, which constitute the auditory division. After many synapses, the impulse reaches the temporal cortex, where the appreciation of the sound occurs. A cross section through the cochlear duct is shown in Figure 9–7.

The sense of *balance* is achieved by visual, vestibular, and proprioceptive* senses. The loss of one of these senses frequently goes unnoticed. The vestibular apparatus appears to be the most important. Motion within the endolymphatic fluid stimulates the hair cells within the ampulla of the semicircular canals. Electrical impulses are transmit-

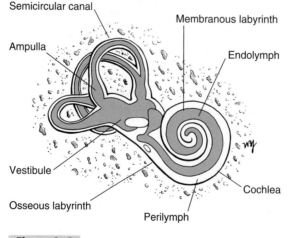

Figure 9–6

A cross-sectional view through the cochlea.

---

* Sensory stimulation from within the tissues of the body concerning their movement or position.

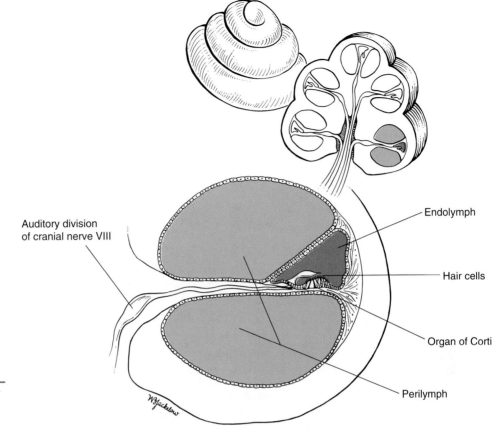

Figure 9–7

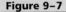

A cross-sectional view through the cochlear duct.

ted to the vestibular portion of the eighth cranial nerve. Synapses occur in the vestibular and oculomotor nuclei, which send efferent fibers to the extraocular and skeletal muscles. This produces a deviation of the eyes with rapid compensatory motions to maintain gaze and increased tone in the skeletal muscles.

Any alteration in the endolymphatic mechanism may affect the control of the eyes. *Nystagmus* is an involuntary rapid back-and-forth motion of the eyes, which can be horizontal, vertical, rotatory, or mixed. The direction of the nystagmus is determined by the direction of the quick component. Abnormalities of the labyrinth tend to produce *horizontal* nystagmus; brain stem disorders often produce *vertical* nystagmus; and retinal lesions may produce *ocular* nystagmus, which is slow and gives an irregular searching quality to the eyes.

The Nose

The external nasal skeleton consists of the *nasal bones,* part of the *maxilla,* and the *cartilage.* The upper third of the skeleton is composed of nasal bones, which articulate with the maxilla and frontal bones. The lower two thirds are made of cartilage.

The internal portion of the nose consists of two cavities divided by the *nasal septum,* which forms the medial wall of the nasal cavity. Projecting from the lateral wall are three *turbinates,* or *conchae.* The *inferior turbinate* is the largest and contains semierectile tissue. Inferior to each turbinate are openings to the *paranasal sinuses,* each opening known as a *meatus.* Each meatus is named for the turbinate above it. The *nasolacrimal duct* empties into the *inferior meatus.* The *middle meatus,* below the *middle turbinate,* contains the openings of the frontal, maxillary, and anterior ethmoid *sinuses.* The posterior ethmoid sinus drains into the *superior meatus.* The *olfactory region* is located high in the nose between the nasal septum and the *superior turbinate.* Figure 9–8 illustrates the lateral wall of the nose.

The blood supply to the nose is derived from the internal and external carotid arteries. The turbinates are vascular and contain large vascular spaces. The blood

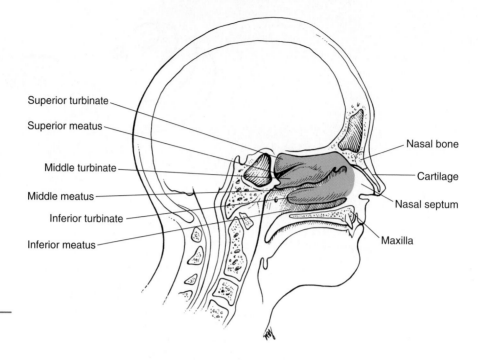

Figure 9–8

Lateral wall of the nose.

vessels of the anterior nasal septum meet at an area about 1 inch from the mucocutaneous junction, known as *Little's area*. This is the area usually responsible for *epistaxis,* or nosebleed. The blood vessels are under autonomic nervous system control. If there is an excess of *sympathetic* stimulation, the blood vessels constrict, and the vascular spaces in the turbinates shrink. If there is an increase in *parasympathetic* tone, the blood pools in the turbinates, resulting in their swelling, obstruction to air flow, and elaboration of a watery discharge.

The nerve supply to the internal nose is from branches of the trigeminal nerve. The olfactory epithelium is supplied by the *olfactory,* or first cranial, nerve. Moist air with the dissolved odorous particles acts as a stimulus. The nerve fibers from this area pierce the *cribriform plate* to the olfactory bulb in the brain. The ability of the olfactory receptors in humans to discern a stimulus diminishes rapidly with exposure to the stimulus.

The main functions of the nose are to provide the following:

- An airway
- Olfaction
- Humidification of inspired air
- Warming of inspired air
- Filtering of inspired air

The inspired air flows above and below the middle turbinate. This produces eddy currents that serve to protect the olfactory epithelium in the superior portion of the nose. The nasal mucosa produces mucus, which increases the relative humidity to nearly 100%. This prevents drying out of the epithelium and possible infection. The air, by its circulation around the conchae, is warmed to nearly body temperature by the time it enters the nasopharynx. The mucus and the nasal hairs, or *vibrissae,* prevent particulate matter from entering the distal respiratory tract. The mucous blanket is swept posteriorly by the *cilia* and is swallowed. The mucus also contains immunoglobulins and enzymes, which serve as a line of defense.

The four *paranasal sinuses* of the head are the *maxillary,* the *ethmoid,* the *frontal,* and the *sphenoid.* These are air-filled cavities lined with mucous membranes. The maxillary sinus is the largest and is bounded by the eye, the cheek, the nasal cavity, and the hard palate. The ethmoid sinuses are multiple and are present in the *ethmoid bone,* which lies medial to the orbit and extends to the pituitary fossa. The frontal sinus is located above the ethmoid sinuses and is bounded by the forehead, the orbit, and the anterior cranial fossa. Behind the ethmoid sinuses is the sphenoid sinus. There are no known functions for the paranasal sinuses. The maxillary, frontal, and ethmoid sinuses and their connections to the nose are illustrated in Figure 9–9.

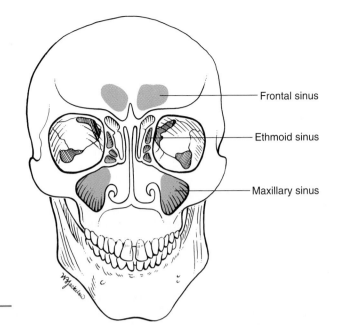

Figure 9–9

The nasal sinuses.

Review of Specific Symptoms

The Ear

The major symptoms of ear disease are the following:

- Hearing loss
- Vertigo
- Tinnitus
- Otorrhea
- Otalgia
- Itching

■ Hearing Loss

Hearing loss may be unilateral or bilateral and may develop slowly or occur suddenly. For any patient with a hearing loss, ask the following questions:

"Is the hearing loss in one ear?"
"For how long have you been aware of a loss of hearing?"
"Was the loss sudden?"
"Is there a family history of hearing loss?"
"What type of work do you do?" "What have you done?"
"What types of hobbies do you have?"
"Have you noticed that you can hear better when it is noisy?"
"What kind of medications are you presently taking?"
"Do you know if you have ever been given an antibiotic called streptomycin or
*   gentamicin?"*

Occupational history is extremely important to ascertain. Patients with otosclerosis* can often hear better in a noisy environment. Drugs are well known to cause sudden bilateral hearing loss. Salicylates and diuretics such as furosemide and ethacrynic acid may produce transient loss of hearing when given in high doses. The aminoglycoside antibiotics such as streptomycin and gentamicin can destroy the hair cells of the organ of Corti and cause permanent hearing loss. An anticancer medication, cisplatin, is also linked to severe ototoxicity.

---

* Otosclerosis is the formation of new bone in the labyrinth, causing progressive fixation of the footplate of the stapes to the oval window.

There are two main types of hearing loss: *conductive* and *sensorineural*. Any condition that interferes with or blocks the transmission of sound waves from the external ear to the inner ear may result in a conductive hearing loss. Blockage may occur as a result of cerumen (earwax), foreign bodies, infection, or congenital abnormalities. Often the position of the cerumen is more important than the amount present. Not infrequently, a small amount of cerumen lying against the tympanic membrane can produce significant hearing loss. Blockage by foreign bodies occurs primarily in 2 to 5 year old children. Once children discover the external canal, they may experiment and place beads or other objects inside. Figure 9–10 shows a clear plastic bead in the external canal of a young child. Effusions from infections in the middle ear represent one of the most common causes of conductive deafness among 4 to 15 year old people. The fluid impedes the transmission of the sound impulses by the tympanic membrane and the ossicles. Otosclerosis is the main cause of conductive hearing loss in individuals 15 to 50 years of age. With the exception of otosclerosis, conditions causing a conductive hearing loss produce alterations in the appearance of the tympanic membrane.

Sensorineural hearing loss is due to a disease process in the inner ear structures or auditory nerve. These conditions may be congenital or acquired, with delayed onset. Congenital deafness accounts for 50% of all deafness in children. In many cases of congenital sensorineural hearing loss, no other congenital abnormality may be noted. At other times, deafness may accompany other defects, especially in the kidney. Infection with rubella in a woman during pregnancy accounts for most of the cases of sensorineural deafness that are due to anomalous development of the cochlea. The acquired, delayed-onset types may or may not be genetic in origin. There are many syndromes, too numerous to mention, as well as viral infections and ototoxic drugs that may cause acquired, delayed-onset sensorineural deafness. Systemic diseases, tumors, and noise are also associated with this type of hearing loss.

A patient's voice may give some ideas as to the nature of his or her deafness. The speaking voice is regulated by the way one hears oneself. Patients with a conductive hearing loss hear their own voices better by bone conduction than by air conduction. They therefore think their voices are loud and speak more softly. In contrast, patients with a sensorineural hearing defect hear less by *both* air and bone conduction; therefore, they tend to speak louder.

■ Vertigo

Vertigo is a sense of spinning or turning while in a resting position. It is frequently associated with a loss of vestibular function, such as unsteadiness of gait. For any patient with vertigo, ask the following questions:

"How long have you had this sensation?"
"Have you had repeated attacks?"
"How long does an attack last? . . . seconds? . . . minutes? . . .
   hours? . . . days?"

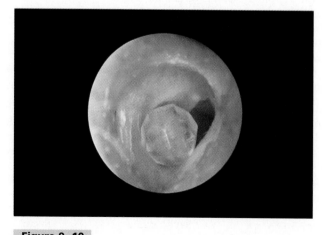

Figure 9–10

Clear plastic bead in the external ear canal.

"Is the onset of an attack abrupt?"
"Was the sensation brought on by, or worsened by, changes in position?"
"Does the spinning sensation progress during an attack?"
"Are there any positions that make you feel better?"
"During an attack, have you had double vision? . . . loss of strength? . . . decreased hearing? . . . a disturbance of gait? . . . nausea? . . . vomiting? . . . ringing in your ears?"
"What kind of medications are you presently taking?"
"Do you know if you have ever been given an antibiotic called streptomycin or gentamicin?"

Vertigo may result from otologic, neurologic, psychological, or iatrogenic causes. *Ménière's disease* causes severe paroxysmal vertigo as a result of labyrinthine lesions. The vertigo has an abrupt onset and may last several hours. It is often associated with nausea, vomiting, headache, a ringing sensation in the ear, and decreased hearing. The auditory abnormalities frequently antedate the vertigo. Vertigo associated with an acoustic neuroma is generally mild. Some antibiotics, such as gentamicin, streptomycin, and kanamycin, are vestibulotoxic and cause vertigo. The neurologic causes of vertigo are discussed further in Chapter 19, The Nervous System.

▨ Tinnitus

Tinnitus is the sensation of hearing sound, such as buzzing or ringing, in the absence of environmental input. It is often associated with a conductive or sensorineural hearing loss. Usually the description of the type of tinnitus (e.g., "ringing" or "buzzing") is of little help in determining its cause. The most common causes result from inner ear disease such as from Ménière's disease, noise trauma, ototoxic drugs, and otosclerosis. Occasionally, patients describe *pulsatile tinnitus*. This type of tinnitus beats at the same rate as the heart and may be a symptom of a vascular tumor of the head or neck. See Table 9–1 for a list of some of the common causes of tinnitus.

▨ Otorrhea

Otorrhea, or discharge from the ear, generally indicates acute or chronic infection. Any patient complaining of an ear discharge should be asked the following:

"Can you describe the discharge?"
"Have you had similar episodes?"
"Do you experience dizziness?"
"Do you have ear pain?"
"Have you had a recent ear or throat infection?"
"Have you had any change in your hearing?"
"Have you used ear drops?"
"Have you been swimming recently?"
"Have you had any recent head or ear injury?"

Table 9–1	Common Causes of Tinnitus	
Location	Pulsatile/Clicking	Nonpulsatile
External ear	External otitis Bullous myringitis Foreign body	Cerumen Tympanic membrane perforation Foreign body
Middle ear	Otitis media Vascular anomalies Neoplasm Eustachian tube dysfunction	Otosclerosis Serous otitis
Inner ear	Vascular anomalies	Cochlear otosclerosis Ménière's disease Labyrinthitis Noise trauma Drug toxicity Presbycusis
Central nervous system	Vascular anomalies Hypertension	Syphilis Degenerative disease Cerebral atherosclerosis

A bloody discharge may be associated with carcinoma or trauma. A clear, watery discharge may indicate a leakage of cerebrospinal fluid. Determine how long the discharge has been present as well as its color, its smell, and its relationship to itching, pain, or trauma.

Otalgia

Otalgia, or ear pain, may be related to inflammatory conditions in or around the ear or may be referred* from distant anatomic sites in the head and neck. External otitis and otitis media are infections of the external and middle ear, respectively, and are common causes of locally produced pain. Pain from the teeth, pharynx, and cervical spine is commonly referred to the ear. Inflammation, trauma, and neoplasms anywhere along the course of the trigeminal, facial, glossopharyngeal, and vagus cranial nerves or cervical nerves C2 or C3 may be responsible for referred pain to the ipsilateral ear.

Itching

Pruritus (itching) of the ear may result from a primary disorder of the external ear or from a discharge from the middle ear. A systemic disease, such as diabetes, hepatitis, and lymphoma, may also be the cause.

The Nose

The specific symptoms related to the nose are the following:

- Obstruction
- Discharge
- Bleeding

Obstruction

The most common symptom of nasal disease is obstruction. If the symptom of nasal obstruction is present, ask the following questions:

"Is the obstruction on one side?"
"Have you ever had an injury to your nose?"
"How long has the obstruction been present?"
"Do you have any allergies?"
"Does the obstruction worsen with stress?"
"Is there a history of nasal polyps?"
"Is the obstruction associated with other symptoms?"
"Is there a seasonal change in your symptoms?" If so, *"Which season is the worst?"*

Rhinitis, which is inflammation of the nasal mucosa, can be allergic or nonallergic in cause. *Allergic rhinitis* is congestion of the nasal mucosa, triggered by an allergen such as pollen. The main symptoms include nasal obstruction, sneezing, and a clear, watery nasal discharge. It is helpful to try to determine the allergen. Weeds pollinate in the spring and fall, trees in the spring, and grasses in the summer. Nonseasonal allergic rhinitis may be due to animal dander, mold, or dust. *Nonallergic rhinitis* produces the same symptoms but is nonseasonal and is not triggered by allergens. An example of nonallergic rhinitis is vasomotor rhinitis. Vasomotor rhinitis occurs at stressful times and results in venous engorgement of the conchae, causing obstruction. There are many other causes of vasomotor rhinitis, such as nasal spray abuse (also known as *rhinitis medicamentosa*), pregnancy, and hypothyroidism.

Nasal *polyps,* usually bilateral, also cause obstruction and are the most common cause of *anosmia,* or loss of smell.

Nasal obstruction may be responsible for symptoms referable to other organs. Eye tearing may result from obstruction of the nasolacrimal duct beneath the inferior turbinate. Sinus symptoms may result from obstruction to their drainage. Ear pain or a "clogged" sensation is commonly associated with eustachian tube obstruction.

---

* Referred pain is pain felt in an area that is separate from the area that is actually the source of the pain. For example, pain from gallbladder disease is frequently felt in the right shoulder. Chapter 15, The Abdomen, discusses further aspects of referred pain.

Discharge

Nasal discharge can be unilateral or bilateral. It usually accompanies nasal obstruction. The discharge may be characterized as

- Thin and watery
- Thick and purulent
- Bloody
- Foul-smelling

A *thin and watery* discharge is usually due to excess mucus production resulting from a viral infection or allergic condition. A *thick, purulent* nasal discharge results from bacterial infection. A *bloody* discharge can result from a neoplasm, trauma, or an opportunistic infection such as mucormycosis (fungal disease). A *foul-smelling* discharge is often associated with foreign bodies in the nose, chronic sinusitis, or malignant disease. A clear, watery discharge that is increased by bending the head forward or by coughing suggests cerebrospinal fluid leakage.

Bleeding

Epistaxis, or bleeding, usually results from the traumatic or spontaneous rupture of the superficial mucosal vessels in Little's area. In order to exclude other causes, determine whether the epistaxis is related to trauma or to a bleeding disorder. It may also result from chronic sinusitis or malignancy within the sinuses. The most common cause of epistaxis is nose-picking. Another prevalent etiologic factor is cocaine abuse.

Sinus Disease Symptoms

The symptoms of sinus disease are similar to the symptoms of nasal disease. Fever, malaise, cough, nasal congestion, maxillary toothache, purulent nasal discharge, headache, and little improvement of symptoms with decongestants increase the likelihood of sinus disease. Pain, often made worse by bending forward, is an important symptom. Pain from localized sinus disease is generally present in the area overlying the involved sinus. The only exception is sphenoid sinus disease, which is felt diffusely. Maxillary sinus pain is felt behind the eye and near the second premolar and first and second molar teeth. Frontal sinus pain is localized to above the eye. Ethmoid sinus pain is usually periorbital. Sometimes sinus pain can be referred to another area. In addition to pain, ocular abnormalities may also be present with diseases of the sinuses.

Williams and Simel (1992, 1993) evaluated the accuracy of symptoms and signs of sinusitis. Colored nasal discharge, cough, and sneezing were the most sensitive symptoms, with sensitivities of 72%, 70%, and 70%, respectively; these symptoms were, however, not very specific. Maxillary toothache was the most specific symptom for sinusitis, with a specificity of 93%; however, only 11% of patients reported this symptom. This symptom had the highest positive likelihood ratio (LR+) of 2.5. They concluded that the presence in combination of maxillary toothache, poor response to decongestants, colored nasal discharge, and abnormal sinus transillumination, discussed later in this chapter, were the strongest predictors of sinusitis in primary care populations. If all of these were present, the LR+ was 6.4, and it was likely that the patient had sinusitis; if none were present, sinusitis was ruled out.

Table 9–2 summarizes the location of pain associated with sinus disease. Table 9–3 lists the other clinical signs and symptoms associated with sinus disease.

Table 9–2   Location of Pain Associated with Sinus Disease

Sinus Involved	Local Pain	Referred Pain
Maxillary	Behind eye Cheek Nose Upper teeth Upper lip	Teeth Retrobulbar
Ethmoid	Periorbital Retronasal Retrobulbar	Occipital Upper cervical
Frontal	Supraorbital Frontal	Bitemporal and occipital headache

Table 9–3   Clinical Signs and Symptoms in Sinus Disease

Sinus Involved	Signs and Symptoms
Maxillary	Ocular abnormalities
	Diplopia
	Proptosis
	Epiphora (tearing)
	Nasal obstruction and rhinorrhea
	Epistaxis
	Loosening of teeth
Ethmoid	Orbital swelling
	Nasal obstruction and purulent rhinorrhea
	Ocular abnormalities
	Proptosis
	Diplopia
	Tenderness over inner canthus of eye
Frontal	Nasal obstruction and rhinorrhea
	Tenderness over frontal sinus
	Pus in middle meatus
	Signs of meningitis

Impact of Deafness on the Patient

The ear is the sensory organ of hearing. Audition is one of the main avenues of communication. Any disturbance in the reception of sound waves by the external ear to the transmission of the electrical impulses to the brain may result in an abnormal interpretation of language.

In 1977, it was estimated that more than 14.2 million persons in the United States had some degree of hearing loss that interfered with their ability to understand speech (Ries, 1982). About half of these individuals, 7.2 million, had bilateral hearing problems. Although persons older than the age of 70 years account for 30% of all deaf individuals, in 1971 there were over 202,000 deaf children younger than 3 years of age (Schein and Delk, 1974). Since the late 1970s, the overall prevalence rate has increased substantially.

In order to understand the impact of deafness on an individual, it is necessary to consider the *age at onset,* the *severity* of the loss, the *rapidity* of the loss, and any *residual* hearing. Persons with insidious or sudden hearing loss experience grief and depression. Consider, for example, the grief expressed in the quotation by Beethoven at the beginning of this chapter.

The psychological effects of deafness include *paranoia, depression, withdrawal, irritability,* and *anxiety.* Although it is not entirely resolved, it appears that deaf persons have an increased tendency toward paranoia. Most deaf individuals tend to be suspicious of others' conversations.

The most profound responses to a severe hearing deficit are depression and withdrawal. The following quotation by Beethoven dramatizes these responses:

> Oh you men who think that I am malevolent, stubborn, or misanthropic, how greatly do you wrong me. You do not know the secret cause which makes me seem that way to you. . . . For me there can be no relaxation with my fellow men, no refined conversations, no mutual exchange of ideas. I must live alone, like one who has been banished. . . . What a humiliation for me when someone standing next to me heard a flute in the distance, and I heard nothing . . . a little more of that and I would have ended my life—it was only my art that held me back.

Hearing-impaired persons have social identity problems as well. They are frequently set aside from previous associations. If they use sign language, they can no longer enjoy the company of individuals who do not know sign language. Work or career may have to be altered. The stigma associated with wearing a hearing aid serves to reinforce the feeling of alienation from others. A patient may avoid wearing a hearing aid for fear of being stigmatized.

Deaf children present even more severe problems. Their lack of auditory input influences character, early childhood experiences, attitudes, and interpersonal relationships. They are deprived of many of the reassuring, loving, and comforting sounds that facilitate the development of personality. They are unable to obtain verbal cues of a parent's affection. They are also unable to be alerted by auditory signs of danger.

Psychological problems, social inadequacy, and educational retardation are common among deaf children. The worse the handicap, the worse are the psychological and educational implications.

The young hearing-impaired child who shows a delay in language development may be diagnosed as *retarded*. In general, children who are congenitally deaf or suffer from severe hearing impairment before 3 years of age suffer the most. As the type of lesion causing deafness progresses from the periphery inward, the deleterious effects increase.

Physical Examination

> The equipment necessary for the examination of the ear and nose is as follows: an otoscope, choice of specula, penlight, and a 512 Hz tuning fork. A nasal illuminator attachment for the otoscope and a nasal speculum are optional.

The physical examination of the ear and the nose is performed with the examiner seated in front of the patient.

The Ear

If the patient has symptoms referable to one ear, examine the uninvolved ear first. The physical examination of the ear includes the following:

- External examination
- Auditory acuity testing
- Otoscopic examination

External Examination

Inspect the pinna and postauricular skin. Note the position, size, and shape of the pinna. The pinna should be positioned centrally and should be in proportion to the face and head. Any obvious abnormalities or surgical scars should be noted.

Inspect the External Ear Structures

A small dimple in front of the tragus is usually a remnant of the first branchial arch.

The external ear is inspected for deformities, nodules, inflammation, or lesions. The presence of *tophi* is a highly specific but nonsensitive sign of gout. Tophi are deposits of uric acid crystals. They appear as hard nodules in the helix or antihelix. In rare cases, a white discharge may be seen in association with them. A "cauliflower ear" is a pinna that is gnarled as a result of repeated trauma.

Inspect for discharge. If discharge is present, note its characteristics, such as color, consistency, and clarity.

Palpate the External Ear Structures

The pinna is palpated for tenderness, swelling, or nodules. If pain is elicited by pulling up and down on the pinna or by pressing in on the tragus, an infection of the external canal is likely present.

The posterior auricular region should be inspected for scars or swelling. The examiner should apply pressure to the mastoid tip, which should be painless. Tenderness may indicate a suppurative process of the mastoid bone.

Auditory Acuity Testing

Testing for auditory acuity is the next part of the physical examination. The easiest method for testing for a gross hearing loss is for the examiner to occlude one external canal by pressing inward on the tragus and to speak softly into the other ear. The examiner should hide his or her mouth to prevent lip reading by the patient. The examiner should whisper words such as "park," "dark," or "daydream" in the nonoc-cluded ear and determine whether the patient can hear them. This procedure is then repeated with the other ear. Asking a patient whether he or she hears a watch ticking when held to the ear is generally meaningless, because the patient knows what to expect.

The use of *tuning fork testing* for hearing loss is more accurate and should be performed regardless of the results of the whisper test. Although there are several tuning fork frequencies available, the best for evaluation of hearing is the 512 Hz fork.* A tuning fork is held by its stem, and its tip is briskly struck against the palm of the hand. It is never to be struck on a solid wooden or metal object. The two tuning fork tests to assess hearing are the following:

- The Rinne test
- The Weber test

The Rinne Test

The Rinne test compares air conduction with bone conduction. Each ear is tested separately. The examiner should strike a 512 Hz tuning fork and place its handle on the mastoid tip near the external auditory meatus. The patient is then asked whether he or she hears the sound and to indicate when it is no longer heard. When the patient can no longer hear the sound, the tines of the vibrating tuning fork are placed in front of the external auditory meatus of the same ear, and the patient is asked whether he or she can still hear the sound. The tines of the vibrating tuning fork should not touch any hair, because the patient may have a hearing impairment but may still feel the vibration. The Rinne test is demonstrated in Figure 9–11.

Normally, air conduction (AC) is better than bone conduction (BC), and patients are able to hear the tuning fork at the external auditory meatus after they can no longer hear it on the mastoid tip; this is a *Rinne positive* test (AC > BC). Patients with a conductive hearing loss, however, have bone conduction that is better than air conduction: a *Rinne negative* test (BC > AC). Patients with sensorineural deafness have impaired air *and* bone conduction but maintain the normal AC > BC response. The middle ear amplifies the sound in both positions.

If there is total deafness in one ear, the patient may hear the tuning fork even when it is placed on the mastoid process of the deaf ear. This is due to the transmis-sion of vibrations by bone across the skull to the opposite side where they are sensed by the healthy ear. This is termed a *false-negative Rinne*.

The Weber Test

The Weber test compares bone conduction in both ears and determines whether monaural impairment is neural or conductive in origin. Stand in front of the patient and place a vibrating 512 Hz tuning fork firmly against the center of the patient's forehead. Ask the patient to indicate whether he or she hears or feels the sound in the right ear, in the left ear, or in the middle of the forehead. Hearing the sound, or feeling the vibration, in the middle is the normal response. If the sound is not heard in the middle, the sound is said to be *lateralized,* and a hearing loss is present. Sound is lateralized to the *affected* side in conductive deafness. Try it on yourself. Occlude your right ear and place a vibrating tuning fork in the center of your forehead. Where do you hear it? On the *right.* You have created a conductive hearing loss on the right by blocking the right canal; the sound is lateralized to the right side. The Weber test is illustrated in Figure 9–12.

The explanation for the Weber test is based on the masking effect of background noise. In normal conditions, there is considerable background noise, which reaches the tympanic membrane by air conduction. This tends to mask the sound of the tuning fork heard by bone conduction. In an ear with a conductive hearing loss, the air conduction is decreased, and the masking effect is therefore diminished. Thus, the affected ear hears and feels the vibrating tuning fork better than does the normal ear.

In patients with unilateral sensorineural deafness, the sound is not heard on the affected side but is heard by, or localized to, the *unaffected* ear.

---

* Different examiners prefer tuning forks of different frequencies for determining auditory acuity. A tuning fork of too high a frequency will fade too quickly.

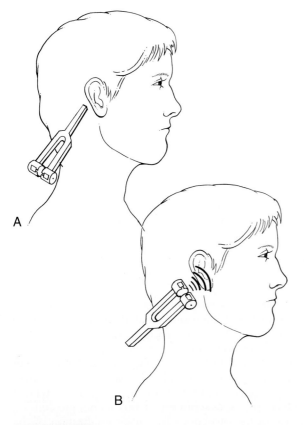

Figure 9–11

The Rinne test. The tuning fork is first placed on the mastoid process as shown in *A*. When the sound can no longer be heard, the tuning fork is placed in front of the external auditory meatus as shown in *B*. Normally, air conduction is better than bone conduction.

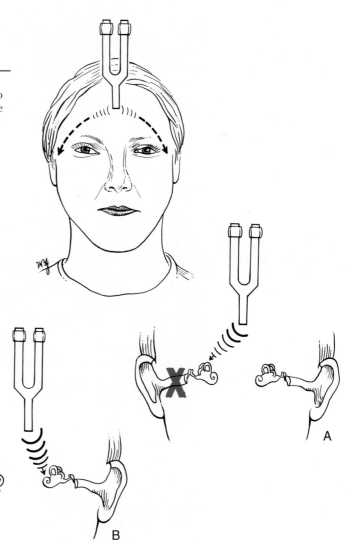

Figure 9–12

The Weber test. When a vibrating tuning fork is placed on the center of the forehead, the sound will be heard in the center without lateralization to either side (normal response). *A,* In the presence of a conductive hearing loss, the sound will be heard on the side of the conductive loss. *B,* In the presence of a sensorineural loss, the sound will be heard better on the opposite (unaffected) side.

In order to test the reliability of the patient's responses, it is useful to occasionally strike the tuning fork against the palm of the hand and hold it briefly to silence it. The two tests are then carried out as indicated, using the silent tuning fork. This serves as a good control.

In summary, consider the following two examples:

Example 1:

Right ear	*Left ear*
AC > BC (Rinne positive)	BC > AC (Rinne negative)

Weber: lateralization to the left ear →
Diagnosis: Left conductive deafness

Example 2:

Right ear	*Left ear*
AC > BC (Rinne positive)	AC > BC (Rinne positive)

Weber: lateralization to the right ear ←
Diagnosis: Left sensorineural deafness

■ Otoscopic Examination

The remainder of the examination of the ear is performed with the otoscope. The otoscope incorporates a halogen light source and fiberoptic circumferential distribution of the light. This provides a 360° ring of light-conducting fibers within the shell of the otoscope through which the observer views the inner structures of the ear. Most otoscopes are illuminated by a bright quartz halogen bulb requiring a 3.5 V power supply. Specially designed speculae, polypropylene reusable or disposable, slip over the tip of the instrument. Most otoscopic heads have the ability to be used with a rubber squeeze bulb for pneumatic otoscopy. A description of this technique follows later in this chapter. Take care in the use of the otoscope. The best visualization of the structure does not require the speculum of the otoscope to be wedged into the canal. Be gentle, in order to achieve the best visualization of the anatomy.

Choose the correct speculum size: small enough to prevent discomfort to the patient and large enough to provide an adequate beam of light. Generally a 4–6 mm tip diameter is used for adults, 3–4 mm for children, and 2 mm for infants.

The Techniques

To examine the patient's *right* ear, the examiner holds the otoscope in the *right* hand. The canal is straightened by the examiner's *left* hand pulling the pinna *up, out,* and *back.* The straighter the canal, the easier the visualization and the more comfortable the examination will be for the patient.

In the child, the canal should be straightened by pulling the pinna *down* and *back.*

The patient is asked to turn his or her head to the side slightly so that the examiner can examine the ear more comfortably. The otoscope may be held in either of two positions. The first, and preferred, position involves holding the otoscope like a pencil, between the thumb and index fingers, in a *downward* position with the ulnar aspect of the examiner's hand braced against the side of the patient's face. This positioning provides a buffer against sudden movement by the patient. By holding the end of the otoscope's handle, the examiner then angles the speculum into the external canal. This technique at first feels more cumbersome than the alternative technique, but it is safer, especially for children. This technique is shown in Figure 9–13.

The second position involves holding the otoscope *upward* as the speculum is introduced into the canal. This technique feels more comfortable, but a sudden movement of the patient can cause pain and injury to the patient. This technique is shown in Figure 9–14.

Inspect the External Canal

Gently insert the speculum and inspect the external canal. The external auditory canal is 24 mm long in the adult and is the only skin-lined, blind-ended canal in the body. The canal follows a tortuous course from the external meatus to the tympanic membrane. The techniques previously described are used to straighten the canal. There should be no evidence of redness, swelling, or tenderness, which indicates inflammation. The walls of the canal should be free of foreign bodies, scaliness, and discharge.

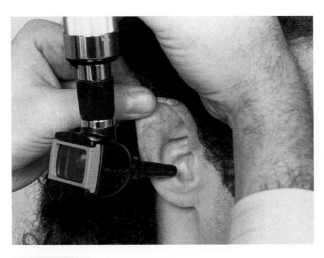

Figure 9–13

Technique for otoscopic examination. Notice that the ear is pulled up, out, and back.

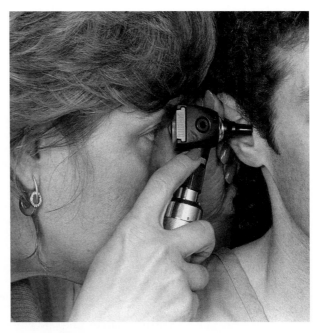

Figure 9–14

Alternative technique for otoscopic examination. The ear is pulled up, out, and back.

If a foreign body is seen, pay particular attention to inspecting the opposite ear canal, nose, and other accessible body orifices.

Any cerumen should be left as is, unless it interferes with the visualization of the rest of the canal and tympanic membrane. Removal of cerumen is best left to the experienced examiner, because any manipulation may result in trauma or abrasions. Figure 9–15 shows an external ear canal with a large hematoma secondary to aggressive use of a cotton-tipped applicator stick. Notice the tympanic membrane in the background.

If a discharge is present, look for the site of origin.

Inspect the Tympanic Membrane

As the speculum is introduced further into the canal in a downward and forward direction, the tympanic membrane will be visualized. The tympanic membrane should appear as an intact, ovoid, semitransparent, pearly-gray membrane at the end of the canal. The lower four fifths of the tympanic membrane is called the *pars tensa;* the

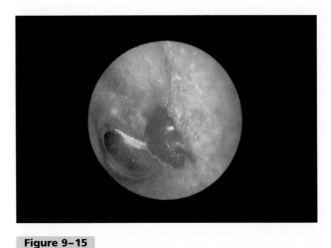

Figure 9–15

External ear canal with large hematoma.

upper fifth, the *pars flaccida*. The handle of the malleus should be seen near the center of the pars tensa. From the lower end of the handle, there is frequently a bright triangular cone of light reflected from the pars tensa. This is called the *light reflex,* which is directed anteroinferiorly. The pars flaccida, the short process of the malleus, and the anterior and posterior folds should be identified. Figure 9–16 shows a normal tympanic membrane with the important landmarks identified.

The presence or absence of the light reflex should not be considered indicative of normality or disease. The sensitivity of the presence of the light reflex indicating disease is low. There are as many normal tympanic membranes without a light reflex as there are abnormal membranes with a light reflex.

Describe the color, integrity, transparency, position, and landmarks of the tympanic membrane.

Healthy tympanic membranes are usually pearly gray. Diseased tympanic membranes may be dull and become red or yellow. Is the drum injected? *Injection* refers to the dilatation of blood vessels, making them more apparent. The blood vessels should be visible only around the perimeter of the membrane. Dense, white plaques on the tympanic membrane may be caused by tympanosclerosis. Tympanosclerosis is caused by a deposition of hyaline material and calcification within the layers of the tympanic membrane. This condition is commonly (50–60%) secondary to insertion of ventilation tubes. The classic horseshoe shape of tympanosclerosis is seen on the tympanic membrane shown in Figure 9–17. Despite the size of these lesions, they usually do not impair hearing and are rarely of clinical importance. If the lesion extends into the middle ear, however, conductive deafness may result.

Is the tympanic membrane bulging or retracted? Bulging of the membrane may indicate fluid or pus in the middle ear. No bubbles or fluid should be seen behind the tympanic membrane in the middle ear. A tympanic membrane becomes retracted when intratympanic cavity pressures are reduced—for example, when the eustachian tube is obstructed. Figure 9–18 shows a "retraction pocket" just above the lateral process of the malleus, a condition known as *attic retraction.* Occasionally, the entire tympanic membrane may become retracted onto the ossicles of the middle ear. The ossicles may become eroded with the development of a conductive hearing loss.

If the tympanic membrane is perforated, describe the characteristics. Perforation of the tympanic membrane can occur after trauma or infection.

The normal position of the tympanic membrane is oblique to the external canal. The superior margin is closer to the examiner's eye. This is frequently better seen in infants than in adults.

In the normal ear, the handle of the malleus attached to the tympanic membrane is the primary landmark. Frequently, the long process of the incus may be seen posterior to the malleus. The chorda tympani nerve, which supplies taste to the anterior two thirds of the tongue, is frequently visible in the upper posterior quadrant; it passes horizontally across the middle ear behind the tympanic membrane between the long process of the incus and the handle of the malleus. Keratin patches appear as multiple,

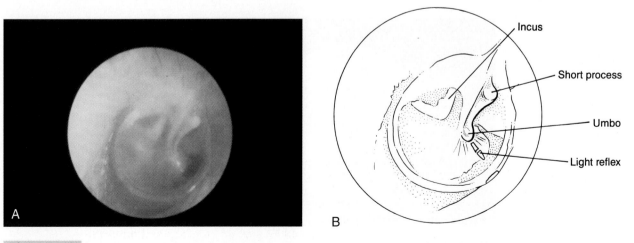

Figure 9–16

A and *B,* Photograph and labeled schematic showing a normal right tympanic membrane.

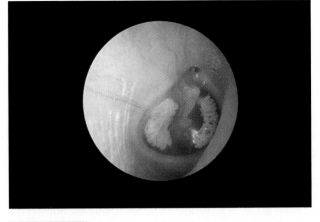

Figure 9–17

Tympanosclerosis.

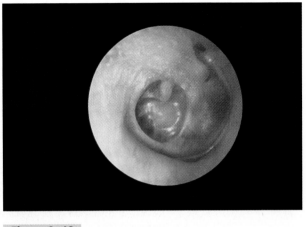

Figure 9–18

Retraction pocket.

discrete, white patches on the tympanic membrane of all normal membranes; if illumination is not sufficient, however, they may not be visualized. In the presence of a retracted tympanic membrane, the malleus is seen in sharp outline.

There are many differences in the color, shape, and contour of the tympanic membrane, which will be recognized only with experience.

After examining the right ear, examine the *left* ear by holding the otoscope in the *left* hand and straightening the canal with the *right* hand.

Determine the Mobility of the Tympanic Membrane

If there is a question of middle-ear infection, pneumatic otoscopy should be performed.

This technique requires the use of a speculum large enough to fit snugly into the external canal in order to establish a closed air chamber between the canal and the interior of the otoscopic head. A rubber squeeze bulb is attached to the otoscopic head. By squeezing the bulb, the pressure of the air in the canal can be increased. Pneumatic otoscopy must be performed gently, and the patient should be informed that he or she may experience a blowing noise during the procedure. When the pressure in the otoscopic head is increased by squeezing the bulb, the normal tympanic membrane will show a prompt inward movement. In patients with an obstructed eustachian tube, the tympanic membrane will move sluggishly inward. If fluid is present in the middle ear, a marked decrease or absence of movement will be detected. The reduction of movement of the tympanic membrane increases the probability of middle-ear infection by as much as 40%. This simple technique can provide invaluable assistance in the early diagnosis of many middle-ear problems.

The Nose

The examination of the nose consists of the following:

- External examination
- Internal examination

■ External Examination

Inspect the Nose

The external examination consists of inspection of the nose for any *swelling, trauma,* or *congenital anomalies.* Is the nose straight? Does a deviation involve the upper, bony portion or the lower, cartilaginous portion?

Inspect the external nares. Are they symmetric?

Test the patency of each nostril. Occlude one nostril by gently placing the finger across the opening of the nostril. Ask the patient to sniff. Do not compress the contralateral nostril by aggressive pressure.

Any swelling or deformity should be palpated for pain and firmness.

Rhinophyma is a common condition in which there is prominent hypertrophy of the sebaceous glands of the nose with overgrowth of the soft tissue. This condition is more common in males (Fig. 9–19). The patient shown also has *acne rosacea,* which is another common associated condition consisting of papules, pustules, and erythema of the face. The cause is unknown. The rash is worsened by hot drinks, highly spiced food, and alcohol.

Palpate the Sinuses

Palpation over the frontal and maxillary sinuses may reveal tenderness that is indicative of sinusitis.

■ Internal Examination

The key to the internal examination is the proper positioning of the head. Ask the patient to hold his or her head back. The examiner places the left hand firmly on top of the patient's head and uses the left thumb to elevate the tip of the patient's nose. In this manner, change the position of the patient's head to visualize intranasal structures. Use a light source to illuminate the internal structures. This technique is shown in Figure 9–20.

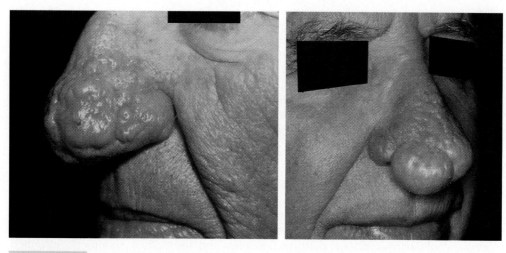

Figure 9–19

Rhinophyma.

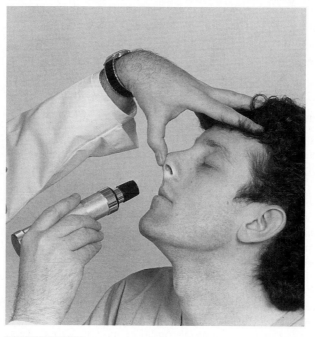

Figure 9–20

Inspection of the internal structures of the nose.

Inspect the position of the septum to the lateral cartilages on each side. Examine the vestibule for inflammation and the anterior septum for deviation or perforation. The *color* of the nasal mucous membrane should be evaluated. Normal nasal mucous membranes are dull red and moist and have a smooth, clean surface. Nasal mucosae are usually darker in color than oral mucosae. Inspect for exudate, swelling, bleeding, and trauma. If epistaxis has occurred, Little's area should be examined for vascular engorgement or crusting.

Is a discharge present? If so, it should be described as purulent, watery, cloudy or bloody. Is crusting present? Are any masses or polyps present?

By tipping the patient's head farther back, check the posterior septum for deviation or perforation. The size and color of the inferior turbinates should be noted. The two inferior turbinates are rarely symmetric.

Inspect the size, color, and mucosal condition of the middle turbinates. Are polyps present? Most polyps are found in the middle meatus.

Use a Nasal Illuminator

If a nasal illuminator is used, the examiner places the left thumb on the tip of the patient's nose while the palm of the examiner's hand steadies the patient's head. The patient's neck is slightly extended as the tip of the speculum of the illuminator is inserted into the nostril. After one nostril is evaluated, the illuminator is placed in the other nostril. The technique of using a nasal illuminator is shown in Figure 9–21.

Use a Nasal Speculum

If a nasal speculum is used, the instrument is held in the examiner's left hand, and the speculum is introduced into the patient's nostril in a vertical position (blades facing up and down). The speculum should not rest on the nasal septum. The blades are inserted about 1 cm into the vestibule, and the patient's neck should be slightly extended. The examiner's left index finger is placed on the ala of the patient's nose to anchor the upper blade of the speculum while the right hand of the examiner steadies the patient's head. The right hand is used to change the head position for better visibility of the internal structures. After one nostril has been examined, the speculum, still being held in the examiner's left hand, is introduced into the patient's other nostril. The technique of holding the speculum is shown in Figure 9–22. Although the nasal speculum provides the best method of inspection, internists rarely use this instrument.

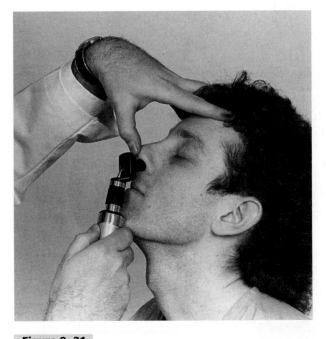

Figure 9–21

Using a nasal illuminator to inspect the internal structures of the nose.

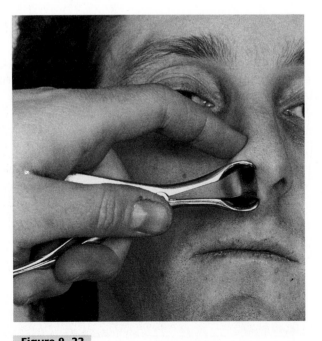

Figure 9–22

Using a nasal speculum to inspect the internal structures of the nose. Note the position of the left index finger.

Transilluminate the Sinuses

If a patient has symptoms referable to sinus problems, transillumination of the sinuses is performed. This examination is performed in a darkened room where a bright light source is placed in the mouth of the patient on one side of the hard palate. The light is transmitted through the maxillary sinus cavity and is seen as a crescent-shaped dull glow under the eye. The other side is then examined. Normally, the glow on each side is equal. If one sinus contains fluid, a mass, or mucosal thickening, there will be a decrease in its glow, indicating loss of aeration on that side. An alternate method of examining the maxillary sinus is to direct a light downward from under the medial aspect of the eye. The patient is asked to open the mouth, and the glow is observed in the hard palate. This technique is illustrated in Figure 9–23. The frontal sinus can be examined in a similar manner by directing the light upward under the medial aspect of the eyebrow and observing the glow above the eye.

The ethmoid and sphenoid sinuses cannot be examined by transillumination.

The variability of sinus transillumination from patient to patient is tremendous. In the absence of sinus symptoms, these differences in transillumination make the technique nonspecific.

Clinicopathologic Correlations

Infectious, inflammatory, traumatic, and neoplastic diseases are common in the organs of the ear and nose. Some of the more common ear infections are discussed in this section.

Acute otitis externa is a common inflammatory condition of the external ear canal, most often caused by *Pseudomonas aeruginosa*. The prominent symptom is severe ear pain (otalgia) accentuated by manipulation of the pinna and especially by pressure on the tragus. Edema of the external ear canal, erythema, and a yellowish-green discharge are prominent signs of this disease. Commonly, the canal is so tender and swollen that adequate visualization of the entire canal and tympanic membrane is impossible. "Swimmer's ear" is a form of otitis externa in which there is a loss of the protective cerumen, and chronic irritation and maceration by the water and bacteria occur. Itching is a common precursor of the otalgia. Figure 9–24 shows the external ear canal of a

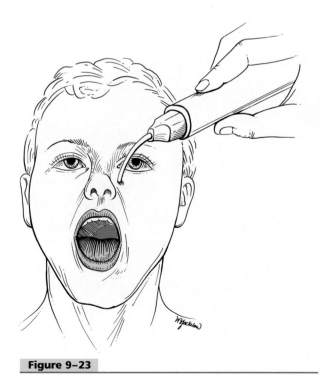

Figure 9–23

Transillumination of the maxillary sinus. Note the red glow seen on the hard palate.

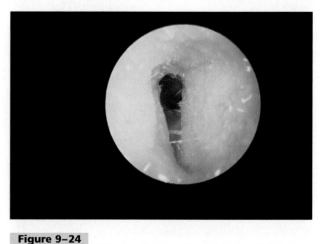

Figure 9–24

Acute otitis externa.

patient with acute otitis externa. Notice the follicular appearance of the canal due to epithelial swelling. As the condition progresses, the lumen may be occluded, producing conductive deafness.

Bullous myringitis is a localized form of external otitis, commonly associated with an acute viral upper respiratory infection. Severe otalgia is present. This is due to bullous, often hemorrhagic, lesions on the skin in the deep external ear canal and on the tympanic membrane. A blood-tinged discharge may also occur. Fortunately, bullous myringitis is a self-limited condition. Figure 9–25 shows the tympanic membrane of a patient with bullous myringitis. Notice the blood-filled bullae on the membrane. Figure 9–26 shows another patient with bullous myringitis. The left ear is shown. Notice the huge bulla filled with serosanguineous fluid arising from the floor of the bony external auditory canal. The bulla is so large that it obscures the tympanic membrane from view.

Acute otitis media is a bacterial infection of the middle ear, seen most commonly in children. Up to 50% of all children experience an attack of acute otitis media before they reach 1 year of age, and 75% of children are affected before the second birthday. After the age of 5 years, the incidence declines rapidly. Affected patients suffer ear pain and have constitutional symptoms of fever and malaise, often associated with gastrointestinal problems and a conductive hearing loss. The tympanic membrane becomes injected, and the entire membrane becomes fiery red. A mucopurulent exudate in the middle ear causes the membrane to bulge outward. In most cases, antibiotic therapy will resolve the condition and restore normal hearing. Figure 9–27 shows the tympanic

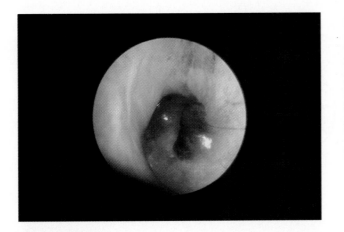

Figure 9–25

Bullous myringitis.

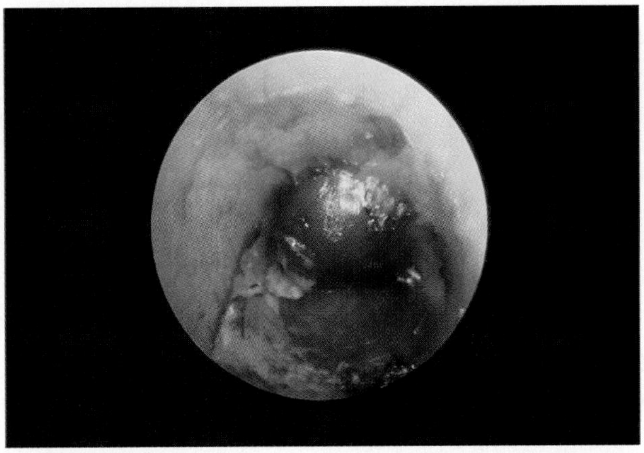

Figure 9–26

Bullous myringitis.

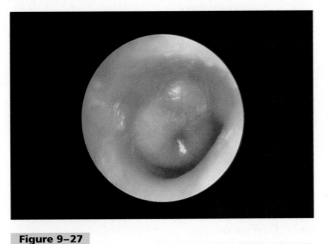

Figure 9–27

Acute otitis media.

membrane of a young child with the classic features of acute otitis media. Notice the erythema, due to the acute inflammation, and the cloudiness and bulging of the tympanic membrane, due to the middle ear exudate. Spontaneous rupture of the tympanic membrane may occur, with the discharge of the mucopurulent exudate into the external ear canal. Unlike in external otitis, in which pulling on the auricle and tragus will cause pain, no pain is elicited when these maneuvers are performed on a patient with acute otitis media.

If the tympanic membrane ruptures from the increased pressure, *advanced acute otitis media* is said to be present. The purulent exudate is then discharged into the external canal. Figure 9–28 shows a tympanic membrane that has perforated as a result of otitis media.

Perforations may be *central* or *marginal* and may result from either otitis or trauma. A central perforation does not involve the margin or annulus of the tympanic membrane; a marginal perforation involves the margin. Marginal perforations are more serious because they predispose the patient to the development of a *cholesteatoma,* which is a chronic condition of the middle ear. A marginal perforation allows squamous epithelium from the external canal to grow into the middle ear. As these cells invade, they desquamate, and debris accumulates in the middle ear, forming a cholesteatoma. Slow enlargement of the cholesteatoma leads to erosion of the ossicles and expansion into the mastoid antrum. (Fig. 9–29*A* shows a cholesteatoma; Fig. 9–29*B* is the schematic.)

A congenital cholesteatoma of the right middle ear is shown in Figure 9–30. A smooth, white cholesteatoma is seen in the anterior middle ear, medial to a normal tympanic membrane.

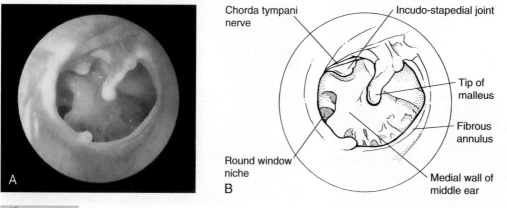

Figure 9–28

A and *B,* Photograph and labeled schematic showing a central perforation of the right tympanic membrane.

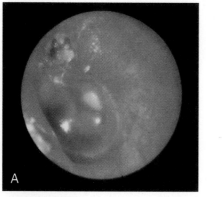
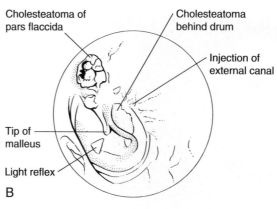

Figure 9–29

A and *B,* Photograph and labeled schematic showing a cholesteatoma of the left ear that resulted from a marginal perforation of the tympanic membrane. Note the injection of the distal external canal.

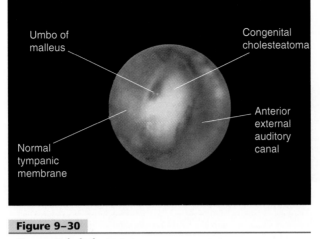

Figure 9–30

Congenital cholesteatoma.

Figure 9–31 shows a patient with a chronic tympanic membrane perforation of the right ear. Notice the smooth, epithelium-covered margin of chronic perforation as well as patches of tympanosclerosis.

Serous otitis media occurs primarily in adults with a viral upper respiratory infection or during sudden atmospheric pressure changes. In the presence of a blocked eustachian tube, air becomes trapped within. The tiny blood vessels in the middle ear absorb much of the air, producing a vacuum that draws in or retracts the tympanic membrane. The sensation of "plugged ears" occurs. If the pressure is not relieved, this vacuum draws serous, nonpurulent fluid from the blood vessels into the middle ear. The tympanic membrane appears yellowish orange as a result of the amber-colored fluid, and the landmarks are clearly seen as the membrane is retracted against these structures. Partial obstruction of the eustachian tube produces air bubbles or an air-fluid level in the middle ear. Figure 9–32 shows a tympanic membrane of a patient with serous otitis media.

Recurrent middle ear infections and tympanic membrane rupture may lead to *chronic otitis media*. Chronic infections may produce a foul-smelling discharge, which is the main symptom of chronic otitis media; pain is usually not present. Erosion of the ossicles and scar tissue may develop, causing a conductive hearing loss.

Figure 9–33 shows the right tympanic membrane from an adult patient with chronic eustachian tube dysfunction. An early pars flaccida retraction pocket is seen.

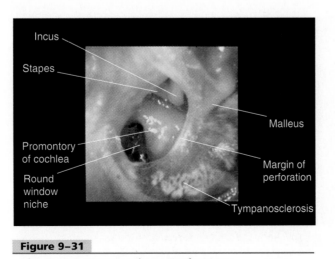

Figure 9–31

Chronic tympanic membrane perforation.

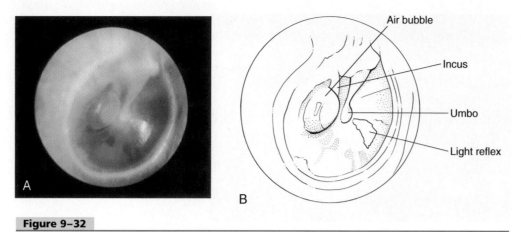

Figure 9–32

A and *B,* Photograph and labeled schematic showing serous otitis media of the right ear. Note the air bubble in the middle ear behind the tympanic membrane.

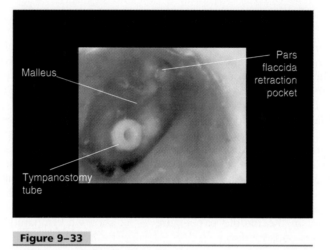

Figure 9–33

Chronic eustachian tube dysfunction.

These retraction pockets result from chronic negative pressure within the middle ear and may progress to form an acquired cholesteatoma. A pressure-equalizing tube, a tympanostomy tube, has been placed to eliminate the negative middle-ear pressure. Figure 9–34 shows the right tympanic membrane from another patient with long-standing eustachian tube dysfunction whose middle ear is ventilated with a chronic

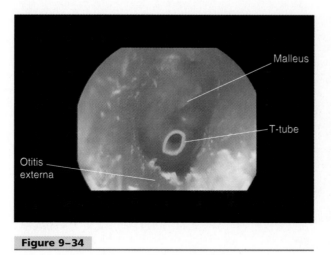

Figure 9–34

Tympanic membrane ventilated with T-tube.

tympanostomy tube, or T-tube. Resolving mild otitis externa is seen with canal skin erythema and desquamation of the epithelium.

Table 9–4 summarizes the comparative features of conductive and sensorineural deafness. Table 9–5 enumerates the common causes of deafness. Table 9–6 is a differentiation of acute external otitis from acute otitis media.

Table 9–4   Comparative Features of Conductive and Sensorineural Hearing Loss

	Conductive Hearing Loss	Sensorineural Hearing Loss
Pathology	External canal Middle ear	Cochlea Cochlear nerve Brain stem
Loudness of speech	Softer than normal	Louder than normal
External canal	May be abnormal	Normal
Tympanic membrane	Usually abnormal	Normal
Rinne's test	Negative	Positive
Weber's test	Heard on "deaf" side	Heard on better side (only in severe unilateral loss)

Table 9–5   Common Causes of Deafness

Patient	Conductive Deafness	Sensorineural Deafness
Child	Congenital Acute otitis media Chronic otitis media Cerumen Trauma	Congenital Mumps labyrinthitis Maternal rubella during first trimester Birth trauma Congenital syphilis
Adult	Serous otitis media Chronic otitis media External otitis Cerumen Eustachian tube blockage Viral myringitis Cholesteatoma Otosclerosis	Delayed-onset congenital Ménière's disease Ototoxic drugs Viral labyrinthitis Acoustic neuroma Presbycusis (age-related deafness)

Table 9–6   Differentiation of Acute External Otitis from Acute Otitis Media

Signs and Symptoms	Acute External Otitis*	Acute Otitis Media†
Pressure on tragus	Painful	No pain
Lymphadenopathy	Frequent	Absent
External canal	Edematous	Normal
Season	Summer	Winter
Tympanic membrane	Normal	Fluid behind drum, possibly perforated
Fever	Yes	Yes
Hearing loss	Slight or normal	Decreased

*See Figure 9–24.
†See Figure 9–27.

Useful Vocabulary

Listed here are the specific roots that are important in order to understand the terminology related to diseases of the ear and nose.

Root	Pertaining to	Example	Definition
audio-	to hear	*audio*meter	Device to measure hearing
aur-	ear	*aur*icle	Portion of the external ear not contained within the head
-cusis	hearing	presby*cusis*	Progressive decrease in hearing with age
-lalia	speech	echo*lalia*	Meaningless repetition by a patient of words addressed to him or her
myringo-	tympanic membrane	*myringo*tomy	Surgical incision of the tympanic membrane
ot(o)-	ear	*ot*itis	Inflammation of the ear
phon-	sound; the sound of a voice	*phon*asthenia	Weakness of the voice
rhino-	nose	*rhino*plasty	Plastic surgery of the nose
tympan(o)-	middle ear	*tympan*otomy	Surgical puncture of the tympanic membrane

Writing Up the Physical Examination

Listed here are examples of the write-up for the examinations of the ear and nose.

- The external ear appears normal without evidence of inflammation or lesions. The patient has no difficulty hearing the whispered word. The Weber test result is midline. AC > BC. The external canals are normal as are the tympanic membranes. There is no injection of the external canals or the tympanic membranes. No discharge is present.
- A 1 cm, round, hard, painless mass is present on the right pinna. The patient has no problem with hearing. The Weber test result shows no lateralization. The external canals and tympanic membranes are normal.
- The external structures of the ears are within normal limits. There is a hearing loss in the left ear. The Weber test lateralizes to the left ear. The left tympanic membrane appears opaque. The ossicles are not seen on the left. The right tympanic membrane appears normal. The ossicles appear normal on the right.
- The nose is not deviated. No swellings are seen. The anterior septum appears pink without discharge or vascular engorgement. The septum is midline. No sinus tenderness is present.
- The nose appears deviated to the right. The nasal mucous membranes are bright red and moist. A whitish-yellow discharge is present on a deviated septum to the right. The sinuses are not tender.

Bibliography

Ballantyne J: Deafness. Edinburgh, Churchill Livingstone, 1977.

Dayal VS: Clinical Otolaryngology. Philadelphia, J.B. Lippincott, 1981.

English GM: Otolaryngology. New York, Harper & Row, 1976.

Furth HG: Thinking Without Language: Psychological Implications of Deafness. New York, Free Press, 1966.

Hawke M, Keene M, Alberti PW: Clinical Otoscopy, 2nd ed. Edinburgh, Churchill Livingstone, 1990.

Hawke M, Kwok P: A mini-atlas of ear-drum pathology. Can Fam Physician 33:1501, 1987.

Hawke M, McCombe A: Diseases of the Ear: A Pocket Atlas. Toronto, Manticore Communication Inc., 1995.

Lucente FE, Sobol SM: Essentials of Otolaryngology. New York, Raven Press, 1983.

Orlans H (ed): Adjustment to Adult Hearing Loss. San Diego, College-Hill Press, 1985.

Ries PW: Hearing ability of persons by sociodemographic and health characteristics: United States (Series 10, No. 140). Washington, DC, U.S. Government Printing Office, 1982.

Schein J, Delk M Jr: The Deaf Population in the United States. Silver Spring, MD, National Association of the Deaf, 1974.

Williams JW, Simel DL: Does this patient have sinusitis? Diagnosing acute sinusitis by history and physical examination. JAMA 270:1242, 1993.

Williams JW, Simel DL, Roberts L, et al: Clinical evaluation for sinusitis: Making the diagnosis by history and physical examination. Ann Intern Med 117:705, 1992.

Zemlin WR: Speech and Hearing Science. Englewood Cliffs, NJ, Prentice-Hall, 1981.

CHAPTER 10

The Oral Cavity and Pharynx

Look to thy mouth; diseases enter here.

George Herbert
1593–1632

General Considerations

The mouth and oral cavity are used by individuals to express the entire range of emotions. As early as infancy, the mouth provides gratification and sensory pleasure.

Approximately 20% of all visits to the primary care physician are related to problems of the oral cavity and throat. The majority of patients with these problems present with throat pain, which may be acute and associated with fever or difficulty in swallowing. A sore throat may be the result of local disease or may be an early manifestation of a systemic problem.

It has been estimated that more than 90% of patients infected with human immunodeficiency virus (HIV) will have at least one oral manifestation of their disease. It appears that as further immunologic impairment develops, the risk of oral lesions increases. There are several important oral manifestations that are highly associated with early HIV infection. The presence of any of them demands HIV testing.

Many visits are also associated with psychiatric disturbances. Often, psychosomatic disease symptoms center on the mouth. Patients with psychosomatic disease may complain of "burning" or "dryness" of the mouth or tongue. *Bruxism,* or grinding of one's teeth other than for chewing, occurs especially during sleep. This overuse of the muscles of mastication has often been interpreted as a manifestation of rage or aggression that is not overtly displayed. Bruxism may be an infantile response to reduce psychic tension. Bruxism may produce facial pain, which causes further spasm of the muscles and continued bruxism, all of which constitute a vicious circle. Individuals who habitually have something in their mouths, such as a pipe, a thumb, or a pencil, may actually cause damage to their oral cavities.

Although it is often thought that the oral cavity examination is performed only by a dentist, the health-care professional must be competent to evaluate this important region of the body. The health-care provider must be able to do the following:

1. Appraise oral hygiene
2. Recognize dental caries and periodontal disease
3. Recognize the presence of oral lesions as well as disorders of the regional lymph nodes, salivary glands, and the bony structures of the region
4. Recognize oral manifestations of systemic disease
5. Recognize systemic problems caused by oral disease and procedures
6. Assess physical findings concerning the range and smoothness of jaw motion
7. Identify dental appliances
8. Know when a dental consultation is required or should be postponed due to a medical problem

Structure and Physiology

The Oral Cavity

The oral cavity consists of the following:

- Buccal mucosa
- Lips
- Tongue

- Hard and soft palate
- Teeth
- Salivary glands

The oral cavity extends from the inner surface of the teeth to the oral pharynx. Forming the roof of the mouth are the hard and soft palates. The soft palate terminates posteriorly at the *uvula*. The *tongue* forms the floor of the mouth. At the most posterior aspect of the oral cavity lie the *tonsils* between the anterior and posterior *pillars*. The oral cavity is shown in Figure 10–1.

The *buccal mucosa* is a mucous membrane that is continuous with the gingivae and lines the inside of the cheeks.

Lips are red as a result of the increased number of vascular dermal papillae and the thinness of the epidermis in this area. An increase in desaturated hemoglobin, *cyanosis*, is therefore apparent as blue lips. The common blue discoloration of the lips in a cold environment is related to the decreased blood supply and increased extraction of oxygen.

The tongue lies at the floor of the mouth and is attached to the *hyoid bone*. It is the main organ of taste, aids in speech, and serves an important function in mastication. The body of the tongue contains intrinsic and extrinsic muscles and contains the strongest muscle of the body. The tongue is supplied by the *hypoglossal*, or twelfth cranial, nerve.

The dorsum of the tongue has a convex surface with a *median sulcus*. At the posterior portion of the sulcus is the *foramen cecum*, which marks the area of the origin of the *thyroid gland*. Behind the foramen cecum are mucin-secreting glands and an aggregate of lymphatic tissue called the *lingual tonsils*. The rough texture of the tongue is due to the presence of papillae, the largest of which are the *circumvallate papillae*. There are approximately 10 of these round papillae, which are located just in front of the foramen cecum and divide the tongue into the anterior two thirds and the posterior one third. *Filiform papillae* are the most common papillae, being present over the surface of the anterior portion of the tongue. The *fungiform papillae* are located at the tip and the sides of the tongue. These papillae can be recognized from their red color and broad surface. Figure 10–2 shows the tongue viewed from above.

The *taste buds* are located on the sides of the circumvallate and fungiform papillae. Taste is perceived from the anterior two thirds of the tongue by the *chorda tympani* nerve, a division of the facial nerve. The *glossopharyngeal*, or ninth cranial, nerve perceives taste sensation from the posterior third of the tongue. There are four basic taste sensations: sweet, salty, sour, and bitter. Sweetness is detected at the tip of the

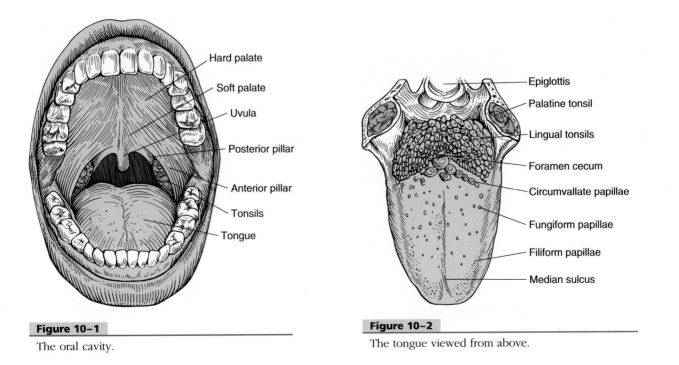

Figure 10–1

The oral cavity.

Labels (Figure 10–1): Hard palate, Soft palate, Uvula, Posterior pillar, Anterior pillar, Tonsils, Tongue

Figure 10–2

The tongue viewed from above.

Labels (Figure 10–2): Epiglottis, Palatine tonsil, Lingual tonsils, Foramen cecum, Circumvallate papillae, Fungiform papillae, Filiform papillae, Median sulcus

tongue. Saltiness is sensed at the lateral margins of the tongue. Sourness and bitterness are perceived at the posterior aspect of the tongue and are carried by the glossopharyngeal nerve.

When the tongue is elevated, a mucosal attachment, the *frenulum,* may be seen underneath the tongue in the midline connecting the tongue to the floor of the mouth.

The *hard palate* is a concave bone structure. The anterior portion has raised folds, or *rugae.* The *soft palate* is a muscular flexible area posterior to the hard palate. The posterior margin ends at the *uvula.* The uvula aids in closing off the nasopharynx during swallowing.

Teeth are composed of several tissues: *enamel, dentin, pulp,* and *cementum.* Enamel covers the tooth and is the most highly calcified tissue in the body. The bulk of the tooth is the dentin. Under the dentin is the pulp, which contains branches of the trigeminal, or fifth cranial, nerve and blood vessels. The cementum covers the root of the tooth and attaches it to the bone. Figure 10–3 shows a cross section through a molar tooth.

The *primary dentition,* or the deciduous teeth, consists of 20 teeth that erupt between 6 and 30 months of age. The primary dentition per quadrant of jaw consists of two incisors, one canine, and two premolars. These teeth are shed from the ages of 6 to 13 years. The *secondary dentition,* or the permanent teeth, consists of 32 teeth that erupt from the ages of 6 to 22 years. The secondary dentition per quadrant of jaw consists of two incisors, one canine, two premolars, and three molars. Figure 10–4 illustrates the primary and secondary dentition, and Table 22–5 summarizes the chronology of dentition.

Although not part of the oral cavity proper, the *salivary glands* are considered part of the mouth. There are three major salivary glands: the *parotid,* the *submandibular,* and the *sublingual* glands. The parotid gland is the largest of the salivary glands. It lies anterior to the ear on the side of the face. The facial, or seventh cranial, nerve courses through the gland. The duct of the parotid gland is called *Stensen's duct* and enters the oral cavity through a small papilla opposite the upper first or second molar tooth. The submandibular gland is the second largest salivary gland. It is located below and in front of the angle of the mandible. The duct of the submandibular gland is called *Wharton's duct* and terminates in a papilla on either side of the frenulum at the base of the tongue. The sublingual gland is the smallest of the major salivary glands. It is located in the floor of the mouth beneath the tongue. There are numerous ducts of the sublingual gland, some of which open into Wharton's duct. In addition to these major salivary glands, there are hundreds of very small salivary glands located throughout the oral cavity.

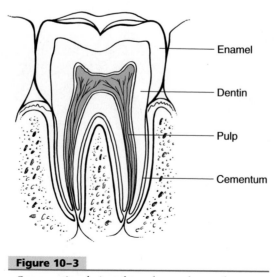

Figure 10–3

Cross-sectional view through a molar tooth.

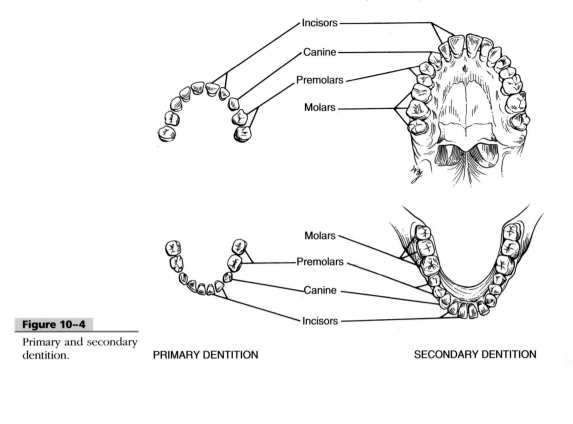

Figure 10–4

Primary and secondary dentition.

PRIMARY DENTITION   SECONDARY DENTITION

The Pharynx

The pharynx is divided into the *nasopharynx,* the *oropharynx,* and the *hypopharynx,* which is also known as the *laryngopharynx.* The nasopharynx lies above the soft palate and is posterior to the nasal cavities. On its posterolateral wall is the opening of the *eustachian tube.* The *adenoids* are pharyngeal tonsils and hang from the posterosuperior wall near the opening of the eustachian tube. The oropharynx lies below the soft palate, behind the mouth, and superior to the hyoid bone. Posteriorly it is bounded by the superior constrictor muscle and the cervical vertebrae. Below the oropharynx is the area known as the hypopharynx. The hypopharynx is surrounded by three constrictor muscles, which are innervated by the glossopharyngeal and vagus nerves. The hypopharynx ends at the level of the cricoid cartilage, where it communicates with the esophagus through the upper esophageal sphincter. Figure 10–5 illustrates the functional parts of the pharynx.

The muscular walls of the pharynx are formed by the constrictor muscles, which function during the act of swallowing. The blood supply is derived from the external carotid artery.

Lymphatic tissue is abundant in the pharynx. The lymphoid tissue consists of the *palatine tonsils,* the *adenoids,* and the *lingual tonsils.* These tissues form *Waldeyer's ring.* The palatine tonsils lie in the tonsillar fossa, between the anterior and posterior pillars. The palatine tonsils are almond-shaped and vary considerably in size. The adenoids lie on the posterior wall of the nasopharynx, and the lingual tonsils are located at the base of the tongue. The upper portion of the pharynx drains to the retropharyngeal nodes, and the lower part drains to the deep cervical lymph nodes.

The functions of the pharynx are to provide

- Swallowing
- Speech
- An airway

Swallowing, or *deglutition,* is divided into three stages. The voluntary stage occurs when a bolus of food is forced by the tongue past the tonsils to the posterior pharyn-

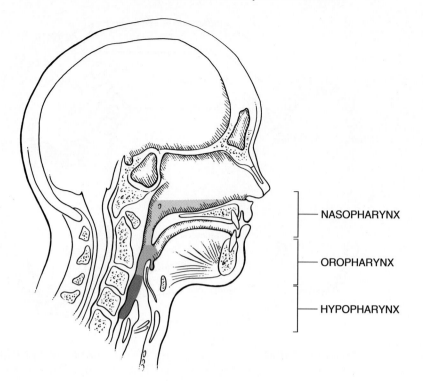

Figure 10–5

Functional parts of the pharynx.

geal wall. The second stage is involuntary constriction by the pharyngeal muscles, propelling the bolus from the pharynx to the esophagus. The third stage is also involuntary, in which the esophageal muscles push the bolus down into the stomach. The larynx is first raised and then closed during the first two stages of swallowing. The eustachian tubes open during swallowing when the nasopharynx closes.

The pharynx also acts as a structure of resonation and articulation. *Resonation* refers to the vibration of a structure. *Articulation* is the change of shape of a structure to produce speech. By contracting the pharyngeal muscles, a change in the acoustic quality of speech results. Changes in the size and shape of the pharynx affect resonance. The soft palate affects resonance by opening and closing the partition between the oral and nasal cavities. If closure is incomplete, nasal speech will result.

The pharynx is part of the airway from the nose and mouth to the trachea.

The Larynx

The larynx is located at the superior margin of the trachea and below the hyoid bone, which is located at the base of the tongue. The larynx is at the level of the fourth to sixth cervical vertebrae. The larynx functions as a guard against the entrance of solids and liquids into the trachea as well as the organ of voice production.

The *epiglottis* is attached above the larynx. The function of the epiglottis is generally held to be protection of the airways during swallowing.

The body of the larynx consists of a series of cartilaginous structures: the *cricoid*, the *thyroid*, and the *arytenoid* cartilages. The thyroid cartilage forms the bulk of the structure of the larynx and produces the prominence in the neck known as the *Adam's apple*. Toward the top of the thyroid cartilage is the *thyroid notch*. Farther down on the thyroid cartilage, there is a space, the *cricothyroid space* and *membrane*. This separates the thyroid cartilage from the cricoid cartilage. The cricoid cartilage articulates with the cricothyroid membrane superiorly and the trachea inferiorly. It is the only complete ring of cartilage in the larynx. The paired arytenoid cartilages provide an important area for attachment of the vocal cords. A projection of the thyroid and cricoid cartilages onto the neck is shown in Figure 10–6, and the laryngeal skeleton is shown in Figure 10–7.

The *vocal cords* vibrate in order to generate speech. Sound is produced by the rapid vibration of the vocal cords excited by the exhaled stream of air. The vocal cords

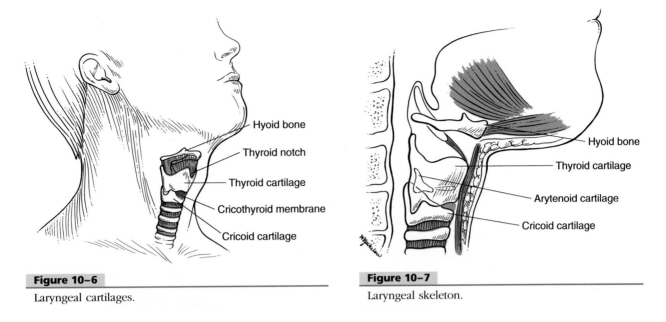

Figure 10–6

Laryngeal cartilages.

Figure 10–7

Laryngeal skeleton.

are approximated, and their tension is changed by the action of various laryngeal muscles. The nerve supply to the larynx is derived from the superior and recurrent laryngeal branches of the *vagus,* or tenth cranial, nerve. Voice produced at the larynx is then modified by the pharynx and oronasal cavity.

Review of Specific Symptoms

The Oral Cavity

All patients should be asked the following:

"When did you last see a dentist?"
"What did the dentist do?"
"Do your gums bleed?"
"Have you any pain, sores, or masses in your mouth?"
"Have you had any problems after extraction of a tooth?"

The most important symptoms of disease of the oral cavity are

- Pain
- Ulceration
- Bleeding
- Mass
- Halitosis (bad breath)

■ **Pain**

When a patient complains of oral pain, it is important to ask the following:

"Where is the pain?"
"Describe the pain."
"Do you feel the pain anywhere else?"
"How long has the pain been present?"
"What brings the pain on?"
"What makes it better? worse?"
"When you have the pain, do you have any other symptoms?"

Tooth pain may be a symptom of underlying gingival disease. A history of dental procedures and recent dental work should be taken.

Pain in the teeth may sometimes be referred from the chest. Patients with angina may actually complain of pain in their teeth associated with exertion. Careful and thoughtful questioning is indicated.

Ulceration

Oral ulcerative lesions are commonly seen and may represent manifestations of local or systemic disease of immunogenic, infectious, malignant, or traumatic causes. The patient's history is most important because it indicates whether the lesions are acute or chronic, single or multiple, and primary or recurrent.

Pain is frequently related to ulceration of the lips or tongue. Cancer is not the most common cause of oral cavity ulceration, but it must always be considered. When a patient complains of ulceration, ask the following questions:

"Have you had a lesion like this before?"
"Are there multiple lesions?"
"How long have the lesions been present?"
"Are there lesions anywhere else on the body, such as in the vagina? in the urethra? in the anus?"
"Are the lesions painful?"
"Do you smoke?" If so, *"How much?"*
"Do you have a history of veneral disease?"

Ask about a patient's sexual habits. These questions were discussed in Chapter 1, The Interviewer's Questions. Smoking and drinking alcohol predispose an individual to precancerous lesions of the mouth, such as leukoplakia and erythroplakia.

Bleeding

Bleeding may result from a primary hematologic disorder or from a local inflammation or neoplasm. Many medications may also cause or predispose a patient to bleeding. Always ask whether the patient is taking any medications.

Mass

If a patient complains of, or is found to have on physical examination, an intraoral mass or a mass in the region of a salivary gland, determine its duration and whether the mass is painful. Are there associated symptoms such as excessive salivation, known as *ptyalism,* or dryness of the mouth, known as *xerostomia?* Is dysphagia (difficulty in swallowing) present? A painless mass usually is a sign of a tumor.

Halitosis*

Halitosis affects about 50% of all adults. Fortunately, only a small percentage of these adults have the problem persisting the entire day. Most individuals with halitosis are told by others that they have bad breath, although they themselves may be unaware of the problem. In some cases, the odor in the mouth is so objectionable that it can compromise the patient's social and professional life.

The source of the bad breath is in the oral cavity in 90% of cases; the other 10% have disorders in the nasal passages or lungs or a systemic disease. It is questionable whether the gastrointestinal tract is a source of halitosis.

It is believed that halitosis is caused by volatile sulfur and other compounds exhaled into the air by the patient during speech and respiration. These compounds are produced by putrefactive, gram-negative anaerobic bacteria colonizing on the posterior dorsum of the tongue, periodontal pockets, and around some dental restorations and prostheses. The volatile sulfur compounds are generated by the bacterial metabolism of sulfur-containing amino acids. Xerostomia increases the level of volatile sulfur compounds.

Patients with systemic diseases, such as diabetes mellitus, cirrhosis, uremia, and cancer; infections of the perioral regions; and trimethylaminuria (fish-odor syndrome) can suffer from bad breath. These conditions must be considered in the absence of oral and sinonasal disease.

Treatment of halitosis should be directed toward the underlying cause. Once it has been determined that the source of the bad breath is the oral region, the patient should be instructed in procedures of good oral hygiene, including proper tooth brushing,

*The author thanks Harry Lumerman, D.D.S., of the Division of Oral and Maxillofacial Pathology at Mount Sinai Medical Center in New York, for his assistance in this section.

flossing, and most important, cleaning of the posterior dorsum of the tongue with a special scraping device or toothbrush. Appropriate mouthwash may also be utilized. These procedures must be performed at least twice a day to remove the bacteria and accumulated metabolic products.

The Pharynx

The most common symptoms of disease of the pharynx include the following:

- Nasal obstruction
- Pain
- Dysphagia
- Deafness
- Snoring

Nasal Obstruction

Nasal obstruction can result from enlarged adenoids or from tumor formation in the nasopharynx. It is important to determine whether the patient has any allergies or sinus trouble or has sustained nasal trauma.

Pain

Pain can result from inflammation of the tonsils or posterior pharynx as well as from a tumor in this area. Acute throat pain may be caused by inflammatory processes or injury. A foreign body in the pharynx often produces severe pain that is worsened by swallowing. Often, throat pain may be referred to the ipsilateral ear. Chronic throat pain may be caused by inflammatory processes as well as by neoplasms. Enlarged thyroid lobes or diffuse thyroid enlargement may cause throat pain associated with dysphagia. Hysteria is another cause of chronic throat pain.

Dysphagia

Dysphagia is difficulty in swallowing. Determine the site of obstruction. Does the dysphagia occur with liquids, solids, or tablets? Questions related to tonsillar infections are relevant because enlarged tonsils may interfere with swallowing. It is prudent to ask whether *regurgitation* of food occurs. This results from an abnormal pharyngeal pouch. The patient may describe that the "food gets stuck." This is often associated with significant disease.

Deafness

A tumor at the distal end of the eustachian tube in the nasopharynx can produce *conductive deafness*. Benign masses such as hypertrophied adenoids may be responsible. Nasopharyngeal malignancies may also be the cause of conductive deafness. In many cases, serous effusions in the middle-ear space cause eustachian tube dysfunction.

Snoring

Snoring is a common complaint. The important problem often associated with heavy snoring is obstructive sleep apnea. Many affected patients are overweight and have a history of excessive daytime sleepiness. A bed partner may describe the patient as sleeping quietly; then a transition occurs to louder snoring, followed by a period of cessation of snoring, during which time the patient becomes restless, has gasping motions, and appears to be struggling for breath. This period is then terminated by a loud snort, and the sequence may begin again. It is common for patients with sleep apnea to have many of these episodes each night.

The Larynx

Dysphonia

The major symptom of laryngeal disease is a change in the voice, especially the development of dysphonia, or hoarseness. Ask the following questions:

"For how long have you had the hoarseness?"
"What seems to make it better? worse?"

"Is there any time of day at which it is worse?"
"Have you had any surgery requiring general anesthesia?"
"Have you had any injury to your neck?"

Determine whether the patient is or was a smoker. Recent onset of hoarseness may result from impingement on the recurrent laryngeal nerve as it hooks around the left bronchus. This may be caused by a tumor or by an enlarged left atrium. Voice overuse or a vocal cord neoplasm are other causes of hoarseness. Procedures involving general anesthesia require the use of an endotracheal tube, which could potentially damage a vocal cord and cause hoarseness.

Impact of a Voice Disorder on the Patient

Phonation is the process of sound production by the interaction of airflow through the glottis and the opening and closing of the vocal cords of the larynx. Voice loudness is proportional to the air pressure below the glottis; pitch is related to this pressure and to the length of the vocal cords. Voice quality may change when there is interference with the vocal cords or pharyngeal cavity vibration, i.e., resonance.

A voice disorder may be related to an increased size of the vocal cord, a laryngeal mass, or a neurologic or psychological problem. A voice disorder is defined as a voice that is different in pitch, quality, loudness, or flexibility in comparison with the voices of other persons of similar age, sex, and ethnic group. An abnormal voice may be a symptom or sign of illness, and its cause should be determined.

In one study of a school-aged population, voice disorders were found in up to 23% of children (Silverman and Zimmer, 1975). Most of these disorders were related to voice abuse and not to organic problems. In another study, 7% of men and 5% of women from the ages of 18 to 82 years were found to have voice disorders (Laguaite, 1972). Most of these disorders were related to organic problems.

Many patients with an organic speech disorder are rejected by other people. Their speech may be high-pitched or nasal, a cause for embarrassment. Their self-esteem is low. They are rejected by others because their voice patterns are objectionable.

Just as a voice disorder has an impact on the person, so can a person use the voice to have an impact on others. The manner in which a person speaks—the quality, pitch, loudness, stress patterns, rate—reflects his or her personality. The psychogenic voice disorders are functional disorders that are manifestations of psychological imbalance. Voice is useful as an indicator of *affective disorders,* such as depression, manic states, and mood swings, as well as of *schizophrenia.* A voice disorder may also be an indication of a sexual identity problem.

Physical Examination

The equipment necessary for the examination of the oral cavity consists of a penlight, gauze pads, gloves, applicator sticks, and tongue depressors.

The Oral Cavity

The physical examination of the oral cavity includes inspection and palpation of the

- Lips
- Buccal mucosa
- Gingivae
- Teeth
- Tongue
- Floor of the mouth
- Hard and soft palates
- Salivary glands
- Cranial nerve XII

The patient should be seated with the examiner seated or standing directly in front of him or her. The patient's face should be well illuminated. The examiner should work systematically from the front to the back so that no areas are omitted. The examiner should put on a pair of gloves when palpating any structure in the mouth. When any lesion is noted, its consistency and tenderness should be noted. If the patient is wearing dentures, he or she should be asked to remove them. Inspect the face and mouth for asymmetries and abnormalities.

Evaluate the breath. Is there any distinctive odor to the patient's breath? This may suggest poor oral hygiene or systemic disease.

Inspect the Lips

Inspect the lips for localized or generalized swellings and the ability of the patient to open the mouth.

The *color* of the lips should be assessed. Is cyanosis present? Are there any lesions on the lips? If a lesion is detected, palpation should be performed to characterize the lesion's texture and consistency. Figure 10–8 shows a patient with multiple herpetic ulcers, commonly known as *cold sores,* on the lips and external nares. Figure 10–9 shows a patient with multiple telangiectatic lesions on the tongue that are secondary to *Osler-Weber-Rendu syndrome.* In this syndrome, multiple telangiectasias are present throughout the gastrointestinal tract. These may bleed insidiously, causing anemia. Figure 10–10 shows the classic brown pigmentary changes on the lips of a patient with *Peutz-Jeghers syndrome.* This is an autosomal dominant disorder that is characterized by generalized gastrointestinal, hamartomatous polyposis and mucocutaneous pigmentation.

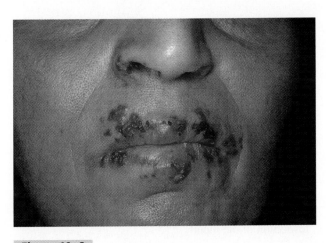

Figure 10–8

Herpes simplex labialis.

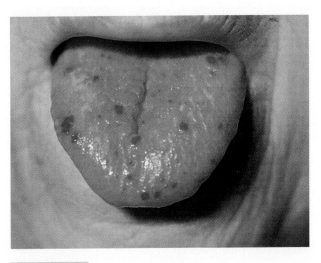

Figure 10–9

Osler-Rendu-Weber syndrome: telangiectatic lesions.

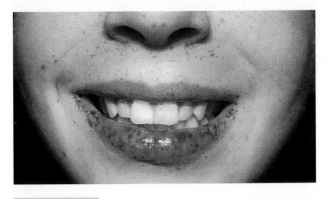

Figure 10–10

Peutz-Jeghers syndrome.

A *mucocele* of the lip is a firm, indentable, painless, translucent swelling with prominent blood vessels seen on its surface. Mucoceles, which occur mostly on the lower lip, develop when the duct to one of the mucus-secreting glands within the lip is traumatized. If ruptured, it releases a clear, thick fluid. Figure 10–11 shows a patient with a mucocele of the lower lip.

Inspect the Buccal Mucosa

The patient should be asked to open the mouth widely. The mouth should be illuminated with a light source. The buccal mucosa must be evaluated for any lesions or color changes, and the buccal cavity is inspected for any evidence of asymmetry or areas of injection (dilated vessels are usually indicative of inflammation). The buccal mucosa, teeth, and gingivae are easily evaluated by using a tongue depressor to pull the cheek away from the gums, as shown in Figure 10–12. Inspect for discolorations, evidence of trauma, and the condition of the parotid duct orifice. Are there any ulcerations of the buccal mucosa? Are there *white lesions* on the buccal mucosa? A common painless white lesion in the mouth is *lichen planus,* which appears as a reticulated, or lace-like, eruption bilaterally on the buccal mucosa. An erosive, painful, variant is similar in appearance except for the presence of hemorrhagic and ulcerated lesions. Nonerosive lichen planus is shown in Figure 10–13. Is *leukoplakia* present? In the mouth, leukoplakia can present as a painless, precancerous white plaque on the cheeks, gingivae, and tongue. Figure 10–14 shows a patient with leukoplakia of the

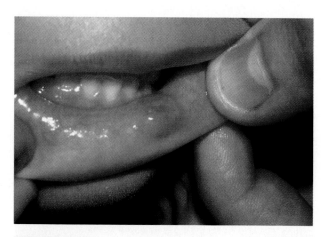

Figure 10–11

Mucocele of the lower lip.

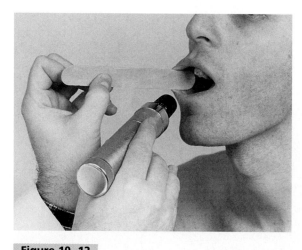

Figure 10–12

Inspection of the mouth.

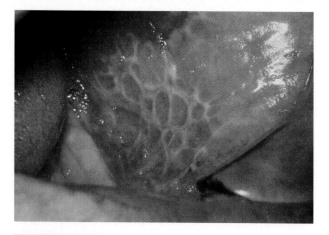

Figure 10–13

Oral lichen planus of the buccal mucosa.

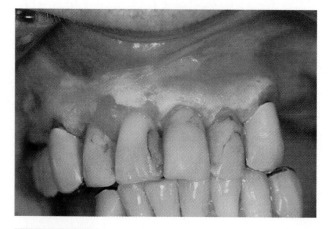

Figure 10–14

Leukoplakia of the gingiva.

gingiva. For 15 years, this lesion developed into verrucous hyperplasia, verrucous carcinoma, and finally into squamous cell carcinoma. A resection of the maxilla and palate was required. Figure 10–15 shows another patient with leukoplakia of the tongue. Notice the thick, white, adherent patches that are sharply demarcated and cannot be denuded from the tongue.

Small yellow papules on the buccal mucous membrane may be *Fordyce spots.* These are normal, prominent sebaceous glands of the lips or buccal mucosa and are frequently seen around the exit of the parotid duct. Figure 10–16 shows Fordyce spots on the buccal mucosa.

Figure 10–17 shows angiokeratomas of the buccal mucosa in a patient with *Fabry's disease,* or angiokeratoma corporis diffusum. See Figure 16–12, which shows angiokeratomas on the scrotum of the same patient.

■ Inspect the Gingivae

Does the gingival tissue completely occupy the interdental space? Are the roots of the teeth visible, indicating recession of the periodontal tissue? Is there pus or blood along the gingival margin? Are the gingivae swollen? Is there evidence of bleeding? Is gingival inflammation present? Is abnormal coloration present? *Erythroplakia* is an area of mucous membrane on which there are granular, erythematous papules that bleed. Erythroplakia has a greater malignant potential than does leukoplakia. Figure 10–18 shows a

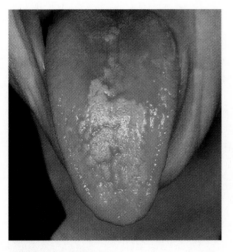

Figure 10–15

Leukoplakia of the tongue.

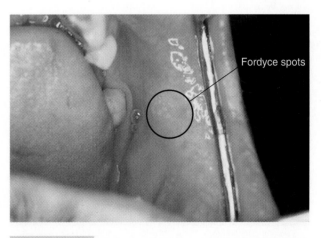

Figure 10–16

Fordyce's spots of the buccal mucosa.

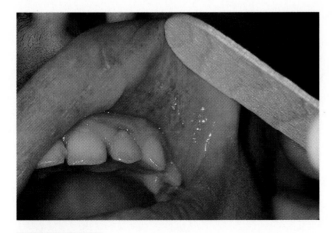

Figure 10–17

Angiokeratomas of the buccal mucosa.

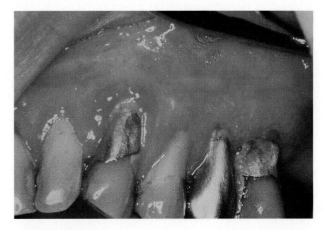

Figure 10–18

Erythroplakia of the gingiva.

patient with erythroplakia of the gingiva, shown on the right, and inflammatory gingivitis shown on the left.

There are many causes of *gingival hypertrophy*, including heredity, hormonal imbalances of puberty and pregnancy, medications, and leukemia. Gingival hypertrophy is commonly seen in patients taking phenytoin (Dilantin), an antiepilepsy medication, and nifedipine, a calcium channel blocker. The hypertrophic gingival changes of hormonal imbalances usually recede once the hormones have returned to their normal, lower level. Figure 10–19 shows marked gingival hypertrophy in a patient who was taking Dilantin. Figure 10–20 shows the gingival changes induced by nifedipine. Figure 10–21 shows gingival enlargement due to acute monomyelocytic leukemic infiltration.

Inspect the Teeth

There are 32 teeth in full adult dentition. Is dentition appropriate for the patient's age? The teeth should be inspected for caries and malocclusion. Are the teeth clean, especially around the gum line? Is there discoloration of the teeth? Is there tooth loss? Inspection of the teeth often provides insight into the patient's attitude toward general hygiene.

Are the teeth aligned properly? Ask the patient to bite normally while you retract the buccal mucosa with a tongue depressor. Repeat on the other side. Do the maxillary teeth overlap the mandibular ones, and are they in contact with them? If so, the bite is probably normal.

If the patient is wearing dental appliances such as dentures or bridges, have the patient remove them for complete evaluation.

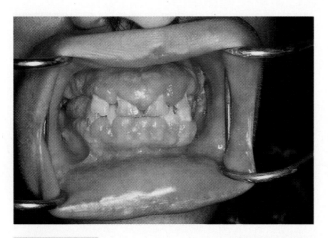

Figure 10–19

Gingival hypertrophy in patient taking Dilantin.

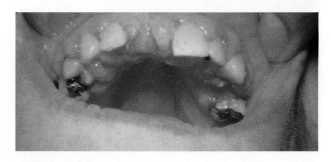

Figure 10–20

Gingival hypertrophy in patient taking nifedipine.

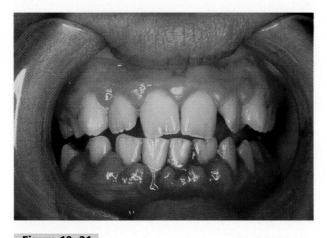

Figure 10–21

Gingival hypertrophy in a patient with acute leukemia.
Notice the bleeding gingivae.

Inspect the Tongue

Inspect the mucosa and note any masses or ulceration. Is the tongue moist? Are there any mass lesions on the sides or undersurface of the tongue? Ask the patient to lift the tongue to the roof of the mouth so that the inferior aspect of the tongue may be inspected. In older individuals, the large veins on the ventral aspect of the tongue may have become tortuous. These varicosities never bleed and have no clinical significance. Figure 10–22 shows a patient with sublingual varices. Figure 10–23 shows a patient with a benign lipoma of the tongue.

A *geographic tongue* is a benign condition in which the dorsum of the tongue shows smooth, localized, red areas, denuded of filiform papillae, surrounded by well-defined raised yellowish-white margins and normal filiform papillae. These areas together give the tongue a "map-like" appearance. The appearance of the tongue gradually changes as the depapillated areas heal while new areas of depapillation occur. A *black hairy tongue* is another benign condition in which the filiform papillae on the dorsum of the tongue are greatly elongated and resemble hairs; these enlarged "hairy" papillae become pigmented with a brownish-black color due to staining from food or tobacco or proliferating chromogenic microorganisms. This condition may commonly be a sequela to antibiotic therapy. A *scrotal,* or *fissured, tongue* is another normal variant; approximately 5% of the population has abnormal fissures in the tongue. The fissures first develop in late childhood and become deeper with age. The fissure pattern is quite variable. Food debris may collect in the fissures, causing inflammation, but the condition is otherwise benign. Halitosis may be a problem. Figure 10–24 shows these three normal tongue variants.

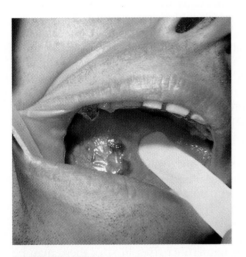

Figure 10–22

Sublingual varices of the tongue.

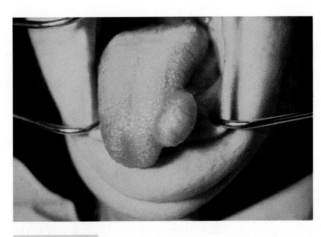

Figure 10–23

Benign lipoma of the tongue.

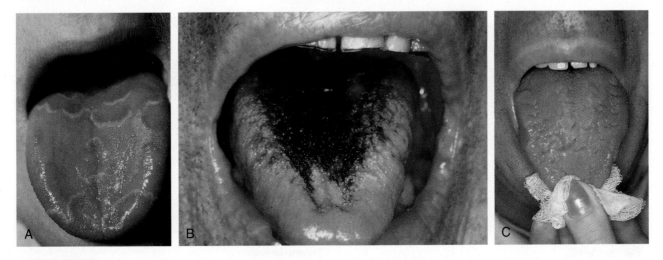

Figure 10–24

Three normal tongue variants. *A,* Geographic tongue; *B,* Black hairy tongue; *C,* Scrotal, or fissured, tongue.

Is *candidiasis* present? Candidiasis, also known as *moniliasis* or *thrush*, is an opportunistic mycotic infection. It frequently involves the oral cavity, gastrointestinal tract, perineum, or vagina. The lesions appear as white, loosely adherent membranes, beneath which the mucosa is fiery red. Oral candidiasis is the most common cause of white lesions in the mouth. It is uncommon in healthy individuals who have not been receiving broad-spectrum antibiotic or steroid-based therapies. The presence of thrush in such a patient may be an initial manifestation of acquired immunodeficiency syndrome (AIDS). Candidiasis is the most common oral infection in AIDS patients. The tongue of a patient with AIDS and oral candidiasis is shown in Figure 10–25.

Is leukoplakia present? A new form of leukoplakia, termed *oral hairy leukoplakia,* is associated with the subsequent development of AIDS. These raised, white lesions appear corrugated or "hairy" and range in size from a few millimeters to 2 to 3 cm. They are most commonly found on the lateral margins of the tongue but may also be seen on the buccal mucosa. In the absence of other causes of immunosuppresion, oral hairy leukoplakia is diagnostic of HIV infection. It is seen in more than 40% of patients with HIV infection. Figure 10–26 shows the tongue of an AIDS patient with oral hairy leukoplakia.

Look for indurated ulcers or masses in the middle, lateral aspect of the tongue. This is the most common site for intraoral squamous cell carcinoma.

Palpate the Tongue

After a thorough inspection of the tongue, the examination proceeds with palpation. In order to palpate the tongue, the patient sticks out the tongue onto a piece of gauze. The tongue is then held by the examiner's left hand as the sides of the tongue are inspected and palpated with the right hand. This is illustrated in Figure 10–27.

The anterior two thirds and the lateral margins of the tongue can be evaluated without causing a gag reflex. Palpate the lateral margins of the tongue, because more than 85% of all lingual cancers arise in this area. All white lesions should be palpated. Is there evidence of induration (hardness)? Induration or ulceration strongly suggests carcinoma. After palpating the tongue, the tongue is unwrapped, and the gauze is discarded. Any intraoral lesion, ulcer, or mass present for more than 2 weeks should be examined by biopsy and evaluated by an oral pathologist.

▧ Inspect the Floor of the Mouth

The floor of the mouth is inspected by asking the patient to lift the tongue to the roof of the mouth. Is there edema on the floor of the mouth? The opening of the submandibular gland, Wharton's duct, should be observed. Look for leukoplakia, erythroplakia, or a mass.

A *ranula* is a large mucocele on the floor of the mouth. It may occur from obstruction to the duct of one of the minor sublingual salivary glands, creating a painless, bluish, mucus-filled cystic mass. As the ranula increases in size, there may be

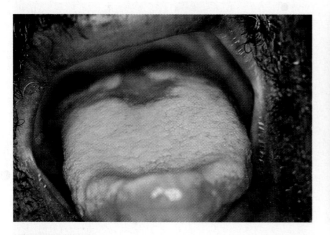

Figure 10–25

Oral candidiasis.

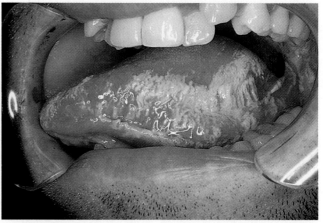

Figure 10–26

Oral hairy leukoplakia.

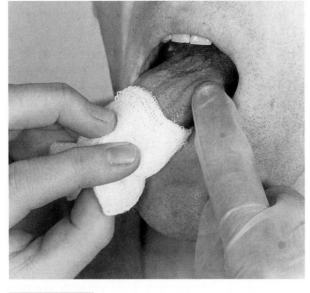

Palpation of the tongue.

reduction in tongue movement and difficulty in speech and swallowing. Figure 10–28 shows a patient with a ranula.

Palpate the Floor of the Mouth

The floor of the mouth should be examined by bimanual palpation. This is performed by placing one finger under the tongue and another finger under the chin to assess any thickening or masses. Whenever palpating in a patient's mouth, the examiner should hold the patient's cheeks, as shown in Figure 10–29. This is a means of precaution in case the patient suddenly tries to speak or bite down on the examiner's finger. Notice that the right index finger is placed under the tongue; the left thumb and index fingers are holding the patient's cheeks; and the left third or fourth finger palpates under the patient's chin.

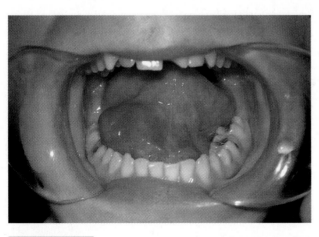

Figure 10–28

A ranula.

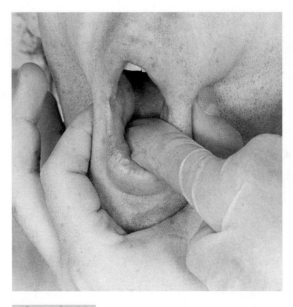

Figure 10–29

Technique for palpating oral structures.

■ **Inspect the Hard and Soft Palates**

The palate should be inspected for ulceration and masses. Masses are usually minor salivary gland tumors, mostly malignant. Are any white plaques present? Is the soft palate edematous? Is the uvula in the midline? Figure 10–30 shows a patient with AIDS and *pseudomembranous candidiasis* of the palate and uvula. *Candida albicans* is a normal commensal organism of the gastrointestinal tract. In patients with impaired immunity, or in those whose microbial flora has been altered by antibiotics, this organism can become highly invasive, as can be seen in this patient.

Are *petechiae* present? Petechiae (Fig. 10–31) are commonly seen in association with endocarditis, leukemia, oral sex, and viral infections such as infectious mononucleosis.

A common finding is a *torus palatinus.* It is painless and asymptomatic and occurs twice as often in women as in men. A torus palatinus is a discrete, hard, lobulated swelling in the midline of the posterior portion of the hard palate. This benign lesion is an overgrowth of the palatine bone. It may remain undetected until middle age, when it may interfere with the fit of a denture. Figure 10–32 shows a patient with a torus palatinus. A *torus mandibularis* is a hard, bony, often bilateral, swelling that protrudes from the lingual surface of the mandible in the premolar region. It is much less common than a torus palatinus.

Figure 10–33 shows a patient with early invasive *erythroplakia* (red plaque) of the palate.

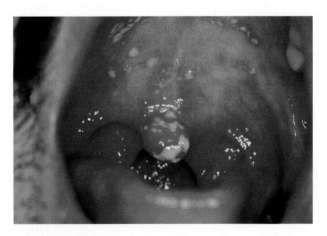

Figure 10–30

Pseudomembranous candidiasis.

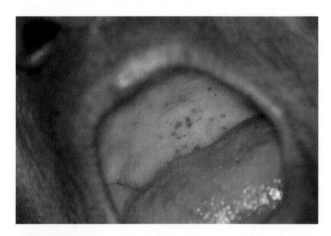

Figure 10–31

Palatal petechiae.

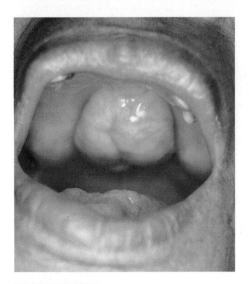

Figure 10–32

A torus palatinus.

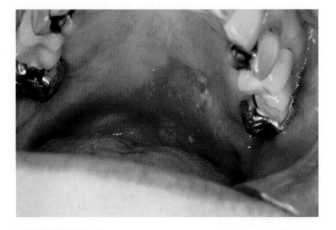

Figure 10–33

Erythroplakia of the palate.

■ Inspect the Salivary Glands

The ductal orifices of the parotid gland and the submandibular gland should be visualized. Inspect the condition of the papillae. Is there a flow of saliva? This is best evaluated by drying the papilla with a cotton applicator and observing the flow of saliva produced by exerting external pressure on the gland itself.

The salivary glands are usually not visible. Careful observation of the face will determine any asymmetry that is due to unilateral salivary gland enlargement. Obstruction to flow or infiltration of the gland results in glandular enlargement. Figure 10–34 illustrates a patient with left parotid enlargement as a result of obstruction to flow.

Palpate the parotid and submandibular glands. Determine the consistency of each gland. Is tenderness present?

■ Inspect Cranial Nerve XII

Ask the patient to stick out the tongue. Does the tongue deviate to one side? A *hypoglossal,* or twelfth cranial, nerve palsy does not allow the lingual muscles on the affected side to contract normally. Consequently, the contralateral side "pushes" the tongue to the side of the lesion.

The Pharynx

■ Inspect the Pharynx

Examination of the pharynx is limited to inspection. In order to visualize the palate and oropharynx adequately, the examiner usually must depress the tongue with a tongue depressor stick. The patient is asked to open the mouth widely, stick out the tongue, and breathe slowly through the mouth. Occasionally, leaving the tongue in the floor of the mouth provides better visibility. The examiner should hold the tongue depressor in the right hand and a light source in the left. The tongue blade should be placed on the middle third of the tongue. The tongue is depressed and scooped forward. The examiner should be careful not to press the patient's lower lip or tongue against the teeth with the tongue depressor stick. If the tongue depressor is placed too anteriorly, the posterior portion of the tongue will mound up, making inspection of the pharynx difficult; if placed too posteriorly, a gag reflex may result.

Is injection present? Is candidiasis present?

An accessory for the oto-ophthalmoscope handle is a light source that holds the tongue depressor stick and makes the examination easier. Both techniques of holding the tongue depressor are shown in Figure 10–35.

■ Inspect the Tonsils

Evaluate tonsillar size. Tonsillar enlargement results from infection or tumor. In chronic tonsillar infection, the deep tonsillar crypts may contain cheese-like debris. Is there a

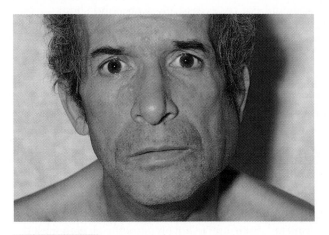

Figure 10–34

Left parotid enlargement.

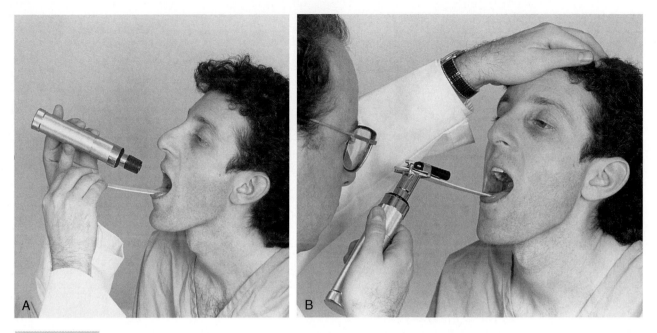

Figure 10-35

A, Use of the tongue depressor stick in inspecting the pharynx. *B,* Use of the tongue depressor attachment for inspecting the oral pharynx. Notice that the tongue depressor is placed on the middle third of the tongue.

membrane over the tonsils? A membrane is associated with acute tonsillitis, infectious mononucleosis, and diphtheria.

Inspect the Posterior Pharyngeal Wall

Is there a discharge, mass, ulceration, or injection present? Ask the patient to say "aahhh" as you observe for soft-palate elevation.

Inspect the Gag Reflex

At the end of the inspection, tell the patient that you are now going to test the gag reflex. The tip of the tongue depressor stick should gently touch the posterior surface of the tongue or the posterior pharyngeal wall. A rapid gag reflex should follow.

The Larynx

Using the Laryngeal Mirror

The tongue is held while a small, slightly warmed mirror is introduced into the mouth. The mirror should not be excessively warm and should avoid contact with the tongue. The patient is asked to breathe normally through the mouth. The mirror should be pushed upward against the uvula and positioned in the oropharynx. A beam of light can then be reflected off the mirror onto the internal laryngeal structures. This technique is shown in Figure 10-36.

Although the examination of the larynx is important, indirect laryngoscopy as just indicated is, in general, performed only by specialists. Certainly, any patient exhibiting symptoms of laryngeal disease should be evaluated further.

Clinicopathologic Correlations

Lesions of the oral cavity are common. The most common acute oral ulcer is the *traumatic ulcer;* the *aphthous ulcer,* or *canker sore,* is the next most common. Traumatic and aphthous lesions vary widely in size, although the latter are usually less than 1 cm in diameter. Both are relatively superficial with raised borders. Aphthous ulcers are usually located on the loose buccal or labial mucosa, whereas traumatic ulcers can occur anywhere. Despite the small size of many of these ulcers, they can be extremely

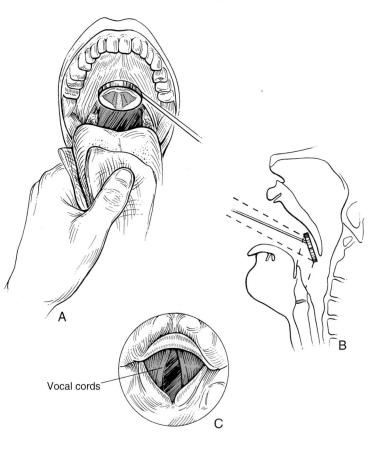

Figure 10–36

Mirror laryngoscopy. *A* illustrates how the tongue is held and the placement of the mirror. *B* shows a cross-sectional view through the pharynx, illustrating placement of the mirror. *C* shows the mirror reflection of the vocal cords.

Vocal cords

painful. In addition, aphthous ulcers may recur in many patients. Both types of ulcers usually heal within 2 to 3 weeks without scarring. A *solitary,* or *giant,* aphthous ulcer of the palate is shown in Figure 10–37. This patient has *periadenitis mucosa necrotica recurrens,* also known as major aphthous ulcer. These lesions are larger than the multiple aphthous ulcer and start as a submucosal lesion that breaks down to form an ulcer that may persist for many weeks prior to healing by secondary intention. Any part of the oropharynx may be affected, but the tonsils and soft palate are the most common sites.

Acute multiple ulcers that are preceded or associated with vesicles may be infective or immunologic in etiology. Primary herpes simplex, herpes zoster, Coxsackie virus,

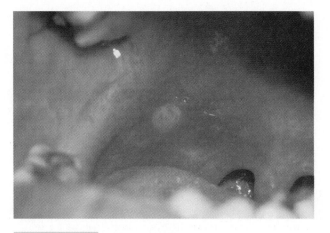

Figure 10–37

A solitary aphthous ulcer.

and the human immunodeficiency virus (HIV) are causative agents in the infective category. Allergic stomatitis, benign mucous membrane pemphigoid, pemphigus vulgaris, Behçet's disease, and erythema multiforme are common immunologic causes. Radiotherapy or chemotherapy may predispose an individual to the development of acute multiple ulcers. Figure 10–38 shows a patient with *benign mucous membrane pemphigoid,* which is a chronic mucocutaneous bullous disease. In this disease, the lesions are commonly limited to the oral cavity and conjunctiva. Subepidermal bullae, up to 2 cm, are present; erosion may be present. Autoantibodies to the basement membrane are present. Skin involvement is rare and usually not severe. Nikolsky's sign is usually positive; in this sign, the bulla or external layer of mucous membrane or skin is easily separated from the underlying tissue by slight friction.

Pemphigus vulgaris affects the oral cavity in 65% of cases. Autoantibodies are present to the epithelial intercellular substance. Nikolsky's sign is negative. Figure 10–39 shows a patient with pemphigus vulgaris; notice the lesions on the tongue and lips.

Large chronic single ulcers may result from fungal infections such as aspergillosis or histoplasmosis. Infections by herpes simplex virus, cytomegalovirus, *Mycobacterium* (which causes tuberculosis), and *Treponema pallidum* (which causes syphilis) are also well-known causes of this type of ulcer. Immunologic disorders such as pemphigus, systemic lupus erythematosus, bullous pemphigoid, and erosive lichen planus are often the cause of chronic multiple ulcers.

Cancer of the oral cavity is common. *Carcinoma of the lip* accounts for 30% of all cancers in this area and approximately 0.6% of all cancers. Most of these malignant tumors are squamous cell carcinomas. The lower lip is the site most frequently involved (95%). The patients are usually 50–70 years of age, with a strong male predominance (95%). Squamous cell carcinoma is characterized by a hard, infiltrative, usually painless, ulcer. The risk factors that predispose to squamous cell carcinoma of the oral cavity are the same as with leukoplakia—smoking, spirits (alcohol), spices, syphilis, and spikes (ill-fitting dentures)—the "5 S's." Figure 10–40 shows a patient with squamous cell carcinoma of the lower lip. *Lingual carcinoma* is often easily missed because, in its early stages, it is usually painless. It occurs on the lateral aspects of the tongue or on its undersurface; commonly there may be extension onto the tongue from a lesion on the floor of the mouth. Figure 10–41 shows a patient with carcinoma of the right lateral border of the tongue. Figure 10–42 shows another patient with squamous cell carcinoma of the right lateral border of the tongue, with extension on the floor of the mouth. *Carcinoma of the floor of the mouth* accounts for 10–15% of all oral cancers and is the most common site of oral cancer in African-Americans. It occurs primarily in males who are an average age of 65 years. Approximately 20% of patients with carcinoma of the floor of the mouth have a second primary tumor. An area of particular importance to examine is the area behind the last molar tooth and the associated floor of the mouth and base of the tongue; this area is often referred to as the "coffin corner." Figure 10–43 shows a patient with a squamous cell carcinoma of the floor of the mouth.

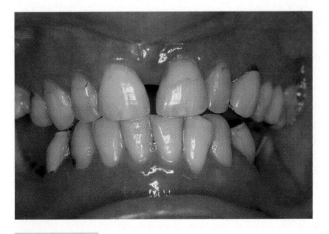

Figure 10–38

Benign mucous membrane pemphigoid.

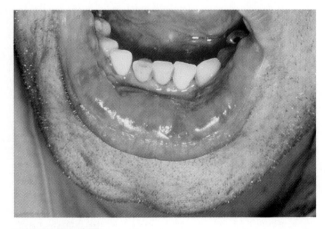

Figure 10–39

Pemphigus vulgaris.

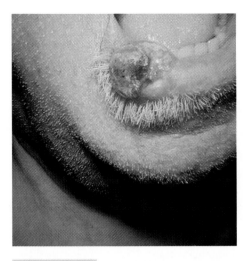

Figure 10-40

Squamous cell carcinoma of the lower lip.

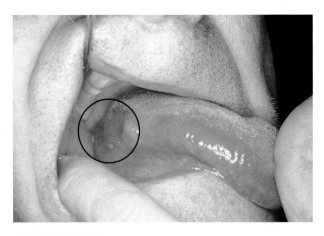

Figure 10-41

Carcinoma of the tongue.

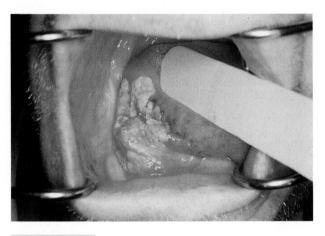

Figure 10-42

Squamous cell carcinoma of the tongue and floor of the mouth.

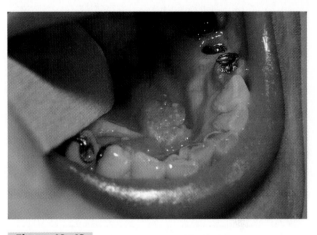

Figure 10-43

Squamous cell carcinoma of the floor of the mouth.

Herpetic gingivostomatitis is the infection of the gums and oral mucosa by herpes simplex virus. Small vesicles form the oral mucous membrane and rapidly break down into painful ulcers on an intensely erythematous base. A patient with herpetic gingivostomatitis is shown in Figure 10–44. Figure 10–45 shows another patient with herpetic lesions on the palate with ulceration.

Acute necrotizing, or *ulcerative,* gingivostomatitis is a severe, noncommunicable disease of young adults resulting from infection by *Fusobacterium nucleatum* or *Borrelia vincentii.* Most cases occur suddenly in the spring or autumn. The patients, commonly men with poor oral hygiene, present with gingival bleeding, alteration of taste, gingival pain, malaise, fever, and halitosis. As the disease progresses, a gray pseudomembrane develops along the gingival margins with ulceration in the interdental papillae. Acute necrotizing gingivitis may be an early feature of HIV infection. Figure 10–46 shows a patient with acute necrotizing gingivitis, also known as *Vincent's disease.*

It has been estimated by the World Health Organization that more than 4 million people in the world have HIV. By the end of 1997, the Centers for Disease Control and Prevention predict that there will be nearly 500,000 cases in the United States. Although first seen in the homosexual population, HIV is spreading mostly in the heterosexual population. These cases are related to the use of illegal drugs, contaminated needles, prostitution, and unprotected sex. It has been estimated that more than 90% of patients

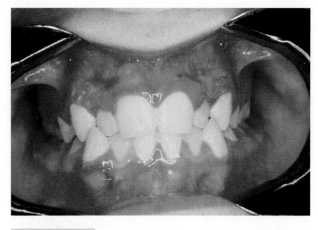

Figure 10–44

Herpetic gingivostomatitis.

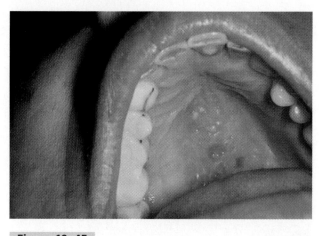

Figure 10–45

Herpetic lesions on the palate.

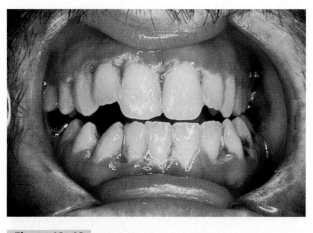

Figure 10–46

Acute necrotizing gingivitis.

infected with HIV will have at least one oral manifestation of their disease. It appears that as further immunologic impairment develops, the risk of oral lesions increases. It has also been shown that the oral manifestations may be used as a marker of immune compromise, which is independent of the CD4+ lymphocyte count. If left untreated, the oral lesions may interfere with chewing, swallowing, and talking. Many patients may have such severe pain that they may reduce their oral intake, which results in additional weight loss, malnutrition, and further wasting. A common oral manifestation of HIV infection is *angular cheilitis,* also known as *perlèche.* This painful condition is characterized by macerated, fissured, eroded, encrusted, whitish (occasionally erythematous) lesions in the corners of the mouth. Accumulations of saliva gather in the skin folds and are subsequently colonized by yeast organisms such as *C. albicans.* Angular cheilitis is often associated with intraoral candidiasis. Patients with normal immunity who wear ill-fitting dentures or dentures during the night may also develop angular cheilitis. A patient with angular cheilitis is shown in Figure 10–47.

Figure 10–26 shows a patient with *oral hairy leukoplakia* (OHL). As mentioned previously, this lesion is seen most frequently either unilaterally or bilaterally on the lateral margins of the tongue. The lesion is white, does not rub off, and occurs occasionally elsewhere in the mouth and oropharynx. Although not correlated with the stage of HIV infection, OHL may be the first sign of infection. OHL is seen most commonly in homosexual and bisexual men infected with HIV. It has been suggested

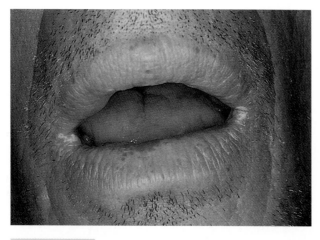

Figure 10–47

Angular cheilitis.

that Epstein-Barr virus may be a cofactor in the development of OHL. The finding of OHL demands HIV testing.

Figure 10–25 shows a patient with *oral candidiasis,* another extremely common condition associated with HIV infection. Oral candidiasis is characterized by chronic severe pain in the throat that worsens on swallowing or eating. The curd-like white plaques are soft and friable and can easily be wiped off, leaving an area of intensely erythematous mucosa.

As discussed in Chapter 6, The Skin, the oral lesions of Kaposi's sarcoma are common. Figure 6–72 shows some of the typical oral lesions. Lesions of Kaposi's sarcoma of the tongue (Figure 10–48) and hard palate (Figure 10–49) are also frequently seen.

Table 10–1 summarizes the important signs and symptoms of some of the more common oral lesions. Table 10–2 reviews the most common oral lesions seen during the stages of HIV infection. Table 22–5 lists the chronology of dentition.

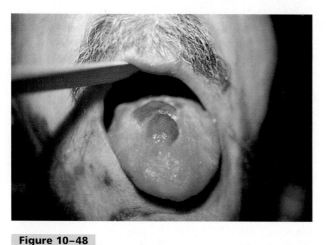

Figure 10–48

Kaposi's sarcoma of the tongue.

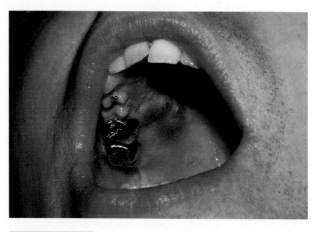

Figure 10–49

Kaposi's sarcoma of the hard palate.

Table 10–1 Symptoms and Signs of Oral Lesions

Lesion	Symptoms	Signs	Other Information
Aphthous ulcer (canker sore) (see Fig. 10–37)	Painful, recurrent white sore with red border on lips, inner side of cheeks, tip and sides of tongue, or palate	Single lesion 0.5–2 cm in diameter that is first maculopapular but then ulcerates and has an area of erythema at its border; lesions usually only on movable mucosal areas	60% of population has periodic canker sores lasting up to 2 weeks; cause is unknown
Herpetic ulcer (cold sore; fever blister) (see Figs. 10–8, 10–44)	Painful, recurrent sores on the lips	Multiple vesicles, papules, or ulcers on the mucocutaneous junction, hard palate, or gingivae; as the bullae break, crusting occurs	*Primary* herpetic infection in children; multiple lesions in clusters on fixed mucous membranes; small, discrete, whitish vesicles before ulceration; ulcers about 1 mm in diameter, which may coalesce; tender lymphadenopathy, fever, and malaise present; lip lesions represent the *recurrent* form, common in adults; self-limited illness, 1–2 weeks, in the primary and recurrent forms
Chancre	Painless sore on lips or tongue lasting 2 weeks to 3 months	Single ulcerated lesion with indurated border; lesion without central necrotic material; tender lymphadenitis may be present	Look for genital lesions
Squamous cell carcinoma (see Figs. 10–40, 10–41, 10–42, 10–43)	Ulcerated sore of the lips, floor of mouth, or tongue (especially lateral borders) / Erythroplakia of floor of mouth, soft palate	Single indurated lesion with indurated and raised border; often in an area of leukoplakia or erythroplakia; absence of necrotic material in crater; base often erythematous; speech alterations may result if lesion is large; painless lymphadenopathy may be present in neck; evidence of distant metastasis may be present	Frequently in alcoholics and/or smokers
Erythema multiforme	Sudden onset of multiple painful ulcers in mouth or lips	Hemorrhagic areas of ulceration with erythematous bases often with pseudomembrane; lesions start as bullae; skin involvement common (target lesions)	Many precipitating factors include drug reactions, herpesvirus infections, endocrine changes, and an underlying malignancy; most common in winter and spring in young adults; frequently recurring
Denture hyperplasia	Painless excess tissue at border of denture	Spongy, redundant, often erythematous tissue with impression of edge of denture; frequently seen on anterior maxillary mucosa	
Candidiasis (moniliasis; thrush) (see Figs. 10–25, 10–30)	Burning areas of tongue, inside of cheek, or throat	Whitish pseudomembrane, resembling milk curd, that can be peeled off, leaving a raw, erythematous area that may bleed; erythematous variant is seen secondary to broad-spectrum antibiotics	Often seen in individuals who are chronically debilitated, patients who are immunosuppressed, or patients on long-term antibiotic therapy; commonly seen in persons with AIDS

Table 10–1   Symptoms and Signs of Oral Lesions *(Continued)*

Lesion	Symptoms	Signs	Other Information
Erythroplakia (see Figs. 10-18, 10-33)	Painless red area on inside of cheek, tongue, or floor of mouth	Granular, erythematous papules that bleed	High malignant potential
Leukoplakia (see Figs. 10-14, 10-15, 10-26)	Painless white area on inside of cheek, tongue, lower lip, or floor of mouth	Hyperkeratinized, whitish lesion that cannot be scraped off; looks similar to flaking white paint; often speckled with reddish areas; associated adenopathy may indicate malignant changes of lesion	Patients are usually men over the age of 40; linked to smoking, AIDS, alcoholism, and chewing tobacco
Lipoma (see Fig. 10-23)	Slow-growing painless mass on inner surface of cheek or tongue	Yellowish, nontender, soft mass; freely mobile	
Lichen planus (see Fig. 10-13)	Usually no symptoms; erosive form causes painful, burning sores of inner side of cheeks or tongue	White lesions on buccal mucosa bilaterally in the form of reticulated papules in lace-like pattern; erosive form appears as hemorrhagic, ulcerated lesion with possible white areas or bullae; pseudomembrane may be present over lesion	Non-erosive form is a common cause of white lesions in the mouth; skin involvement in 10–35% of patients; more frequently seen in patients with emotional stress
Traumatic ulcer	Pain in an area of a sore; short duration (1–2 weeks)	Single lesion with raised erythema at its border; center often with necrotic debris; occasionally purulent; mild lymphadenitis may be present	Patient can frequently relate the cause (e.g., biting cheek while eating)
Mucocele (see Fig. 10-11)	Intermittent, painless swelling of the lower lip or inside of cheek; slightly bluish; occasionally ruptures	Dome-shaped, 1–2 cm in diameter, freely mobile cystic lesion	Is related to trauma to ductal system of minor labial salivary glands
Hairy tongue (see Fig. 10-24B)	Gagging sensation associated with "hairy" sensation of tongue; large, brown or blackish, painless lesion on top of tongue	Elongation of filiform papillae on the dorsum of tongue with a change in their color to almost black or brown	History of excessive antibiotic use, excessive use of mouthwash, poor oral hygiene, smoking, or alcohol are common
Fordyce's spots (see Fig. 10-16)	None	Clusters of small, yellowish, raised lesions best seen on the buccal mucosa opposite the molar teeth	Common in older individuals; they are normal, hyperplastic sebaceous glands

Table 10–2   Occurrence of Oral Lesions During the Stages of HIV Infection

Oral Lesion	Occurrence During Primary HIV Infection	Occurrence During Early HIV Disease*	Occurrence During Advanced HIV Disease†
Candidiasis (see Figs. 10–25, 10–30)	Common	Occasional	Very common
Oral hairy leukoplakia (see Fig. 10–26)	No	Occasional	Very common
Kaposi's sarcoma (see Figs. 10–48, 10–49)	No	Rare	Very common
Linear gingival erythema	No	Common	Very common
Necrotizing gingivitis (see Fig. 10–46)	No	Rare	Common
Necrotizing stomatitis	No	No	Common
Herpes simplex (see Figs. 10–8, 10–44, 10–45)	No	Occasional	Common
Aphthous ulcers (see Fig. 10–37)	Common	Occasional	Very common

Adapted from Weinert M, Grimes RM, Lynch DP: Oral manifestations of HIV infection. Ann Intern Med 125:485, 1996.
* CD4+ count > 500 cells/mm³
† CD4+ count < 200 cells/mm³

Useful Vocabulary

Listed here are the specific roots that are important in order to understand the terminology related to diseases of the mouth and pharynx.

Root	Pertaining to	Example	Definition
arytenoid-	pitcher-shaped	*arytenoid*itis	Inflammation of the arytenoid cartilage
bucco-	cheek	*bucco*pharyngeal	Pertaining to the cheek and pharynx
cheil(o)-	lip	*cheil*itis	Inflammation of the lip
dent-	tooth	*dent*al	Pertaining to the teeth
gingiv-	gingiva(e)	*gingiv*ectomy	Surgical excision of diseased gingiva(e)
gloss(o)-	tongue	*glosso*plegia	Paralysis of the tongue
-labi-	lips	naso*labi*al	Pertaining to the nose and lip
leuko-	white	*leuko*plakia	White patch on mucous membrane; often pre-malignant
linguo-	tongue	*linguo*papillitis	Painful ulcers around the papillae of the tongue
-plakia	patch	erythro*plakia*	Red patch on mucous membrane; often premalignant
ptyal-	saliva	*ptyal*ism	Excessive salivation
stoma-	mouth; opening	*stoma*titis	Inflammation of the mouth

Writing Up the Physical Examination

Listed here are examples of the write-up for the examinations of the oral cavity and pharynx.

■ The lips appear normal. The mucosa of the oral cavity is red and without masses, leukoplakia, or other lesions. There is good dentition and good dental hygiene. The tongue is midline and does not deviate to either side. The tonsils are absent. The pharynx appears normal. The palate is normal without ulcers or masses.

■ There is a 1–2 cm, painful vesicular lesion at the mucocutaneous junction on the right side of the mouth. There is tonsillar hypertrophy with a purulent discharge in the crypts of both tonsils. There is bilateral anterior triangle lymphadenopathy, greater on the right. The remainder of the examination of the oral cavity is unremarkable.

- There is a whitish pseudomembrane over the hard and soft palate as well as over the tongue. When lifted, its erythematous base is friable and bleeds. The rest of the mouth and throat appears normal.
- The lateral border of the tongue has an ulcerated, indurated lesion 2 × 1 cm.
- The palate shows a dome-shaped 3 cm mass to the right of midline. Biopsy is recommended.

Bibliography

Aronson AE: Clinical Voice Disorders: An Interdisciplinary Approach. New York, Thieme-Stratton, 1980.

Benjamin B, Bingham B, Hawke M, et al: A Color Atlas of Otorhinolaryngology. Philadelphia, J.B. Lippincott Co., 1995.

Bingham BJG, Hawke M, Kwok P, et al: Atlas of Clinical Otolaryngology. St. Louis, Mosby-Year Book, Inc., 1992.

Dayal VS: Clinical Otolaryngology. Philadelphia, J.B. Lippincott, 1981.

DeBoever EH, Loesche W: Assessing the contribution of anaerobic microflora of the tongue to oral malodor. J Am Dent Assoc 126:1384, 1995.

Kirby AJ, Munoz A, Detels R, et al: Thrush and fever as measures of immunocompetence in HIV-1-infected men. J Acquir Immune Defic Syndr Hum Retrovirol 7:1242, 1994.

Laguaite JK: Adult voice screening. J Speech Hear Disord 37:147, 1972.

McCarthy GM: Host factors associated with HIV-related oral candidiasis. Oral Surg Oral Med Oral Pathol Oral Radiol Endod 73:181, 1992.

Moore PS, Chang Y: Detection of herpesvirus-like DNA sequences in Kaposi's sarcoma in patients with and without HIV infection. N Engl J Med 332:1181, 1995.

Nielsen H, Bentsen KD, Hojtved L, et al: Oral candidiasis and immune status of HIV-infected patients. Pathol Med 23:140, 1994.

Pindborg JJ: Classification of oral lesions associated with HIV infection. Oral Surg Oral Med Oral Pathol Oral Radiol Endod 67:292, 1989.

Rosenberg M: Clinical assessment of bad breath: Current concepts. J Am Dent Assoc 127:475, 1996.

Scully C, Laskaris G, Pindborg J, et al: Oral manifestations of HIV infection and their management. I: More common lesions. Oral Surg Oral Med Oral Pathol Oral Radiol Endod 71:158, 1991.

Scully C, Laskaris G, Pindborg J, et al: Oral manifestations of HIV infection and their management. II: Less common lesions. Oral Surg Oral Med Oral Pathol Oral Radiol Endod 71:167, 1991.

Silverman EM, Zimmer CH: Incidence of chronic hoarseness among school-age children. J Speech Hear Disord 40:211, 1975.

Silverman S: Color Atlas of Oral Manifestations of AIDS, 2nd ed. St. Louis, Mosby-Year Book, Inc., 1996.

Silverman S Jr, Migliorati CA, Lozada-Nur F, et al: Oral findings in people with or at high risk for AIDS: A study of 375 homosexual males. J Am Dent Assoc 112:187, 1986.

Speilman AL, Bivona P, Rifkin BR: Halitosis: A common oral problem. N Y State Dent J 62:36, 1996.

Tonzetich J: Production and origin of oral malodor: A review of mechanisms and methods of analysis. J Periodontol 48:13, 1977.

Weinert M, Grimes RM, Lynch DP: Oral manifestations of HIV infection. Ann Intern Med 125:485, 1996.

Zemlin WR: Speech and Hearing Science. Englewood Cliffs, NJ, Prentice-Hall, 1981.

CHAPTER 11

The Chest

In the beginning the malady (tuberculosis) is easier to cure but difficult to detect, but later it becomes easy to detect but difficult to cure.

Niccolò Machiavelli
1469–1527

General Considerations

Oxygen enables the breath of life; without adequate lung function, lives cannot be sustained. Patients with pulmonary disease must work harder for adequate oxygenation. These patients complain of "air hunger" or "too little air." Anyone who has traveled to areas of high altitude, where the oxygen concentration is reduced, has experienced shortness of breath.

The magnitude of pulmonary disease is enormous. It had been estimated that, annually, more than 80,000 individuals in the United States die of chronic lung disease, more than 5 million have some degree of pulmonary disability, and more than 20 million have pulmonary symptoms (National Institutes of Health Task Force Report, 1980). In 1967, the estimated cost of morbidity and mortality from lung disease was 1.8 billion dollars (National Heart and Lung Institute, 1972). It is estimated that as of the year 2000, this figure will skyrocket to more than 60 billion dollars.

Cancer of the lung is the leading cause of death from cancer in the United States. In 1990, nearly 200,000 new cases of lung cancer were diagnosed, with more than 150,000 deaths. In 1985, cancer of the lung was equal to cancer of the breast as the leading causes of death from cancer in women.

Pulmonary diseases arise when the lungs are unable to provide adequate oxygenation or to eliminate carbon dioxide. Any derangement of these functions indicates abnormal respiratory function.

During a 24 hour period, the lungs oxygenate more than 5700 liters of blood with more than 11,400 liters of air in the lungs. The total surface area of the alveoli of the lungs comprises an area larger than that of a tennis court.

Structure and Physiology

The chest forms the bony case that houses and protects the lungs, the heart, and the esophagus as it passes into the stomach. The bony chest skeleton consists of 12 thoracic vertebrae, 12 pairs of ribs, the clavicle, and the sternum. The bony structure is shown in Figure 11–1.

The lungs continuously provide oxygen to and remove carbon dioxide from the circulatory system. The power required for breathing comes from the intercostal muscles and the diaphragm. The integrated action of these muscles acts as a bellows to suck air into the lungs. Expiration is passive. The control of breathing is complex and is controlled by the *breathing center* in the medulla of the brain.

Inspired air is warmed, filtered, and humidified by the upper respiratory passages. After passing through the cricoid cartilage of the larynx, air travels through a system of flexible tubes, the *trachea*. At the level of the fourth or fifth thoracic vertebra, the trachea bifurcates into the *left* and *right bronchi*. The right bronchus is shorter, wider, and straighter than the left bronchus. The bronchi continue to subdivide into smaller bronchi and then into *bronchioles* within the lungs. Each respiratory bronchiole terminates in an *alveolar duct,* from which many *alveolar sacs* branch off. It is estimated that there are more than 500 million alveoli in the lungs. Each alveolar wall contains

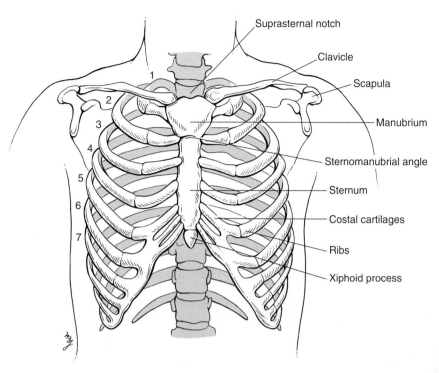

Suprasternal notch

Clavicle

Scapula

Manubrium

Sternomanubrial angle

Sternum

Costal cartilages

Ribs

Xiphoid process

Figure 11–1

Bony chest skeleton.

elastin fibers that allow the sac to expand with inspiration and to contract with expiration by *elastic recoil*. This system of air conducting passages is shown in Figure 11–2.

The lungs are subdivided into lobes: the *upper, middle,* and *lower* on the *right,* and the *upper* and *lower* on the left. The lungs are enveloped in a thin sac, the *pleura*. The *visceral* pleura overlies the lung parenchyma, whereas the *parietal* pleura lines the

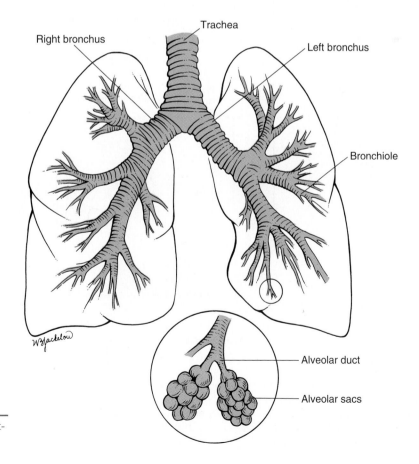

Trachea

Right bronchus

Left bronchus

Bronchiole

Alveolar duct

Alveolar sacs

Figure 11–2

System of air-conducting passages.

chest wall. The two pleural surfaces glide over each other during inspiration and expiration. The space between the pleura is the pleural cavity.

In order to describe physical signs within the chest accurately, the examiner must understand the topographic landmarks of the chest wall. The landmarks of clinical importance are as follows:

- Sternum
- Clavicle
- Suprasternal notch
- Sternomanubrial angle
- Midsternal line
- Midclavicular lines
- Anterior axillary lines
- Midaxillary lines
- Posterior axillary lines
- Scapular lines
- Midspinal line

Figure 11–3 shows the anterior thorax and lateral views, and Figure 11–4 shows the posterior thorax.

The *suprasternal notch* is located at the top of the sternum and can be felt as a depression at the base of the neck. The *sternomanubrial angle* is often referred to as

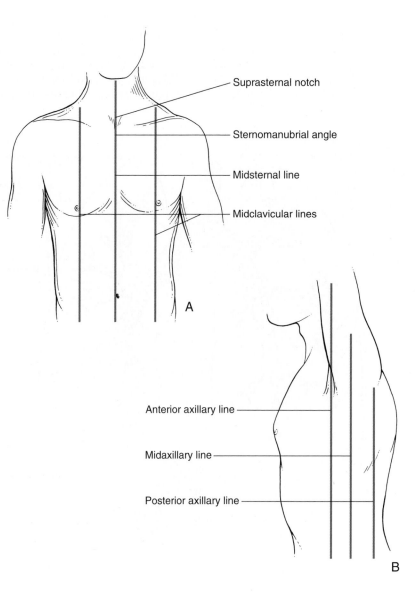

Figure 11–3

Thoracic cage landmarks. *A,* The topographic landmarks of the anterior thorax. *B,* The landmarks on the lateral view.

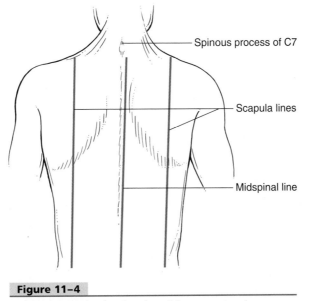

Spinous process of C7

Scapula lines

Midspinal line

Figure 11–4

The topographic landmarks of the posterior thorax.

the angle of Louis. This bony ridge lies approximately 5 cm below the suprasternal notch. When you move your fingers off the ridge laterally, the adjacent rib that you feel is the second rib. The interspace below the second rib is the *second intercostal space*. Using this as a reference point, you should be able to identify the ribs and interspaces anteriorly. Try it on yourself.

In order to identify areas, several imaginary lines are drawn on the anterior and posterior chest. The *midsternal line* is drawn through the middle of the sternum. The *midclavicular lines* are drawn through the middle points of the clavicles and parallel to the midsternal line. The *anterior axillary lines* are vertical lines drawn along the anterior axillary folds parallel to the midsternal line. The *midaxillary lines* are drawn from each vertex of the axillae parallel to the midsternal line. The *posterior axillary lines* are parallel to the midsternal line and extend vertically along the posterior axillary folds. The *scapular lines* are parallel to the midspinal line and pass through the inferior angles of the scapulae. The *midspinal line* is a vertical line that passes through the posterior spinous processes of the vertebrae.

Rib counting from the posterior chest is slightly more complicated. The inferior wing of the *scapula* lies at the level of the seventh rib or interspace. Another useful landmark can be found by having the patient flex the neck; the most prominent cervical spinous process, the *vertebra prominens,* protrudes from the seventh cervical vertebra.

Only the first seven ribs articulate with the sternum. The eighth, ninth, and tenth ribs articulate with the cartilage above. The eleventh and twelfth ribs are floating ribs and have a free anterior portion.

The *interlobar fissures,* shown in Figure 11–5, are situated between the lobes of the lungs. Both the right and left lungs have an *oblique fissure,* which begins on the anterior chest at the level of the sixth rib at the midclavicular line and extends laterally upward to the fifth rib in the midaxillary line, ending at the posterior chest at the spinous process of T3. The right lower lobe is located below the right oblique fissure; the right upper and middle lobes are superior to the right oblique fissure. The left lower lobe is below the left oblique fissure; the left upper lobe is superior to the left oblique fissure. The *horizontal fissure* is present only on the right and divides the right upper lobe from the right middle lobe. It extends from the fourth rib at the sternal border to the fifth rib at the midaxillary line.

The lungs extend superiorly about 3–4 cm above the medial end of the clavicles. The inferior margins of the lungs extend to the sixth rib at the midclavicular line, the eighth rib at the midaxillary line, and between T9 and T12 posteriorly. This variation is related to respiration. The bifurcation of the trachea, the *carina,* is located behind the angle of Louis at approximately level T4 on the posterior chest. The *right hemidia-*

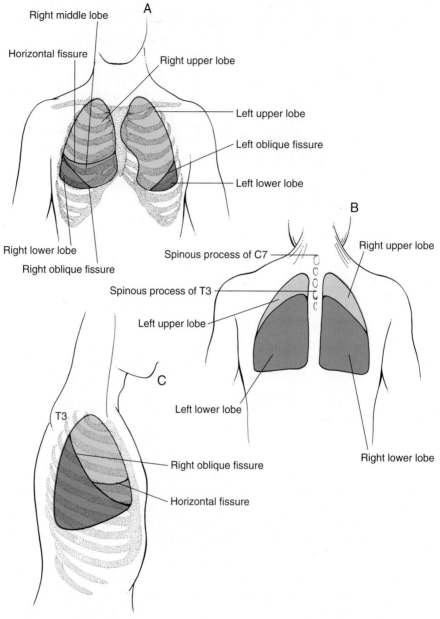

Figure 11–5

Surface topography and the underlying interlobar fissures. *A,* Anterior view, *B,* Posterior view. *C,* Lateral view.

phragm at the end of the expiration is located at the level of the fifth rib anteriorly and T9 posteriorly. The presence of the liver on the right side makes the right hemidiaphragm slightly higher than the left.

During quiet breathing, muscle contraction occurs only during inspiration. Expiration is passive, resulting from the elastic recoil of the lungs and chest.

Review of Specific Symptoms

The main symptoms of pulmonary disease are the following:

- Cough
- Sputum production
- Hemoptysis (coughing up blood)
- Dyspnea (shortness of breath)
- Wheezing
- Cyanosis (bluish discoloration of the skin)
- Chest pain

Cough

The most common symptom of lung disease is the *cough*. Coughing is so common that it is frequently regarded as a trivial complaint. The cough reflex is a normal defense mechanism of the lungs that serves to protect the lungs from foreign bodies and excessive secretions. Infections of the upper respiratory tract are associated with coughing that usually improves in 2–3 weeks. A persistent cough necessitates further investigation.

Coughing is a coordinated, forced expiration, interrupted by repeated closure of the glottis. The expiratory muscles contract against the partially closed glottis, creating high pressure within the lungs. When the glottis suddenly opens, there is an explosive rush of air that clears the air passages. When a patient complains of coughing, ask these questions:

"Can you describe your cough?"
"How long have you had a cough?"
"Was there a sudden onset of coughing?"
"Do you smoke?" If so, *"How much, and for how long?"*
"Does your cough produce sputum?" If so, *"Can you estimate the amount of your expectorations? What is the color of the sputum? Does the sputum have a foul odor?"*
"Does the cough occur for prolonged periods?"
"Does the cough occur after eating?"
"Is the coughing worse in any position?"
"What relieves the cough?"
"Are there any other symptoms associated with the cough? fever? headaches? night sweats? chest pain? runny nose? shortness of breath? weight loss? hoarseness? loss of consciousness?"
"Do you have any birds as pets? Do you feed pigeons?"
"Have you ever been exposed to anyone with tuberculosis?"

Coughing may be voluntary or involuntary, productive or nonproductive. In a *productive* cough, mucus or other materials are expelled. A *dry* cough does not produce any secretions.

Smoking is probably the most common cause of the chronic cough. *Smoker's cough* results from inhalation of irritants in tobacco and is most marked in the morning. Coughing is normally decreased during sleep. When the smoker awakens in the morning, productive coughing tends to clear the respiratory passages. Coughing decreases and may disappear in patients who stop smoking.

Coughing may also be *psychogenic*. This nonproductive cough occurs in individuals with emotional stress. When attention is drawn to it, the cough increases. During sleep, or when the patient is distracted, the coughing stops. Psychogenic coughing is a *diagnosis of exclusion:* only after all other causes have been eliminated can this diagnosis be made.

There are many terms used by patients and physicians to describe a cough. Table 11–1 provides a list of some of the more common descriptors and their possible causes.

Table 11–1	Descriptors of Coughing
Description	**Possible Causes**
Dry, hacking	Viral infections, interstitial lung disease, tumor, allergies, anxiety
Chronic, productive	Bronchiectasis, chronic bronchitis, abscess, bacterial pneumonia, tuberculosis
Wheezing	Bronchospasm, asthma, allergies, congestive heart failure
Barking	Epiglottal disease (e.g., croup)
Stridor	Tracheal obstruction
Morning	Smoking
Nocturnal	Postnasal drip, congestive heart failure
Associated with eating or drinking	Neuromuscular disease of the upper esophagus
Inadequate	Debility, weakness

Sputum Production

Sputum is the substance expelled by coughing. Approximately 75–100 mL of sputum is secreted daily by the bronchi. By ciliary action, it is brought up to the throat and then swallowed unconsciously with the saliva. An increase in the quantity of sputum production is the earliest manifestations of bronchitis. Sputum may contain cellular debris, mucus, blood, pus, or microorganisms.

Sputum should be described according to color, consistency, quantity, number of times it is brought up during the day and night, and the presence or absence of blood. An adequate description may indicate a cause of the disease process. Uninfected sputum is odorless, transparent, and whitish-gray, resembling mucus; it is termed *mucoid*. Infected sputum contains pus and is termed *purulent;* the sputum may be yellow, greenish, or red. Table 11–2 lists the appearances of sputum and their possible causes.

Hemoptysis

Hemoptysis is the coughing up of blood. Few symptoms produce as much alarm in patients as does hemoptysis. Careful description of the hemoptysis is crucial, because it can include clots of blood as well as blood-tinged sputum. The implications of each are very different. Coughing up clots of blood is a symptom of extreme importance because it often heralds a serious illness. Clots of blood are generally indicative of a cavitary lung lesion, a tumor of the lung, certain cardiac diseases, or pulmonary embolism. Blood-tinged sputum is usually associated with smoking or minor infections, but it can be seen with tumors and more serious diseases as well. When a patient complains of coughing up blood, ask the following questions:

"Do you smoke?"
"Did the coughing up of blood occur suddenly?"
"Have there been recurrent episodes of coughing up blood?"
"Is the sputum blood-tinged, or are there actual clots of blood?"
"How long have you noticed the blood?"
"What seems to bring on the coughing up of blood? vomiting? coughing? nausea?"
"Have you ever had tuberculosis?"
"Is there a family history of coughing up blood?"
"Have you had recent surgery?"
"Do you take any 'blood thinners'?"
"Are you aware of any bleeding tendency?"
"Have you had night sweats? shortness of breath? palpitations? irregular heartbeats? hoarseness? weight loss? swelling or pain in your legs?"
"Have you felt any unusual sensation in your chest after coughing up blood?" If so, *"Where?"*

For the woman with hemoptysis, *"Do you use oral contraceptives?"*

Table 11–2   Appearances of Sputum

Appearance	Possible Causes
Mucoid	Asthma, tumors, tuberculosis, emphysema, pneumonia
Mucopurulent	Asthma, tumors, tuberculosis, emphysema, pneumonia
Yellow-green, purulent	Bronchiectasis, chronic bronchitis
Rust-colored, purulent	Pneumococcal pneumonia
Red currant jelly	*Klebsiella pneumoniae* infection
Foul odor	Lung abscess
Pink, blood-tinged	Streptococcal or staphylococcal pneumonia
Gravel	Broncholithiasis
Pink, frothy	Pulmonary edema
Profuse, colorless (also known as bronchorrhea)	Alveolar cell carcinoma
Bloody	Pulmonary emboli, bronchiectasis, abscess, tuberculosis, tumor, cardiac causes, bleeding disorders

Any suppurative (associated with the production of pus) process of the airways or lungs can produce hemoptysis. Bronchitis is probably the most common cause of hemoptysis. Bronchiectasis and bronchogenic carcinoma are also major causes. Hemoptysis results from mucosal invasion, tumor necrosis, and pneumonia distal to bronchial obstruction by tumor. Pneumococcal pneumonia characteristically produces rust-colored sputum. Pink and frothy sputum can result from pulmonary edema.

Occasionally, patients have a warm sensation within their chest at the location from which the hemoptysis has originated. Therefore, it is useful to ask patients who have had recent hemoptysis whether they have experienced such a sensation. This information may lead to a more careful review of the physical examination and x-ray films of that area.

Patients who have undergone recent surgery are at risk for deep vein thrombophlebitis with pulmonary embolism. Women taking oral contraceptives are likewise at risk for pulmonary embolic disease. Hemoptysis occurs when pulmonary emboli result in infarction with necrosis of the pulmonary parenchyma.

Recurrent episodes of hemoptysis may result from bronchiectasis, tuberculosis, or mitral stenosis. Atrial fibrillation is a common cause of "irregular heartbeats" and embolic phenomena.

At times, it may be difficult to ascertain whether the patient coughed up or vomited blood. Most patients can provide a sufficiently clear history. Table 11–3 lists characteristics that help distinguish hemoptysis from *hematemesis* (vomiting up blood).

Dyspnea

The *subjective* sensation of "shortness of breath" is *dyspnea*. Dyspnea is an important manifestation of cardiopulmonary disease, although it is found in other states such as neurologic, metabolic, and psychological conditions. It is important to differentiate dyspnea from the *objective* finding of *tachypnea,* or rapid breathing. A patient may be observed to be breathing rapidly while stating that he or she is not short of breath. The converse is also true: a patient may be breathing slowly but may have dyspnea. Never assume that a patient with a rapid respiratory rate is dyspneic.

It is important for the examiner to inquire when dyspnea occurs and in which position. *Paroxysmal nocturnal dyspnea* is the sudden onset of shortness of breath occurring at night during sleep. Patients suddenly are seized with an intense strangling sensation. They frantically sit up and, classically, run to the window for "air." As soon as they assume an upright position, the dyspnea usually improves. *Orthopnea* is difficulty in breathing while lying flat. Patients require two or more pillows to breathe comfortably. *Platypnea* is a rare symptom of difficulty in breathing while sitting up and is relieved by a recumbent position. *Trepopnea* is a condition in which patients are more comfortable breathing while lying on one side. (Some of the more common causes of positional dyspnea are listed in Table 11–4.) Ask all patients complaining of dyspnea the following questions:

"How long have you had shortness of breath?"
"Did the shortness of breath occur suddenly?"
"Is the shortness of breath constant?"
"Does the shortness of breath occur with exertion? at rest? lying flat? sitting up?"
"What makes the shortness of breath worse? What relieves it?"
"How many level blocks can you walk without becoming short of breath?"
    "How many could you walk 6 months ago?"

Table 11–3   Characteristics Distinguishing Hemoptysis from Hematemesis

Features	Hemoptysis	Hematemesis
Prodrome	Coughing	Nausea and vomiting
Past history	Possible history of cardiopulmonary disease	Possible history of gastrointestinal disease
Appearance	Frothy	Not frothy
Color	Bright red	Dark red, brown, or "coffee grounds"
Manifestation	Mixed with pus	Mixed with food
Associated symptoms	Dyspnea	Nausea

Table 11–4   Positional Dyspnea

Type	Possible Causes
Orthopnea	Congestive heart failure
	Mitral valvular disease
	Severe asthma (rarely)
	Emphysema (rarely)
	Chronic bronchitis (rarely)
	Neurologic diseases (rarely)
Trepopnea	Congestive heart failure
Platypnea	Status post-pneumonectomy
	Neurologic diseases
	Cirrhosis (intrapulmonary shunts)
	Hypovolemia

"Is the shortness of breath accompanied by wheezing? fever? cough? coughing up blood? chest pain? palpitations? hoarseness?"
"Do you smoke?" If so, *"How much? For how long?"*
"Have you had any exposure to absestos? sandblasting? pigeon breeding?"
"Have you had any exposure to individuals with tuberculosis?"
"Have you ever lived near the San Joaquin Valley? midwestern or southeastern United States?"

It is essential to try to quantify the dyspnea. Questions such as "How many level blocks can you walk?" provide a framework for *exercise tolerance.* For example, if the patient answers, "two blocks," he is said to have *2 block dyspnea on exertion* (DOE). The interviewer can then ask, "How many level blocks were you able to walk 6 months ago?" The interviewer can thus make a rough assessment of the progression of the disease or the efficacy of therapy.

Careful questioning regarding *industrial exposure* is paramount in any patient with unexplained dyspnea. Examples of further questions regarding occupational and environmental history are discussed in Chapter 1, The Interviewer's Questions. Exposure to pigeons may result in psittacosis. Outbreaks of coccidioidomycosis have occurred in individuals living in the southwestern United States. Living in the midwestern and southeastern United States has been linked to outbreaks of histoplasmosis.

Wheezing

Wheezing is an abnormally high-pitched noise resulting from a partially obstructed airway. It is usually present during expiration when slight bronchoconstriction occurs physiologically. Bronchospasm, mucosal edema, loss of elastic support, and tortuosity of the airways are the usual causes. Asthma causes bronchospasm, which is the cause of the wheezing associated with this condition. Obstruction by intraluminal material, such as aspirated foreign bodies or secretions, is another important cause of wheezing. A well-localized wheeze, unchanged by coughing, may indicate a partially obstructed bronchus by a foreign body or tumor. When a patient complains of wheezing, the examiner must determine the following:

"At what age did the wheezing begin?"
"How often does it occur?"
"Are there any precipitating factors, such as foods, odors, emotions, animals, etc.?"
"What usually stops the attack?"
"Have the symptoms worsened over the years?"
"Are there any associated symptoms?"
"Is there a history of nasal polyps?"
"What is your smoking history?"
"Is there a history of heart disease?"

An important axiom to remember is

Asthma is associated with wheezing, but not all wheezing is asthma.

Do not equate wheezing with asthma. As will be indicated subsequently, congestive heart failure is usually associated with abnormal breath sounds called crackles. Sometimes there is such severe bronchospasm in heart failure that the main physical finding is a wheeze and not a crackle.

A decrease in wheezing may result from either an opening of the airway or a progressive closing off of the air passage. A "silent" chest in a patient with an acute asthmatic attack is generally a bad sign: it indicates worsening of the obstruction.

Cyanosis

Cyanosis is commonly detected by a family member. The subtle bluish discoloration may go completely unnoticed by the patient. *Central* cyanosis occurs with inadequate gas exchange in the lungs that results in a significant reduction in arterial oxygenation. Primary pulmonary problems or diseases that cause mixed venous blood to bypass the lungs (e.g., intracardiac shunt) are frequently the etiologic factors. The bluish discoloration is best seen in the mucous membranes of the mouth (e.g., the frenulum) and lips. *Peripheral* cyanosis results from an excessive extraction of oxygen at the periphery. It is limited to cyanosis of the extremities (e.g., the fingers, toes, nose). Ask the following questions:

> *"Where is the cyanosis present?"*
> *"How long has the cyanosis been present?"*
> *"Are you aware of any lung problem? heart problem? blood problem?"*
> *"What makes the cyanosis worse?"*
> *"Is there associated shortness of breath? cough? bleeding?"*
> *"What types of work have you performed?"*
> *"Is there anyone else in your family who has cyanosis?"*

Cyanosis from birth is associated with congenital heart lesions. The acute development of cyanosis can occur in severe respiratory disease, especially acute airway obstruction. Peripheral cyanosis is due to increased oxygen extraction in states of low cardiac output and is seen in cooler areas of the body such as the nail beds and the outer surfaces of the lips. Peripheral cyanosis disappears as the area is warmed. Cyanosis of the nails and warmth in the hands suggest that the cyanosis is central. Central cyanosis occurs only after the oxygen saturation has fallen to below 80%. Central cyanosis diffusely involves the skin and mucous membranes and does not disappear with warming of the area. At least 2–3 g of unsaturated hemoglobin per 100 mL of blood must be present for the patient to manifest central cyanosis. Exercise worsens central cyanosis because the exercising muscles require an increased extraction of oxygen from the blood. In patients with severe anemia, in whom hemoglobin levels are markedly decreased, cyanosis may not be seen. Clubbing is seen in association with central cyanosis and significant cardiopulmonary disorders.

Some workers, such as arc welders, inhale toxic levels of nitrous gases that can produce cyanosis by methemoglobinemia. Hereditary methemoglobinemia is a primary hemoglobin abnormality causing congenital cyanosis.

Chest Pain

Chest pain related to pulmonary disease generally results from involvement of the chest wall or parietal pleura. Nerve fibers are abundant in this area. *Pleuritic pain* is a common symptom of inflammation of the parietal pleura. It is described as a sharp, stabbing pain, which is usually felt in inspiration. It may be localized to one side, and the patient may *splint** to avoid the pain. Chapter 12, The Heart, summarizes the important questions to ask a patient complaining of chest pain.

Acute dilatation of the main pulmonary artery may also produce a dull pressure sensation, often indistinguishable from angina pectoris. This results from nerve endings responding to the stretch on the main pulmonary artery.

Although chest pain occurs in pulmonary disease, chest pain is the cardinal symptom of cardiac disease and is discussed more completely in Chapter 12.

---

* Splinting is making the chest muscles rigid to avoid motion of that part of the chest.

Other Symptoms

In addition to the main symptoms of pulmonary disease, there are other, less common symptoms. These include the following:

- Stridor (noisy breathing)
- Voice changes
- Swelling of the ankles (dependent edema)

Stridor is a harsh type of noisy breathing and is generally associated with obstruction of a major bronchus that occurs with aspiration. Voice changes can occur with inflammation of the vocal cords or interference with the recurrent laryngeal nerve. Swelling of the ankles is a manifestation of dependent edema, which is associated with right-heart failure, renal disease, liver disease, and obstruction of venous flow. As the condition worsens, abnormal accumulations of fluid produce generalized edema, known as *anasarca*.

Impact of Lung Disease on the Patient

The impact of lung disease on the patient varies greatly with the nature of the ailment as does the subjective sensation of air hunger. Some patients with lung disease are hardly aware of the dyspnea. The decrease in exercise tolerance is so insidious that these patients may not be aware of any problem. Only when asked to try to quantify the dyspnea do these patients realize their deficiency. In other patients, dyspnea is so rapidly progressive that they experience severe depression. They recognize that little can be done to improve their lung conditions and thus markedly alter their lifestyle. They become incapacitated, and many are forced to retire from work. They can no longer experience the slightest exertion without becoming dyspneic.

Often, chronic lung disease develops as a result of occupational hazards. These patients are embittered and hostile. There has been much publicity about occupational exposure, but some industries still provide little protection for their employees.

Chronic obstructive pulmonary disease (COPD) is a form of lung disease that can be subdivided into two types: *emphysema* and *chronic bronchitis*. Both are characterized by a slowly progressive course, obstruction of airflow, and destruction of the lung parenchyma. Classically, patients with emphysema are the "pink puffers." They are thin and weak from severe dyspnea associated with little cough and sputum production. The classic "blue bloaters" suffer primarily from bronchitis. They are cyanotic and have a productive cough but are less troubled by dyspnea, and they are short and stocky. These classic descriptions are interesting, but most patients with COPD have characteristics of both types.

Since ancient times, clinicians have recognized that emotional factors play a role in the onset and maintenance of symptoms in bronchial asthma. Attacks of asthma can be provoked by a range of emotions: fear, anger, anxiety, depression, guilt, frustration, and joy. It is the patient's attempt to suppress the emotion, rather than the emotion itself, that precipitates the asthmatic attack (Rees, 1956).

The patient having an asthmatic attack becomes anxious and fearful, which tends to perpetuate the attack. Hyperventilation may contribute to the breathlessness of the frightened patient. Despite being given adequate medical therapy, these patients remain dyspneic. In such patients, it is the *anxiety* and its causes that require attention. They need continuing medical *and* psychological support after the acute attack. As early as the 12th century, Maimonides recognized that "mere diet and medical treatment cannot fully cure this disorder."

Children with asthma present a special problem. Anxiety, underachievement, peer pressure, and noncompliance with medications contribute to exacerbate episodes of asthma. These children are absent from school more than their nonasthmatic peers, which causes schoolwork to suffer; this creates another vicious cycle. The incidence of emotional disorders is greater than twofold in asthmatic school-aged children in comparison with the general population (Mattson, 1975).

Asthma can affect a person's sexual function physiologically as well as psychologically. Asthmatic patients may become more dyspneic as a result of the increased physical demands of sexual intercourse. Bronchospasm may occur, owing to excitement, anxiety, or panic (Conine and Evans, 1981). Anxiety about precipitating an asthmatic attack during sexual intercourse worsens the patient's dyspnea and sexual performance; another vicious cycle is set into motion. Patients may then tend to avoid sexual intercourse.

Physical Examination

> The equipment necessary for the examination of the chest is a stethoscope.

After a general assessment of the patient, the examination of the posterior chest is performed while the patient is still seated. The patient's arms should be folded in his or her lap. After the completion of the examination of the posterior chest, the patient is asked to lie down, and the examination of the anterior chest is begun. During the examination, the examiner should try to imagine the underlying lung areas.

If the patient is a man, his gown should be removed to his waist. If the patient is a woman, the gown should be positioned to prevent unnecessary or embarrassing exposure of the breasts. The examiner should stand facing the patient.

The examination of the anterior and posterior aspects of the chest includes the following:

- Inspection
- Palpation
- Percussion
- Auscultation

General Assessment

Inspect the Patient's Facial Expression

Is the patient in acute distress? Is there nasal flaring or pursed lip breathing? Nasal flaring is the outward motion of the nares during inhalation. This is seen in any condition that causes an increase in the work of breathing. Are there audible signs of breathing, such as stridor and wheezing? These are related to obstruction to airflow. Is cyanosis present?

Inspect the Patient's Posture

Patients with airway obstructive disease tend to prefer a position in which they can support their arms and fix the muscles of the shoulder and neck to aid in respiration. A common technique used by patients with bronchial obstruction is to clasp the sides of the bed and use the latissimus dorsi muscle to help overcome the increased resistance to outflow during expiration. Patients with orthopnea remain seated or lie on several pillows.

Inspect the Neck

Is the patient's breathing aided by the action of the *accessory muscles?* Use of the accessory muscles is one of the earliest signs of airway obstruction. In respiratory distress, the trapezius and sternocleidomastoid muscles contract during inspiration. The accessory muscles assist in ventilation; they raise the clavicle and anterior chest to increase the lung volume and produce an increased negative intrathoracic pressure. This results in retraction of the supraclavicular fossae and intercostal muscles. An upward motion of the clavicle of more than 5 mm during respiration has been associated with severe obstructive lung disease (Anderson et al, 1980).

Inspect the Configuration of the Chest

A variety of conditions may interfere with adequate ventilation, and the configuration of the chest may indicate lung disease. An increase in the *anteroposterior* (AP) *diameter* is seen in advanced COPD. The AP diameter tends to equal the lateral diameter, and a *barrel chest* results. The ribs lose their 45° angle and become more horizontal. A *flail chest* is a chest configuration in which one chest wall moves paradoxically inward during inspiration. This condition is seen with multiple rib fractures. *Kyphoscoliosis* is a spinal deformity in which there are an abnormal AP diameter and lateral curvature of the spine that produces a severe restriction of chest and lung expansion. Figure 11–6 shows a patient with severe kyphoscoliosis. A *pectus excavatum,* or funnel chest, is a depression of the sternum that produces a restrictive lung problem only if the depression is marked. Patients with a pectus excavatum may have abnormalities of their mitral valve, especially mitral valve prolapse. Figure 11–7 shows a patient with a pectus excavatum. *Pectus carinatum,* or pigeon breast, which results from an anterior protrusion of the sternum, is a common deformity but does not compromise ventilation. Figure 11–8 shows a patient with a pectus carinatum. Notice the prominent sternal ridge and the ribs falling steeply away on either side. Figure 11–9 illustrates the various configurations of the chest.

Assess the Respiratory Rate and Pattern

When assessing respiratory rate never ask the patient to breathe "normally." Individuals voluntarily change their breathing pattern and rate once they are aware of it. A better way is, after taking the radial pulse, to direct your eyes to the chest and evaluate the respirations while still holding the wrist. The patient is unaware that you are no longer taking the pulse, and voluntary changes in breathing rate will not occur. Counting the number of respirations in a 30 second period and multiplying this number by 2 will provide an accurate respiratory rate.

The normal adult takes about 10–14 breaths a minute. *Bradypnea* is an abnormal slowing of respiration; *tachypnea* is an abnormal increase. *Apnea* is the temporary cessation of breathing. *Hyperpnea* is an increased depth of breathing, usually associated with metabolic acidosis. It is also known as *Kussmaul's breathing.* There are many types of abnormal breathing patterns. Figure 11–10 illustrates and lists the more common types of abnormal breathing.

Inspect the Hands

Is *clubbing* present? The technique for the evaluation of clubbing is described in Chapter 6, The Skin. The earliest finding of clubbing is the loss of the angle between

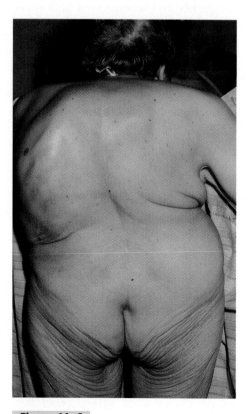

Figure 11–6

Severe kyphoscoliosis.

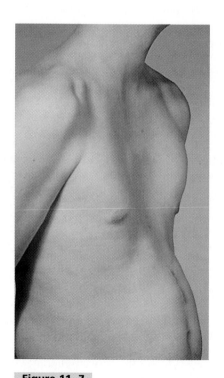

Figure 11–7

Pectus excavatum.

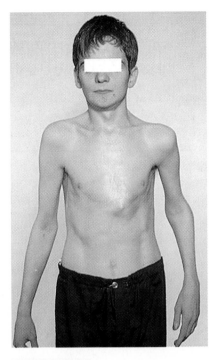

Figure 11–8

Pectus carinatum.

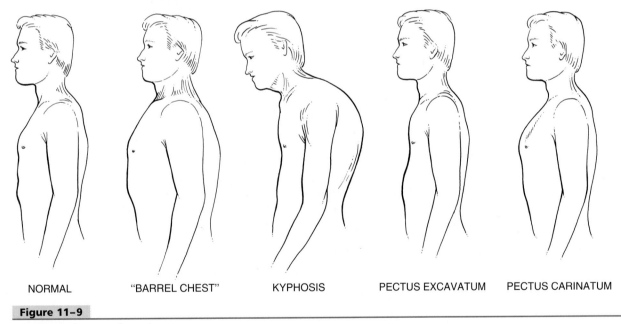

| NORMAL | "BARREL CHEST" | KYPHOSIS | PECTUS EXCAVATUM | PECTUS CARINATUM |

Figure 11–9

Common chest configurations.

the nail and the terminal phalanx. Look at Figure 6–10, in which a normal index finger is compared with a severely clubbed index finger of a patient with bronchogenic carcinoma.

Clubbing has been associated with a number of clinical disorders, such as the following:

- Intrathoracic tumors
- Mixed venous-to-arterial shunts
- Chronic pulmonary disease
- Chronic hepatic fibrosis

The pathogenesis of clubbing is unclear. In many conditions, however, arterial desaturation occurs. This, in some way, may be the underlying problem.

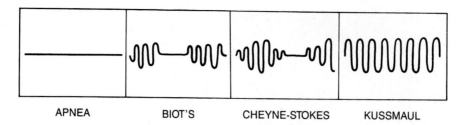

APNEA	BIOT'S	CHEYNE-STOKES	KUSSMAUL

Pattern	Characteristic	Cause
Apnea	Absence of breathing	Cardiac arrest
Biot's	Irregular breathing with long periods of apnea	Increased intracranial pressure Drug-induced respiratory depression Brain damage (usually at the medullary level)
Cheyne-Stokes	Irregular breathing with intermittent periods of increased and decreased rates and depths of breaths alternating with periods of apnea	Drug-induced respiratory depression Congestive heart failure Brain damage (usually at the cerebral level)
Kussmaul's	Fast and deep	Metabolic acidosis

Figure 11–10

Patterns of abnormal breathing.

Posterior Chest

Now move to the back of the patient to examine the posterior chest. Palpation is used in examination of the chest to assess the following:

- Areas of tenderness
- Symmetry of chest excursion
- Tactile fremitus

Palpate for Tenderness

Palpate firmly with your fingers any chest areas where tenderness is experienced by the patient. A complaint of "chest pain" may be related only to local musculoskeletal disease and not to disease of the heart or lungs. Be meticulous in assessing for areas of tenderness.

Evaluate Posterior Chest Excursion

The degree of symmetry of chest excursion may be determined by placing the hands flat against the patient's back with the thumbs parallel to the midline at approximately the level of the tenth ribs and pulling the underlying skin slightly toward the midline. The patient is asked to inhale deeply, and the movement of the hands is noted. Symmetry of hand movement should be noted. Localized pulmonary disease may cause one side of the chest to move less than the opposite side. The placement of the hands is shown in Figure 11–11.

The Principle of Tactile Fremitus

Speech creates vibrations that can be heard when one listens to the chest and lungs. These vibrations are termed *vocal fremitus*. When one palpates the chest wall while an individual is speaking, these vibrations can be felt and are termed *tactile fremitus*. Sound is conducted from the larynx through the bronchial tree to the lung parenchyma and the chest wall. Tactile fremitus provides useful information about the density of the underlying lung tissue and chest cavity. Conditions that increase the density of the lung and make it more solid, such as consolidation, increase the transmission of tactile fremitus. Clinical states that decrease the transmission of these sound waves will reduce

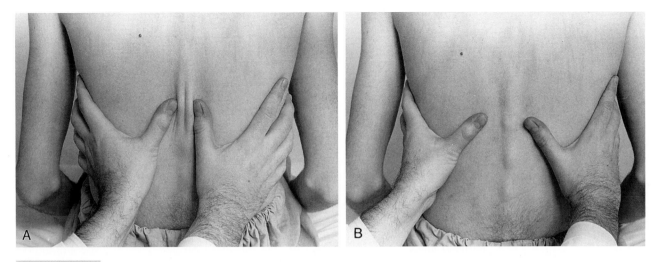

Figure 11–11

Technique for evaluating posterior chest excursion. *A,* Placement of the hands during normal expiration. *B,* Placement of the hands after normal inspiration.

tactile fremitus. If there is excess fat tissue on the chest, air or fluid in the chest cavity, or overexpansion of the lung, tactile fremitus will be diminished.

■ Evaluate Tactile Fremitus

Tactile fremitus can be evaluated in two ways. In the first technique, the examiner places the ulnar side of the right hand against the patient's chest wall, as shown in Figure 11–12, and asks the patient to say "ninety-nine." Tactile fremitus is evaluated, and the examiner's hand is moved to the corresponding position on the other side. Tactile fremitus is then compared with the opposite side. By moving the hand from side to side and from top to bottom, the examiner can detect differences in the transmission of the sound to the chest wall. "Ninety-nine" is one of the phrases used because it causes good vibratory tones. If the patient speaks either louder or deeper, the tactile sensation is enhanced. Tactile fremitus should be evaluated in the six locations shown in Figure 11–13.

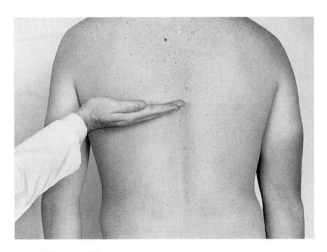

Figure 11–12

Technique for evaluating tactile fremitus.

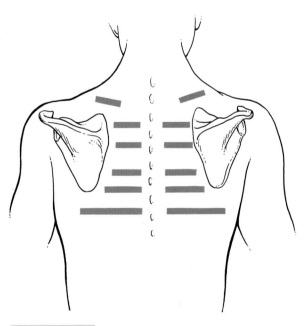

Figure 11–13

Locations on the posterior chest for evaluating tactile fremitus.

The other method of evaluating tactile fremitus is to use the fingertips instead of the ulnar side of the hand. The same side-to-side and top-to-bottom positions as shown in Figure 11–13 are used. It is necessary to perform this evaluation with only one of these techniques. The examiner should try both methods initially to determine which one is preferable.

Table 11–5 provides a list of some of the important pathologic causes for changes in tactile fremitus.

The Principle of Percussion

Percussion refers to tapping on a surface to determine the underlying structure. It is similar to a radar or echo detection system. Tapping on the chest wall is transmitted to the underlying tissue, reflected back, and picked up by the examiner's tactile and auditory senses. The sound heard and the tactile sensation felt are dependent on the air-tissue ratio. The vibrations set up by the percussion of the chest enable the examiner to evaluate the lung tissue only to a depth of 5–6 cm, but percussion is valuable because many changes in the air-tissue ratio are readily apparent.

Percussion over a solid organ, such as the liver, produces a *dull,* low-amplitude, short-duration note without resonance. Percussion over a structure containing air within a tissue, such as the lung, produces a *resonant,* higher-amplitude, lower-pitched note. Percussion over a hollow air-containing structure, such as the stomach, produces a *tympanic,* high-pitched, hollow-quality note. Percussion over a large muscle mass, such as the thigh, produces a *flat,* high-pitched note.

Normally, in the chest, dullness over the heart and resonance over the lung fields are heard and felt. As the lungs are filled with fluid and become more dense, as in pneumonia, resonance is replaced by dullness. The term *hyperresonance* has been applied to the percussion note obtained from a lung of decreased density, as is found in emphysema. Hyperresonance is a low-pitched, hollow-quality, sustained resonant note bordering on tympany.

Perform Percussion

In percussion of the chest, the examiner uses the middle finger of the left hand placed firmly against the patient's chest wall parallel to the ribs in an interspace, with the palm and other fingers held off the chest. The tip of the right middle finger strikes a quick, sharp blow to the terminal phalanx of the left finger on the chest wall. The motion of the striking finger should come from the wrist and not from the elbow. Paddle ball players use this motion, whereas tennis players must learn to concentrate on using this wrist motion. The technique of percussion is diagrammed in Figure 11–14 and shown in Figure 11–15.

Try percussion on yourself. Percuss over your right lung (resonant), stomach (tympanic), liver (dull), and thigh (flat).

Percuss the Posterior Chest

The sites on the posterior chest for percussion are above, between, and below the scapulae in the intercostal spaces, as shown in Figure 11–16. The bony scapulae are not percussed. The examiner should start at the top and work downward, proceeding from side to side, comparing one side with the other.

Evaluate Diaphragmatic Movement

Percussion is also used to detect diaphragmatic movement. The patient is asked to take a deep breath and hold it. Percussion at the right lung base determines the lowest area

Table 11–5	Tactile Fremitus	
	Increased	Decreased
	Pneumonia	Unilateral
		Pneumothorax
		Pleural effusion
		Bronchial obstruction
		Atelectasis (incomplete expansion of lung tissue)
		Bilateral
		Chronic obstructive lung disease
		Chest wall thickening (muscle, fat)

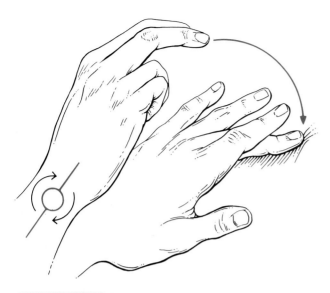

Figure 11–14

Technique of percussion.

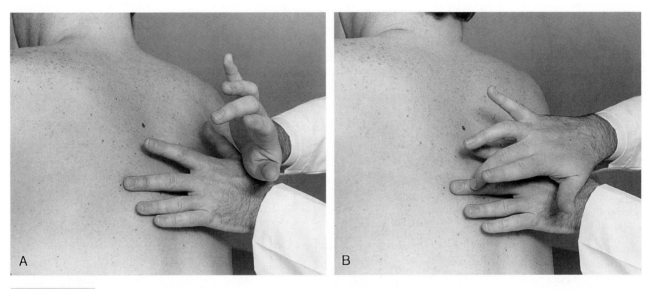

Figure 11–15

A, Position of the right hand ready to percuss. *B,* Location of the fingers after striking. Notice that the motion is from the wrist.

of resonance, which represents the lowest level of the diaphragm. Below this level is dullness from the liver. The patient is then instructed to exhale as much as possible, and the percussion is repeated. With expiration, the lung will contract, the liver will move up, and the same area will become dull. The level of dullness has moved upward. The difference between the inspiration and expiration levels represents diaphragmatic motion, which is normally 4–5 cm. In patients with emphysema, the motion is reduced. In patients with a phrenic nerve palsy, diaphragmatic motion is absent. This test is illustrated in Figure 11–17.

Perform Auscultation

Auscultation is the technique of listening for sounds produced in the body. Auscultation of the chest is used to identify lung sounds. The stethoscope usually has two heads: the bell and the diaphragm. The bell is used to detect low-pitched sounds, and the diaphragm is better at detecting higher-pitched sounds. The bell must be loosely applied to the skin; if it is pressed too tightly, the skin will act as a diaphragm and the lower-pitched sounds will be filtered out. In contrast, the diaphragm is applied firmly

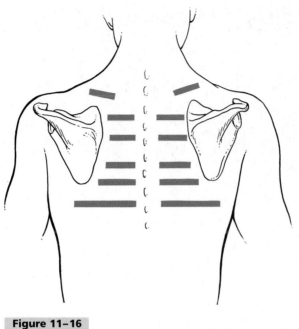

Figure 11–16

Locations on the posterior chest for percussion.

Figure 11–17

Technique for evaluating diaphragmatic motion. During inspiration, in the example on the left, percussion in the right seventh posterior interspace at the midscapular line would be resonant as a result of the presence of the underlying lung. During expiration, in the example on the right, the liver and diaphragm move up. Percussion in the same area would now be dull, owing to the presence of the underlying liver.

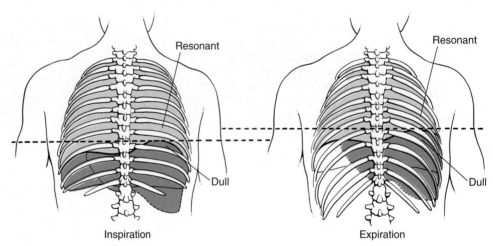

to the skin. In very cachectic individuals the bell may be more useful, as placement of the diaphragm is more difficult in these patients because of the protrusion of their ribs. The correct placement of the heads of the stethoscope is shown in Figure 11–18.

It is *never* acceptable to listen through clothing. The bell or the diaphragm of the stethoscope must *always* be in contact with the skin.

■ **Types of Breath Sounds**

Breath sounds are heard over most of the lung fields. They consist of an inspiratory phase followed by an expiratory phase. There are four types of normal breath sounds:

- ■ Tracheal
- ■ Bronchial
- ■ Bronchovesicular
- ■ Vesicular

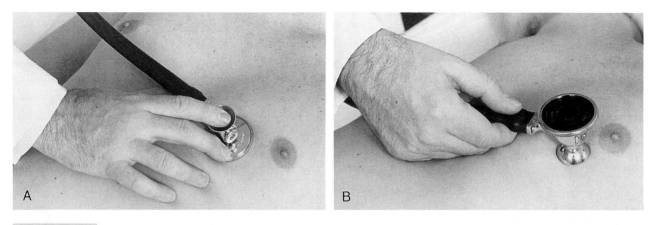

Figure 11–18

Placement of stethoscope heads. *A,* Correct placement of the diaphragm. Notice that the head is applied tightly to the skin. *B,* Placement of the bell. Notice that the bell is applied lightly to the skin.

Tracheal breath sounds are harsh, loud, and high-pitched sounds heard over the extrathoracic portion of the trachea. The inspiratory and expiratory components are approximately equal in length. Although always heard when one listens over the trachea, they are rarely evaluated because they do not represent any clinical lung problems.

Bronchial breath sounds are loud and high pitched and sound like air rushing through a tube. The expiratory component is louder and longer than the inspiratory component. These sounds are normally heard when one is listening over the manubrium. A definite pause is heard between the two phases.

Bronchovesicular breath sounds are a mixture of bronchial and vesicular sounds. The inspiratory and expiratory components are equal in length. They are normally heard only in the first and second interspaces anteriorly and between the scapulae posteriorly. This is the area overlying the carina and mainstem bronchi.

Vesicular breath sounds are the soft, low-pitched sounds heard over most of the lung fields. The inspiratory component is much longer than the expiratory component, which is also much softer and frequently inaudible.

The four types of breath sounds are shown and summarized in Figure 11–19.

Auscultate the Posterior Chest

Auscultation should be performed in a quiet environment. The patient is asked to breathe in and out through the mouth. The examiner should first concentrate on the length of inspiration and then on expiration. Very soft breath sounds are referred to as *distant.* Distant breath sounds are commonly found in patients with hyperinflated lungs, as in emphysema.

The examination should proceed from side to side and from top to bottom, one side being compared with the other. The positions are illustrated in Figure 11–20. Because most breath sounds are high pitched, the diaphragm is used to evaluate lung sounds.

Anterior Chest

The examiner should now move to the front of the patient. The first part of the examination of the anterior chest is performed with the patient seated, after which the patient is asked to lie down.

Evaluate Position of the Trachea

The position of the trachea can be determined by placing the right index finger in the suprasternal notch and moving slightly lateral to feel the location of the trachea. This technique is repeated, moving the finger from the suprasternal notch to the other side. The space between the trachea and the clavicle should be equal. A shift of the mediastinum can displace the trachea to one side. This technique is shown in Figure 11–21.

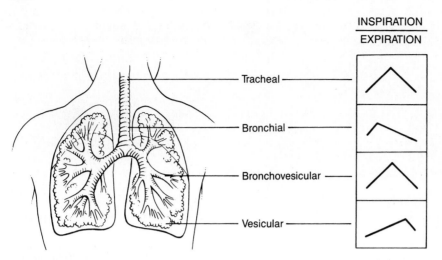

Characteristic	Tracheal	Bronchial	Bronchovesicular	Vesicular
Intensity	Very loud	Loud	Moderate	Soft
Pitch	Very high	High	Moderate	Low
I : E Ratio*	1 : 1	1 : 3	1 : 1	3 : 1
Description	Harsh	Tubular	Rustling but tubular	Gentle rustling
Normal locations	Extrathoracic trachea	Manubrium	Over mainstem bronchi	Most of peripheral lung

* Ratio of duration of inspiration to expiration.

Figure 11–19

Characteristics of breath sounds.

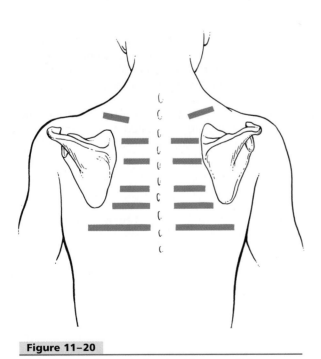

Figure 11–20

Locations on the posterior chest for auscultation.

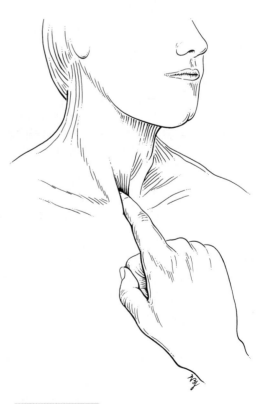

Figure 11–21

Technique for determining the position of the trachea.

Look at the patient shown in Figure 11–22. Notice that the trachea is markedly displaced to the right in this very cachectic woman. The diagnosis of a mass either pushing or pulling the trachea to the right is suggested.

Evaluate the Mobility of the Trachea

The upward motion of the trachea is used to ascertain whether the trachea is *fixed* in the mediastinum. The technique is called the *tracheal tug*. The patient's head should be slightly flexed, and the examiner's left hand should support the back of the patient's head. The examiner's right hand should be placed parallel against the patient's trachea with the palm facing out. The middle fingers should slide into the cricothyroid space, and the larynx is pushed upward. The larynx and trachea normally move about 1–2 cm. After moving the larynx upward, lower it slowly before removing your fingers. Do not suddenly release it from its superior position. A fixed trachea indicates mediastinal fixation, which can occur with neoplasm or tuberculosis. Be careful not to place the examining fingers horizontally, push backward, or drop the trachea. These maneuvers can cause the patient much discomfort. The correct position is shown in Figure 11–23.

Now ask the patient to lie on his or her back for the rest of the examination of the anterior chest. The patient's arms are at the sides. If the patient is a woman, either have her elevate her breasts or displace them yourself as necessary during palpation, percussion, and auscultation. These examinations should not be performed over breast tissue.

Evaluate Tactile Fremitus

Tactile fremitus is assessed in the supraclavicular fossae and in alternate anterior interspaces, beginning at the clavicle. The techniques for evaluating tactile fremitus have been discussed. Proceed from the supraclavicular fossae downward, comparing one side with the other.

Percuss the Anterior Chest

Percussion of the anterior chest includes the supraclavicular fossae, the axillae, and the anterior interspaces, as shown in Figure 11–24. The percussion note on one side is always compared with that on the corresponding position on the other side. Dullness may be elicited in the third to fifth intercostal spaces to the left of the sternum, which is related to the presence of the heart. Percuss high in the axillae because the upper lobes are best evaluated at these positions. Axillary percussion is sometimes easier to perform while the patient is sitting.

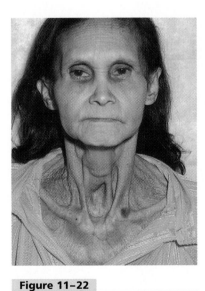

Figure 11–22

Tracheal deviation. Notice the marked trachial deviation to the right.

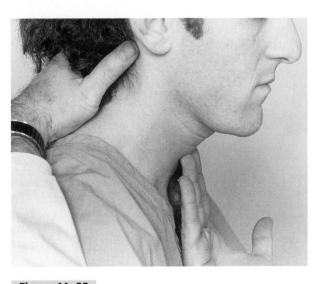

Figure 11–23

Technique for the tracheal tug.

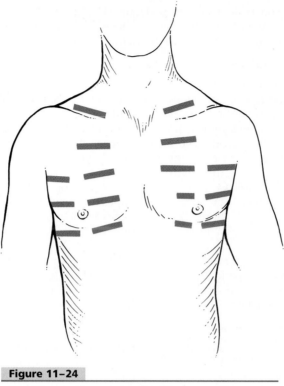

Figure 11–24

Locations on the anterior chest for percussion.

Auscultate the Anterior Chest

Auscultation of the anterior chest is performed in the supraclavicular fossae, the axillae, and the anterior chest interspaces, as illustrated in Figure 11–25. The techniques of auscultation have been discussed. The breath sounds of one side are compared with the breath sounds in the corresponding position on the other side.

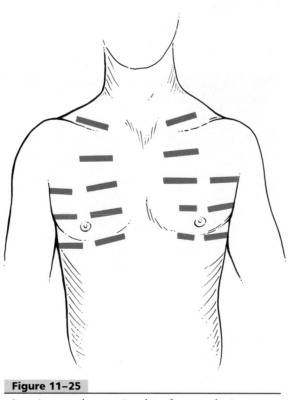

Figure 11–25

Locations on the anterior chest for auscultation.

Clinicopathologic Correlations

In addition to the normal breath sounds discussed, other lung sounds may be produced in abnormal clinical states. These abnormal sounds heard during auscultation are called *adventitious* sounds. Adventitious sounds include the following:

- Crackles
- Wheezes
- Rhonchi
- Pleural rubs

Crackles are short, discontinuous, nonmusical sounds heard mostly during inspiration. Also known as rales or crepitation, crackles are caused by the opening of collapsed distal airways and alveoli. A sudden equalization of pressure seems to result in a crackle. Coarser crackles are related to larger airways. Crackles are likened to the sound made by rubbing hair next to the ear or the sound made when Velcro is opened. They may be described as early or late, depending on when they are heard during inspiraton. The timing of common inspiratory crackles is summarized in Table 11–6. The most common causes of crackles are pulmonary edema, congestive heart failure, and pulmonary fibrosis.

Wheezes are continuous, musical, high-pitched sounds heard mostly during expiration. They are produced by airflow through narrowed bronchi. This narrowing may be due to swelling, secretions, spasm, a tumor, or a foreign body. Wheezes are commonly associated with the bronchospasm of asthma.

Rhonchi are lower-pitched, more sonorous lung sounds. They are believed to be more common with transient mucus plugging and poor movement of airway secretions.

A *pleural rub* is a grating sound produced by motion of the pleura, which is impeded by frictional resistance. It is best heard at the end of inspiration and at the beginning of expiration. The sound of a pleural rub has been described as like that made by creaking leather. Pleural rubs are heard when pleural surfaces are roughened or thickened by inflammatory or neoplastic cells or by fibrin deposits.

All of the adventitious sounds should be described as to their location, timing, and intensity.

There is much confusion regarding the terminology of adventitious sounds. Table 11–7 summarizes the adventitious sounds.

Table 11–6   Timing of Common Inspiratory Crackles

Disease	Early Crackle	Late Crackle
Congestive heart failure	Very common	Common
Obstructive lung disease	Present	Absent
Interstitial fibrosis	Absent	Present
Pneumonia	Absent	Present

Table 11–7   Adventitious Sounds

Recommended Term	Older Term	Mechanism	Causes
Crackle	Rale Crepitation	Excess airway secretions	Bronchitis, respiratory infections, pulmonary edema, atelectasis, fibrosis, congestive heart failure
Wheeze	Sibilant rale Musical rale Sonorous rale Low-pitched wheeze	Rapid airflow through obstructed airway	Asthma, pulmonary edema, bronchitis, congestive heart failure
Rhonchus		Transient airway plugging	Bronchitis
Pleural rub		Inflammation of the pleura	Pneumonia, pulmonary infarction

Occasionally, breath sounds are transmitted abnormally. This may result in auscultatory changes known as

- Egophony
- Whispered pectoriloquy
- Bronchophony

Egophony (egobronchophony) is said to be present when the spoken word heard through the lungs is increased in intensity and takes on a nasal or bleating quality. The patient is asked to say "eeee" while the examiner listens to an area in which consolidation is suspected. If egophony is present, the "eeee" will be heard as "aaaa." This "e to a" change is seen in consolidation of lung tissue. The area of compressed lung above a pleural effusion often produces egophony.

Whispered pectoriloquy is the term given to the intensification of the whispered word heard in consolidation of the lung. The patient is instructed to whisper "one-two-three" while the examiner listens to the area suspected of having consolidation. Normally, whispering produces high-pitched sounds that tend to be filtered out by the lungs. Little or nothing may be heard when one listens to a normal chest. However, if consolidation is present, the transmission of the spoken words will be increased, and the words will be clearly heard.

Bronchophony is the increased transmission of spoken words heard in consolidation of the lungs. The patient is asked to say "ninety-nine" while the examiner listens to the chest. If bronchophony is present, the words will be transmitted louder than normally.

One of the most important principles concerning the examination of the chest is to correlate the findings of percussion, palpation, and auscultation. Dullness, crackles, increased breath sounds, and increased tactile fremitus suggest consolidation. Dullness, decreased breath sounds, and decreased tactile fremitus suggest a pleural effusion.

Many physical signs are associated with obstructive lung disease. These include *impaired breath sounds, barrel chest, decreased chest expansion,* impaired cardiac dullness, use of accessory muscles, absent cardiac impulse, cyanosis, and diminished diaphragmatic excursion. Although all these are important physical findings, the first three have the greatest intrinsic value as diagnostic tools.

Table 11–8 lists some of the common causes of dyspnea and their associated symptoms. Table 11–9 summarizes some important manifestations of common pulmonary conditions.

Useful Vocabulary

Listed here are the specific roots that are important in order to understand the terminology related to diseases of the chest.

Root	Pertaining to	Example	Definition
broncho-	bronchus	*bronch*itis	Inflammation of the bronchus
-capnia	carbon dioxide	hyper*capnia*	Excessive carbon dioxide in the blood
chondro-	cartilage	*chondr*oma	Hyperplastic growth of cartilage
costo-	ribs	*costo*chondritis	Inflammation of the rib cartilage
muc(o)-	mucus	*muc*olytic	Agent that dissolves mucus
phren-	diaphragm	*phreno*hepatic	Pertaining to the diaphragm and liver
pleur(o)-	pleura	*pleur*itic	Pertaining to inflammation of the pleura
-pne(o)-	breath	dys*pne*a	Difficulty in breathing; shortness of breath
pneumo-	lungs	*pneumo*nectomy	Surgical removal of lung tissue
spiro-	to breathe	*spiro*gram	A tracing of respiratory movements
-stern(o)-	sternum	costo*stern*al	Pertaining to the ribs and sternum

Table 11–8   Common Conditions Associated with Dyspnea

Condition	Dyspnea	Other Symptoms
Asthma	Episodic, symptom-free between attacks	Wheezing, chest pain, productive cough
Pneumonia	Insidious onset	Cough
Pulmonary edema	Abrupt	Tachypnea, cough, orthopnea, and paroxysmal nocturnal dyspnea with chronic state
Pulmonary fibrosis	Progressive	Tachypnea, dry cough
Pneumonia	Exertional	Productive cough, pleuritic pain
Pneumothorax	Sudden, moderate to severe	Sudden pleuritic pain
Emphysema	Insidious onset, severe	Cough as disease progresses
Chronic bronchitis	As disease progresses and with infection	Chronic, productive cough
Obesity	Exertional	

Table 11–9   Differentiation of Common Pulmonary Conditions

Condition	Vital Signs	Inspection	Palpation	Percussion	Auscultation
Asthma*	Tachypnea; tachycardia	Dyspnea; use of accessory muscles; possible cyanosis; hyperinflation	Often normal; decreased fremitus	Often normal; hyperresonant; low diaphragm	Prolonged expiration; wheezes; decreased lung sounds
Emphysema	Stable	Increased anteroposterior diameter; use of accessory muscles; thin individual	Decreased tactile fremitus	Increased resonance; decreased excursion of diaphragm	Decreased lung sounds; decreased vocal fremitus
Chronic bronchitis	Tachycardia	Possible cyanosis; short, stocky individual	Often normal	Often normal	Early crackles; rhonchi
Pneumonia	Tachycardia; fever; tachypnea	Possible cyanosis; possible splinting on affected side	Increased tactile fremitus	Dull	Late crackles; bronchial breath sounds†
Pulmonary embolism	Tachycardia; tachypnea	Often normal	Usually normal	Usually normal	Usually normal
Pulmonary edema	Tachycardia; tachypnea	Possible signs of elevated right heart pressures‡	Often normal	Often normal	Early crackles; wheezes
Pneumothroax	Tachypnea; tachycardia	Often normal lag on affected side	Absent fremitus; trachea may be shifted to other side	Hyperresonant	Absent breath sounds
Pleural effusion	Tachypnea; tachycardia	Often normal; lag on affected side	Decreased fremitus; trachea shifted to other side	Dullness	Absent breath sounds
Atelectasis	Tachypnea	Often normal; lag on affected side	Decreased fremitus; trachea shifted to same side	Dullness	Absent breath sounds
Adult respiratory distress syndrome	Tachycardia; tachypnea	Use of accessory muscles; cyanosis	Usually normal	Often normal	Normal initially; crackles and decreased lung sounds, late

* Often the physical findings in asthma are not reliable in predicting its severity.
† Bronchophony, pectoriloquy, and egophony are also often present.
‡ Elevated jugular venous distention, pedal edema, hepatomegaly.

Writing Up the Physical Examination

Listed here are examples of the write-up for the examination of the chest.

- The trachea is midline and is not fixed. The chest is normal in appearance. Palpation is normal. The chest is clear to percussion and auscultation.
- The trachea is midline. A mild pectus excavatum is present. There is increased tactile fremitus at the left posterior chest, up one third from the base. This area is also dull to percussion. Bronchial breath sounds and crackles are present in the area of dullness. Bronchophony and whispered pectoriloquy are also present in this area.
- The trachea is deviated to the left. The chest structure is within normal limits. There is decreased tactile fremitus on the right chest posteriorly, up three quarters from the base. The percussion note is dull in the area of decreased fremitus. There are no breath sounds heard in this area. An area of egophony is present above the area of dullness.
- The trachea is midline. Tactile fremitus is normal, as is percussion. Auscultation reveals normal breath sounds with bilateral basilar crackles present.

Bibliography

Anderson CL, Shankar PS, Scott JH: Physiological significance of sternomastoid muscle contraction in chronic obstructive pulmonary disease. Respir Care 25:937, 1980.

Conine TA, Evans JH: Sexual adjustment in chronic obstructive pulmonary disease. Respir Care 26: 871, 1981.

Forgacs P: The functional basis of pulmonary sounds. Chest 73:399, 1978.

Glauser FL: Signs and Symptoms in Pulmonary Medicine. Philadelphia, J.B. Lippincott, 1983.

Hinshaw HC, Murray JF: Diseases of the Chest, 4th ed. Philadelphia, W.B. Saunders, 1980.

Mattson A: Psychologic aspects of childhood asthma. Pediatr Clin North Am 2:77, 1975.

National Heart and Lung Institute. NIH Publication No. 72-516, 1972.

National Institutes of Health. Epidemiology of Respiratory Diseases—Task Force Report. NIH Publication No. 81-2019, 1980.

Raffin TA: Separating cardiac from pulmonary dyspnea. JAMA 238:206, 1977.

Rees L: Physical and emotional factors in bronchial asthma. J Psychosomatic Res 1:98, 1956.

Stubbing DG, Mathur PN, Roberts RS: Some physical signs in patients with chronic airway obstruction. Am Rev Respir Dis 125:549, 1982.

CHAPTER 12

The Heart

. . . For it is the heart by whose virtue and pulse the blood is moved, perfected, made apt to nourish and is preserved from corruption and coagulation. . . . It is indeed the fountain of life, the source of all action.

William Harvey
1578–1657

General Considerations

The heart does not rest for more than a fraction of a second at a time. During a lifetime, it contracts more than 4 billion times. To support this active state, the coronary arteries supply more than 10 million liters of blood to the myocardium and more than 200 million liters to the systemic circulation. Cardiac output can vary under physiologic conditions from 3 to 30 L/min, and regional blood flow can vary by 200%. This wide range occurs without any loss of efficiency in the normal state.

Diseases of the heart are common. The major disease categories are coronary artery disease, hypertension, rheumatic heart disease, bacterial endocarditis, and congenital heart disease. The clinical consequences of these conditions are generally serious.

Coronary artery disease is the leading cause of death in the United States. By the age of 60 years, nearly one in five American men has symptomatic coronary artery disease caused by coronary atherosclerosis. Autopsy studies during the Korean War showed that 40% of all American soldiers who were killed in their early twenties had atheromatous involvement of one or more of their coronary arteries.

In the United States, more than 1 million myocardial infarctions are suffered annually, resulting in more than 650,000 deaths, half of which are sudden. An additional 200,000 individuals die of strokes and related vascular diseases. The cost of diseases related to the cardiovascular system exceeds 40 billion dollars per year. Unlike other forms of cardiac disease, coronary atherosclerotic disease may be severe and life-threatening despite a normal physical examination, electrocardiogram, and chest x-ray film.

Systemic arterial hypertension affects approximately 20% of the American population. It is a major risk factor for coronary artery disease as well as a prime cause of congestive heart failure and strokes. It has been well established that among patients with higher systolic or diastolic pressures, there is a greater incidence of morbidity and mortality.

Since the implementation of antibiotic therapy, the incidence of rheumatic heart disease has been decreasing in the more affluent countries. In areas of overcrowding and in less affluent areas, rheumatic fever and the valvular heart disease that results from it are still a major cause of cardiac morbidity and mortality.

Bacterial endocarditis remains a significant medical problem despite the wide use of antibiotics. The increasing number of cases is related to intravenous use of street drugs. The diagnosis of endocarditis is often not suspected until serious sequelae develop. In addition to causing valvular damage, the persistent bacteremia can spread the infection to the brain, myocardium, spleen, kidneys, and other sites in the body.

The incidence of congenital heart disease averages 5 per 1000 live births. If other commonly found congenital conditions, such as bicuspid aortic valve and mitral valve prolapse, are included, the incidence approaches 1 per 100 live births.

It is clear that the magnitude of cardiac disease is enormous, and the cost of the morbidity and mortality is directly proportional.

Structure and Physiology

The principal function of the cardiovascular system is to deliver nutrients to and remove metabolites from every cell in the body. This metabolic exchange system is produced by a high-pressure delivery system, an area of exchange, and a low-pressure return system. The high-pressure delivery system is the *left* side of the heart and *arteries,* and the low-pressure return system includes the *veins* and the *right* side of the heart. The circulation of blood through the heart is illustrated in Figure 12–1.

The heart is enveloped by a thin *pericardial sac.* The bottom of this sac is adherent to the diaphragm, and the top is loosely attached to the upper portion of the sternum. The *visceral* pericardium is the epicardial, or outermost, layer of cells of the heart. The *parietal* pericardium is the outer sac. Between these two surfaces, a small amount of pericardial fluid in the pericardial sac provides a lubricating interface for the constantly moving heart. The parietal pericardium is innervated by the phrenic nerve, which contains pain fibers. The visceral pericardium is insensitive to pain.

The synchronous contraction of the heart results from the conduction of impulses generated by the *sinoatrial* (SA) *node* and propagated through the *conduction system.* The SA node is located at the juncture of the superior vena cava and the right atrium. The SA impulse spreads from its point of origin concentrically. When the impulse reaches the *atrioventricular* (AV) *node,* in the interatrial septum near the entrance of the coronary sinus, the impulse is slowed. It is then transmitted to the specialized conducting tissue known as the *right* and *left bundle branches,* which conduct the impulse to the specialized conducting pathways within the ventricles, *Purkinje's fibers.* The impulse spreads from the endocardial to the epicardial surface of the heart. These conducting pathways are illustrated in Figure 12–2.

The heart is innervated extensively by branches of the autonomic nervous system. Both sympathetic and parasympathetic fibers are present in the SA and AV nodes. The atrial muscle is also innervated by both types of fibers. The ventricular musculature is innervated predominantly by the sympathetic nervous system.

The *parasympathetic* fibers travel along the vagus, or tenth cranial, nerve. The *sympathetic* fibers descend in the spinal cord to the level of T1–T5, where they emerge through the ventral roots to form a synapse in the thoracic and cervical *sympathetic ganglia.* The postganglionic fibers travel through the cervical *cardiac nerves* to join the parasympathetic fibers in forming the *cardiac plexus,* which is located near the aortic arch and the tracheal bifurcation. These neural pathways are shown in Figure 12–3.

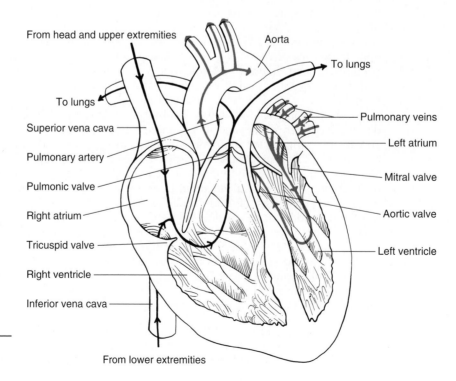

Figure 12–1

Circulation of blood through the heart.

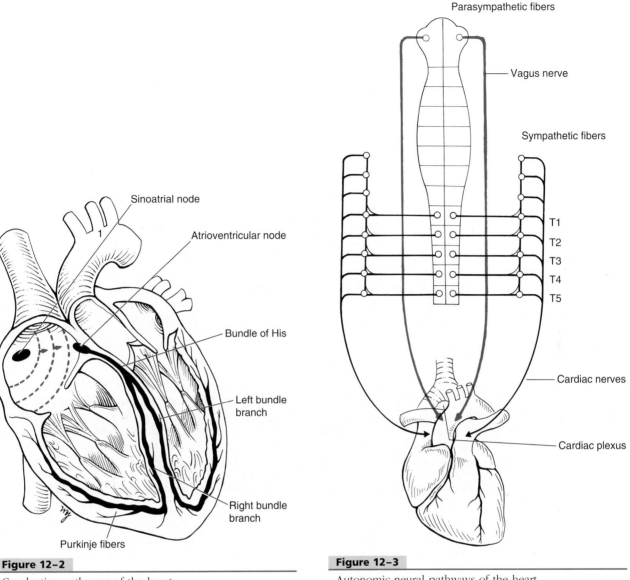

Figure 12-2

Conducting pathways of the heart.

Figure 12-3

Autonomic neural pathways of the heart.

Sympathetic stimulation by *norepinephrine* produces marked increases in heart rate and contractility. Parasympathetic stimulation mediated by *acetylcholine* slows the heart rate and decreases contractility.

In addition, several receptor sites provide circulatory information to the *medullary cardiovascular center* in the brain. This center has cardioexcitatory and cardioinhibitory areas that regulate the neural output to the sympathetic and parasympathetic fibers. *Stretch receptors* in the aortic arch and in the carotid sinus monitor blood pressure. These *baroreceptors* respond to a decrease in blood pressure by decreasing their impulses to the medullary center. The center senses this decreased activity and increases its sympathetic efferent activity and decreases its parasympathetic efferent activity. The net result is to increase the heart rate and contractility. An increase in blood pressure causes an increase in afferent activity to the center, and the opposite changes occur.

To describe physical signs, the examiner must be able to identify the important surface topographic landmarks. Chapter 11, The Chest, describes the major areas. These areas should be reviewed at this time.

The surface projection of the heart and great vessels is shown in Figure 12–4. Most of the anterior cardiac surface is the right ventricle. The right atrium forms a narrow border from the third to the fifth rib to the right of the sternum. The left ventricle lies

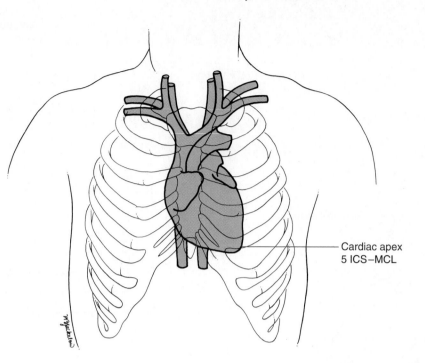

Cardiac apex
5 ICS–MCL

Figure 12–4

Surface topography of
the heart. (5 ICS-MCL
= fifth intercostal
space at the midclavic-
ular line.)

to the left and behind the right ventricle. The left ventricular *apex* is normally in the *fifth* intercostal space at the *mid*clavicular *line*. This location is commonly written as 5ICS-MCL. This *apical impulse* is called the *point of maximum impulse (PMI)*. The other chambers and vessels of the heart are usually not identifiable on examination.

The four classic *auscultatory areas* correspond to points over the precordium, at which events originating at each valve are best heart. The areas are not necessarily related to the anatomic position of the valve, nor are all sounds heard in the area directly produced by the valve that names the area. The normal areas are as follows:

Aortic   Second intercostal space, right sternal border (2ICS-RSB)
Pulmonic   Second intercostal space, left sternal border (2ICS-LSB)
Tricuspid   Left lower sternal border (LLSB)
Mitral   Cardiac apex (5ICS-MCL)

In addition to these four areas, the third left interspace, known as *Erb's point,* is frequently the area to which pulmonic or aortic sounds radiate. The five areas are illustrated in Figure 12–5. The second intercostal space to the right and left of the sternum is called the *base*.

It should be remembered that the left atrium is the most posterior portion of the heart. When the left atrium enlarges, it extends posteriorly and to the right.

The Cardiac Cycle

To understand the cardiac cycle, the motion of the valves and the pressures within the chambers should be reviewed. The interrelationships of valve motion are critically important and must be understood. Only with the knowledge of these cycles can you fully comprehend the cardiac physical examination and heart sounds. The pressure tracings and valve motions are shown in Figure 12–6.

Normally, only the closing of the heart valves can be heard. The closure of the *atrioventricular valves,* the tricuspid and the mitral, produces the *first heart sound (S_1)*. The closure of the *semilunar valves,* the aortic and the pulmonic, produces the *second heart sound (S_2)*.

The opening of the valves can be heard only if they are damaged. When an atrioventricular valve is narrowed, or *stenotic,* the opening of the valve may be heard and is termed an *opening snap*. If a semilunar valve is stenotic, the opening may be heard and is termed an *ejection click*. It should be noted from Figure 12–6 that the

uals older than the age of 30 years, it indicates a *noncompliant,* or "stiff," ventricle. Pressure overload on a ventricle causes concentric hypertrophy, which produces a noncompliant ventricle. In addition, coronary artery disease is a major cause of a stiff ventricle.

Two useful mnemonics for remembering the cadence and pathophysiology of the third and fourth heart sounds are

SLOSH′-ing-in   SLOSH′-ing-in   SLOSH′-ing-in
S_1 S_2 S_3 S_1 S_2 S_3 S_1 S_2 S_3

a-STIFF′-wall   a-STIFF′-wall   a-STIFF′-wall
S_4 S_1 S_2 S_4 S_1 S_2 S_4 S_1 S_2

The presence of an S_3 or an S_4 creates a cadence resembling the gallop of a horse. These sounds are, therefore, called *gallop* sounds or rhythms.

The first heart sound is loudest at the cardiac apex. *Splitting* of the first heart sound may be heard in the tricuspid area. The second heart sound is loudest at the base.

The terms A_2 and P_2 indicate the aortic component and the pulmonic component of S_2, respectively. A_2 normally precedes P_2, meaning that the aortic valve closes before the pulmonic valve. With inspiration, the intrathoracic pressure lowers. This causes more blood to be drawn from the superior and inferior venae cavae into the right heart. The right ventricle enlarges, and it takes longer for all the blood to be ejected into the pulmonary artery; thus the pulmonic valve stays open longer. P_2 occurs later in inspiration, and the split between A_2 and P_2 is widened during inspiration in comparison with expiration. This is the cause of *physiologic splitting* of S_2, which is diagrammed in Figure 12–7.

The blood in the right ventricle is then pumped into the large capacitance bed of the lungs. Therefore, the return of blood from the lungs to the left heart is decreased, and the left atrium and left ventricle become smaller. Atrial receptors trigger a reflex tachycardia that compensates for the decreased left ventricular volume. This increase in heart rate with inspiration is termed *sinus arrhythmia*. It is a misnomer, because it is not really an arrhythmia but a normal physiologic response to a decreased left ventricular volume during inspiration.

The Arterial Pulse

The arterial pulse is produced by the ejection of blood into the aorta. The normal configuration of the pulse consists of a smooth and rapid upstroke that begins about 80 msec after the first component of S_1. There is sometimes a slight notch in the arterial pulsation toward the end of the rapid ejection period. This is called the *anacrotic notch*. The peak of the pulse is smooth, is dome shaped, and occurs about 100 msec after the onset of the pulse. The descending limb from the peak is less steep. There is a gradual descent to the dicrotic notch, which represents the closure of the aortic valve. The contour and volume of the arterial pulse are determined by several

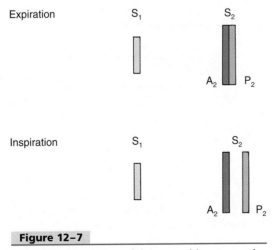

Figure 12–7

Physiologic splitting of the second heart sound.

factors, including the left ventricular stroke volume, the ejection velocity, the relative compliance and capacity of the arteries, and the pressure waves that result from the antegrade flow of blood. Figure 12–8 shows a characteristic arterial pulse.

As the arterial pulse travels to the periphery, there are several changes. The initial upstroke becomes steeper, the systolic peak is higher, and the anacrotic notch becomes less evident. In addition, the dicrotic notch occurs later in the peripheral pulse. This occurs approximately 300 msec after the onset of the pulse. The positive wave that follows the dicrotic notch is called the *dicrotic wave*.

Commonly, two waves may be present in the arterial pulse, which precedes the dicrotic notch. The *percussion wave* is the earlier wave and is associated with the rate of flow in the artery. The percussion wave occurs during peak velocity of flow. The *tidal wave* is the second wave, is related to pressure in the vessel, and occurs during peak systolic pressure. The tidal wave is usually smaller than the percussion wave, but it may be increased in hypertensive or elderly patients.

Blood Pressure

Arterial blood pressure is the lateral pressure exerted by a column of blood against the arterial wall. It is the result of cardiac output and peripheral vascular resistance. Blood pressure is dependent on the volume of blood ejected, its velocity, the distensibility of the arterial wall, the viscosity of the blood, and the pressure within the vessel after the last ejection.

Systolic blood pressure is the peak pressure in the arteries. It is regulated by the stroke volume and the compliance of the blood vessels. Diastolic blood pressure is the lowest pressure in the arteries and is dependent on peripheral resistance. The difference in the systolic and diastolic pressure is the *pulse pressure*. Systolic blood pressure in the legs is 15–20 mm Hg greater than in the arms, even while the individual is lying flat. This is in part related to Poiseuille's law, which states that the total resistance of vessels connected in parallel is greater than the resistance of a single large vessel. The blood pressure in the aorta is less than the blood pressure in the branched arteries of the lower extremities.

Blood pressure varies greatly, according to the patient's degree of excitement, degree of activity, smoking habits, pain, bladder distention, and dietary pattern. There is normally an inspiratory decline of up to 10 mm Hg in systolic blood pressure during quiet respiration.

Jugular Venous Pulse

The jugular venous pulse provides direct information about the pressures in the right side of the heart, because the jugular system is in direct continuity with the right atrium. During diastole, when the tricuspid valve is open, the jugular veins are continuous with the right ventricle as well. If there is no stenotic lesion at the pulmonic or

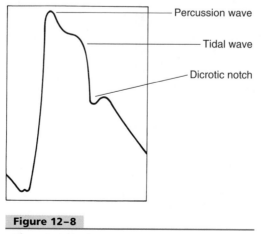

Percussion wave

Tidal wave

Dicrotic notch

Figure 12–8

The arterial pulse.

mitral valves, the right ventricle will indirectly monitor the pressures in the left atrium and left ventricle. The most common cause of *right*-sided heart failure is *left*-sided heart failure. Examination of the neck veins also provides information about the cardiac rhythm.

The understanding of the normal physiology is important in the consideration of the jugular venous pulsation. Figure 12–9 is an enlargement of the atrial and ventricular pressure curves shown in Figure 12–6.

The *"a" wave* of the jugular venous pulse is produced by right atrial contraction. When the "a" wave is timed with the electrocardiogram, it is found to occur about 90 msec after the onset of the P wave. This time delay is related to the time from electrical stimulation of the atria, to atrial contraction, and to the resultant wave propagated in the neck. The *x descent* is caused by atrial relaxation, which occurs just before ventricular contraction. This drop in right atrial pressure is terminated by the *"c" wave*. This increase in right atrial pressure is due to tricuspid valve closure secondary to right ventricular contraction. The descent of the atrioventricular valve rings produces the next change in right atrial pressure, called the *x prime descent*. As the free wall of the right ventricle approaches the septum during contraction, the atrioventricular valve rings descend toward the apex as contraction progresses. This increases the size of the atrium, causing a fall in its pressure (hence the "x prime" descent). During ventricular systole, the right atrium begins to fill with blood returning via the venae cavae. This increase in right atrial pressure as a result of its filling produces the ascending limb of the *"v" wave*. At the end of ventricular systole, right ventricular pressure falls rapidly. At the point at which it falls below the right atrial pressure, the tricuspid valve opens. This drop in right atrial pressure produces the *y descent*.

Normally, only the "a" and "v" waves are visible on examination. Because the "c" wave is frequently not observed, the x and x prime descents are summated into a single x descent. Occasionally the later portion of the "c" wave may be enlarged by a carotid artery pulsation artifact.

Evaluation of the jugular venous pulse provides information about the level of venous pressure and the type of venous wave pattern. These are described in a later section.

Review of Specific Symptoms

The important symptoms of cardiac disease are the following:

- Chest pain
- Palpitations
- Dyspnea
- Syncope
- Fatigue
- Dependent edema
- Hemoptysis
- Cyanosis

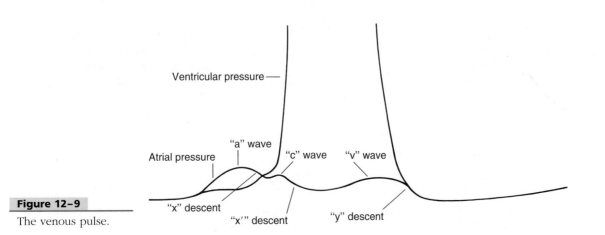

Figure 12–9

The venous pulse.

Chest Pain

Chest pain is probably the most important symptom of cardiac disease. It is, however, not pathognomonic for heart disease. It is well known that chest pain may result from pulmonary, intestinal, gallbladder, and musculoskeletal disorders. Ask the following questions of any patients complaining of chest pain.

> *"Where is the pain?"*
> *"How long have you had the pain?"*
> *"Do you have recurrent episodes of pain?"*
> *"What is the duration of the pain?"*
> *"How often do you get the pain?"*
> *"What do you do to make it better?"*
> *"What makes the pain worse? breathing? lying flat? moving your arms or neck?"*
> *"How would you describe the pain?* burning? pressing? crushing? dull? aching? throbbing? knife-like? sharp? constricting? sticking?"*
> *"Does the pain occur at rest? with exertion? after eating? when moving your arms? with emotional strain? while sleeping? during sexual intercourse?"*
> *"Is the pain associated with shortness of breath? palpitations? nausea or vomiting? coughing? fever? coughing up blood? leg pain?"*

Angina pectoris is the true symptom of coronary artery disease. Angina is commonly the consequence of hypoxia of the myocardium resulting from an imbalance of coronary supply and myocardial demand. Table 12–1 lists the characteristics that differentiate angina pectoris from the other types of chest pain.

Commonly, a patient may describe the angina by clenching the fist and placing it over the sternum. This is a pathognomonic sign of angina commonly referred to as *Levine's sign*. Figure 12–10 demonstrates this body language.

When chest pain is related to a cardiac cause, coronary atherosclerosis and aortic valvular disease are the most common ones. Table 12–2 lists some common causes of chest pain.

Palpitations

Palpitations are the uncomfortable sensations in the chest associated with a range of arrhythmias. Patients may describe palpitations as "fluttering," "skipped beats," "pounding," "jumping," "stopping," or "irregularity." Determine whether the patient has had similar episodes and what was done to extinguish them. Palpitations are common and do not necessarily indicate serious heart disease. Any condition in which there is an increased stroke volume, as in aortic regurgitation, may be associated with a sensation

Table 12–1   Characteristics of Chest Pain†

	Angina	Not Angina
Location	Retrosternal, diffuse	Left inframammary, localized
Radiation	Left arm, jaw, back	Right arm
Description	"Aching," "dull," "pressing," "squeezing," "vise-like"	"Sharp," "shooting," "cutting"
Intensity	Mild to severe	Excruciating
Duration	Minutes	Seconds, hours, days
Precipitated by	Effort, emotion, eating, cold	Respiration, posture, motion
Relieved by	Rest, nitroglycerin	Nonspecific

† Angina and other chest pain may present in a variety of ways. The characteristics listed here are the common presentations. This list, however, is not exhaustive. This list should be used only as a guide.

---

* In general, it is best to allow the patient to describe the character of the pain. These descriptions are provided for the interviewer to use only when the patient is unable to characterize the pain.

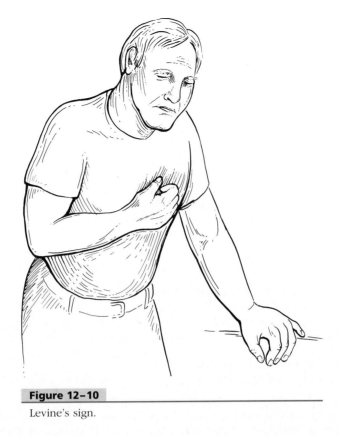

Figure 12–10

Levine's sign.

Table 12–2	**Common Causes of Chest Pain**
Organ System	**Cause**
Cardiac	Coronary artery disease
	Aortic valvular disease
	Pulmonary hypertension
	Mitral valve prolapse
	Pericarditis
	Idiopathic hypertrophic subaortic stenosis
Vascular	Dissection of the aorta
Pulmonary	Pulmonary embolism
	Pneumonia
	Pleuritis
	Pneumothorax
Musculoskeletal	Costochondritis*
	Arthritis
	Muscular spasm
	Bone tumor
Neural	Herpes zoster†
Gastrointestinal	Ulcer disease
	Bowel disease
	Hiatal hernia
	Pancreatitis
	Cholecystitis
Emotional	Anxiety
	Depression

* Tietze's syndrome, which is an inflammation of the costal cartilages.
† Shingles, which is a viral invasion of the peripheral nerves in a dermatomal distribution.

of "forceful contraction." When a patient complains of palpitations, ask the following questions:

> *"How long have you had palpitations?"*
> *"Do you have recurrent attacks?"* If so, *"How frequently do they occur?"*
> *"When did the current attack begin?"*
> *"How long did it last?"*
> *"What did it feel like?"*
> *"Did any maneuvers or positions stop it?"*
> *"Did it stop abruptly?"*
> *"Could you count your pulse during the attack?"*
> *"Can you tap out on the table what the rhythm was like?"*
> *"Have you noticed palpitations after strenuous exercise? on exertion? while lying on your left side? after a meal? when tired?"*
> *"During the palpitations, have you ever fainted? had chest pain?"*
> *"Was there an associated flush, headache, or sweating associated with the palpitations?"* *
> *"Have you noticed an intolerance to heat? cold?"*
> *"What kind of medications are you taking?"*
> *"Do you take any medications for your lungs?"*
> *"Are you taking any thyroid medications?"*
> *"Have you ever been told that you had a problem with your thyroid?"*
> *"How much tea, coffee, chocolate, or cola sodas do you consume a day?"*
> *"Do you smoke?"*
> *"Do you drink alcoholic beverages?"*
> *"Did you notice that after the palpitations you had to urinate?"* †

In addition to primary cardiovascular causes, thyrotoxicosis, hypoglycemia, fever, anemia, pheochromocytoma, and anxiety states are commonly associated with palpitations. Hyperthyroidism is an important cause of rhythm disturbances that originate outside the cardiovascular system. Caffeine, tobacco, and drugs are also important factors in arrhythmogenicity. Sympathomimetic amines used in the treatment of bronchoconstriction are potent stimuli for arrhythmia as well. In patients with panic disorders and other anxiety states, the sensation of palpitations may occur during periods of normal rate and rhythm.

Patients who have had previous attacks of palpitations should be asked the following:

> *"How was your previous attack terminated?"*
> *"How often do you get the attacks?"*
> *"Are you able to terminate them?"* If so, *"How?"*
> *"Have you ever been told that you have Wolff-Parkinson-White syndrome?"* ‡

Table 12–3 outlines the common causes of palpitations.

Dyspnea

The complaint of dyspnea is important. Patients report that they have "shortness of breath" or that they "can't get enough air." Dyspnea is commonly related to cardiac or pulmonary conditions. The questions relating to dyspnea are discussed in Chapter 11, The Chest. This section further delineates dyspnea as a *cardiac* symptom.

Paroxysmal nocturnal dyspnea (PND) occurs at night or when the patient is supine. This position increases the intrathoracic blood volume, and a weakened heart may be unable to handle this increased load; congestive heart failure may result. The patient is awakened about 2 hours after having fallen asleep, is markedly dyspneic, is

---

* Symptoms associated with a pheochromocytoma.
† After an attack of paroxysmal atrial tachycardia, patients often have an urge to urinate. The pathophysiology is not well understood, but the association is present.
‡ The use of this technical term is appropriate, because a patient having this form of pre-excitation may have been told of this condition and may recognize the name.

Table 12–3   **Common Causes of Palpitations**

Extrasystoles
    Atrial premature beats*
    Nodal premature beats
    Ventricular premature beats†
Tachyarrhythmias
    Paroxysmal supraventricular tachycardia
    Atrial flutter
    Atrial fibrillation
    Multifocal atrial tachycardia
    Ventricular tachycardia
Bradyarrhythmias
    Heart block
    Sinus arrest
Drugs
    Bronchodilators
    Digitalis
    Antidepressants
Smoking
Caffeine
Thyrotoxicosis

* Also known as an atrial premature contraction or a premature atrial contraction.
† Also known as a ventricular premature contraction or a premature ventricular contraction.

often coughing, and seeks relief by running to a window to "get more air." Episodes of PND are relatively specific for congestive heart failure.

The symptom of PND is often associated with the symptom of *orthopnea,* the need for using more pillows on which to sleep. Inquire of all patients, "How many pillows do you need in order to sleep?" To help quantify the orthopnea, you can state, for example, "3-pillow orthopnea for the past 4 months."

Dyspnea on exertion (DOE) is usually due to chronic congestive heart failure or severe pulmonary disease. Quantify the severity of the dyspnea by asking, "How many level blocks can you walk now?" "How many level blocks could you walk 6 months ago?" The examiner can now attempt to quantify the dyspnea: for example, "The patient has had 1-block DOE for the past 6 months. Before 6 months ago, the patient was able to walk 4 blocks without becoming short of breath. In addition, during the last 3 months the patient has noted 4-pillow orthopnea."

Trepopnea is a rare form of positional dyspnea in which the dyspneic patient has less dyspnea while lying on the left or right side. The pathophysiology of trepopnea is not well understood.

Table 12–4 lists the common causes of dyspnea.

Table 12–4   **Common Causes of Dyspnea**

Organ System or Condition	Cause
Cardiac	Left ventricular failure
	Mitral stenosis
Pulmonary	Obstructive lung disease
	Asthma
	Restrictive lung disease
	Pulmonary embolism
	Pulmonary hypertension
Emotional	Anxiety
High-altitude exposure	Decreased oxygen pressure
Anemia	Decreased oxygen-carrying capacity

Syncope

Fainting, or syncope, is the transient loss of consciousness that is due to inadequate cerebral perfusion. Ask patients what *they* mean by "fainting" or "dizziness." Syncope may be related to cardiac as well as noncardiac causes. When a patient describes fainting, ask the following questions:

> *"What were you doing just before you fainted?"*
> *"Have you had recurrent fainting spells?"* If so, *"How often do you have these attacks?"*
> *"Was there an abrupt onset to the fainting?"*
> *"Did you lose consciousness?"*
> *"In what position were you when you fainted?"*
> *"Was the fainting preceded by any other symptom? nausea? chest pain? palpitations? confusion? numbness? hunger?"*
> *"Did you have any warning that you were going to faint?"*
> *"Did you have any black, tarry bowel movements after the faint?"*

The activity that preceded the syncope is important because some cardiac causes are associated with syncope during exercise (e.g., valvular aortic stenosis, idiopathic hypertrophic subaortic stenosis, and primary pulmonary hypertension). If a patient describes palpitations before the syncope, an arrhythmogenic cause may be present. Cardiac output may be reduced by arrhythmias or obstructive lesions.

The position of the patient just before fainting is important because this information may help determine the cause of the syncope. For example, if a patient fainted after rising suddenly from bed in the middle of the night to run to answer the telephone, *orthostatic hypotension* may be the cause. Orthostatic hypotension is a common form of postural syncope and is the result of a peripheral autonomic limitation. There is a sudden fall in systemic blood pressure resulting from a failure of adaptive reflexes to compensate for an erect posture. Symptoms due to orthostatic hypotension include dizziness, blurring of vision, profound weakness, and syncope. Many drugs can cause orthostatic hypotension by leading to changes in intravascular volume or tone. The geriatric patient is most prone to orthostatic hypotension. *Micturition syncope* usually occurs in men during straining with nocturnal urination. It usually occurs after considerable alcohol consumption.

Vasovagal syncope is the most common type of fainting. Vasovagal syncope occurs during periods of emotional strain, such as receiving bad news, experiencing a stressful situation, or donating blood. It is often preceded by nausea, weakness, perspiration, epigastric discomfort, or a "sinking feeling." There is a sudden fall in systemic vascular resistance without a compensatory increase in cardiac output as a result of an increased vagotonia. *Carotid sinus syncope* is associated with a hypersensitive carotid sinus and is seen more commonly in the aged population. Whenever a patient with carotid sinus syncope wears a tight shirt collar or turns the neck in a certain way, there is an increased stimulation of the carotid sinus. This causes a sudden fall in systemic pressure, and syncope results. Two types of carotid sinus hypersensitivity exist: a cardioinhibitory (bradycardia) type and a vasodepressor (hypotension without bradycardia) type. *Post-tussive syncope* generally occurs in patients with chronic obstructive lung disease. Several mechanisms have been postulated to explain its occurrence. It is generally accepted that coughing produces an increase in intrathoracic pressure, which decreases venous return and decreases cardiac output. There may also be a rise in cerebrospinal fluid pressure, producing a decreased perfusion to the brain.

There are other suggested questions to ask a patient with syncope that direct attention to a neurologic cause. These are summarized in Chapter 19, The Nervous System. Table 12–5 lists the common causes of syncope.

Fatigue

Fatigue is a common symptom of decreased cardiac output. Patients with congestive heart failure and mitral valvular disease frequently complain of fatigue. Fatigue, however, is not specific for cardiac problems. The most common causes of fatigue are anxiety and depression. Other conditions associated with fatigue include anemia and

Table 12–5   Common Causes of Syncope

Organ System or Condition	Cause
Cardiac	Decreased cerebral perfusion secondary to cardiac rhythm disturbance
	Left ventricular output obstruction
Metabolic	Hypoglycemia
	Hyperventilation
	Hypoxia
Psychiatric	Hysteria
Neurologic	Epilepsy
	Cerebrovascular disease
Orthostatic hypotension	Volume depletion
	Antidepressant medications
	Antihypertensive medications
Vasovagal	Vasodepression
Micturition	Visceral reflex (vasodepressor)
Cough	Chronic lung disease
Carotid sinus	Vasodepressor response to carotid sinus sensitivity

chronic diseases. The examiner must attempt to differentiate organic from psychogenic fatigue. As the following questions:

"How long have you been tired?"
"Was the onset abrupt?"
"Do you feel tired all day? in the morning? in the evening?"
"When do you feel least tired?"
"Do you feel more tired at home than at work?"
"Is the fatigue relieved by rest?"

Patients with psychogenic fatigue are tired "all the time." They are often more tired at home than at work but occasionally describe being more tired in the morning. They may feel their best at the *end* of the day, which is when most patients with organic causes feel the worst.

Dependent Edema

Swelling of the legs, a form of *dependent edema,* is a frequent complaint of patients. The interviewer should ask:

"When was the swelling first noted?"
"Are both legs swollen equally?"
"Did the swelling appear suddenly?"
"Is the swelling worse at any time of the day?"
"Does it disappear after a night's sleep?"
"Does elevation of your feet reduce the swelling?"
"What kind of medications are you taking?"
"Is there a history of kidney, heart, or liver disease?"
"Do you have shortness of breath?" If so, *"Which came first, the edema or the shortness of breath?"*
"Do you have pain in the legs?"
"Do you have any ulcers on your legs?"
If the patient is a woman, *"Are you taking oral contraceptives?" "Is the edema associated with menstrual changes?"*

The patient with congestive heart failure has symmetric edema of the lower extremities that worsens as the day progresses. It is least in the morning after sleeping with elevation of the legs in bed. If the patient also complains of dyspnea, it is helpful to determine which symptom came first. In patients with dyspnea and edema secondary to cardiac causes, the dyspnea usually precedes the edema. Bedridden patients may have dependent edema in the sacral area.

Hemoptysis

Hemoptysis is discussed in Chapter 11, The Chest. In addition to the pulmonary causes, mitral stenosis should not be forgotten as an important cause of hemoptysis. Rupture of the bronchial veins, which are under high back pressure, produces the hemoptysis.

Cyanosis

Cyanosis is also discussed in Chapter 11, The Chest. The important questions regarding cyanosis are indicated in that chapter.

Occasionally, cyanosis is noted in only the lower extremities. This is termed *differential cyanosis*. It is related to a right-to-left shunt through a patent ductus arteriosus (PDA). In a right-to-left shunt resulting from pulmonary hypertension, blood in the pulmonary artery crosses the PDA, which is located below the level of the carotid and left subclavian arteries; deoxygenated blood is pumped only to the lower extremity, producing cyanosis in only that location. Some blood does get to the lungs for oxygenation and is ultimately pumped out through the aorta to produce normal skin color in the upper extremity.

Look at Figure 12–11. The patient is a 30 year old Russian immigrant who was evaluated in the United States for cyanosis. Until the age of 20 years, he had marked "bluish discoloration" of his lower extremities and relatively normal color in his upper extremities. During the 1970s, there was a gradual darkening of his upper extremities. Notice marked cyanosis of the extremities and nail beds of the fingers and toes. The patient had a PDA with marked pulmonary hypertension.

Impact of Cardiac Disease on the Patient

Cardiac patients are intensely fearful. Once cardiac disease has been diagnosed, a series of reactions occur. Fear, depression, and anxiety are the outcomes. The patients, who were totally asymptomatic until their episode of "sudden death" resulting from a coronary occlusion, are scared. They were resuscitated the first time; will it happen again? When? During recovery in the hospital, they are afraid to leave the intensive care unit for fear that "no one will be watching." At the time of discharge from the hospital, they are filled with anxiety. Although they desperately want to go home, they ask themselves, "What will happen if I have chest pain at home? Who will provide medical assistance?" They go through a period of depression, recognizing what they

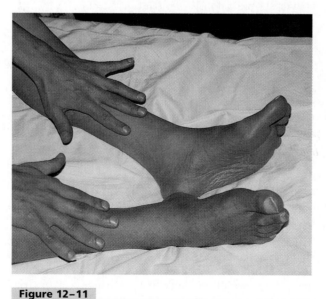

Figure 12–11

Differential cyanosis of the extremities: patent ductus arteriosus.

have gone through. After convalescence, they become fearful of daily situations that may provoke another attack. Can they go back to the daily "hassles" at work? Is it safe to have sexual intercourse? Despite appropriate reassurances from the physician, their anxiety level may remain high. The "cardiac cripple" has developed.

Cardiac patients who have witnessed a fatal cardiac arrest of another patient in their room often refuse to admit how stressful this event really was. The patients freely discuss the efficiency of the cardiac arrest team or complain that the noise kept them from sleeping. They refuse to identify with the deceased patient.

The cardiac patient approaching surgery has the same fears as all surgical patients; these fears are discussed in Chapter 2, The Patient's Responses. However, surgical procedures for the cardiac patient involve the "nucleus" of the body. The conscientious clinician will take time to explain the nature of the problem and the surgical approach. Before the procedure, the physician should allow the patient, and especially the family, to visit the intensive care unit where the patient will be for a few days after surgery. Patients should be reassured that everything possible will be done in their behalf. *Their* courage and determination and *the physician's* support are essential.

Physical Examination

> The equipment necessary for the examination of the heart is a stethoscope, a penlight, and an applicator stick.

The physical examination of the heart includes the following:

- Inspection of the patient
- Blood pressure assessment
- Assessment of the arterial pulse
- Assessment of the jugular venous pulse
- Percussion of the heart
- Palpation of the heart
- Auscultation of the heart
- Examination for dependent edema

The patient should be supine, and the examiner should stand on the right side of the bed. The head of the bed may be elevated slightly if the patient is more comfortable in this position.

Inspection

Evaluate General Appearance

The general inspection of the patient offers clues to cardiac diagnosis. Is the patient in acute distress? What is the patient's breathing like? Is it labored? Are accessory muscles being used?

Inspect the Skin

The skin can reveal many changes associated with cardiac disease. Inspect the skin color. Is cyanosis present? If so, does it appear central or peripheral? Is pallor present?

The *temperature* of the skin may reflect cardiac disease. Severe anemia, beriberi, and thyrotoxicosis tend to make the skin warmer; intermittent claudication is associated with coolness of the lower extremity compared with the upper extremity.

Are *xanthomata* present? Tendon xanthomata are stony hard, slightly yellowish masses that are commonly bound on the extensor tendons of the fingers and are pathognomonic for familial hypercholesterolemia. The Achilles tendon and plantar tendons of the soles are also common locations for tendon xanthomata. Figure 12–12 shows tendon xanthomata on the extensor surfaces of the fingers of a patient with a total cholesterol concentration of greater than 450 mg/dL.*

---

* The total cholesterol concentration for an adult is normally less than 220 mg/dL.

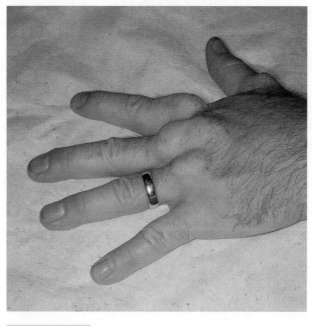

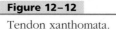
Figure 12–12

Tendon xanthomata.

Figure 12–13 shows another patient with multiple tuberous xanthomata of the hand. This patient had *primary biliary cirrhosis* and extremely elevated cholesterol levels. Primary biliary cirrhosis is a rare, progressive, and often fatal liver disease seen mostly in women. Pruritus is a common symptom. Xanthomata develop on approximately 15–20% of patients and are typically found on the palms, soles, knees, elbows, and hands. The cholesterol, usually in high-density lipoprotein, is often as high as 1000–1500 mg/dL. Antimitochondrial antibody is present in nearly 90% of patients.

Figure 12–14 shows *eruptive xanthomata* on the abdomen of a patient with uncontrolled diabetes mellitus and hypertriglyceridemia. Eruptive xanthomata result from acute elevations in plasma triglycerides, usually more than 1500 mg/dL.* Following excessive alcohol consumption, this patient developed these lesions; his serum triglycerides exceeded 2,000 mg/dL. The lesions, frequently found on the abdomen,

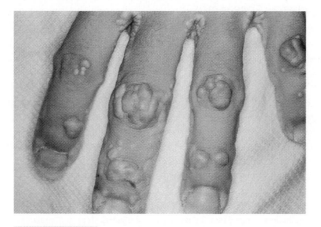

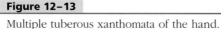
Figure 12–13

Multiple tuberous xanthomata of the hand.

---

* The serum triglyceride concentration for an adult is normally less than 200 mg/dL.

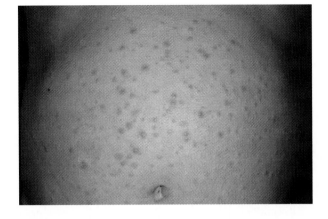

Figure 12–14

Eruptive xanthomata on the abdomen.

buttocks, elbows, knees, and back, are small, 1–3 mm in diameter, yellowish papules on an erythematous base. With reduction in the level of triglycerides, the lesions may recede.

Is a rash present? The presence of *erythema marginatum* (erythema in which the reddened areas are disc-shaped with raised edges) in a febrile patient suggests acute rheumatic fever.

Inspect the Nails

Frequently, *splinter hemorrhages* are visible as small reddish-brown lines in the nail bed. These hemorrhages run from the free margin proximally and are classically associated with subacute bacterial endocarditis. However, the finding is nonspecific because it is found in many other conditions, including even local trauma to the nail. Splinter hemorrhages in a finger of a patient with endocarditis are shown in Figure 12–15.

Inspect the Facies

Abnormalities of the heart may also be associated with peculiarities of the face and head. Supravalvular aortic stenosis, a congenital problem, occurs in association with widely set eyes, strabismus, low-set ears, an upturned nose, and hypoplasia of the mandible. Moon facies and widely spaced eyes are suggestive of pulmonic stenosis. Expressionless facies with puffy eyelids and loss of the outer third of the eyebrow is seen in hypothyroidism. Affected individuals may have a cardiomyopathy. The *earlobe crease,* or Lichtstein's sign, is an oblique crease, often bilateral, seen frequently in

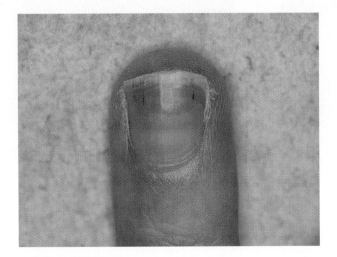

Figure 12–15

Splinter hemorrhages.

patients older than the age of 50 years with significant coronary artery disease. This sign is shown in Figure 12–16. Although it is a useful sign, there are too many false-positive and false-negative findings for this sign to be very reliable.

■ Inspect the Eyes

The presence of yellowish plaques on the eyelids, called *xanthelasma,* should raise the suspicion of an underlying hyperlipoproteinemia, even though this lesion is less specific than the xanthoma. A patient with xanthelasma and hypercholesterolemia is shown in Figure 12–17.

Examination of the eyes may reveal an *arcus senilis.* An arcus (see Fig. 8–24) seen in a patient *younger than* the age of 40 years should raise the suspicion of *hypercholesterolemia.* Opacities in the cornea may be evidence for sarcoidosis, which may be responsible for cor pulmonale or myocardial involvement. Displacement of the lens is frequently seen in patients with *Marfan's syndrome,* an important cause of aortic regurgitation. Conjunctival hemorrhages are commonly seen in infective endocarditis. *Hypertelorism,* or widely set eyes, is associated with congenital heart disease, especially pulmonic stenosis and supravalvular aortic stenosis. Retinal evaluation may furnish valuable information about diabetes, hypertension, and atherosclerosis.

■ Inspect the Mouth

Have the patient open the mouth widely. Inspect the palate. Is the palate highly arched? A high-arched palate may be associated with congenital heart problems such as mitral valve prolapse.

Are there *petechiae* on the palate? Subacute bacterial endocarditis is often associated with palatal petechiae, as seen in the patient in Figure 12–18.

■ Inspect the Neck

Examination of the neck may reveal webbing. Webbing is seen in individuals with *Turner's syndrome,** who may have coarctation of the aorta, and in patients with

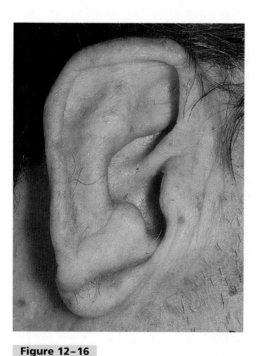

Figure 12–16

Earlobe creases.

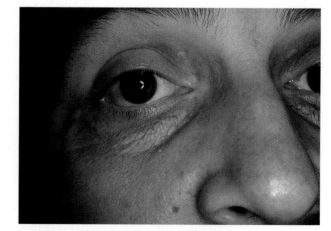

Figure 12–17

Xanthelasma.

---

* Short stature, retarded sexual development, and webbed neck in a female, associated with an abnormality of the sex chromosomes (45,XO).

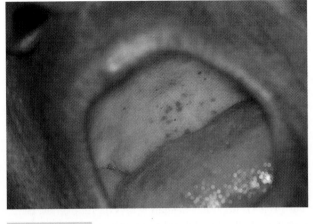

Figure 12–18

Palatal petechiae.

Noonan's syndrome.* Pulmonic stenosis is the associated cardiac abnormality in this condition.

Inspect the Chest Configuration

Inspection of the chest often reveals information about the heart. Because the chest and the heart develop at about the same time during embryogenesis, it is not surprising that anything interfering with the development of the chest may interfere with the heart. A *pectus excavatum,* or caved-in chest, is seen in Marfan's syndrome and in mitral valve prolapse (see Figure 11–7). *Pectus carinatum,* or pigeon breast, is also associated with Marfan's syndrome (see Figure 11–8).

Are there any visible cardiac motions?

Inspect the Extremities

Some congenital abnormalities of the heart are associated with abnormalities of the extremities. Patients with atrial septal defects may have an extra phalanx, an extra finger, or an extra toe. Long, slender fingers suggest Marfan's syndrome and possible aortic regurgitation. Short stature, cubitus valgus, and medial deviation of the extended forearm are typical of patients with Turner's syndrome.

Blood Pressure Assessment

The Principles

Blood pressure can be measured directly with an intra-arterial catheter or indirectly with a *sphygmomanometer.* The sphygmomanometer consists of an inflatable rubber bladder within a cloth cover, a rubber bulb to inflate the bladder, and a manometer to measure the pressure in the bladder. Indirect measurement of blood pressure involves the auscultatory detection of the appearance and disappearance of the *Korotkoff sounds* over the compressed artery. Korotkoff sounds are low-pitched sounds originating in the vessel that are related to turbulence produced by partially occluding an artery with a blood pressure cuff. Several phases occur in sequence as the occluding pressure drops. Phase 1 occurs when the occluding pressure falls to the systolic blood pressure. The tapping sounds are clear and gradually increase in intensity as the occluding pressure falls. Phase 2 occurs at a pressure about 10–15 mm Hg lower than phase 1 and consists of tapping sounds followed by murmurs.† Phase 3 occurs when the occluding pressure falls enough to allow a large amount of volume to cross the partially occluded artery. The sounds are similar to the sounds of phase 2, except that only the tapping

---

* Male Turner's syndrome (46,XY).

† A murmur is a blowing auscultatory sign produced by turbulence in blood flow. These vibrations can originate in the heart or in blood vessels as a result of hemodynamic changes.

sounds are heard. Phase 4 is the abrupt muffling and decreased intensity of the sounds as the pressure approaches the diastolic blood pressure. Phase 5 is the complete disappearance of the sounds. The vessel is no longer compressed by the occluding cuff. Turbulent flow is no longer present.

The normal blood pressure for adults is up to 140 mm Hg systolic and up to 95 mm Hg diastolic. The point of disappearance of the Korotkoff sounds is probably more accurate than the point of muffling for the diastolic blood pressure reading (London and London, 1976). However, if the point of disappearance is more than 10 mm Hg lower than the point of muffling, the point of muffling is probably more accurate (Freis, 1968). Recording both the point of muffling and disappearance frequently helps in communication. A blood pressure might be recorded as 125/75–65: the systolic blood pressure is 125; the point of muffling is 75; the point of disappearance is 65 (the diastolic blood pressure).

Blood pressure should be recorded only to the nearest 5 mm Hg, because there is a ± 3 mm Hg limit of accuracy for all sphygmomanometers. In addition, normal blood pressure changes occur from moment to moment, and measuring to less than 5 mm Hg provides a false sense of accuracy.

The size of the cuff is important for the accurate determination of blood pressure. It is recommended that the cuff be snugly applied around the arm, with its lowest edge 1 inch above the antecubital fossa. The cuff should be approximately 20% wider than the diameter of the extremity. The bladder should overlie the artery. The use of a cuff that is too small for a large arm will result in an erroneously high reading of blood pressure.

Another cause of falsely elevated blood pressure readings is lack of support of the patient's arm. To obtain an accurate measurement, the cuff must be at heart level. If the arm is not supported, the patient will be performing isometric exercise, which will raise the recorded pressure. In contrast, excessive pressure on the diaphragm of the stethoscope produces a spuriously lower reading of the diastolic blood pressure without any significant alteration of systolic pressure. If the arm is held correctly, no skin indentations should occur.

The *auscultatory gap* is the silence caused by the disappearance of the Korotkoff sounds after the initial appearance and the reappearance at a lower pressure. The auscultatory gap is present when there is a decreased blood flow to the extremities, as is found in hypertension and in aortic stenosis. The clinical importance lies in the fact that the systolic blood pressure may be mistaken for the lower blood pressure, the point of reappearance.

Determine Blood Pressure by Palpation

Blood pressure assessment is performed with the patient lying comfortably in the supine position. The cuff bladder is centered over the right brachial artery. If the arm is obese, a thigh cuff should be used. The arm should be slightly flexed, and it should be supported at approximately the level of the heart. To determine the systolic blood pressure adequately and to exclude an error as a result of an auscultatory gap, blood pressure is first assessed by palpation. In this procedure, the right brachial or right radial artery is palpated while the cuff is inflated above the pressure required to obliterate the pulse. The adjustable screw is opened slowly for slow deflation. The systolic pressure is identified by the reappearance of the brachial pulse. As soon as the pulse is felt, the adjustable screw is opened for rapid deflation. This is the systolic blood pressure. This is shown in Figure 12–19.

Determine Blood Pressure by Auscultation

Blood pressure by auscultation is assessed in the right arm by inflating the cuff to about 20 mm Hg above the systolic pressure that was determined by palpation. The diaphragm of the stethoscope should be placed over the artery as close to the edge of the cuff as possible, preferably just under the edge. The cuff is deflated *slowly* while the Korotkoff sounds are evaluated. The systolic blood pressure, the point of muffling, and the point of disappearance are determined. The systolic blood pressure is the point at which the initial tapping sounds are heard. The technique of determining auscultatory blood pressure is shown in Figure 12–20. If the blood pressure is high, it is useful to retake the blood pressure at the end of the examination, when the patient may be calmer.

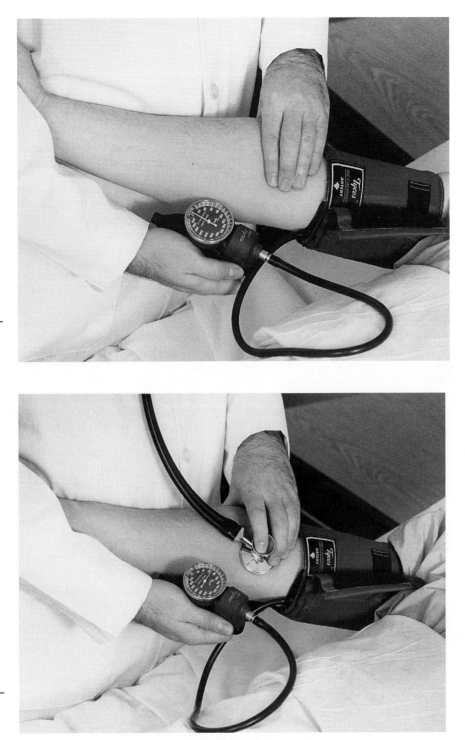

Figure 12–19

Technique for blood pressure assessment by palpation.

Figure 12–20

Technique for blood pressure assessment by auscultation.

▮ Rule Out Orthostatic Hypotension

After the patient has been recumbent for at least 5 minutes, measure the baseline blood pressure and pulse. Then have the patient stand, and repeat the measurements immediately and 2 minutes later.

Orthostatic hypotension is defined as a drop in systolic blood pressure of 20 mm Hg or more upon assuming the standing position in association with the development of symptoms such as dizziness or syncope. In most patients, there is also an increase in heart rate.

■ Rule Out Supravalvular Aortic Stenosis

If hypertension is detected in the right arm, perform the following test. Place the cuff on the patient's left arm, and determine the auscultatory pressure. It is not necessary to retake the palpatory pressure or re-evaluate for orthostatic changes. In supravalvular aortic stenosis, there is a difference in the blood pressures in the arms; hypertension may be detected in the right arm, whereas hypotension will be present in the left arm.

■ Rule Out Coarctation of the Aorta

If the blood pressure is elevated in the arms, determination of the blood pressure in the lower extremities is important for ruling out coarctation of the aorta. The patient is asked to lie on the abdomen while the thigh cuff, which is 6 cm wider than the arm cuff, is placed around the posterior aspect of the midthigh. The stethoscope is placed over the artery in the popliteal fossa. The Korotkoff sounds are determined as in the upper extremity. If a thigh cuff is not available, the regular cuff can be applied to the lower leg with the distal border just at the malleoli. The stethoscope is placed over either the posterior tibial or the dorsalis pedis artery, and the auscultatory blood pressure is taken. A leg systolic blood pressure that is lower than that in the arm should raise suspicion of coarctation of the aorta.

■ Rule Out Cardiac Tamponade

In the presence of low arterial blood pressure and a rapid and feeble pulse, it is necessary to rule out the presence of cardiac tamponade. A valuable clinical sign suggesting cardiac tamponade is the presence of a marked *paradoxical pulse* (also known as a *pulsus paradoxus*), which is characterized by an exaggeration of the normal inspiratory fall in systolic pressure. There is much confusion about the definition of a normal paradoxical pulse. A normal paradoxical pulse should be defined as the *normal* fall (about 5 mm Hg) in systolic arterial pressure during inspiration (Henkind et al, 1987). It is the *magnitude* of the phenomenon that should determine whether the pulsus paradoxus is normal or abnormal.

The technique for assessing the magnitude of a paradoxical pulse is as follows: Have the patient breathe as normally as possible. Inflate the blood pressure cuff until no sounds are heard. Gradually deflate the cuff until sounds are heard in expiration only. Note this pressure. Continue to deflate the cuff slowly until sounds are heard during inspiration. Note this pressure. If the difference in these two pressures exceeds 10 mm Hg, a marked (abnormal) pulsus paradoxus is present; cardiac tamponade may be the cause. Cardiac tamponade results when there is an increase in intrapericardial pressure that interferes with normal diastolic filling. A marked paradoxical pulse is not a specific phenomenon for tamponade because it is also seen in large pericardial effusions, in constrictive pericarditis, and in conditions associated with increased ventilatory effort, such as asthma and emphysema.

The Arterial Pulse

The following information is gained from palpation of the arterial pulse:

- ■ The rate and rhythm of the heart
- ■ The contour of the pulse
- ■ The amplitude of the pulse

■ Determine the Cardiac Rate

Cardiac rate is routinely assessed by the radial pulse. The examiner should stand in front of the patient and grasp both radial arteries. The second, third, and fourth fingers should overlie the radial artery, as shown in Figure 12–21. The examiner should count the pulse for 30 seconds and multiply the number of beats by 2 to obtain the beats per minute. This method is accurate for most *regular* rhythms. If the patient has an *irregularly irregular* rhythm, as is found in atrial fibrillation, a *pulse deficit* may be present. In atrial fibrillation, many impulses bombard the AV node and ventricles. Owing to the varying lengths of diastolic filling periods, some of the contractions may be very weak and unable to produce an adequate pulse wave despite ventricular contraction. A pulse deficit, which is the difference between the apical (precordial) and radial pulses, will occur. In such cases, only auscultation of the heart, not the radial pulse, will provide an accurate assessment of the cardiac rate.

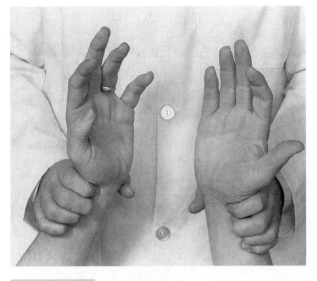

Figure 12-21

Technique for evaluating the radial artery pulses.

■ Determine the Cardiac Rhythm

When palpating the pulse, carefully evaluate the regularity of the rhythm. The slower the rate, the longer you should palpate. If the rhythm is irregular, is there a pattern to the irregularity?

Cardiac rhythm may be described as *regular, regularly irregular,* or *irregularly irregular.* A regularly irregular rhythm is a pulse with an irregularity that occurs in a definite pattern. An irregularly irregular pulse has no pattern.

The electrocardiogram is really the best medium for diagnosing the rhythm, but the physical examination may provide some clues. *Premature beats* may be recognized by the presence of isolated extra beats during a regular rhythm. *Bigeminy* is a coupled rhythm of beats in pairs. The first beat is the sinus beat, which is followed by a premature, usually ventricular, beat. If the premature beat is very early in the diastolic period, the pulse from this beat may be missed if the examiner evaluates the rhythm by palpation alone. A rhythm that is grossly irregular with no pattern is irregularly irregular and is the pulse in patients with *atrial fibrillation.*

■ Palpate the Carotid Artery

Assess the carotid artery pulse by standing at the patient's right side, with the patient lying on the back. Auscultate the carotid arteries for bruits *first* (see Chapter 13, The Peripheral Vascular System). If a bruit is present, do not palpate the carotid artery. If a cholesterol plaque is present, palpation may produce an embolus.

To palpate the carotid artery, place your index and third fingers on the thyroid cartilage and slip them laterally between the trachea and the sternocleidomastoid muscle. You should be able to feel the carotid pulsations just medial to the sternocleidomastoid muscle. Palpation should be performed low in the neck to avoid pressure on the carotid sinus, which would cause a reflex drop in blood pressure and heart rate. Each carotid artery is evaluated separately. *Never* press on both carotid arteries at the same time. After the right carotid artery is evaluated, stand in the same position, and place the same fingers back on the trachea and slip them laterally to the left to feel the left carotid artery. This technique is shown in Figure 12–22.

■ Evaluate the Characteristics of the Pulse

The carotid artery is used for the assessment of the contour and amplitude of the pulse. Contour is the shape of the wave. It is frequently described as the speed of the upslope, downslope, and duration of the wave. The examiner should place a hand firmly against the carotid artery until maximal force is felt. At this moment, the wave form should be discernible. The pulse may be described as *normal, diminished, increased,* or *double-peaked.* The normal carotid pulse wave is smooth, with the upstroke

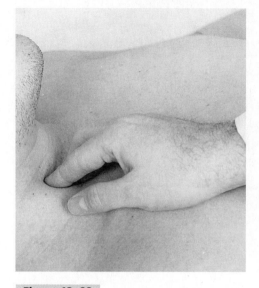

Figure 12-22

Technique for evaluating the carotid artery pulsations.

steeper and more rapid than the downstroke. A diminished pulse is a small, weak pulse. The palpating finger feels a gentle pressure rise with a distinct peak. An increased pulse is a large, strong, hyperkinetic pulse. The palpating finger feels an increased rate of rise of the ascending limb of the pulse and a brisk tap at its peak. A double-peaked pulse has a prominent percussion and tidal wave with or without a dicrotic wave. A summary of arterial pulse abnormalities is in Figure 12-23.

The Jugular Venous Pulse

The *internal jugular vein* provides information about the wave forms and right atrial pressure. The pulsations of the internal jugular vein are beneath the sternocleidomastoid muscle and are visible as they are transmitted through the surrounding tissue. The vein itself is not visible. Because the right internal jugular vein is straighter than the left, only the right internal jugular vein is evaluated. The external jugular system, which is easier to visualize, is much less accurate and should not be used.

Determine the Jugular Wave Forms

To visualize the *jugular wave forms,* the examiner should have the patient lie flat without a pillow so that the neck will not be flexed and interfere with the pulsations. The patient's trunk should be at approximately 25° to the horizontal. The higher the venous pressure, the greater the elevation that will be required; the lower the pressure, the lower the elevation needed. The patient's head should be turned slightly to the right and slightly down to relax the right sternocleidomastoid muscle. Standing on the patient's right side, the examiner should place the right hand, holding a small pocket flashlight, on the patient's sternum and shine the light tangentially across the right side of the patient's neck. Shadows of the pulsations will be cast on the sheet behind the patient. The light and shadows magnify the wave forms. This technique is shown in Figure 12-24. If no wave forms are seen, the angle of elevation of the head of the bed should be reduced. To help identify the wave forms, the examiner can time the cardiac cycle by palpating the cardiac impulse beneath the right hand or by feeling the left carotid impulse with the left hand. The descents, rather than the waves themselves, tend to be more obvious. If the neck veins are visible at the jaw margin while the patient is seated, the examiner should watch for the wave forms at the angle of the jaw with the patient seated upright.

The jugular pulse must be differentiated from the pulsation of the carotid artery. Table 12-6 lists the most important characteristic differences of these pulses.

Type	Description	Cause
Anacrotic*	Small, slow rising, delayed pulse with a notch or shoulder on the ascending limb	Aortic stenosis
Waterhammer	Rapid and sudden systolic expansion	Aortic regurgitation
Bisferiens	Double-peaked pulse with a midsystolic dip	Aortic regurgitation Combined aortic stenosis and aortic regurgitation Idiopathic hypertrophic subaortic stenosis (IHSS)
Alternans	Alternating amplitude of pulse pressure	Congestive heart failure
Paradoxical (marked)	Detected by blood pressure assessment. An exaggerated drop in systolic blood pressure during inspiration	Tamponade Constrictive pericarditis Chronic obstructive lung disease

* Also known as plateau pulse or *pulsus parvus et tardus*.

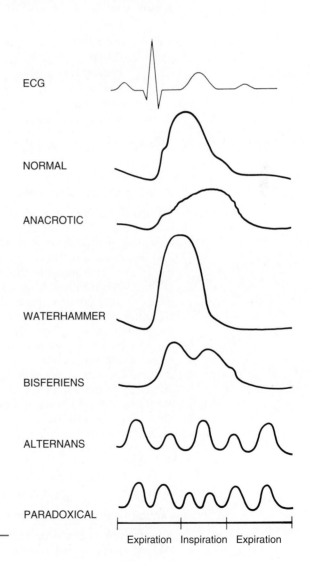

ECG

NORMAL

ANACROTIC

WATERHAMMER

BISFERIENS

ALTERNANS

PARADOXICAL

Expiration Inspiration Expiration

Figure 12–23

Arterial pulse abnormalities.

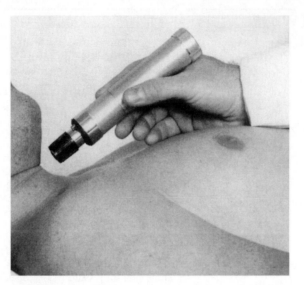

Figure 12-24

Technique for evaluating the jugular wave forms.

Table 12-6   Differentiation of Jugular and Carotid Wave Forms

	Internal Jugular Pulse	Carotid Pulse
Palpation	Not palpable	Palpable
Wave forms	Multiform: 2 or 3 components	Single
Quality	Soft, undulating	Vigorous
Pressure*	Wave forms obliterated	No effect
Inspiration	Decreased height of wave forms	No effect
Sitting up	Decreased height of wave forms	No effect
Valsalva's maneuver	Increased height of wave forms	No effect

* Light pressure on the vessel above the sternal end of clavicle.

Estimate the Jugular Venous Pressure

To assess the pressure in the right side of the heart, it is necessary to establish a reference level. The standard reference is the *manubriosternal angle*. At any degree of elevation, this position is used to measure the pressure in the internal jugular system. The examiner must first determine the height of the venous distention by noting the top of the wave forms in the internal jugular venous pulsations. An imaginary horizontal line is then drawn from this height to the sternal angle. The examiner should then measure the distance from the sternal angle to this imaginary line. The angle of elevation of the head of the bed is also estimated. It might be stated, "At 45° elevation, the jugular pulse is 7 cm above the sternal angle." At 45°, the upper limit of normal is 4–5 cm above the sternal angle; if the patient is at 30°, the upper limit of normal is 6 cm. When the height of the venous column is equal to or lower than the sternal angle in the supine position, venous pressure is usually normal.

There is tremendous inaccuracy in attempting to determine the pressure in the right atrium by the jugular manometer, as just indicated. It has been demonstrated numerous times that the sensitivity and specificity of this test are low, thus rendering this test inaccurate in predicting elevated pressures. The only accurate statement is that right atrial pressure is high when there is neck vein distention up to the jaw margin while the patient is seated at 90°. At this time, the right atrial pressure generally exceeds 15 mm Hg. The patient shown in Figure 12–25 had neck veins distended to the angle of the jaw while seated upright. His right atrial pressure was 21 mm Hg.

Evaluate the Hepatojugular Reflux

A useful test in assessing high jugular venous pressure is the *hepatojugular reflux,* also known as abdominal compression. By applying pressure over the liver, the examiner can grossly assess right ventricular function. Patients with right ventricular failure have dilated sinusoids in the liver. Pressure on the liver pushes blood out of these sinusoids

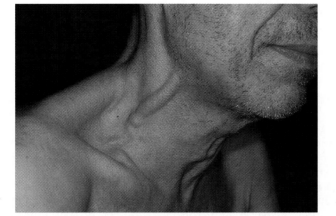

Figure 12–25

Neck vein distention.

and into the inferior vena cava and right heart, causing further distention of the neck veins. The procedure is performed with the patient lying in bed, mouth open, breathing normally; this prevents a Valsalva maneuver. The examiner places the right hand over the liver in the right upper quadrant and applies a firm, progressive pressure. Compression is maintained for 10 seconds. The normal response is for the internal and external jugular veins to show a transient increase in distention during the first few cardiac cycles, which is followed by a fall to baseline levels during the later part of the compression. In patients with right ventricular failure or elevated pulmonary artery wedge pressure, the neck veins remain distended during the entire period of compression; this distention falls rapidly (at least 4 cm) on sudden release of the compressing hand. If the examination is incorrectly performed with the patient's mouth closed, a Valsalva maneuver will result and will produce inaccurate results of the hepatojugular reflux test.

Like most other clinical maneuvers, the hepatojugular reflux must be performed in a standardized manner. If performed correctly, this test can be of considerable value in the bedside assessment of the patient. The test result correlates best with the pulmonary artery wedge pressure and, as such, is a reflection of increased central blood volume. Ewy (1988) evaluated this test and showed that in the absence of right ventricular failure, a positive test result suggests a pulmonary artery wedge pressure of 15 mm Hg or greater.

Percussion

Percuss the Heart's Borders

The technique of percussion was discussed in Chapter 11, The Chest. Percussion of the heart is performed at the third, fourth, and fifth intercostal spaces from the left anterior axillary line to the right anterior axillary line. Normally, there will be a change in the percussion note from resonance to dullness about 6 cm lateral to the left of the sternum. This dullness is due to the presence of the heart.

According to Heckerling et al (1993, 1991), a percussion dullness distance of greater than 10.5 cm in the left fifth intercostal space had a sensitivity of 91.3% and a specificity of 30.3% for detecting increased left ventricular end-diastolic volume (LVEDV) or left ventricular mass (LVM). Percussion dullness of more than 10.5 cm in the fifth intercostal space had a sensitivity of 94.4% and a specificity of 67.2% in detecting cardiomegaly. In patients with a palpable apical impulse of greater than 3.0 cm in the left decubitus position, the sensitivity of detecting increased LVEDV or LVM increased to 100% and the specificity to 40%. In the study, however, only 53% of cases had a palpable apical impulse, and there was poor interobserver reliability.

Palpation

Palpation is performed to evaluate the apical impulse, the right ventricle, the pulmonary artery, and the left ventricular motions. The presence or absence of *thrills** is also

---

* Low-frequency cutaneous vibrations associated with loud heart murmurs.

determined by palpation. The point of maximum impulse (PMI) describes the outward motion of the cardiac apex as it rotates counterclockwise, as viewed from below, to strike the anterior chest wall during isovolumetric contraction.

Palpate the PMI

The examiner should stand on the right side of the patient, with the bed at a level comfortable for the examiner. Palpation for the PMI is most easily performed with the patient in a sitting position. Only the fingertips should be applied to the chest in the fifth intercostal space, midclavicular line, because they are the most sensitive for assessing localized motion. The PMI should be noted. This technique is demonstrated in Figure 12–26. If the apical impulse is not felt, the examiner should move the fingertips in the area of the cardiac apex. The PMI is usually within 10 cm from the midsternal line and is no larger than 2–3 cm in diameter. A PMI that is laterally displaced or is felt in two interspaces during the same phase of respiration suggests cardiomegaly.

The PMI is felt in approximately 70% of normal individuals while sitting. If it cannot be felt in the sitting position, the patient should be re-evaluated while supine and in the left lateral decubitus position. The position of the PMI in the left lateral decubitus position must be assessed with the understanding that the normal cardiac impulse will now be shifted slightly to the left. If in the left lateral decubitus position the PMI is not laterally displaced, the examiner can suspect that cardiomegaly is not present.

In a patient without conditions predisposing to left ventricular hypertrophy, a palpable apical impulse felt in the left lateral decubitus position that is greater than 3 cm is said to be a specific (91%) and sensitive (92%) indicator of left ventricular enlargement. An apical diameter of greater than 3 cm is predictive (86%) of an increased left ventricular end-diastolic volume. In patients with an apical diameter of less than 3 cm and a normal left ventricular end-diastolic volume, the negative predictive value is 95%.

Although the PMI usually corresponds to the *left* ventricular apex, in patients with an enlarged right ventricle the heart rotates clockwise, as viewed from below, and the PMI may actually be produced by the *right* ventricle. This rotation turns the left ventricle posteriorly and makes it difficult to palpate. The apical impulse by the right ventricle is more diffuse than that of the left ventricle, which tends to be more localized.

In patients with chronic obstructive lung disease, the overinflation of the lungs displaces the PMI downward and to the right. The PMI in such patients is felt in the *epigastric* area, at the lower end of the sternum. In patients with chronic obstructive lung disease, a PMI in the normal location suggests cardiomegaly.

Palpate for Localized Motion

The patient should now be instructed to lie down so that palpation of all four main cardiac areas can be performed. The examiner uses the fingertips to assess any localized motion. This technique is shown in Figure 12–27.

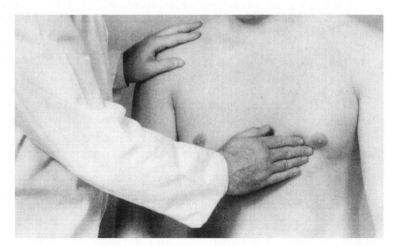

Figure 12–26

Technique for assessing point of maximum impulse.

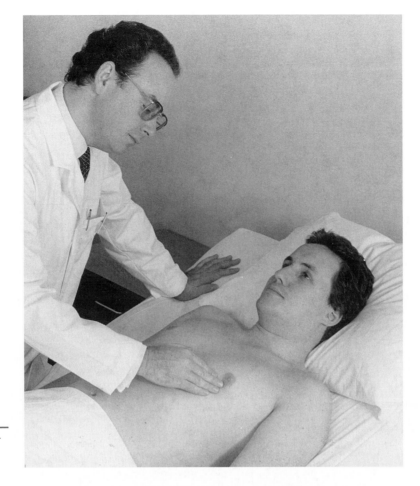

Figure 12–27

Technique for assessing localized cardiac movement.

The presence of a systolic impulse in the second intercostal space to the left of the sternum is suspicious for pulmonary hypertension. This impulse is due to the closure of the pulmonic valve under increased pressure. The presence of this impulse suggests a dilated pulmonary artery, but it may also be felt in thin individuals without pulmonary hypertension.

Palpate for Generalized Motion

After the chest has been palpated with the fingertips, the examiner uses the proximal portion of the hand to palpate for any large area of sustained outward motion, called a *heave* or *lift*. The examiner again palpates each of the four main cardiac areas. The technique for assessing heaves is shown in Figure 12–28. The presence of an *RV rock,* which is a sustained left parasternal impulse associated with lateral retraction, suggests a large right ventricle.

Any condition that increases the rate of ventricular filling during early diastole can produce a palpable impulse that occurs *after* the main left ventricular impulse. This second impulse in the area of the point of maximum impulse is usually felt in association with an S_3. Frequently, an S_3 is more easily felt than heard.

The use of a tongue blade or an applicator stick can be helpful to visually reinforce what has been palpated. The tip of the stick is placed directly over the area and held in place by the examiner's finger. This acts as a fulcrum, and the motions tend to be magnified by the movement of the stick. The technique is shown in Figure 12–29.

Palpate for Thrills

Thrills are the superficial vibratory sensations felt on the skin overlying an area of turbulence. The presence of a thrill indicates a loud murmur. Thrills are best felt by using the heads of the metacarpal bones rather than the fingertips and applying very

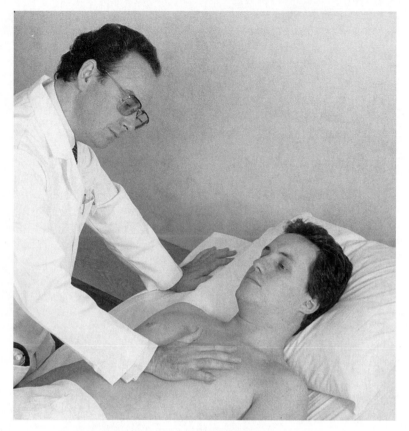

Figure 12–28

Technique for assessing generalized cardiac movement.

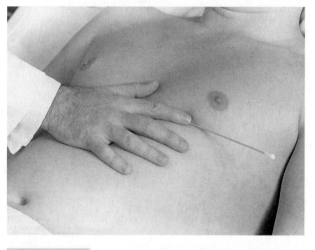

Figure 12–29

Technique for amplifying detection of cardiac movement.

gentle pressure on the skin. If too much pressure is applied, thrills will not be felt. The palpation of thrills is generally of little importance, because auscultation will reveal the presence of the loud murmur that has produced the thrill. Therefore, the finding of a thrill adds little to the diagnosis, but it is an interesting physical sign to alert the examiner as to what will be heard.

Auscultation

The Technique

Proper auscultation requires a quiet area. Every attempt should be made to eliminate extraneous noise from radios, televisions, and so forth. The earpieces of the stethoscope are directed anteriorly or parallel to the direction of the external auditory canal. If the earpieces are put in backward, the openings of the earpieces will impinge on the wall of the external canal and lower the intensity of the sounds. The earpieces should fit properly so as to be comfortable but tight enough to exclude external noises.

It is often useful for you to close your eyes when listening to the heart. Sounds that are more difficult to hear will actually sound louder. This is related to the fact that our brains are flooded with all types of sensory input. The input from our eyes appears to be the most important. The next important sensory input is auditory, which is followed by tactile input. If you eliminate the distraction of visual stimuli, more concentration by the brain will be placed on the auditory input, and the sounds will become more evident.

As indicated in the previous chapter, the bell of the stethoscope should be applied lightly to the skin, whereas the diaphragm should be pressed tightly to the skin. High-pitched sounds, such as valve closure, systolic events, and regurgitant murmurs, are better heard with the diaphragm. Low-pitched sounds, such as gallop rhythms or the murmur of atrioventricular stenosis, are better heard with the bell.

Never listen through *any* type of clothing.

There are several other pitfalls in auscultation. Make sure that the stethoscope is in good shape. Cracked tubing will certainly interfere with good listening. Both the examiner and the patient must be comfortable for the best hearing. An examiner who is straining over the patient and is uncomfortable will want to finish the examination quickly without a proper assessment. Always inspect and palpate *before* auscultation. Accumulate as much information as possible before listening!

■ Auscultate the Cardiac Areas

The examiner should be on the right side of the patient while the patient lies flat on the back. If not already at the proper height, the bed should be adjusted so that the examiner will be comfortable. The examiner should listen in the aortic, pulmonic, tricuspid, and mitral areas. However, the examiner should not limit auscultation to these areas alone. The examiner should start at any area and "inch" the stethoscope over the precordium from area to area. The areas have been established to provide some degree of standardization.

While listening at the apex and left lower sternal border with the bell, the examiner should determine whether an S_3 or an S_4 is present.

Cardiac murmurs may radiate widely. Determine where the sounds are loudest or best heard. There are no acoustic walls in the chest. A murmur typically heard at the apex with radiation to the axilla may be heard in the neck, if it is loud enough. The murmur in this example is probably loudest at the apex and axilla.

■ The Standard Auscultation Positions

The four standard positions for auscultation are shown in Figure 12–30. They are as follows:

- ■ Supine
- ■ Left lateral decubitus
- ■ Upright
- ■ Upright, leaning forward

All precordial areas are examined while the patient is supine. Using a systematic approach, the examiner starts at either the aortic area or the apex and carefully listens to the heart sounds. After all areas are examined, the patient is then instructed to turn onto the left side. The examiner should now listen at the apex for the low-pitched diastolic murmur of *mitral stenosis,* which is best heard with the bell of the stethoscope. The examiner has the patient sit upright and examines all areas with the diaphragm of the stethoscope. Finally, the patient is asked to sit up and lean forward. The patient is asked to exhale and hold the breath while the examiner, using the diaphragm, listens for the high-pitched diastolic murmur of *aortic regurgitation* at the right and left second and third intercostal spaces.

■ The Influence of Breathing

The examiner should pay special attention to the influence of breathing on the intensity of heart sounds. Most murmurs or sounds originating in the right heart will be accentuated with inspiration. This is related to the increased return of blood that occurs

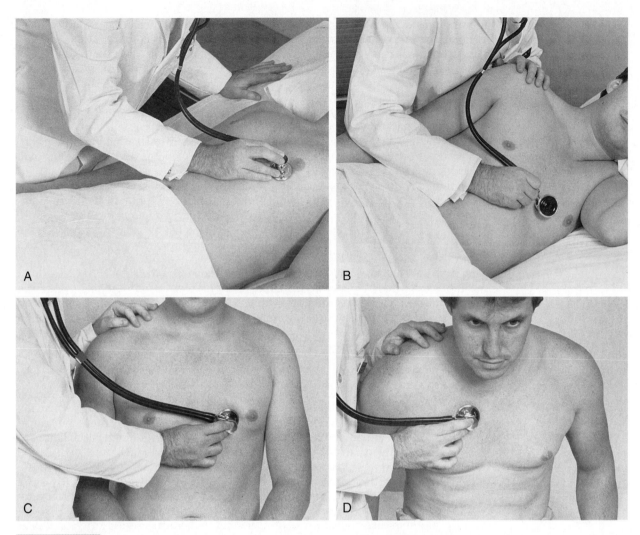

Figure 12–30

Positions for auscultation. *A,* The supine position, used for listening to all areas. *B,* The left lateral decubitus position, used for listening with the bell in the mitral area. *C,* The upright position, used for listening to all areas. *D,* The upright, leaning-forward position, used for listening with the diaphragm at the base positions.

with inspiration and the resultant increased right ventricular output. In addition, an S_3 or an S_4 originating in the right side of the heart will be accentuated during inspiration.

Time the Cardiac Events

To interpret heart sounds accurately, the examiner must be able to time the events of the cardiac cycle. The most reliable way of identifying S_1 and S_2 is to time the sounds by palpating the carotid artery. While the examiner's right hand is positioning the stethoscope, the left hand is placed on the patient's carotid artery. This technique is demonstrated in Figure 12–31. The sound that precedes the carotid pulse is the S_1. The S_2 follows the pulse. The carotid, *not* the radial pulse, must be used. The time delay from S_2 to the radial pulse is significant, and errors in timing will result.

Approach to Careful Auscultation

Until the examiner gains expertise in cardiac examination, heart sounds should be evaluated in the manner suggested in Table 12–7. The examiner should take time in each area before continuing on to the next area. The examiner should listen to several cardiac cycles at each position to be certain of the observations made, which include respiratory effects.

Describe Any Murmurs Present

If a murmur is present, attention should be directed to the following features:

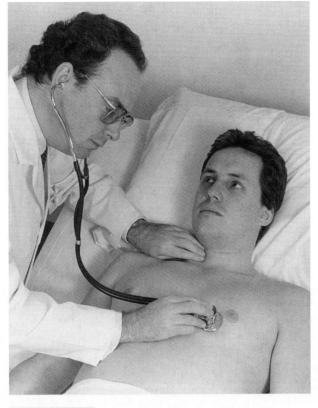

Figure 12–31

Technique for timing the heart sounds.

Table 12–7   Approach to Cardiac Auscultation

Position	Evaluate
Supine	S_1 in all areas
	S_2 in all areas
	Systolic murmurs or sounds in all areas
Left lateral decubitus	Diastolic events at apex with bell of stethoscope
Upright	S_1 in all areas
	S_2 in all areas
	Systolic murmurs or sounds in all areas
	Diastolic murmurs or sounds in all areas
Upright, leaning forward	Diastolic events at base with diaphragm of stethoscope

- Timing in the cardiac cycle
- Location
- Radiation
- Duration
- Intensity
- Pitch
- Quality
- Relationship to respiration
- Relationship to body position

Timing of murmurs as to systole and diastole is paramount. Does the systolic murmur begin with, or after, S_1? Does it end before, with, or after S_2? Does the murmur occupy the entire systolic period? Murmurs occurring throughout systole are termed *holosystolic* or *pansystolic*. These murmurs begin with S_1 and end after S_2. A *systolic ejection* murmur begins after S_1 and ends before S_2. Does the murmur occur only in early systole, midsystole, or late systole? Does the murmur persist throughout the entire diastolic period? Such murmurs are termed *holodiastolic*.

In which area is the murmur best heard?

The *radiation* of the murmur can provide a clue as to its cause. Does it radiate to the axilla? the neck? the back?

The intensity of a murmur is graded from I to VI, based on increasing loudness. The following grading system, though antiquated, serves as a means of communicating to others the intensity of the murmur:

   I Lowest intensity, often not heard by inexperienced listeners
  II Low intensity, usually audible by inexperienced listeners
 III Medium intensity without a thrill
  IV Medium intensity with a thrill
   V Loudest murmur that is audible when the stethoscope is placed on the chest. Associated with a thrill.
  VI Loudest intensity: audible when stethoscope is removed from chest. Associated with a thrill.

Murmurs can be described, for example, as "grade II/VI," "grade IV/VI," or "grade II–III/VI." Any murmur associated with a thrill must be at least a grade IV/VI. A grade IV/VI murmur is louder than a grade II/VI murmur only because there is more turbulence; both or neither may have clinical significance. The "/VI" is used because there is another, less popular, grading system using only four categories. An important axiom to remember is the following:

> In general, the intensity of a murmur tells nothing about the severity of the clinical state.

The *quality* of a murmur can be described as rumbling, blowing, harsh, musical, machinery, or scratchy.

Describe Any Pericardial Rubs

Friction rubs are extracardiac sounds of short duration that have a unique quality similar to the sound of scratching on sandpaper. Rubs may result from irritation of the pleura (i.e., a pleural rub) or of the pericardium (i.e., a pericardial rub). Pericardial rubs typically have three components: one systolic and two diastolic. The systolic component occurs during ejection; the two diastolic components occur during rapid filling and atrial contraction. Pericardial rubs are best heard with the patient sitting while holding breath in expiration. Patients with pericardial rubs commonly have chest pain that is lessened by sitting forward. A rub that disappears while the patient holds the breath originates from the pleura.

The Goals of Auscultation

The goals at the end of auscultation are to be able to describe the following:

- The intensity of S_1 in all areas
- The intensity of S_2 in all areas
- The characterization of any systolic sounds
- The characterization of any diastolic sounds

With experience, the examiner will be able to listen to all parts of the cardiac cycle in one area and compare the sounds and events with those of other areas. Normally, S_1 is loudest at the apex, and S_2 is loudest at the base. Splitting of S_2 into A_2 and P_2 during inspiration is best heard at the pulmonic area with the patient lying on the back. This increases venous return and widens the A_2–P_2 split.

Examination for Edema

When peripheral venous pressure is high, as in congestive heart failure, pressure within the veins is distributed retrograde to the smaller vessels. Transudation of fluid occurs, and edema of dependent areas results. This increase in tissue fluid produces edema that "pits."

Test for Edema

To test for pitting edema, the fingers are pressed into a dependent area, such as the shin, for 2–3 seconds. If pitting edema is present, the fingers will sink into the tissue, and when the fingers are removed, the impression of the fingers will remain. This technique is shown in Figure 12–32.

Pitting edema is usually quantified from 1+ to 4+, depending on how long the indentation persists. The most noticeable is 4+. In patients who are bedridden, the dependent area is usually the sacrum and not the shins. The examiner should evaluate for edema at the sacrum in these patients. Figure 12–33 illustrates 4+ sacral edema in a bedridden patient.

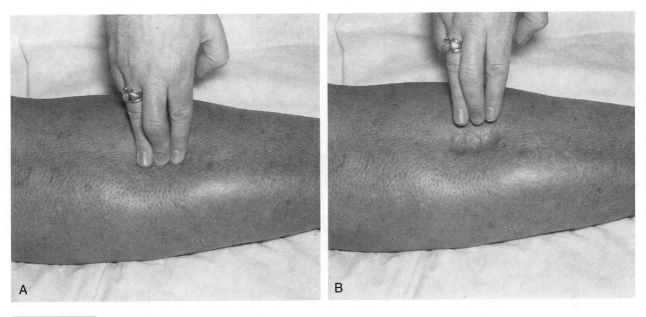

Figure 12–32

Technique for testing for pitting edema. *A* shows the examiner pressing into the shin area. *B* shows the indentation that occurs after the fingers are lifted when pitting edema is present.

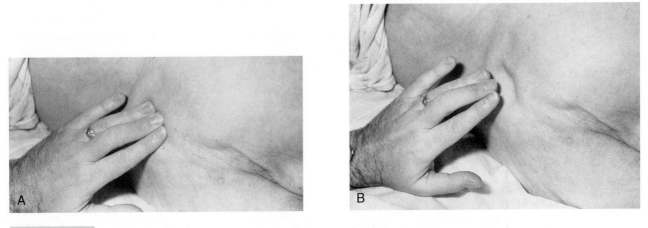

Figure 12–33

Technique for testing for pitting edema of the sacrum. *A* shows the examiner pressing at the sacrum. *B* shows the pitting edema in this bedridden patient.

Clinicopathologic Correlations

Discussion now focuses on the pathologic changes that result in the following:

- Abnormalities of the first heart sound
- Abnormalities of the second heart sound
- Systolic clicks
- Diastolic opening snaps
- Murmurs

Abnormalities of the First Heart Sound

■ Abnormalities of the Intensity of S_1

The factors that are responsible for the intensity of S_2 are as follows:

- The rate of rise of ventricular pressure
- The condition of the valve
- The position of the valve
- The distance of the heart from the chest wall

The faster the *rate of rise* of left ventricular pressure, the louder the mitral component of S_1 will be. Increased contractility will increase the intensity of S_2. Decreased contractility will soften S_1.

When the atrioventricular valve stiffens as a result of fibrosis or calcification, its closure will be louder. The pathologically deformed valve of mitral stenosis will produce an accentuated or louder S_1. After many years, as the valve becomes more and more calcified, it will be unable to move, causing S_1 to soften.

The *position of the valve* at the time of ventricular contraction affects the intensity of S_1. The *arc of coaptation* is the angle through which the valve closes. If the valve is in a midposition, it travels less than when it closes from a widely opened position. The more it is opened, the wider the arc of coaptation, and the louder is S_1. This is directly related to the pressure in the left atrium at the moment that the left ventricular pressure exceeds it and closes the valve. This can be seen in conditions in which there is a shortened PR interval on the electrocardiogram. The mitral valve is opened normally during diastole for ventricular filling. The P wave of the electrocardiogram corresponds to atrial contraction, which elevates left atrial pressure (the "a" wave of the left atrial tracing), further opening the mitral valve in late diastole. If the PR interval is short, ventricular contraction occurs so quickly after atrial contraction that the atrial pressure is still high when the left ventricular pressure exceeds it. The mitral valve stays open longer and closes later than normal, during the rapid rate of rise of pressure of the ventricle, which accentuates S_1.

In general, the longer the PR interval, the softer the S_1. Lengthening of the PR intervals, as is seen in Wenckebach's phenomenon,* produces an S_1 that softens until the dropped beat occurs.

Whenever the heart is *farther from the chest wall,* S_1 will be softer than normal. In patients who are very obese or who have chronic obstructive lung disease, the intensity of S_1 will be softer than normal. In patients with a large pericardial effusion, S_1 will likewise be soft.

Abnormalities of the Second Heart Sound

■ Abnormalities of the Intensity of S_2

The conditions that change the intensity of S_2 are the following:

- Changes in systolic pressure
- Condition of the valve

---

* Gradually increasing PR intervals until a dropped beat occurs.

Any condition that produces an increase in the systolic pressure will increase the intensity of S_2. Conversely, conditions that lower the systolic pressure will soften S_2. Hypertension raises aortic systolic pressure and produces a loud A_2 component of S_2.

Calcification or *fibrosis* of the semilunar valves will produce a softening of their closure, S_2. Because the semilunar valves are a morphologically different type of valve, fibrosis does not cause an increased intensity, as in closure of a fibrotic atrioventricular valve.

▥ Abnormalities of Splitting of S_2

Normal physiologic splitting of S_2 was discussed in the section on anatomy and physiology. This section deals with abnormalities of splitting.

Any condition that delays right ventricular systole, either electrically or mechanically, will delay P_2 and produce a widened splitting of S_2. Right ventricular emptying will be delayed by a right bundle branch block or pulmonic stenosis. The pulmonic component of S_2 will be delayed during both inspiration and expiration, and *wide splitting* of S_2 will occur.

Any condition that shortens left ventricular systole will allow A_2 to occur earlier than normal, and wide splitting will likewise occur. Conditions such as mitral regurgitation, ventricular septal defect, and patent ductus arteriosus shorten left ventricular systole, and the S_1 to A_2 interval will be shorter than normal. In these conditions, there is a "double outlet" to the left ventricle, and systole will therefore be shorter. In a ventricular septal defect, with a left-to-right shunt, not only will left ventricular systole be shorter, but right ventricular systole will also be prolonged, both factors being key in producing the wide splitting of S_2.

Any condition, either electrical or mechanical, that delays left ventricular emptying produces *paradoxical splitting* of S_2. Left bundle branch block or aortic stenosis delays left ventricular emptying. These conditions delay the closure of the aortic valve after right ventricular systole and P_2 have occurred. The normal sequence of A_2–P_2 is reversed. During inspiration, P_2 moves normally away from S_1 toward A_2. The split is said to be *narrowed*. With expiration, P_2 moves normally and approaches S_1: the P_2–A_2 split widens. This widening during expiration is paradoxical. Other conditions, such as left ventricular failure and severe hypertension, delay left ventricular ejection and cause paradoxical splitting of S_2.

Fixed splitting of S_2 is the auscultatory hallmark of an atrial septal defect. In this situation, the split is wide and does not change with respiration. This is because inspiratory increases in venous return to the right atrium normally raise its pressure. During expiration, the right atrial pressure is lower, but the left-to-right atrial shunt keeps the volume in the right atrium constant during respiration; therefore, normal splitting does not occur.

Normal physiologic splitting of the second heart sound and abnormalities of splitting are illustrated in Figure 12–34.

Systolic Clicks

Ejection clicks are high-pitched sounds that occur early in systole at the onset of ejection and are produced by the opening of pathologically deformed semilunar valves. Pulmonic or aortic stenosis may produce ejection clicks. The sounds are short and have the quality of a "click." Pulmonic ejection clicks are best heard at the pulmonic area, and aortic ejection clicks are heard at the aortic area. As calcification progresses, the mobility of the valve decreases, and the ejection click disappears.

Midsystolic clicks are not ejection clicks. They occur in the middle of systole. They may be single or multiple, and they may change in position during the cardiac cycle with various maneuvers that change ventricular geometry. The most common condition associated with a midsystolic click is prolapse of the mitral or tricuspid valve.

Diastolic Opening Snaps

The opening of an atrioventricular valve is normally silent and occurs about 100 msec after S_2. This is about as long as it takes to say "ma-ma" quickly. An *opening snap* is a diastolic event that is the sound of the opening of a pathologically deformed atrioven-

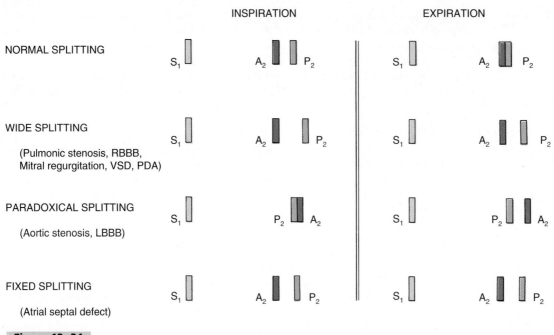

INSPIRATION   EXPIRATION

NORMAL SPLITTING

WIDE SPLITTING

(Pulmonic stenosis, RBBB,
Mitral regurgitation, VSD, PDA)

PARADOXICAL SPLITTING

(Aortic stenosis, LBBB)

FIXED SPLITTING

(Atrial septal defect)

Figure 12–34

Abnormalities of splitting of the second heart sound. (RBBB = right bundle branch block; VSD = ventricular septal defect; PDA = patent ductus arteriosus; LBBB = left bundle branch block.)

tricular valve. The sound is sharp and high-pitched. The mitral opening snap of mitral stenosis occurs after A_2; the tricuspid opening snap of tricuspid stenosis occurs after P_2.

The interval between S_2 and the opening snap is termed the S_2–OS *interval* and has specific significance as to the severity of the stenosis. As mitral stenosis worsens, the resistance and obstruction to flow increase. Pressure in the left atrium increases, and the gradient across the mitral valve increases. The mitral valve, therefore, opens earlier than normal when the left ventricular pressure falls below left atrial pressure. The S_2–OS time shortens as the severity increases. Try saying "ma-da" as quickly as possible. This interval is about 50–60 msec and approximates a very short S_2–OS interval, as heard in severe mitral stenosis.

Murmurs

Murmurs are produced when there is turbulent energy in the walls of the heart and blood vessels. Obstruction to flow or flowing from a narrow- to a larger-diameter vessel produces turbulence. Turbulence sets up eddies that strike the walls to produce vibrations that the examiner recognizes as a murmur. Murmurs can also be produced when there is a large volume of blood through a normal opening. In this circumstance, the normal opening is relatively stenotic for the increased volume. "Blowing" murmurs are produced by large gradients with variable flow volumes. "Rumbling" murmurs result from areas of small gradients that are dependent on flow. "Harsh" murmurs result from large gradients and high flow.

An ejection murmur is a murmur produced by turbulence across a semilunar valve during systole, such as in aortic stenosis or pulmonic stenosis. Ejection murmurs are diamond-shaped and are described as "crescendo-decrescendo." They begin slightly after S_1 and end before S_2. An ejection click from stenosis of the semilunar valve may precede the murmur. These murmurs are medium-pitched and are best heard with the diaphragm of the stethoscope. Because they are based on flow, the intensity of these murmurs does not indicate the degree of severity. Increased flow across a minimally narrowed aortic valve produces a loud murmur; decreased flow across a severely stenotic aortic valve may produce a barely audible murmur. Any increase in flow or volume may produce an ejection murmur even in the presence of a normal valve. An ejection murmur as a sign of aortic stenosis is a finding of high sensitivity but low specificity. Figure 12–35 illustrates an ejection murmur.

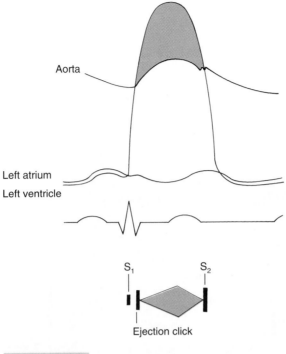

Aorta

Left atrium

Left ventricle

S₁   S₂

Ejection click

Figure 12–35

A systolic ejection murmur such as that occurring in aortic stenosis.

Regurgitant systolic murmurs are produced by retrograde flow from a higher-pressure area to a lower-pressure area during systole, such as in mitral or tricuspid regurgitation. These murmurs are holosystolic or pansystolic. They begin with S_1 and end after S_2. These murmurs extend past S_2 because ventricular pressure is higher than atrial pressure, even after the closure of the semilunar valve. An S_3 indicative of volume overload to the ventricle is often heard. These murmurs are high-pitched and are best heard with the diaphragm. The terms *regurgitation, incompetence,* and *insufficiency* are often used synonymously for this type of murmur. The preferred term is regurgitation, because it implies the retrograde direction of flow. The holosystolic murmur of atrioventricular valve regurgitation is a finding of high sensitivity. Figure 12–36 illustrates a regurgitant murmur.

Diastolic atrioventricular murmurs begin a finite time after S_2 with the opening of the atrioventricular valve. Mitral stenosis and tricuspid stenosis are examples of this type of murmur. There is a pause between S_2 and the beginning of the murmur. Isovolumetric relaxation is occurring during this period. The murmur is decrescendo in shape, beginning with an opening snap, if the valve is mobile. These murmurs are low-pitched and are best heard with the bell of the stethoscope, with the patient lying in the left lateral decubitus position. Because the atrioventricular valve is stenotic, rapid filling does not occur, and a gradient persists throughout diastole. If the patient is in normal sinus rhythm, atrial contraction will increase the gradient at the end of diastole, or presystole, and there will be an increase in the murmur at this time. The diastolic atrioventricular murmur is a sensitive and specific sign of atrioventricular valve stenosis.

The first heart sound is the loudest sound. The cadence and emphasis of the sounds are best heard by saying the following mnemonic:

MIT′—ral-vaaaaalve   MIT′—ral-vaaaaalve
S_1 S_2 OS S_1 S_2 OS

OS is the mitral opening snap. The "aaaalve" is the presystolic accentuation heard when a patient with mitral stenosis is in normal sinus rhythm. Figure 12–37 illustrates a diastolic atrioventricular murmur.

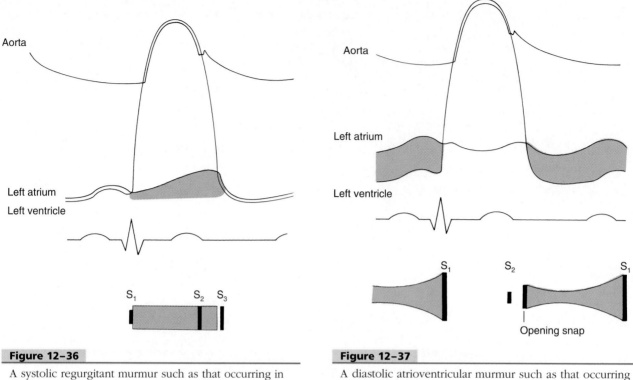

Figure 12–36

A systolic regurgitant murmur such as that occurring in mitral regurgitation.

Figure 12–37

A diastolic atrioventricular murmur such as that occurring in mitral stenosis.

Diastolic semilunar murmurs begin immediately after S_2, as heard in aortic or pulmonic regurgitation. Unlike the diastolic atrioventricular murmurs, there is no delay after S_2 to the beginning of the murmur. The high-pitched murmur is decrescendo in shape and is best heard with the diaphragm of the stethoscope while the patient is sitting up and leaning forward. A diastolic semilunar murmur is a sign of low sensitivity but high specificity. Figure 12–38 illustrates the pressure curves responsible for the generation of a diastolic semilunar murmur.

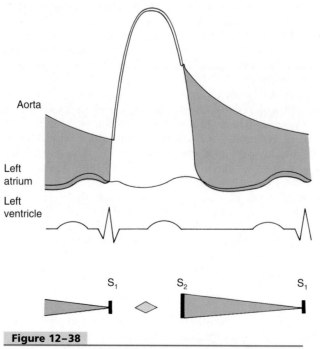

Figure 12–38

A diastolic semilunar murmur such as that occurring in aortic regurgitation. Note the systolic ejection murmur, which is related to the increased volume and flow.

Table 12–8 lists important cardiac sounds according to the cardiac cycle. Figure 12–39 lists important characteristics of the systolic murmurs of aortic stenosis and mitral regurgitation. Table 12–9 summarizes the differentiation of some additional systolic murmurs. Figure 12–40 lists important characteristics of the diastolic murmurs of mitral stenosis and aortic regurgitation.

Table 12–8 Cardiac Sounds

Cardiac Cycle	Sound
Early systolic	Ejection click Aortic prosthetic valve opening sound*
Mid-late systolic	Midsystolic click Rub
Early diastolic	Opening snap S_3 Mitral prosthetic valve opening sound† Tumor plop‡
Middiastolic	S_3 Summation gallop§
Late diastolic (sometimes called *presystolic*)	S_4 Pacemaker sound

* Opening and closure of the prosthetic aortic valve are heard with many prosthetic valves. The opening is comparable to an ejection click; the closing is a "prosthetic" S_2.

† Opening and closure of the prosthetic mitral valve are heard with many prosthetic valves. The opening is comparable to an opening snap; the closing is a "prosthetic" S_1.

‡ An atrial myxoma that is pedunculated may "plop" in and out of the mitral annulus, simulating the auscultatory signs of mitral stenosis.

§ At fast heart rates, the diastolic period shortens. If an S_3 and S_4 are present, the sounds may be summated into a single sound called a *summation gallop*.

Table 12–9 Differentiation of Other Systolic Murmurs

	Pulmonic Stenosis	Tricuspid Regurgitation	Ventricular Septal Defect	Venous Hum	Innocent Murmur
Location	Pulmonic area	Tricuspid area	Tricuspid area	Above clavicle	Widespread*
Radiation	Neck	Right of sternum	Right of sternum	Right neck	Minimal
Shape	Diamond	Holosystolic	Holosystolic	Continuous	Diamond
Pitch	Medium	High	High	High	Medium
Quality	Harsh	Blowing	Harsh	Roaring; humming	Twanging; vibratory

* Usually between the apex and the left lower sternal border.

Useful Vocabulary

Listed here are the specific roots that are important in order to understand the terminology related to cardiac disease.

Root	Pertaining to	Example	Definition
brady-	slow	*brady*cardia	Slow heart rate
-cardio-	heart	*cardio*megaly	Enlargement of the heart
sphygmo-	pulse	*sphygmo*manometer	Instrument for measuring blood pressure
supra-	above	*supra*ventricular	Above the level of the ventricles
tachy-	fast	*tachy*cardia	Rapid heart rate

Systolic Murmurs

	Aortic Stenosis	**Mitral Regurgitation**
Location	Aortic area	Apex
Radiation	Neck	Axilla
Shape	Diamond	Holosystolic
Pitch	Medium	High
Quality	Harsh	Blowing
Associated signs	Decreased A_2	Decreased S_1
	Ejection click	S_3
	S_4	Laterally displaced diffuse PMI
	Narrow pulse pressure	
	Slow rising and delayed pulse	

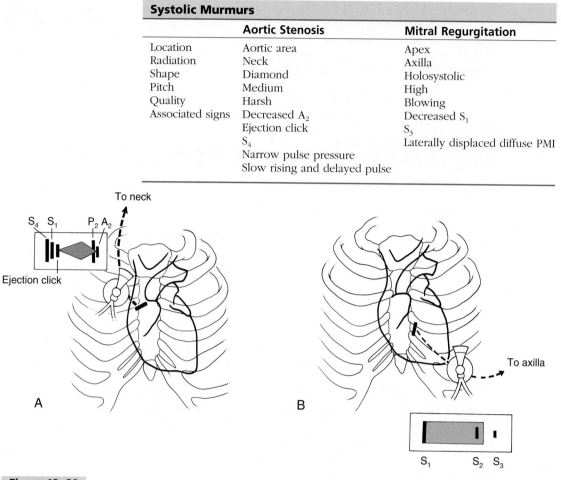

Figure 12–39

Systolic murmurs. *A,* Pathophysiology of aortic stenosis. Note the paradoxical splitting of the second heart sound (S_2), the S_4, and the ejection click. *B,* Mitral regurgitation. Notice that the murmur ends after S_2, and note the presence of the S_3. (PMI = point of maximum impulse.)

Writing Up the Physical Examination

Listed here are examples of the write-up for the examination of the heart.

- The PMI is in the fifth intercostal space, midclavicular line. S_1 and S_2 are normal.* Physiologic splitting is present. No murmurs, gallops, or rubs are heard. There is no clubbing, cyanosis, or edema.
- The PMI is in the sixth intercostal space, anterior axillary line. S_1 is soft. S_2 is widely split on inspiration and expiration. A grade III/VI, high-pitched, holosystolic murmur is heard at the apex with radiation to the axilla. A palpable S_3 is present at the apex. There is 2+ pitting edema on the shins bilaterally. No cyanosis or clubbing is present.
- The PMI is in the fifth intercostal space, midclavicular line. S_1 is normal. S_2 is soft. An S_4 is present at the apex. A grade IV/VI, harsh, medium-pitched, crescendo-decrescendo murmur, beginning slightly after S_1 and ending before S_2, is present at the aortic area. This murmur radiates to both carotids. No clubbing, cyanosis, or edema is present.
- The PMI is in the fifth intercostal space, midclavicular line. S_1 is accentuated. S_2 is normal. An RV rock is present at the left lower sternal border. There is a grade II/VI, low-pitched, diastolic rumble heard at the apex, best heard in the left lateral decubitus position. A grade III/VI, high-pitched, holosystolic murmur is heard at the left lower sternal border, which increases in intensity with inspiration. A right ventricular S_3 may be present at the left lower sternal border.† There is 4+ pitting sacral edema. No cyanosis or clubbing is present.

---

*The descriptors for S_1 and S_2 are *normal, increased, decreased, widely split, narrowly split, fixed split,* or *paradoxically split.* Never indicate that S_1 and S_2 are present.
†Notice that in this example the examiner stated that a finding may be present.

Diastolic Murmurs

	Mitral Stenosis	Aortic Regurgitation
Location	Apex	Aortic area
Radiation	No	No
Shape	Decrescendo	Decrescendo
Pitch	Low	High
Quality	Rumbling	Blowing
Associated signs	Increased S₁	S₃
	Opening snap	Laterally displaced PMI
	PV rock§	Wide pulse pressure*
	Presystolic accentuation	Bounding pulses
		Austin Flint murmur†
		Systolic ejection murmur‡

*The wide pulse pressure is the cause of the many physical signs of aortic regurgitation: Quincke's pulse, de Musset's sign, Duroziez' sign, Corrigan's pulse, etc.
†An apical diastolic murmur heard in association with aortic regurgitation mimicking mitral stenosis.
‡A flow murmur across a valve that is relatively narrow for the increased blood volume as a result of aortic regurgitation. It is relatively stenotic and need not be anatomically stenotic, as in true aortic stenosis.
§Right ventricular impulse at lower left sternal border.

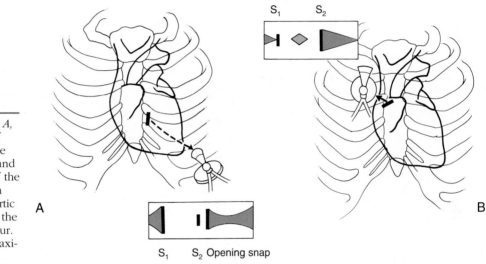

Figure 12–40

Diastolic murmurs. *A,* Pathophysiology of mitral stenosis. Note the intensity of S₁ and the accentuation of the diastolic murmur in late diastole. *B,* Aortic regurgitation. Note the systolic flow murmur. (PMI = point of maximum impulse.)

Bibliography

Braunwald E: Heart Disease: A Textbook of Cardiovascular Medicine, 5th ed. Philadelphia, W.B. Saunders, 1997.

Cochran PT: Bedside aids to auscultation of the heart. JAMA 239:54, 1978.

Constant J: Bedside Cardiology. Boston, Little, Brown, 1985.

Cook DJ, Simel DL: Does this patient have abnormal central venous pressure? JAMA 275:630, 1996.

Criscitiello MG: Pitfalls in auscultation. Proc N Engl Cardiovasc Soc 29:19, 1977.

Ducas J, Magder S, McGregor M: Validity of the hepatojugular reflux as a clinical test for congestive heart failure. Am J Cardiol 52:1299, 1983.

Eilen SD, Crawford MH, O'Rourke RA: Accuracy of precordial palpation for detecting increased left ventricular volume. Ann Intern Med 99:628, 1983.

Elliott WJ: Ear lobe crease and coronary artery disease. Am J Med 75:1024, 1983.

Ewy G: The abdominojugular test: Technique and hemodynamic correlates. Ann Intern Med 109: 456, 1988.

Freis ED: Auscultatory indication of diastolic blood pressure. Cardiol Digest 3:13, 1968.

Heckerling PS, Wiener SL, Moses VK, et al: Accuracy of precordial percussion in detecting cardiomegaly. Am J Med 91:328, 1991.

Heckerling PS, Wiener SL, Wolfkiel CJ, et al: Accuracy and reproducibility of precordial percussion and palpation for detecting increased left ventricular end-diastolic volume and mass. JAMA 270:1943, 1993.

Henkind SJ, Benis AM, Teichholz LE: The paradox of pulsus paradoxus. Am Heart J 114:198, 1987.

Johnson R, Swartz MH: A Simplified Approach to Electrocardiography. Philadelphia, W.B. Saunders, 1986.

Kroenke MK: Sphygmomanometry: The correct arm position. West J Med 140:459, 1984.

Lembo NJ, Dell'Italia LJ, Crawford MH, et al.: Bedside diagnosis of systolic murmurs. N Engl J Med 318:1572, 1988.

Londe S, Klitzner TS: Auscultatory blood pressure measurement: Effect of pressure on the head of the stethoscope. West J Med 141:193, 1984.

London SR, London RE: Critique of indirect diastolic end-point. Arch Intern Med 119:39, 1976.

Maisel AS, Atwood JE, Goldberger AL: Hepatojugular reflux: Useful in the bedside diagnosis of tricuspid regurgitation. Ann Intern Med 101:781, 1984.

Prior DB, et al.: Value of the history and physical in identifying patients at increased risk for coronary artery disease. Ann Intern Med 118:81, 1993.

Rothman A, Goldberger AL: Aids to cardiac auscultation. Ann Intern Med 99:346, 1983.

Silverberg DS, Shemesh E, Iaina A: The unsupported arm: A cause of falsely raised blood pressure readings. Br Med J 2:1331, 1977.

Thomas JE, Schirger A, Fealey RD, et al.: Orthostatic hypotension. Mayo Clin Proc 56:117, 1981.

CHAPTER 13

The Peripheral Vascular System

Veins which by the thickening of their tunicles in the old restrict the passage of blood, and by this lack of nourishment destroy their life without any fever, the old coming to fail little by little in slow death.

Leonardo da Vinci
1452–1519

General Considerations

Diseases of the peripheral vascular system are common and may involve the arteries, veins, or lymphatics. The arterial conditions include cerebrovascular, aorto-iliac, femoral-popliteal, renal, and aortic occlusive and aneurysmal disease. The two most important diseases of the peripheral arteries are atherosclerosis of the larger arteries and microvascular disease.

The most common cause of peripheral arterial occlusive disease is atherosclerosis affecting the medium-sized and large vessels of the extremities. The narrowing of the vessel causes a decreased blood supply, resulting in ischemia. In addition, atherosclerosis may become manifest by aneurysmal dilatation. The abdominal aorta is the artery most frequently involved. The aneurysm is commonly below the renal arteries and may extend to as far as the external iliac arteries. Often, this aneurysm produces few, if any, symptoms. The examiner may discover a pulsatile mass as an incidental finding. Frequently, the first manifestation may be the catastrophic rupture of the aneurysm. An abdominal aortic aneurysm larger than 5 cm in diameter carries a 20% risk of rupturing within the first year of discovery and a 50% risk within 5 years. However, not until 1951 was the first abdominal aneurysm surgically treated by resection and grafting. Since 1951, great strides have been made in understanding the natural history of vascular disease as well as in the institution of new technology to help diagnose and treat it.

Microvascular arterial disease occurs in patients with diabetes. Changes develop in the small arterioles that impair circulation to the skin or nerves, especially of the lower extremities, producing symptoms of ischemia. Peripheral neuropathy is a common sequela to microvascular disease. This neuropathy may be manifested as a defect in the sensory, motor, or autonomic system. Microvascular disease affects more than 15 million individuals in the United States.

Peripheral venous disease often progresses to venous stasis and thrombotic disorders. One of the dread complications of thrombotic disease is pulmonary embolism. In the United States, more than 175,000 deaths per year are attributed to acute pulmonary embolism.

Structure and Physiology

Diseases of the peripheral *arterial* system cause ischemia of the extremities. When the body is at rest, collateral blood vessels may be able to provide adequate circulation. During exercise, when oxygen demand increases, this circulation may not be sufficient for the actively contracting muscles, resulting in ischemia.

The *venous* system consists of a series of low-pressure capacitance vessels. Nearly 70% of the blood volume is contained in this system. Although offering little resistance, the veins are controlled by a variety of neural and humoral stimuli that enhance venous return to the right side of the heart. In addition, valves aid in the return of blood.

When an individual is in the upright posture, the venous pressure in the lower extremity is the highest. Over many years, dilation of the veins occurs as a result of the weakening of their walls. As the walls dilate, the veins are unable to close adequately, the reflux of blood occurs. In addition, there is a loss of the efficiency of the venous pump in returning blood to the heart. Both these factors are responsible for the venous stasis seen in patients with chronic venous insufficiency. Complications from venous stasis include pigmentation, dermatitis, cellulitis, ulceration, and thrombus formation.

The *lymphatic* system is an extensive vascular network and is responsible for returning tissue fluid (lymph) back to the venous system. The extremities are richly supplied with lymphatic tissue. Lymph nodes, many of which are located between major proximal joints, aid in filtering the lymphatic fluid before it enters the blood. The most important clinical symptoms of lymphatic obstruction are *lymphedema* and *lymphangitis*.

Review of Specific Symptoms

Many patients with peripheral vascular disease are asymptomatic. When patients are symptomatic, vascular disease causes the following:

- Pain
- Changes in skin temperature and color
- Edema
- Ulceration
- Emboli
- Stroke
- Dizziness

Pain

Pain is the principal symptom of atherosclerosis. Whenever a patient complains of pain while walking in the calf, arch of the foot, thighs, hips, or buttocks, peripheral vascular disease of the arteries must be considered. The symptom of the pain in the lower extremity occurring during exercise is *intermittent claudication.* The site of the pain is always distal to the occlusive disease. As the disease progresses, pain at rest occurs. This is often severe and is aggravated by cool temperatures and elevation, especially during the night in bed. Pain may also occur with deep vein thrombosis.

If a male patient complains of buttock or thigh pain while walking, the examiner should inquire about impotence. *Leriche's syndrome* is chronic aortoiliac obstruction; the patient presents with intermittent claudication and impotence. In this condition, the terminal aorta and iliac arteries are involved by severe atherosclerosis at the aortic bifurcation.

Patients occasionally complain of bilateral leg pain or numbness occurring while walking as well as while resting. This is *pseudoclaudication* and is a symptom of musculoskeletal disease in the lumbar area.

Skin Changes

Color changes are common with vascular disease. Chronic *arterial* insufficiency produces a cool and pale extremity. Chronic *venous* insufficiency produces a warmer than normal extremity. The leg becomes erythematous, and erosions produced by excoriations result. With chronic insufficiency, stasis changes produce increased pigmentation, swelling, and an "aching" or "heaviness" in the legs. These changes are characteristically in the lower third of the extremity and are more prominent medially. When venous insufficiency occurs, edema of dependent areas results.

Patients with acute deep vein thrombosis have secondary inflammation of the tissue surrounding the vein. This produces signs of inflammation: warmth, redness, and fever. Swelling is the most reliable symptom and sign associated with venous obstruction. This finding is indicative of severe deep venous obstruction, because the superficial veins of the lower extremity carry only 20% of the total drainage and are not associated with swelling. The extremities should be compared, and a difference in circumference of 2 cm at the ankle or midcalf should be considered significant.

Edema

Lymphedema results from either a primary abnormality in the development of the lymphatic system or an acquired obstruction to flow. Whether the congenital or the acquired form is involved, the net result is stasis of lymph fluid in the tissues producing a *firm, nonpitting edema*. Over several years, the skin takes on a rough consistency similar to pigskin. Because lymphedema is usually painless, the only symptom is "heaviness" of the extremity.

Ulceration

Persistent ischemia of a limb is associated with ischemic ulceration and gangrene. Ulceration is almost inevitable once skin has thickened and the circulation is compromised. Ulceration related to arterial insufficiency occurs as a result of trauma to the toes and heel. These ulcers are painful, have discrete edges producing a "punched-out" appearance, and are often covered with crust. When infected, the tissue is erythematous.

In contrast to arterial insufficiency ulceration, venous insufficiency leads to stasis ulceration, which is painless and occurs in the ankle area or lower leg just above the medial malleolus. The classic presentation is a diffusely reddened, thickened area over the medial malleolus. The skin has a cobblestone appearance resulting from fibrosis and venous stasis. Ulceration occurs with the slightest trauma. Rapidly developing ulcers are commonly arterial, whereas slowly developing ulceration is usually venous. Figure 13–1 shows a patient with stasis dermatitis and bilateral ulcerations over the medial malleoli.

Emboli

A history of emboli is important. Thrombus formation results from stasis and hypercoagulability. It appears, however, that venous stasis is the most important cause of thrombus formation. Bed rest, congestive heart failure, obesity, pregnancy, and oral contraceptives have been associated with thrombus formation and emboli. Patients with leg ulcers should be asked the following:

> *"What did the ulcer look like when it first appeared?"*
> *"What do you think started the ulcer?"*
> *"How quickly did it develop?"*
> *"How painful is the ulcer?"*
> *"What kind of medication(s) have you been taking?"*
> *"Is there a history of any generalized diseases, such as anemia? rheumatoid arthritis?"*
> *"Is there a family history of leg ulcers?"*

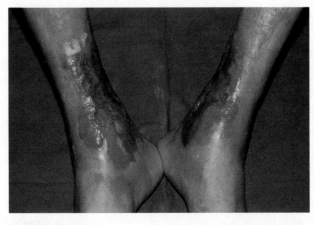

Figure 13–1

Stasis dermatitis and ulceration over the medial malleoli.

Symptoms secondary to emboli can include shortness of breath from pulmonary emboli; abdominal pain from splenic, intestinal, or renal artery emboli; neurologic symptoms from carotid or vertebral-basilar artery emboli; and pain and paresthesias from peripheral artery emboli.

Neurologic Symptoms

Cerebrovascular occlusive disease causes many neurologic symptoms, including strokes,* dizziness, and changes in consciousness. Occlusion of the internal carotid artery produces a syndrome of contralateral hemiplegia, contralateral sensory deficits, and dysphasia. Vertebrobasilar disease is associated with diplopia, cerebellar dysfunction, changes in consciousness, and facial paresis.

Impact of Vascular Disease on the Patient

The patient with chronic arterial insufficiency has progressive pain while walking. As the condition progresses, ulceration of the toes, feet, and areas susceptible to trauma, such as the shin, develops. Pain may become excruciating. Gangrene of a toe may develop, and amputation of it is frequently followed by amputation of the foot and leg. The patient becomes more and more depressed from ongoing mutilation of the body.

Physical Examination

The equipment necessary for the examination of the peripheral vascular system is a stethoscope, a tourniquet, and a tape measure.

The physical examination of the peripheral vascular system consists of inspection, palpation of the arterial pulses, and some additional tests if disease is considered to be present. All these techniques are usually integrated with the rest of the physical examination.

The patient lies supine, with the examiner standing to the right of the bed. The evaluation of the peripheral vascular system includes the following:

- Inspection
- Examination of the arterial pulses
- Examination of the lymphatic system
- Other special techniques

Inspection

▨ Inspect for Symmetry of the Extremities

The extremities should be compared for symmetric differences in size, color, temperature, and venous patterns. Look at the patient in Figure 13–2. This patient has massive lymphedema of her right upper extremity secondary to a right mastectomy 18 years earlier.

▨ Inspect the Lower Extremities

The lower extremities should be inspected for pigmentary abnormalities, ulcers, edema, and venous patterns. Is cyanosis present? Is edema present? If edema is present, does it pit? Look at the bilateral color changes and swelling of the legs of the patient shown in Figure 13–3. This patient had chronic venous insufficiency. She died of a massive pulmonary embolus 1 day after this photograph was taken.

---

* A stroke is also known as a cerebrovascular accident.

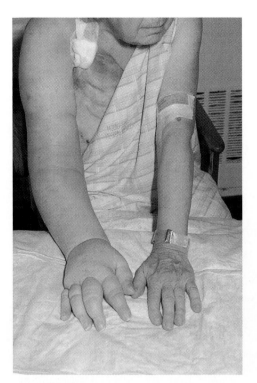

Figure 13-2

Lymphedema.

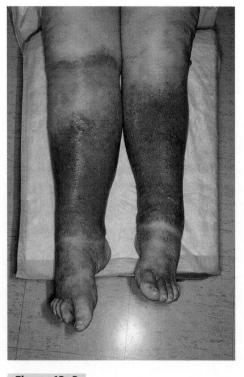

Figure 13-3

Chronic venous stasis.

Assess the Skin Temperature

Evaluate the temperature by using the back of your hand. Compare comparable areas of each extremity. Coolness of an extremity is commonly found with arterial insufficiency.

Inspect for Varicosities

Ask the patient to stand, and inspect the lower extremities for varicosities. Look at the area of the proximal femoral ring as well as in the distal portion of the legs. Varicose veins in these locations may not have been visible when the patient was lying.

Look at Figure 13–4. The patient is a 37 year old woman with severe right-sided heart failure. Notice the marked dilated and tortuous veins in the popliteal fossa. Also notice the increased pigmentation of the skin over the lower legs.

Examination of the Arterial Pulses

The most important finding when one is examining the peripheral arterial tree is a decreased or absent pulse. The peripheral arterial pulses routinely evaluated are the radial, brachial, femoral, popliteal, dorsalis pedis, and posterior tibial.

Palpate the Radial Pulse

The examiner should stand in front of the patient. The radial pulses are evaluated by the examiner grasping both of the patient's wrists and palpating the pulses with the index, middle, and fourth fingers. The examiner holds the patient's right wrist with the left fingers and the patient's left wrist with the examiner's right fingers, as shown in Figure 12–21. The symmetry of the pulses is then evaluated for timing and strength.

Palpate the Brachial Pulse

Because the brachial pulse is stronger than the digital pulses, the examiner may use the thumbs to palpate the patient's brachial pulses. The brachial artery may be felt medially

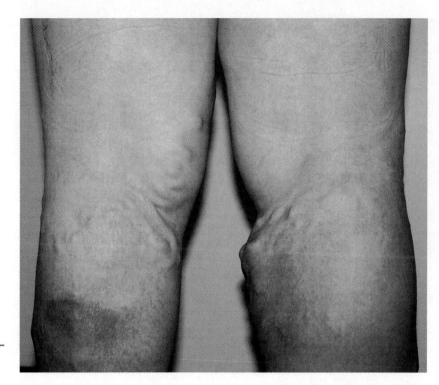

Figure 13-4

Marked varicosities of the popliteal fossa.

just under the belly or tendon of the biceps muscle. With the examiner still standing in front of the patient, both brachial arteries may be felt simultaneously. The examiner's left hand holds the patient's right arm while the right hand holds the patient's left arm. Once the brachial pulsation is felt with the thumbs, the examiner should apply progressive pressure to it until the maximal systolic force is felt. This is shown in Figure 13–5. The examiner should now be able to assess its wave form.

■ Auscultate the Carotid Artery

Auscultation for carotid bruits* is performed by having the examiner place the diaphragm of the stethoscope over the carotid artery while the patient is lying supine.

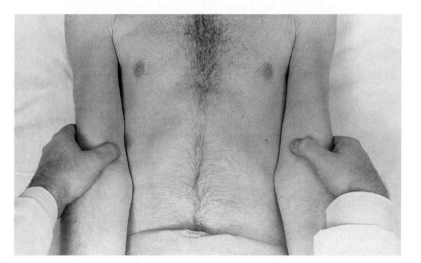

Figure 13-5

Technique for brachial artery palpation.

---

* A bruit is a sound or murmur heard in a vessel as a result of increased turbulence.

This is shown in Figure 13–6. The head of the patient should be slightly elevated on a pillow and turned away slightly from the carotid artery being evaluated. It is often helpful for the examiner to ask the patient to hold the breath during the auscultation. Normally, either nothing or transmitted heart sounds will be heard. After one carotid artery is evaluated, the other carotid artery is examined. After auscultation of the carotid arteries, they are palpated (see Chapter 12, The Heart).

The presence of a murmur is to be noted. This may be a bruit resulting from atherosclerotic disease of the carotid artery. Occasionally, loud murmurs originating from the heart can be transmitted to the neck. With experience, the examiner will be able to determine whether the disorder is local in the neck or distal in the heart.

▣ Palpate the Abdominal Aorta

Abdominal aortic aneurysms kill approximately 10,000 people in the United States each year. Many of these deaths would be preventable if the patient were aware of the presence of this defect. Once recognized, the rate of operative mortality for a nonruptured aneurysm is less than 5%, and, after operation, the survival rate equals that of the general population. If unrecognized, an abdominal aortic aneurysm that ruptures carries a mortality rate of nearly 90%. Even among patients who reach the operating room alive, the surgical mortality rate is 50%.

The examination is performed by palpating deeply, but gently, into the midabdomen. The presence of a mass with laterally expansive pulsation suggests an abdominal aortic aneurysm. Some caution is urged in making this diagnosis in thin individuals in whom the normal pulsatile aorta may be easily palpated. A high false-positive rate on this examination should not cause a problem, however, because confirmation with abdominal ultrasonography is safe and inexpensive.

Other findings associated with an abdominal aortic aneurysm include an abdominal bruit, a femoral bruit, and a femoral pulse deficit. In fewer than 10% of patients with an abdominal aortic aneurysm, a bruit may be present. Acute rupture of an abdominal aortic aneurysm is suggested when a bruit that is present is associated with severe pain in the abdomen or back and when there is an absent or diminished distal pulse that later returns.

Table 13–1 summarizes the characteristics of the physical signs for detection of an abdominal aortic aneurysm.

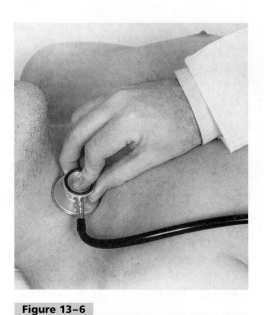

Figure 13–6

Technique for auscultation of the carotid artery.

Table 13–1   Characteristics of Physical Signs for Detection of an Abdominal Aortic Aneurysm

Physical Sign	Sensitivity (%)	Specificity (%)
Definite pulsatile mass	28	97
Definite or suggestive pulsatile mass	50	91
Abdominal bruit	11	95
Femoral bruit	17	87
Femoral pulse deficit	22	91

Data from Lederle FA, Walker JM, Reinke DB: Selective screening for abdominal aortic aneurysms with physical examination and ultrasound. Arch Intern Med 148:1753, 1988.

Rule Out Abdominal Bruits

The patient should be supine. The examiner should place the diaphragm of the stethoscope in the midline of the abdomen about 2 inches above the umbilicus and listen carefully for the presence of an *aortic* bruit. This technique is shown in Figure 13–7.

A *renal* bruit may be the only clue to renal artery stenosis. Auscultation should be performed about 2 inches above the umbilicus and 1–2 inches laterally to the right and to the left of midposition.

Abdominal bruits present only during systole are frequently of little clinical value, because they are found in normal individuals as well as in patients with essential hypertension. The presence of a systolic-diastolic abdominal bruit, however, should raise the suspicion of renal vascular hypertension. Nearly 60% of all patients with renal vascular hypertension have such a bruit.

Grim et al (1979) reported that the presence of a combined systolic-diastolic abdominal bruit had a sensitivity of 39% and a specificity of 99% for detecting renovascular hypertension. The presence of this type of bruit had a positive likelihood ratio (LR+) of 39 and, if absent, a negative likelihood ration (LR−) of 0.6. A study by Fenton et al (1966) evaluated the presence of any epigastric or flank bruit and its association with renovascular hypertension. The sensitivity was 63%, but the specificity dropped to 90%. The presence of any abdominal bruit confers a much lower LR+ for renovascular hypertension, i.e., 6.4.

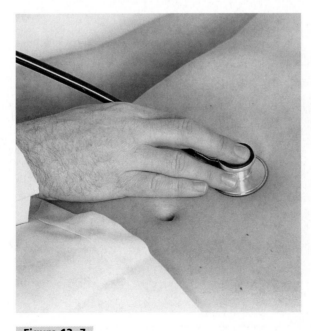

Figure 13–7

Technique for auscultation of the abdominal aorta.

◼ Palpate the Femoral Pulse

The femoral pulse is evaluated with the patient lying on the back and the examiner at the patient's right side. The lateral corners of the pubic hair triangle are observed and palpated. The femoral artery should run obliquely through the corner of the pubic hair triangle below the inguinal ligament and midway between the pubic symphysis and the anterosuperior iliac spine. Both femoral pulses may be compared simultaneously. The technique is shown in Figure 13–8.

If one of the femoral pulses is diminished or absent, auscultation for a bruit is necessary. The diaphragm of the stethoscope is placed over the femoral artery. The presence of a bruit may indicate obstructive aortoiliofemoral disease.

Rule Out Coarctation of the Aorta

The timing of the femoral and radial pulses is important. Normally, these pulses peak either at the same time or with the femoral pulse preceding the radial pulse. By placing one hand on the femoral artery and the other on the radial artery, the examiner can determine the peaking of these pulses. The technique need be performed only on one side. Any delay in the femoral pulse should raise suspicion of coarctation of the aorta, especially in a hypertensive individual. This technique is shown in Figure 13–9.

◼ Palpate the Popliteal Pulse

The popliteal artery is often difficult to assess. Each artery is evaluated separately. While the patient is lying on the back, the examiner places the thumbs on the patella and the remaining fingers of both hands in the popliteal space behind, as shown in Figure 13–10. The examiner should hold the leg in a mild degree of flexion. The patient should not be asked to elevate the leg, because this will tighten the muscles and make feeling the pulse more difficult. Both hands should squeeze in the popliteal fossa. Firm pressure is usually required to feel the pulsation.

◼ Palpate the Dorsalis Pedis Pulse

The dorsalis pedis pulse is best felt by dorsiflexion of the foot. The dorsalis pedis artery passes along a line from the extensor retinaculum of the ankle to a point just lateral to the extensor tendon of the great toe. The dorsalis pedis pulses may be felt simultaneously, as shown in Figure 13–11.

◼ Palpate the Posterior Tibial Pulse

The posterior tibial artery can be felt as it wraps around the medial malleolus during plantar flexion. Both arteries may be evaluated simultaneously. Figure 13–12 shows this procedure. Although posterior tibial pulses are absent in 15% of normal subjects, the most sensitive sign of occlusive peripheral arterial disease in patients older than the age of 60 years is the absence of the posterior tibial pulse.

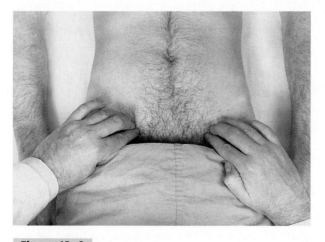

Figure 13–8

Technique for palpation of the femoral arteries.

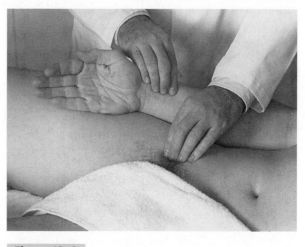

Figure 13–9

Technique for timing the femoral and radial arteries.

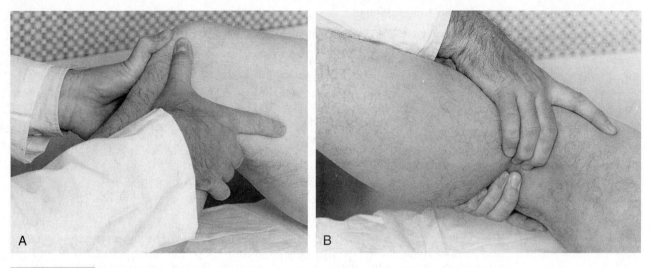

Figure 13–10

Technique for palpation of the popliteal artery. *A,* Correct position of the hands from the front. *B,* View from behind the popliteal fossa.

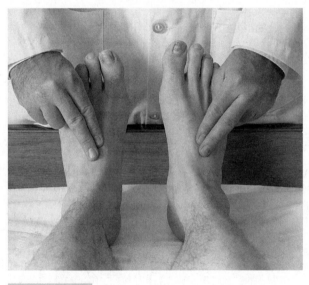

Figure 13–11

Technique for palpation of the dorsalis pedis arteries.

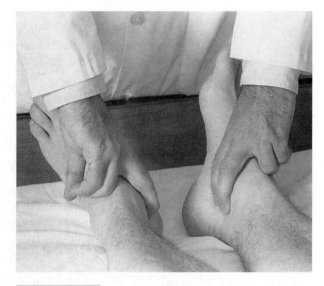

Figure 13–12

Technique for palpation of the posterior tibial arteries.

■ Grading of Pulses

The description of the amplitude of the pulse is most important. The following is the most accepted grading system:

0   Absent
1   Diminished
2   Normal
3   Increased
4   Bounding

It is important that the patient's socks or stockings be removed in order for the examiner to assess the peripheral pulses of the lower extremities. If there is confusion about whether the examiner is feeling the patient's pulse or his or her own, the examiner may wish to palpate the patient's pulse with the right hand and use the left hand to palpate his or her own right radial pulse. If the pulses are different, the examiner is feeling the patient's pulse with the right hand.

Examination of the Lymphatic System

Physical signs of lymphatic system disease include the following:

- Palpable lymph nodes
- Lymphangitis
- Lymphedema

Lymph nodes should be described as painless or tender or as single or matted. Generalized lymphadenopathy suggests diagnoses different from localized adenopathy. *Generalized* lymphadenopathy is the presence of palpable lymph nodes in three or more lymph node chains. Lymphoma, leukemia, collagen vascular disorders, and systemic bacterial, viral, and protozoal infections may be responsible. *Localized* lymphadenopathy is usually the result of localized infection or neoplasm. *Lymphangitis* is lymphatic spread manifested by thin red streaks on the skin. Obstruction to lymphatic flow produces *lymphedema,* which is usually indistinguishable from other types of edema.

The examinations for lymphadenopathy of the head, neck, and supraclavicular areas are described in Chapters 7, The Head and Neck, and 11, The Chest. Chapter 14, The Breast, describes the examination for palpating axillary adenopathy. Chapter 16, Male Genitalia and Hernias, describes the technique for palpating inguinal lymph nodes. The only other important lymph node chain is the epitrochlear nodes, which are discussed in the following section.

Palpate for Epitrochlear Nodes

Epitrochlear nodes are palpated by having the patient flex the elbow about 90°. The examiner should feel for the nodes in the fossa about 3 cm proximal to the medial epicondyle of the humerus, in the groove between the biceps and the triceps muscles. Epitrochlear nodes are rarely palpable but, if present, should be described as to their size, consistency, and tenderness. Acute infections of the ulnar aspect of the forearm and hand may be responsible for epitrochlear adenopathy. Epitrochlear nodes are also seen in non-Hodgkin's lymphomas.

Other Special Techniques

Evaluate Arterial Supply in the Lower Extremity

The most important sign of arterial insufficiency is a decreased pulse. In patients in whom chronic arterial insufficiency of the lower extremity is suspected, another test may be useful. The amount of pallor that develops after elevation and dependency of the ischemic extremity provides an approximate guide to the extent of decreased circulation. The patient is asked to lie on the back, and the examiner elevates the patient's legs at about 45° above the bed. The patient is asked to move the ankles to help drain the blood from the venous system, making the color changes more obvious. After about 30 seconds, the feet are inspected for pallor. Mild pallor is normal. At this point, the patient is asked to sit dangling the feet off the side of the bed, and the examiner quickly assesses the time for color return. Normally, it takes 10 seconds for color to return and 15 seconds for the superficial veins to fill. A prolongation is related to arterial insufficiency, as is the development of a dusky or cyanotic color. This test is useful only if the superficial veins are competent.

Evaluate Arterial Supply in the Upper Extremity

Chronic arterial insufficiency of the upper extremity is much less common than that of the lower extremity. *Allen's test* may be used to determine whether arterial insufficiency exists in the upper extremity. This test takes advantage of the radial-ulnar loop. The ulnar artery is normally not palpable. Allen's test determines the patency of the radial and ulnar arteries. The radial artery is first occluded by the examiner applying firm pressure over it. The patient is then asked to clench the fist tightly. The patient is asked to open the fist, and the color of the palm is observed. The test is repeated with occlusion of the ulnar artery. Pallor of the palm during compression of one artery indicates occlusion of the other.

Test for Incompetent Saphenous Veins

The diagnosis of incompetent saphenous vein valves is easy to demonstrate on examination. The patient is asked to stand, and the dilated varicose vein will become obvious. The examiner compresses the proximal end of the varicose vein with one hand while placing the other hand about 15–20 cm below it at the distal end of the vein. Incompetent saphenous valves present between the portion of the vein examined will produce a transmission of an impulse to the distal fingers.

▩ Test for Retrograde Filling

The *Trendelenburg maneuver* tests for retrograde filling of the superficial venous system. A tourniquet is placed around the upper thigh of a patient's leg after it has been elevated 90° for 15 seconds. The tourniquet should not occlude the arterial pulse. The patient is then instructed to stand, while the examiner watches for venous filling. The saphenous vein should fill slowly from below in about 30 seconds. Filling from above indicates retrograde flow. After 30 seconds, the tourniquet is released. Any sudden filling also indicates incompetent saphenous vein valves.

All the described tests are to be used in conjunction with other forms of testing. Each of these special vascular techniques has been associated with many false-positive and false-negative findings. The results, therefore, must be considered as part of the total evaluation.

Clinicopathologic Correlations

The signs of an acute arterial occlusion are the *five Ps: p*ain, *p*allor, *p*aresthesia, *p*aralysis, and *p*ulselessness.

Chronic progressive small vessel disease is characteristic of diabetes mellitus. It is commonly observed that arterial pulses are present despite a gangrenous extremity. Look at Figure 13–13. The patient, who was diabetic, had dry gangrene of his toes.

Diabetes has been associated with many skin disorders. The cutaneous hallmark of diabetes is a waxy, yellow, reddish-brown, sharply demarcated, plaque-like lesion known as *necrobiosis lipoidica diabeticorum.* These lesions are classically found on the anterior surface of the lower legs. They are shiny and atrophic, with marked telangiectasia over their surface. The lesions have a tendency to ulcerate, and the ulcers, once present, heal very slowly. Necrobiosis lipoidica diabeticorum often predates the frank development of diabetes. The severity of the cutaneous lesion is not related to the severity of the diabetes. Figure 13–14 shows a patient with necrobiosis lipoidica diabeticorum; Figure 13–15 shows a close-up of the lesion in another patient with diabetes.

Deep vein thrombosis of a lower extremity is diagnosed when there is unilateral marked swelling, venous distention, erythema, pain, increased warmth, and tenderness. There is often resistance to dorsiflexion of the ankle. Calf swelling is present in most patients with femoral or popliteal venous involvement, whereas thigh swelling occurs

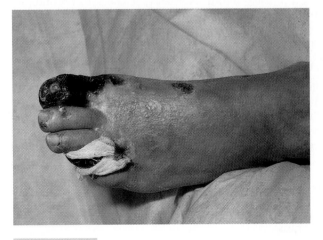

Figure 13–13

Diabetic gangrene.

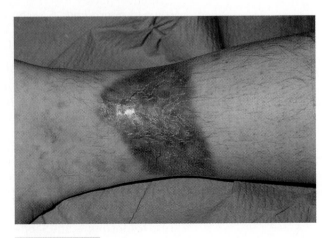

Figure 13–14

Necrobiosis lipoidica diabeticorum.

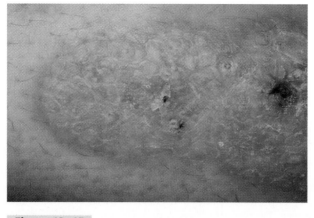

Figure 13–15

Close-up of a necrobiosis lipoidica diabeticorum lesion.

with iliofemoral thrombosis. Figure 13–16 shows left femoral deep vein thrombosis secondary to cancer. Notice the marked swelling of the left leg.

Gentle squeezing of the affected calf or slow dorsiflexion of the ankle may produce calf pain in approximately 50% of patients with femoral vein thrombosis. Pain elicited in this technique is referred to as a *positive Homans' sign*. Unfortunately, owing to the low sensitivity of Homans' sign, this finding should not be used as a single criterion for deep vein thrombophlebitis. A variety of unrelated conditions also may elicit a false-positive response.

As a result of the venous thrombosis, a secondary inflammation around the vein may result. Erythema, warmth, and fever then occur, and *thrombophlebitis* is present.

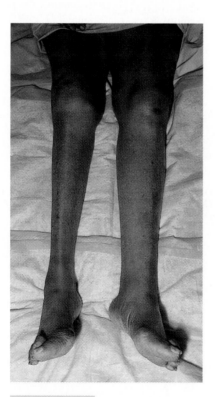

Figure 13–16

Deep vein thrombosis.

Frequency, the examiner can palpate this tender, indurated vein in the groin or medial thigh. This is commonly referred to as a *cord*.

Deep venous thrombophlebitis is associated with symptomatic *pulmonary embolism* in approximately 10% of patients. If the embolus is large, main pulmonary artery obstruction may occur, which can result in death. It is estimated that an additional 45% of patients with thrombophlebitis suffer asymptomatic pulmonary emboli.

Several factors importat in precipitating thromboembolism are outlined in Table 13–2.

An important and common peripheral vascular condition is *Raynaud's disease* or *phenomenon*. Classically, this condition is associated with three color changes of the distal fingers or toes: white *(pallor)*, blue *(cyanosis),* and red *(rubor)*. These color changes are related to arteriospasm and decreased blood supply (pallor), increased peripheral extraction of oxygen (cyanosis), and return of blood supply (rubor). The patient may experience pain or numbness of the involved area as a result of the pallor and cyanosis. During the hyperemic or rubor stage, the patient may complain of burning paresthesias. Between episodes, there may be no symptoms or signs of the condition.

Primary or idiopathic Raynaud's disease must be differentiated from *secondary* Raynaud's phenomenon. Table 13–3 lists some of the differential characteristics of these conditions. *Gangrene* is necrosis of the deep tissues resulting from a decreased blood supply. A summary of the major features of the main vascular diseases causing gangrene of the lower extremities is shown in Table 13–4.

Table 13–2   Precipitating Factors in Thromboembolism

Factor	Cause
Stasis	Arrhythmia
	Heart failure
	Immobilization
	Obesity
	Varicose veins
	Dehydration
Blood vessel injury	Trauma
	Fracture
Increased coagulability	Neoplasm
	Oral contraceptives
	Pregnancy
	Polycythemia
	Previous thromboembolism

Table 13–3   Differential Diagnosis of Raynaud's Disease from Raynaud's Phenomenon

Feature	Raynaud's Disease	Raynaud's Phenomenon
Sex	Female	Female
Bilaterality	Present (often symmetric)	±(asymmetric)
Precipitated by cold	Common	Increases symptoms
Ischemic changes	Rare	Common
Gangrene	Rare	More commonly seen
Disease association*	No	Yes

* Such as scleroderma, systemic lupus erythematosus, dermatomyositis, or rheumatoid arthritis.

Table 13–4   Differential Diagnosis of the Main Vascular Diseases Causing Gangrene

Feature	Diabetes	Atherosclerosis	Thromboangiitis Obliterans	Raynaud's Disease	Arterial Embolism
Age	Any	Older than 60 years	Younger than 40 years	Younger than 40 years	Any
Sex	Either	Either	Male	Female	Either
Onset	Gradual	Gradual	Gradual	Gradual	Sudden
Pain	Moderate	Moderate	Severe	Moderate	Often severe
Distal pulses	May be absent	May be absent	May be absent	Present	Absent*

* Affected artery does not have pulsation.

Useful Vocabulary

Listed here are the specific roots that are important in order to understand the terminology related to vascular disease.

Root	Pertaining to	Example	Definition
angi(o)-	blood vessel	*angio*graphy	X-ray visualization of blood vessels
embolo-	wedge; stopper	*embol*ism	Sudden blocking of a vessel by a clot
phleb(o)-	veins	*phlebo*tomy	Incision into a vein for blood removal
thrombo-	clot	*thrombo*embolism	Obstruction of a blood vessel by a clot that has broken loose from its site of formation
varico-	twisted; swollen	*varico*se	Unnaturally swollen and twisted

Writing Up the Physical Examination

Listed here are examples of the write-up for the examination of the vascular system.

- The extremities are normal in color, size, and temperature. All pulses in the upper and lower extremities are grade 2 and are equal. No bruits are present. No clubbing, cyanosis, or edema is present.
- There are bilateral, yellow, waxy, sharply demarcated lesions on both anterior shins. Both legs appear slightly cool, the left greater than the right. There is a punched-out ulceration on the lateral aspect of the left ankle. The left big toe is blackened, with a sharp demarcation. The femoral pulses are grade 2 bilaterally. No distal pulses are felt. There is 1+ pretibial edema present bilaterally. No clubbing or cyanosis is present.
- The right lower extremity is 3 cm larger than the left, measured 4 cm below the inferior aspect of the patella. The right calf is tender, warm, and erythematous. A cord is palpated in the right groin. Both lower extremities are edematous and hyperpigmented. There is 3+ pretibial edema on the right and 2+ pretibial edema on the left. A small ulceration is present above the left medial malleolus. The arterial pulses are grade 2 at the femorals and grade 1 at the popliteals. No pulses are palpated distal to the popliteals. No clubbing or cyanosis is present.

Bibliography

Fenton S, Lyttle JA, Pantridge JF: Diagnosis and results of surgery in renovascular hypertension. Lancet 2:117, 1966.

Grim CE, Luft FC, Myron H, et al: Sensitivity and specificity of screening tests for renal vascular hypertension. Ann Intern Med 91:617, 1979.

Hunt JC, Strong CG: Renovascular hypertension: Mechanisms, natural history, and treatment. Am J Cardiol 32:562, 1973.

Juergens JL, Spittell JA Jr, Fairbairn JF II: Allen-Barker-Hines Peripheral Vascular Diseases, 5th ed. Philadelphia, W.B. Saunders, 1980.

Kurtz KJ: Dynamic vascular auscultation. Am J Med 76:1066, 1984.

Lederle FA, Walker JM, Reinke DB: Selective screening for abdominal aortic aneurysms with physical examination and ultrasound. Arch Intern Med 148:1753, 1988.

Turnbull JM: Is listening for abdominal bruits useful in the evaluation of hypertension? JAMA 274: 1299, 1995.

CHAPTER 14

The Breast

The shape of the breast is like a gourd. They are round for holding blood to be changed into milk. . . . They have teats, that the new born child may suck therefrom.

Mondino De' Luzzi
1275–1326

General Considerations

In the United States, 1 woman of every 10 will develop breast cancer at some time during her life. Among the malignant diseases, breast cancer is the most common cause of death in women. It accounts for 26% of new cancers in American women and 18% of cancer deaths. In 1995 in the United States, there were more than 150,000 new cases with 50,000 deaths. The incidence of cancer of the breast is higher in the United States than in European or Asian countries. It has been well established that women in underdeveloped nations have lower rates of breast cancer than do women from more affluent societies.

Once breast cancer has occurred in a family, the risk that other women in the same family will develop breast cancer is significantly higher. First degree relatives, such as sisters or daughters, have more than twice the risk of developing breast cancer if the original patient developed cancer in one breast after menopause. Women with a family history of premenopausal breast cancer in one breast have three times the risk. If the original patient had postmenopausal cancer in both breasts, the first degree relatives have more than four times the risk. First degree relatives of patients with cancer in both breasts before menopause have nearly nine times the risk.

The age at onset of menarche and the reproductive cycle seems to play some role in the development of breast cancer. In women with menarche before the age of 12 years, the incidence of breast cancer appears to be higher. Women who had their first child at the age of 30 years or older have three times the risk than those having their first child at a younger age.

Most breast cancers are detected as painless masses noticed by either the patient or the examiner during a routine physical examination. The earlier the diagnosis, the better the prognosis. The most rewarding method of screening for breast cancer is annual clinical breast examination.

Structure and Physiology

The *mammary glands* are the distinguishing feature of all mammals. Human breasts are conical in form but are often unequal in size. The breast extends from the second or third rib to the sixth or seventh rib, from the sternal edge to the anterior axillary line. The "tail" of the breast extends into the axilla and tends to be thicker than the other breast areas. This upper outer quadrant contains the greater bulk of mammary tissue and is frequently the site of neoplasia. Figure 14–1 illustrates the normal breast.

The normal breast consists of glandular tissue, ducts, supporting muscular tissue, fat, blood vessels, nerves, and lymphatics. The glandular tissue consists of 15–25 lobes, each of which drains into a separate excretory duct that terminates in the nipple. Each duct dilates as it enters the base of the nipple to form a *milk sinus*. This serves as a reservoir for milk during lactation. Each lobe is subdivided into 50–75 lobules, which drain into a duct that empties into the excretory duct of the lobe.

Both the nipple and areola contain smooth muscle that serves to contract the areola and compress the nipple. Contraction of the smooth muscle makes the nipple erect and firm, thereby facilitating the emptying of the milk sinuses.

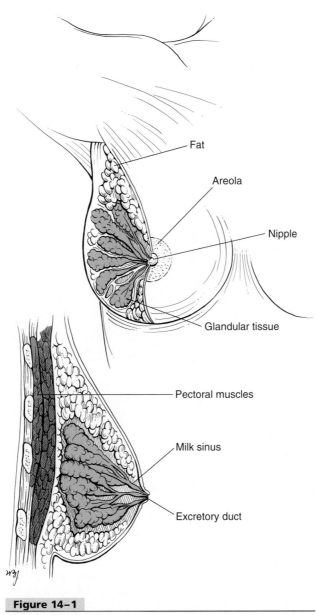

Figure 14–1

Anatomy of a normal breast.

The skin of the nipple is deeply pigmented and hairless. The dermal papillae contain many sebaceous glands, which are grouped near the openings of the milk sinuses. The skin of the areola is also deeply pigmented but, unlike the skin of the nipple, contains occasional hair follicles. Its sebaceous glands are commonly seen as small nodules on the areolar surface and are termed *Montgomery's tubercles.*

Cooper's ligaments are projections of the breast tissue that fuse with the outer layers of the superficial fascia and serve as suspensory structures.

The blood supply to the breast is carried by the internal mammary artery. The breast has an extensive network of venous and lymphatic drainage. Most of the lymphatic drainage empties into the nodes in the axilla. Other nodes lie beneath the lateral margin of the pectoralis major muscle, along the medial side of the axilla, and in the subclavicular region. The main lymph node chains and lymphatic drainage of the breast are shown in Figure 14–2.

Several physiologic changes occur in the breast. These changes are a result of the following factors:

- Growth and aging
- The menstrual cycle
- Pregnancy

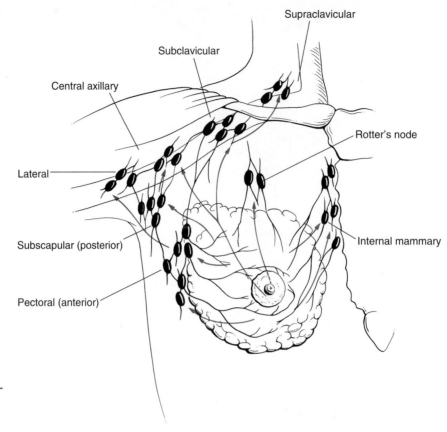

Figure 14–2

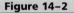

Lymphatic drainage of the breast.

At birth, the breasts contain a branching system of ducts emptying into a developed nipple. There is elevation of only the nipple at this stage. Shortly after birth, there is a slight secretion of milky material. After 5–7 days, this secretory activity stops. Before puberty, there is elevation of the breast and nipple, called the breast bud stage. The areola has increased in size. At the onset of puberty, the areola enlarges further and darkens in color. A distinct mass of glandular tissue begins to develop beneath the areola. By the onset of menstruation, the breasts are well developed, and there is forward projection of the areola and nipple at the apex of the breast. One to 2 years later, when the breast has reached maturity, only the nipple projects forward; the areola has receded to the general contour of the breast. The stages of breast development from birth to adulthood are illustrated in Figure 14–3. Figure 22–25 (Chapter 22, The Pediatric Patient) further illustrates and describes the breast developmental stages.

The nodularity, density, and fullness of the adult breast depend on several factors. Most important is the presence of excess adipose tissue. Because the mammary gland consists mainly of adipose tissue, women who are overweight have larger breasts. Pregnancy and nursing also alter the character of the breasts. Women who have nursed often have softer, less nodular breasts. However, because the glandular tissue is approximately equal in all women, the size of the breast is unrelated to nursing. With menopause, the breasts decrease in size and become less dense. There is an associated increase in elastic tissue as women age.

The major physiologic change related to the menstrual cycle is engorgement, occurring 3–5 days before menstruation. This is an increase in the size, density, and nodularity of the breasts. There is also an increased sensitivity of the breasts at this time. Because the nodularity of the breasts increases, the examiner should not attempt to diagnose a breast mass at this time. The patient should be re-evaluated during the midperiod of the next cycle.

With pregnancy, the breasts become fuller and firmer. The areola darkens, and the nipples become erect as they enlarge. As the woman approaches the 3rd trimester, a thin, yellowish secretion, called *colostrum,* may be noted. After the birth of the child, if the mother begins nursing within 24 hours the secretion of colostrum will stop, and the

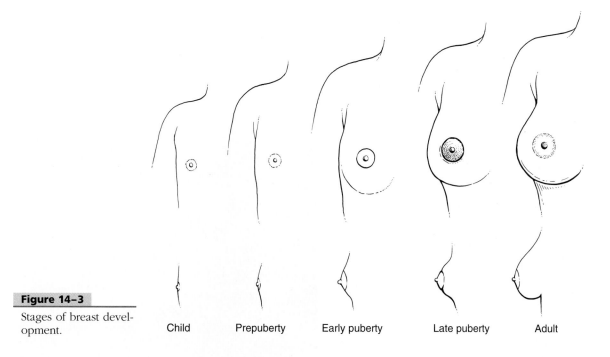

Figure 14–3

Stages of breast development.

Child   Prepuberty   Early puberty   Late puberty   Adult

secretion of milk will begin. During nursing, the breasts become markedly engorged. After the woman has stopped nursing, lactation will continue for a short period.

The neuroendocrine control of the breasts can be outlined as follows. Suckling produces nerve impulses that travel to the hypothalamus. The hypothalamus stimulates the anterior pituitary to secrete *prolactin,* which acts on the glandular tissue of the breast to produce milk. The hypothalamus also stimulates the posterior pituitary to produce *oxytocin,* which stimulates the muscle cells surrounding the glandular tissue to contract and force the milk into the ductular system.

Many abnormalities of the breast are related to its embryology. An epithelial ridge, called the *milk line,* forms along each side of the body from the axilla to the inguinal region. Along this milk line are multiple rudiments for future breast development. In humans, only one rudimentary pair in the pectoral region persists and eventually develops into normal breasts. Accessory breasts or nipples do occur in as many as 2% of white women. Accessory breasts may exist as glandular tissue, nipple, or only the areola. The axilla is the most common site for these anomalous structures, followed by a site just below the normal breast. In more than 50% of all patients with accessory breast tissue, the anomalies are bilateral. In general, accessory breast tissue is of little clinical significance. It usually has no physiologic function and is rarely associated with disease. Figure 14–4 illustrates the milk line. Figure 14–5 shows a woman with an accessory nipple.

Review of Specific Symptoms

The most important symptoms of breast disease are the following:

- Mass or swelling
- Pain
- Nipple discharge
- Change in skin over breast

Mass or Swelling

During self-examination, a patient may discover a breast mass. Ask the following questions:

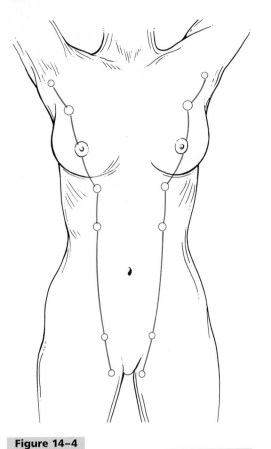

Figure 14–4

The milk line.

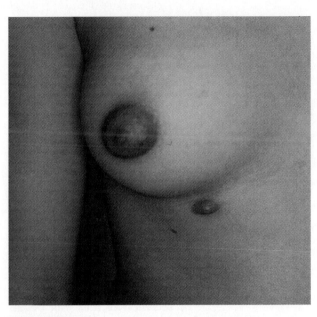

Figure 14–5

Accessory nipple.

"When did you first notice the lump?"
"Have you noticed that the mass changes in size during your menstrual periods?"
"Is the mass tender?"
"Have you ever noticed a mass in your breast before?"
"Have you noticed any skin changes on the breast?"
"Have you had any recent injury to the breast?"
"Is there any nipple discharge? nipple retraction?"

If the lump enlarges during the premenstrual and menstrual stages of the cycle, it is likely that the woman is detecting only physiologic nodularity. The association of nipple discharge, nipple inversion, or skin changes overlying the mass is strongly suggestive of neoplasm. Figure 14–6 shows a patient with a large breast mass found on self-examination.

Pain

Breast pain or tenderness is a common symptom. Most often, these symptoms are due to the normal physiologic cycle. Ask the following questions of any patient with breast pain:

"Can you describe the pain?"
"When did you first experience the pain?"
"Are there any changes in the pain with your menstrual cycle?"
"Do you have pain in both breasts?"
"Have you had any injury to the breast?"
"Is the pain associated with a mass in the breast? nipple discharge? nipple retraction?"
"Has there been a change in your brassiere size?"

Rapidly enlarging cysts may be painful. Cystic disease of the breasts, as well as breast cancer, is usually painless.

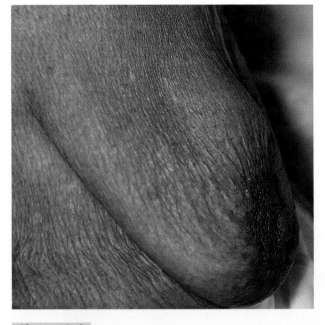

Figure 14–6

Large breast mass found on self-examination.

Nipple Discharge

Nipple discharge is not a common symptom, but it should always raise the suspicion of breast disease, especially if the discharge occurs spontaneously. Any patient who describes a nipple discharge should be asked the following questions:

> *"What is the color of the discharge?"*
> *"Do you have a discharge from both breasts?"*
> *"When did you first notice the discharge?"*
> *"Is the discharge related to your menstrual cycle?"*
> *"When was your last menstrual cycle?"*
> *"Is the discharge associated with nipple retraction? a breast mass? breast tenderness?"*
> *"Do you have headaches?"*
> *"Are you taking any medications?"*
> *"Are you using oral contraceptives?"*
> If the woman has recently delivered a child, *"Were there any problems during the delivery of your last child?"*

The most common types of discharge are serous and bloody. A *serous* discharge is thin and watery and may appear as a yellowish stain on the patient's garments. This commonly results from an intraductal papilloma in one of the large subareolar ducts. Women taking oral contraceptives may complain of bilateral serous discharge. A serous discharge can also occur in women with breast carcinoma.

A *bloody* discharge is associated with an intraductal papilloma, which is common among pregnant and menstruating women. It may, however, be associated with a malignant intraductal papillary carcinoma. The presence of any nipple discharge is more important than its character, because both types of discharge are associated with benign or malignant disease.

A milky discharge is usually milk. It is common for women to continue to secrete milk for a few months after they stop nursing. In rare instances, the secretion may continue for a year. Persistent lactation, also known as *galactorrhea,* can be a result of massive hemorrhage occurring during childbirth and producing pituitary necrosis. Abnormal lactation may also result from a pituitary tumor that interferes with the normal hypothalamic-pituitary feedback loop or from the use of certain tranquilizing medications. Mechanical stimulation or suckling may produce physiologic stimulation.

Change in Skin over Breast

A change in the color or texture of the skin of the breast or areola is an important symptom of breast carcinoma. The presence of dimpling, puckering, or scaliness warrants further investigation. The presence of unusually prominent pores, indicative of edema of the skin, is an important sign of malignancy. This clinical sign is called *peau d'orange* because of its orange-peel appearance. During the early stages of breast carcinoma, the lymphatics of the breast are dilated and contain occasional emboli of carcinoma cells. Limited peau d'orange over the lower half of the areola is present. As the disease progresses, more lymphatics become filled with carcinoma cells that block them, creating more generalized edema. Figure 14–7 shows the classic appearance of peau d'orange.

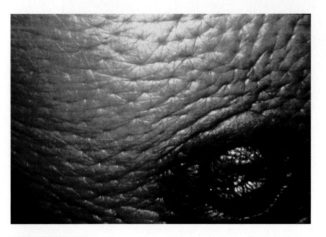

Figure 14–7

Peau d'orange.

General Suggestions

The interviewer should pay special attention to the family history of any woman presenting with symptoms of breast disease. As indicated earlier, breast cancer is a familial disorder. The occurrence of breast disease in a close relative and the age at which it developed are relevant to the patient's disease.

Impact of Breast Disease on the Patient

The psychosocial problems resulting from breast cancer are far-reaching. Although the loss of an extremity is more disabling in everyday life, the loss of a breast produces intense feelings of loss of the feminine identity. Many women who lose a breast become depressed, because they feel their symbol of femininity has been removed. They are afraid that they will no longer be considered "whole" women because their bodies have been maimed. They fear that they can no longer be loved normally and that they can no longer experience sexual satisfaction. They fear looking at themselves in a mirror and perceive themselves as ugly. The asymmetry is often described as "mutilation" or "a bomb crater." After mastectomy, women often suffer from sexual inhibition and sexual frustration.

Once a woman has discovered a mass in her breast, she becomes intensely fearful. The fear of breast cancer is twofold: it is a cancer, often with a bad prognosis, and it is associated with disfigurement. For these reasons, the patient commonly denies the presence of the mass and delays seeking medical attention. It is not uncommon for a patient to seek medical assistance for the first time with a large tumor mass the size of an orange that has eroded through the skin and has become infected. When asked how long the mass has been present, the woman might answer that she "discovered it yesterday."

After a mastectomy, the patient will probably suffer from depression and low self-esteem. The patient should be supported, and counseled if necessary. Open communication and sharing of feelings among the patient, husband, significant other, physician, and family are important factors in the psychological rehabilitation of the woman.

Look at Figure 14–8. The patient has inflammatory carcinoma of her left breast, with massive lymphedema of the left arm. The patient had noticed that her arm had been swelling for the past few months, and she now needed support in order to raise it. She presented to the clinic complaining only about the heaviness of her arm. When examination revealed the breast lesion, she stated that she had noticed the breast changes "only a few days ago." This is the story of denial.

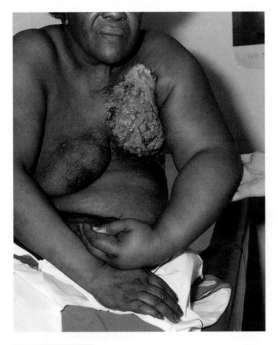

Figure 14–8

Inflammatory breast carcinoma.

Physical Examination

No special equipment is necessary for the examination of the breast.

The examination of the breast consists of the following:

- Inspection
- Axillary examination
- Palpation

The examination of the breast is in two parts. The first is performed with the patient sitting up. Inspection of the breasts and palpation of the lymph nodes are done in this position. The second is performed with the patient lying down. The examiner systematically palpates the entire breast by using firm, gentle pressure exerted by the pulp of the finger rather than the fingertips.

To facilitate communication, the breast is divided into four quadrants. Two imaginary lines are drawn through the nipple at right angles to each other. By visualizing the breast as a face of a clock, one line is the "12 o'clock–6 o'clock" line, and the other is the "3 o'clock–9 o'clock" line. The resulting four quadrants are the upper outer, upper inner, lower outer, and lower inner. The "tail" is an extension of the upper outer quadrant. This is illustrated in Figure 14–9.

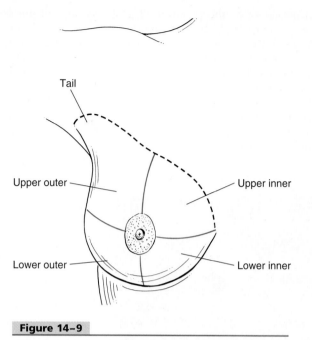

Figure 14–9

The four breast quadrants.

Inspection

The woman should be seated on the edge of the examination table, facing the examiner. The examiner should ask the woman to remove her gown to her waist.

▧ Inspect the Breasts

Inspection is first accomplished with the patient's arms at her side, as shown in Figure 14–10. Tell the patient, "I am inspecting the breasts for any changes in the skin, contour, or symmetry." The breasts are inspected for size, shape, symmetry, contour, color, and edema. The nipples are inspected as to size, shape, inversion, eversion, or discharge. The nipples should be symmetric. Is any abnormal bulging present?

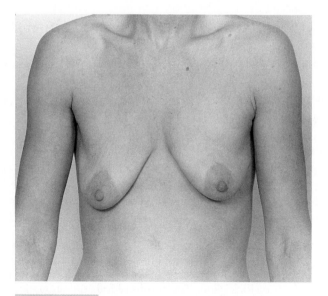

Figure 14–10

Position of patient for inspection of the breasts.

The skin of the breast is observed for edema. Edema of the skin of the breast that overlies a malignancy may show peau d'orange.

Is erythema present? Erythema is associated with infection and with inflammatory carcinoma of the breast. Figure 14–11 shows marked erythema of the breast secondary to inflammatory breast carcinoma. The scar above the areola is from a previous biopsy of a benign breast mass.

Is dimpling present? The examiner must inspect the breasts for the presence of *retraction phenomena*. Dimpling is a sign of the retraction phenomena that are due to an underlying neoplasm and its fibrotic response. Skin retraction is commonly associated with malignancy that causes an abnormal traction on Cooper's ligaments. The shortening of the larger mammary ducts by cancer produces flattening or inversion of the nipple. A change in the position of the nipple is important, because many women have a congenitally inverted nipple on one or both sides. The dimpling of the breast in Figure 14–12 is associated with a bloody nipple discharge; both are secondary to carcinoma.

Is there a red, scaling, crusting plaque around one nipple, areola, or surrounding skin? *Paget's disease* of the breast is a surface manifestation invariably associated with an underlying invasive or intraductal carcinoma. The lesion appears eczematous, but unlike eczema, it is unilateral. The skin may also weep and be eroded. A much less common form is extramammary Paget's disease, which is seen around the anus or genitalia and is usually associated with malignant disease of the adnexae, bowel, or genitourinary tract. Figure 14–13 shows a patient with Paget's disease of the breast; an underlying ductal adenocarcinoma was present.

▪ Inspect the Breasts in Various Postures

Inspection is next performed while the woman assumes several postures that may bring out signs of retraction that were previously less evident. Ask the woman to press her arms against her hips. This maneuver tenses the pectoralis muscles, which may bring out dimpling caused by fixation of the breast to the underlying muscles. This technique is shown in Figure 14–14. If a malignancy is present, the abnormal attachment of the tumor to the fascia and pectoralis muscle will draw on the skin and may produce skin dimpling. Any bulging may also indicate an underlying mass.

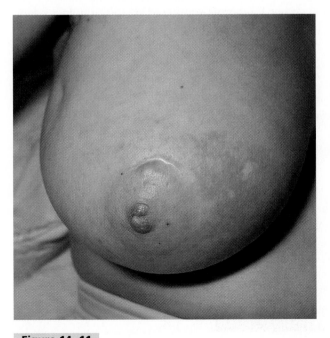

Figure 14–11

Erythema of the breast.

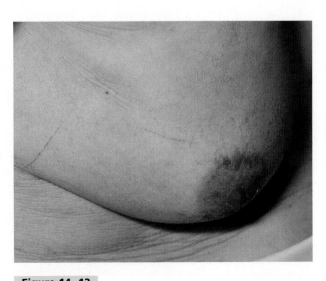

Figure 14–12

Breast carcinoma. Note dimpling of the breast and bloody nipple discharge.

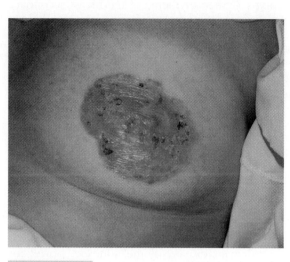

Figure 14–13

Paget's disease of the breast.

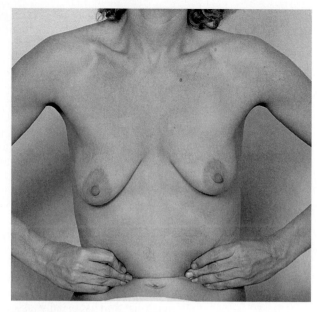

Figure 14–14

Technique for tensing the pectoralis muscles.

Another maneuver, which is useful for a woman with pendulous breasts, involves asking her to bend at the waist and allow her breasts to hang free from the chest wall. This technique is shown in Figure 14–15. A carcinoma causing fibrosis in one breast will produce a change in the contour of that breast.

Axillary Examination

The axillary examination is performed with the patient seated facing the examiner.

■ Palpate Axillary Nodes

Examination of the axilla is best accomplished by relaxing the pectoral muscles. To examine the right axilla, the patient's right forearm is supported by the examiner's right hand. The tips of the fingers of the examiner's left hand start low in the axilla, and, as the patient's right arm is drawn medially, the examiner advances the left hand higher into the axilla. This technique is shown in Figure 14–16. Palpate the supraclavicular, subclavian, and axillary regions.

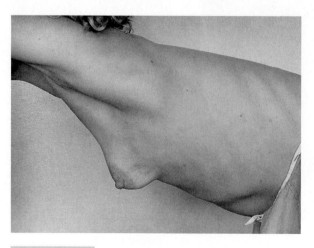

Figure 14–15

Position of patient for inspecting the breasts.

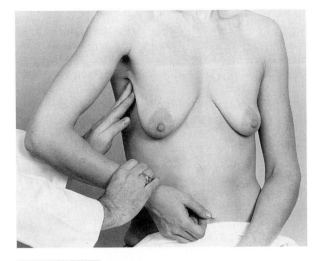

Figure 14–16

Technique for axillary examination.

The technique of using small, circular motions of the fingers riding over the ribs is used for detecting adenopathy. Freely mobile nodes 3–5 mm in diameter are common and are usually indicative of lymphadenitis secondary to minor trauma of the hand and arm. After one axilla is examined, the other is evaluated by the examiner's opposite hand.

Palpation

The woman is asked to lie down and is told that palpation of the breast is next. The examiner stands at the right side of the patient's bed. Although the examiner can usually palpate each breast from the patient's right side, it is often better with large-breasted women to examine the left breast from the left side.

The breast is best palpated by allowing it to lie evenly distributed over the chest wall. Small-breasted women may lie with their arms at their sides; larger-breasted women should be instructed to place their hands behind their head. A pillow placed beneath the shoulder on the side being examined facilitates the examination.

◼ Palpate the Breast

In palpation of the breast, the examiner should use both the flat of the hand and the fingertips, as shown in Figure 14–17. Palpation should be performed by the "spokes of

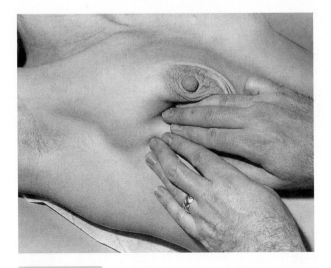

Figure 14–17

Technique for breast palpation.

a wheel," the "concentric circle," or the vertical strip method. The "spokes of a wheel" method starts at the nipple. The examiner should start the palpation by moving outward from the nipple to the 12 o'clock position. The examiner then should return to the nipple and move along the 1 o'clock position and continue the palpation around the breasts. The "concentric circles approach" also starts at the nipple, but the examiner moves from the nipple in a continuous circular manner around the breast. Any lesion found by either technique is described as being a certain distance from the nipple in clock time: for example, 3 cm from the nipple along the 1 o'clock line. These techniques are illustrated in Figure 14–18.

Another method is the vertical strip, or grid, technique. The breast is divided into eight or nine vertical strips, each approximately one finger-width wide. The examiner's three middle fingers are held together and slightly bowed to ensure contact with the skin. The pads, not the tips, of the fingers must be used for palpation. Using dime-sized circles, the examiner evaluates the breast at each of three different levels of pressure—light, medium, and deep. Each strip consists of nine or ten areas of palpation, slightly overlapping the previous area, and each vertical strip is evaluated with the

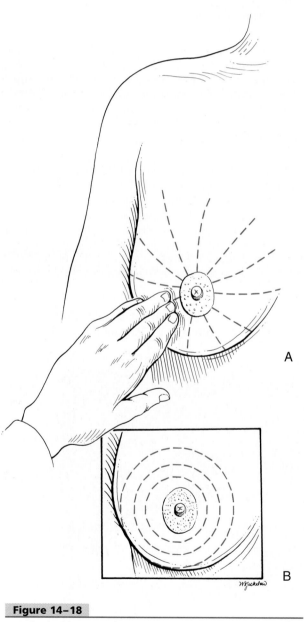

Figure 14–18

Method of breast palpation. *A,* "Spokes of a wheel." *B,* "Concentric circles."

three pressures. Although this method has been shown to be superior to the other traditional types of breast palpation, it is more time-consuming and may be best used by women for breast self-examination.

The examiner should be careful when evaluating the *inframammary fold*. This fold is commonly observed in older women and is the area where the mammary tissue is bound tightly to the chest wall. Often, this ridge is mistaken for a breast disorder.

Describe the Findings

If a mass is palpated, the following characteristics should be described:

1. The *size* of the mass in centimeters and its position.
2. The *shape* of the mass.
3. The *delimitation,* referring to the borders of the mass. Is it well delimited, as with a cyst? Are the edges diffuse, as with a carcinoma?
4. The *consistency,* describing the "hardness" of the mass. A carcinoma is often stony hard. A cyst has some elastic qualities.
5. The *mobility* of the lesion. Is the lesion movable in the tissue that surrounds it? Benign tumors and cysts are freely mobile. Carcinomas are generally fixed to the skin, underlying muscle, or chest wall.

Evaluate for Retraction Phenomenon

If a mass is detected, *molding* of the skin may be useful to determine whether the retraction phenomenon is present. The examiner should elevate the breast around the mass. Dimpling may occur if a carcinoma is present. Figure 14–19 shows the technique of molding and its result in a patient with carcinoma of the breast. Notice the marked dimpling of the breast. This patient also has metastatic lesions of breast carcinoma on her arm together with lymphedema. She presented to the clinic stating that she had discovered the swollen arm the day before.

Palpate the Subareolar Area

The subareolar area, the area directly under the areola, should be palpated while the patient is lying supine. In the subareolar area, the breast tissue is less dense. An abscess of Montgomery's glands in the areola may cause a tender mass in this area.

Examine the Nipple

Examination of the nipple concludes the examination of the breast. Inspect for nipple retraction, fissures, and scaling. To examine for discharge, place each hand on either side of the nipple and gently compress the nipple, noting the character of any discharge. This technique is shown in Figure 14–20. Ask the woman whether she would prefer to do this part of the examination herself.

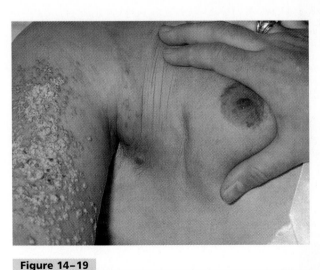

Figure 14–19

Breast dimpling. Note the satellite skin lesions of metastatic breast cancer.

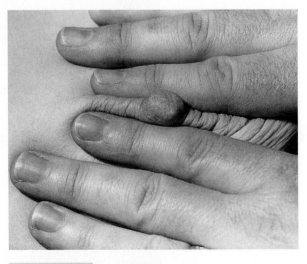

Figure 14–20

Technique for nipple examination.

The Male Breast

Gynecomastia is the enlargement of one or both breasts in a man. It often occurs at puberty, occurs with aging, or is drug-related. Figure 14–21 shows a 90 year old man who was treated with diethylstilbestrol for carcinoma of the prostate and developed gynecomastia.

Carcinoma of the breast affects approximately 1000 men per year in the United States. More than 300 men per year die of metastatic breast cancer. The average age at the time of diagnosis is 59 years. The most common clinical manifestation, occurring in 75% of cases, is a painless, firm, subareolar mass or a mass in the upper outer quadrant of the breast.

The incidence of breast carcinoma in men, as well as in women, is highest in North America and in the British Isles; it is lowest in Japan and Finland. As in women, breast carcinoma in men most commonly metastasizes to the bone, lung, liver, pleura, lymph nodes, skin, and other visceral sites.

Examination of the Male Breast

Examination of the breast should be performed on all men. The nipples should be inspected for swelling, discharge and ulceration. The areola and the subareolar tissue should be palpated for any masses. The axillary examination is as indicated for women.

Clinicopathologic Correlations

Cancer of the Breast

Two genes, BRCA1 and BRCA2, have been identified as *breast cancer susceptibility genes*. Carriers of germ-line mutations in BRCA1, located on chromosome 17, or BRCA2, located on chromosome 13, are associated with an increased incidence of early-onset, familial breast and ovarian cancer. Both genes are autosomal dominant genes. Mutations in these tumor suppressor genes have been found in 12% or more of women with early-onset breast cancers. If a mutation in the BRCA1 gene is present, it is estimated that the woman's risk of developing breast cancer may reach 85–90%.

The finding of a breast mass on palpation, even in the presence of a normal mammogram, requires a biopsy. However, breast palpation has a much lower true positive rate (sensitivity) than mammography. There are many false-negative findings in breast palpation. This is related to the difficulty in palpating a small mass in large breasts, the inherent properties of breast tissue, and poor technique. The limitations of physical examination and mammography are shown in Table 14–1.

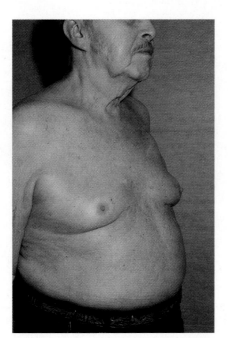

Figure 14–21

Gynecomastia.

The physical examination is of great importance in determining the probability that a mass is cancerous. Any lump detected by either the patient or the examiner carries a 20% risk of cancer (Baker, 1982). As indicated in Table 14–2, benign lesions generally are freely mobile, have well-delimited borders, and feel soft or cystic. However, of all breast cancers, 60% are freely mobile, 40% have well-delimited borders, and 50% feel soft or cystic. A fixed lesion has a 50% chance of malignancy. If this lesion had irregular borders, the likelihood of malignancy rises to 60%. The sensitivity and specificity of certain physical findings in evaluating a breast mass for malignancy are shown in Table 14–3.

Table 14–1   Limitations of Physical Examination and Mammography

Operating Characteristic	Physical Examination	Mammography
Sensitivity (%)	24	62
Specificity (%)	95	90

Data from Bond WH: The treatment of carcinoma of the breast. In Jarrett AS (ed): Proceedings of a Symposium on the Treatment of Carcinoma of the Breast. Amsterdam, Excerpta Medica, 1968.

Table 14–2   Differentiation of Breast Masses

Characteristic	Cystic Disease	Benign Adenoma	Malignant Tumor
Patient age	25–60 years	10–55 years	25–85 years
Number	One or more	One	One
Shape	Round	Round	Irregular
Consistency	Elastic, soft to hard	Firm	Stony hard
Delimitation	Well delimited	Well delimited	Poorly delimited
Mobility	Mobile	Mobile	Fixed
Tenderness	Present	Absent	Absent
Skin retraction	Absent	Absent	Present

Table 14–3   Characteristics of Breast Masses Suspicious for Cancer

Characteristic	Sensitivity (%)	Specificity* (%)
Fixed mass	40	90
Poorly delimited mass	60	90
Hard mass	62	90

* Based on the assumption that nonmalignant breast masses have benign characteristics.
Data from Venet L, Strax P, Venet W, et al: Adequacies and inadequacies of breast examination by physicians in mass screening. Cancer 28:1546, 1971.

Breast Self-Examination*

Women should be encouraged to do a breast self-examination monthly. It is important for a woman to learn what is normal and about the changes in her breasts that occur with her menstrual cycle. Familiarity with breast tissue makes it easier for the woman to notice any changes in the breast from month to month.

---

* The importance of breast self-examination has been recognized for more than 60 years. However, to date, the efficacy of this examination is not definitive. A large, randomized, controlled trial was conducted in 1997 by Thomas et al in Shanghai that included more than 267,040 women, half of whom were given intensive training in breast self-examination; the other half were asked to attend training sessions on the prevention of low back pain. All women were observed for 5 years for the development of breast diseases. The study showed neither a significant difference in mortality in the two groups nor an earlier identification of breast disease in the group trained in breast self-examination. The authors' conclusion was that "there was insufficient evidence to recommend for or against the teaching of breast self-examination."

Advise the woman that the best time to perform breast self-examination is 2 to 3 days after the end of her period. At this time the breasts will be less tender or swollen. A woman past menopause should be advised to pick a particular day of the month and then perform the examination monthly.

Advise the patient that if she discovers anything unusual, such as a lump, discharge from the nipple, or dimpling of the skin, she should seek medical attention. Inform her that 8 of 10 breast lumps are *not* cancer.

The techniques of breast self-examination are included here for the purpose of patient education:

1. Stand with your arms at your sides in front of a mirror. Inspect both breasts for anything unusual, such as dimpling, puckering, discharge from the nipples, or scaling of the skin.
2. Raise your arms and clasp your hands behind your head. Press your hands forward. Look in the mirror for any changes in the breast tissue.
3. Put your hands down and place them on your hips. Bend slightly toward the mirror as you pull your shoulders and elbows forward.
4. Raise your right arm; using the pads of your left fingers, explore your right breast firmly, carefully, and thoroughly. Start at the upper outer edge and move in small circles, moving the circles slowly around the breast. Pay special attention to the breast tissue between the breast and the underarm. Use a massaging motion.
5. Gently squeeze your nipple and look for any discharge.
6. Repeat Steps 4 and 5 while lying down with a small pillow under your right shoulder. Place your right arm over your head.
7. Repeat the examination on your left breast.

There are several errors that patients make in breast self-examination. The first is failure to perform self-examination. Menstruating patients should examine their breasts regularly, ideally just after menstrual period. Women on cyclic estrogen-progesterone replacement therapy should be instructed to examine their breasts on the last day of the interval between cycles. For postmenopausal women who are not on replacement therapy, examination of the breasts should be on the first day of the calendar month. Second, a woman should also examine her breasts in the sitting (or standing) position as well as when lying down. Third, always have the woman use a pillow under the side that is being examined. Fourth, the arm on the side being examined should be raised above the head and relaxed.

Useful Vocabulary

Listed here are the specific roots that are important in order to understand the terminology related to breast disease.

Root	Pertaining to	Example	Definition
gyne(co)-	woman	*gyneco*mastia	Excessive development of the male breast
lact(o)-	milk	*lact*ation	The secretion of milk
mammo-	breast	*mammo*graphy	X-ray visualization of the breast
mast(o)-	breast	*mast*itis	Inflammation of the breast

Writing Up the Physical Examination

Listed here are examples of the write-up for the examination of the breast.

- The breasts are symmetric, with both nipples pointing outward. The overlying skin is normal. No dimpling is present. There are no masses or discharge. Axillary examination reveals no lymphadenopathy.
- The left breast is slightly larger than the right. There is a serosanguineous discharge from the left nipple. When the patient presses her arms against her hips, a dimple is seen 4 cm from the nipple at the 2 o'clock position of the left breast. Palpation reveals a 2 × 3 cm stony mass under the area of dimpling. The mass appears fixed to the underlying muscle and overlying skin. Examination of the left axilla reveals numerous hard, fixed lymph nodes.
- The right breast is larger than the left. The skin is erythematous and warm to the touch, especially around the areola. The right nipple is inverted. No masses are felt. Dimpling cannot be appreciated. No axillary adenopathy is present.
- The breasts are pendulous and symmetric. Both nipples are everted. There are multiple round, freely mobile masses in both breasts, more on the right. The masses are 2–3 cm in diameter, elastic in consistency, and somewhat tender. Skin retraction is absent. No discharge is present. No axillary adenopathy is present.

Bibliography

Baker LH: Breast Cancer Detection Demonstration Project: Five-year summary report. CA 32:194, 1982.

Bond WH: The treatment of carcinoma of the breast. In Jarrett AS (ed): Proceedings of a Symposium on the Treatment of Carcinoma of the Breast. Amsterdam, Excerpta Medica, 1968.

Campbell HS, Fletcher SW, Lin S: Improving physicians' and nurses' clinical breast examination: A randomized controlled trial. Am J Prev Med 7:1, 1991.

Collins FS: BRCA1—Lots of mutations, lots of dilemmas. N Engl J Med 334:186, 1996.

Couch FJ, DeShano ML, Blackwood A, et al: BRCA1 mutations in women attending clinics that evaluate the risk of breast cancer. N Engl J Med 336:1409, 1997.

Easton DF, Ford D, Bishop DT, et al: Breast and ovarian cancer incidence in BRCA1—mutation carriers. Am J Hum Genet 56:265, 1995.

Feig SA, Schwartz GF, Nerlinger R, et al: Prognostic factors of breast neoplasms detected on screening by mammography and physical examination. Radiology 133:577, 1979.

Fletcher SW, O'Malley MS, Earp JL, et al: How best to teach women breast self-examination: A randomized controlled trial. Ann Intern Med 112:772, 1990.

Ford D, Easton DF: The genetics of breast and ovarian cancer. Br J Cancer 72:805, 1995.

Haagensen CD: Diseases of the Breast, 3rd ed. Philadelphia, W.B. Saunders, 1986.

Healy B: BRCA genes—Bookmaking, fortunetelling, and medical care. N Engl J Med 336:1448, 1997.

Hicks MJ, Davis JR, Layton JM, et al: Sensitivity of mammography and physical examination of the breast for detecting breast cancer. JAMA 242:2080, 1979.

Jaiyesimi IA, Buzdar AU, Sahin AA, et al: Carcinoma of the male breast. Ann Intern Med 117:771, 1992.

Krainer M, Silva-Arrieta S, FitzGerald MG, et al: Differential contributions of BRCA1 and BRCA2 to early-onset breast cancer. N Engl J Med 336:1416, 1997.

Pennypacker HS, Pilgrim CA: Achieving competence in clinical breast examination. Nurse Pract 4: 85, 1993.

Saunders KJ, Pilgrim CA, Pennypacker HS: Increased proficiency of search in breast self-examination. Cancer 58:2531, 1986.

Schulman JD, Stern HJ: Genetic predispostion testing for breast cancer. Cancer J Sci Am 2:244, 1996.

Struewing JP, Hartge P, Wacholder S, et al: The risk of developing cancer associated with specific mutations of BRCA1 and BRCA2 among Ashkenazi Jews. N Engl J Med 336:1401, 1997.

Thomas DB, Gao DL, Self SG, et al: Randomized trial of breast self-examination in Shanghai: Methodology and preliminary results. J Natl Cancer Inst 89:355, 1997.

Venet L, Strax P, Venet W, et al: Adequacies and inadequacies of breast examination by physicians in mass screening. Cancer 28:1546, 1971.

CHAPTER 15

The Abdomen

A good eater must be a good man; for a good eater must have good digestion, and good digestion depends upon a good conscience.

Benjamin Disraeli
1804–1881

General Considerations

Diseases of the abdomen are common. In the United States, approximately 10% of the adult male population is affected by peptic ulcer disease. Five percent of the population older than the age of 40 years has diverticular disease. Cancer of the large bowel is the second most common malignant neoplasm affecting Americans (skin cancer is the first). Annually, approximately 120,000 new cases are diagnosed, and nearly 51,000 mortalities occur.

In the general American population, the probability of developing colorectal cancer between birth and age 70 years is approximately 4%. The risk for this type of cancer differs widely among individuals. Some patients, such as those with congenital polyposis or ulcerative colitis, have a predisposition to the development of cancer of the colon, frequently at an early age. The lifetime risk of colonic cancer in patients with polyposis coli is 100% (Mulvihill, 1983). The incidence of polyposis in the population of the United States varies from 1 in 7000 to 1 in 10,000 live births. The risk of developing colonic cancer in patients with ulcerative colitis is 20% per decade.

Diet has been shown to have a relationship to the incidence of colonic cancer. Individuals on a low-fiber and high-fat diet are at higher risk.

Earlier physical diagnosis has been clearly shown to lower the mortality rates for colorectal cancer.

Structure and Physiology

For descriptive purposes, the abdominal cavity is generally divided into four quadrants. Two imaginary lines cross at the umbilicus to divide the abdomen into the *right upper* and *lower quadrants* and the *left upper* and *lower quadrants*. One line extends from the sternum to the pubic bone through the umbilicus. The second line is at right angles to the first at the level of the umbilicus. The four quadrants formed and the abdominal organs within each quadrant are shown in Figure 15–1.

Another method of description divides the abdomen into nine areas: *epigastric, umbilical, suprapubic,* right and left *hypochondriac,* right and left *lumbar,* and right and left *inguinal.* Two imaginary lines are drawn by extending the midclavicular lines to the middle of the inguinal ligaments. These lines form the lateral extent of the rectus abdominus muscles. At right angles to these lines, two parallel lines are drawn: one at the costal margins and the other at the anterosuperior iliac spines. The nine-area system is shown in Figure 15–2.

The examiner should recognize the abdominal structures that are located in each area. Table 15–1 lists the organs present in each of the four quadrants.

Because the kidneys, duodenum, and pancreas are posterior organs, it is unlikely that abnormalities in these organs can be felt in adults. In children, in whom the abdominal muscles are less developed, renal masses can often be felt.

A detailed description of the pathophysiology of the gastrointestinal system is beyond the scope of this text. A brief statement regarding the basic physiology will serve to integrate the signs and symptoms of abdominal disease.

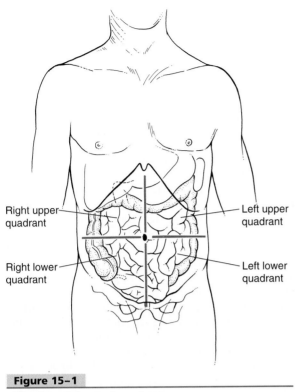

Figure 15–1

The four abdominal quadrants.

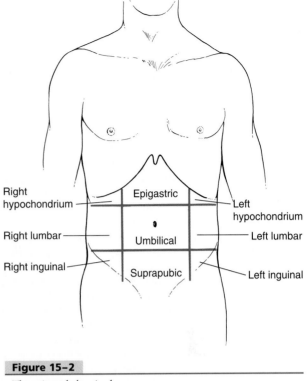

Figure 15–2

The nine abdominal areas.

Table 15–1	Abdominal Structures by Quadrants	
	Right	**Left**
Upper		
	Liver	Liver, left lobe
	Gallbladder	Spleen
	Pylorus	Stomach
	Duodenum	Pancreas: body
	Pancreas: head	Left adrenal gland
	Right adrenal gland	Left kidney: upper pole
	Right kidney: upper pole	Splenic flexure
	Hepatic flexure	Transverse colon: portion
	Ascending colon: portion	Descending colon: portion
	Transverse colon: portion	
Lower		
	Right kidney: lower pole	Left kidney: lower pole
	Cecum	Sigmoid colon
	Appendix	Descending colon: portion
	Ascending colon: portion	Left ovary
	Right ovary	Left fallopian tube
	Right fallopian tube	Left ureter
	Right ureter	Left spermatic cord
	Right spermatic cord	Uterus (if enlarged)
	Uterus (if enlarged)	Bladder (if enlarged)
	Bladder (if enlarged)	

As food passes into the esophagus, an obstructing lesion can produce *dysphagia,* or difficulty swallowing. Gastroesophageal reflux can lead to heartburn. Upon entry of partially digested food into the stomach, relaxation of the stomach occurs. A failure of this relaxation may lead to early satiety or pain. The stomach functions as a food reservoir, secreting gastric juice and providing peristaltic activity with its muscular wall. Two to three liters of gastric juice are produced daily by the stomach lining and affect the digestion of proteins. The semifluid, creamy material produced by gastric digestion of food is called *chyme.* Secretion of gastric juice may produce pain if a gastric ulcer is present. Intermittent emptying of the stomach occurs when intragastric pressure overcomes the resistance of the pyloric sphincter. Emptying is normally complete within 6 hours after eating. Any obstruction to gastric emptying may produce vomiting.

The entry of chyme from the stomach into the duodenum stimulates the secretion of pancreatic enzymes and contraction of the gallbladder. The flow of pancreatic juice is maximal approximately 2 hours after a meal; the daily output is 1–2 liters. Its three enzymes—lipase, amylase, and trypsin—are responsible for the digestion of fats, starches, and proteins, respectively. In cases of pancreatic insufficiency, the stool is pale and bulky and has more of an offensive odor. The chyme and the neutralizing effect of these enzymes reduce the acidity of the duodenal contents and relieve the pain of peptic duodenal ulcer. The pain from an acutely inflamed gallbladder or from pancreatitis worsens at this phase of the digestive cycle.

The digested food continues its course through the small intestine, where further digestion and absorption occur. Failure of bile production or its release from the gallbladder results in decreased digestion and absorption of fats, leading to diarrhea. Gallstones may form as a result of diet or hereditary predisposition.

The liver functions to produce bile, to detoxify the byproducts of the digestion of food, and to metabolize proteins, lipids, and carbohydrates. The daily output of bile is about 1 liter. In the absence of normal liver function, jaundice, ascites, and coma may result.

The jejunum and ileum further digest and absorb the nutients. Bile acids and vitamin B_{12} are absorbed in the ileum. The color of stool is due to the presence of stercobilin, a metabolite of bilirubin, which is secreted in the bile. If bile does not flow into the small intestine, the stools become clay-colored and are called *acholic,* or free from bile.

The colon functions to remove much of the remaining water and electrolytes from the chyme. Approximately 600 mL of fluid enters the colon daily, and only 200 mL of water is excreted in the stool daily. Abnormal colonic function leads to diarrhea or constipation. Aneurysmal pouches of colonic mucosa may cause bleeding; if they are infected, pain results. Colonic obstruction produces severe pain. Tumors may cause obstruction or bleeding.

Review of Specific Symptoms

The most common symptoms of abdominal disease are as follows:

- Pain
- Nausea and vomiting
- Change in bowel movements
- Rectal bleeding
- Jaundice
- Abdominal distention
- Mass
- Pruritus (itching)

Pain

Pain is probably the most important symptom of abdominal disease. Although abdominal neoplasia may be painless, most abdominal disease manifests itself with some amount of pain. Pain can result from mucosal irritation, smooth muscle spasm, peritoneal irritation, capsular swelling, or direct nerve stimulation. Abdominal pain calls for speedy diagnosis and therapy. When a patient complains of abdominal pain, ask the following questions:

"Where is the pain?"
"Has the pain changed its location since it started?"
"Do you feel the pain in any other part of your body?"
"How long have you had the pain?"
"Have you had recurrent episodes of abdominal pain?"
"Did the pain start suddenly?"
"Can you describe the pain? Is it sharp? burning? cramping?"
"Is the pain continuous?"
"Has there been any change in the severity or nature of the pain since it began?"
"What makes it worse?"
"What makes it better?"
"Is the pain associated with nausea? vomiting? sweating? constipation? diarrhea? bloody stools? abdominal distention? fever? chills? eating?"
"Have you ever had gallstones? kidney stones?"
If the patient is a woman, *"When was your last period?"*

Note the exact *time* at which the pain started and what the patient was doing at that time. Sudden, severe pain awakening a patient from sleep may be associated with acute perforation, inflammation, or torsion of an abdominal organ. A stone in the biliary or renal tract also causes intense pain. Note *acuteness* of the pain. Acute rupture of a fallopian tube by an ectopic pregnancy, perforation of a gastric ulcer, peritonitis, and acute pancreatitis cause such severe pain that fainting may result.

It is critical to determine the *location* of the pain at its onset, its *localization,* its *character,* and its *radiation.* Commonly, when an abdominal organ ruptures, pain is felt "all over the belly," without localization to a specific area. Pain arising from the small intestine is commonly felt in the umbilical or epigastric regions: for example, pain from acute appendicitis begins at the umbilicus.

After time, pain may become localized to other areas. Pain from acute appendicitis travels from the umbilicus to the right lower quadrant in about 1–3 hours after the initial event. Pain in the chest followed by abdominal pain should raise the suspicion of a dissecting aortic aneurysm.

Note the nature of the pain. Pain caused by a perforated gastric ulcer is often described as "burning"; dissecting aneurysm, as "tearing"; intestinal obstruction, as "gripping"; pyelonephritis, as "dull, aching"; biliary or renal colic, as "crampy, constricting."

Referred pain often provides insight as to the cause. *Referred pain* is a term used to describe pain originating in the internal organs but described by the patient as being located in the abdominal or chest wall, shoulder, jaw or other areas supplied by the somatic nerves. Pain appears to originate in areas supplied by the somatic nerves entering the spinal cord at the same segment as the sensory nerves from the organ responsible for the pain. For example, right-shoulder pain may result from acute cholecystitis; testicular pain may result from renal colic or from appendicitis. The common sites for referred pain are shown in Figure 15–3. The location of pain in abdominal disease is summarized in Table 15–2.

The time of occurrence and factors that aggravate or alleviate the symptoms (e.g., meals or defecation) are particularly important. Periodic epigastric pain occurring 1/2 to 1 hour after eating is a classic symptom of gastric peptic ulcers. Patients with a duodenal peptic ulcer have pain 2–3 hours after eating or before the next meal. Food tends to lessen the pain, especially in duodenal ulcers. Perforation of a duodenal ulcer to the pancreas may produce backache simulating an orthopedic problem. *Nocturnal pain* is a classic symptom of duodenal peptic ulcer disease. Pain after eating may also be associated with vascular disease of the abdominal viscera. Patients with this condition are older and have postprandial pain, anorexia, and weight loss. This triad is seen in *abdominal angina* resulting from obstructive vascular disease in the celiac axis or the superior mesenteric artery. Table 15–3 provides a summary of the important maneuvers for ameliorating abdominal pain.

Nausea and Vomiting

Vomiting may be caused by severe irritation of the peritoneum resulting from the perforation of an abdominal organ; obstruction of the bile duct, ureter, or intestine; or toxins. Vomiting resulting from a *perforation* is rarely massive. *Obstruction* of the bile

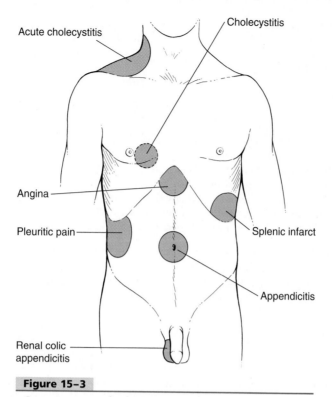

Figure 15-3

Common areas of referred pain. The dotted area is on the posterior chest.

Table 15-2   Location of Pain in Abdominal Disease

Area of Pain	Affected Organ	Clinical Example
Substernal	Esophagus	Esophagitis
Shoulder	Diaphragm	Subphrenic abscess
Epigastric	Stomach	Peptic gastric ulcer
	Duodenum	Peptic duodenal ulcer
	Gallbladder	Cholecystitis
	Liver	Hepatitis
	Bile ducts	Cholangitis
	Pancreas	Pancreatitis
Right scapula	Biliary tract	Biliary colic
Midback	Aorta	Aortic dissection
	Pancreas	Pancreatitis
Periumbilical	Small intestine	Obstruction
Hypogastrium	Colon	Ulcerative colitis
		Diverticulitis
Sacrum	Rectum	Proctitis
		Perirectal abscess

Table 15-3   Maneuvers for Ameliorating Abdominal Pain

Maneuver	Affected Organ	Clinical Example
Belching	Stomach	Gastric distention
Eating	Stomach, duodenum	Peptic ulcer
Vomiting	Stomach, duodenum	Pyloric obstruction
Leaning forward	Retroperitoneal structures	Pancreatic cancer
		Pancreatitis
Flexion of knees	Peritoneum	Peritonitis
Flexion of right thigh	Right psoas muscle	Appendicitis
Flexion of left thigh	Left psoas muscle	Diverticulitis

duct or other tube produces stretching of the muscular wall, resulting in episodic vomiting that occurs at the height of the pain. Intestinal obstruction prevents the intestinal contents from passing distally; consequently, vomiting may result in the expulsion of intestinal contents. *Toxins* generally cause persistent vomiting. Not all abdominal emergencies cause vomiting. Intraperitoneal bleeding may occur in the absence of vomiting. Vomiting is frequently also caused by inflammation of intra-abdominal structures as well as by extra-abdominal conditions, including drug toxicity, central nervous system disorders, myocardial infarction and pregnancy. Ask the following questions if a patient complains of nausea, vomiting, or both:

"How long have you had nausea or vomiting?"
"What is the color of the vomitus?"
"Is there any unusually foul odor to the vomitus?"
"How often do you vomit?"
"Is vomiting related to eating?" If so, *"How soon after eating do you vomit? Do you vomit only after eating certain foods?"*
"Do you have nausea without vomiting?"
"Is the nausea or vomiting associated with abdominal pain? constipation? diarrhea? a loss of appetite? a change in the color of your stools? a change in the color of your urine? fever? chest pain?"
"Have you noticed a change in your hearing ability?"
"Have you noticed ringing in your ears?"
If the patient is a woman, *"When was your last period?"*

The relationship of the pain to vomiting is important and may help in providing the diagnosis. In acute appendicitis, pain precedes the vomiting usually by a few hours. The character of the vomit may aid in determining its cause. Acute gastritis causes the patient to vomit stomach contents. Biliary colic produces bilious, or greenish-yellow, vomitus. Intestinal obstruction often causes the patient to vomit bilious vomitus followed by feculent smelling fluid. *Feculent vomitus* is usually due to intestinal obstruction.

Nausea without vomiting is a common symptom in patients with hepatocellular disease, pregnancy, and metastatic disease. Nausea may be associated with a hearing loss and tinnitus in patients with Ménière's disease.

Change in Bowel Movements

Take a careful history of bowel habits. A change in bowel movements requires further elaboration. Ask these questions of the patient with *acute* onset of diarrhea:

"How long have you had the diarrhea?"
"How many bowel movements do you have a day?"
"Did the diarrhea start suddenly?"
"Did the diarrhea begin after a meal?" If so, *"What did you eat?"*
"Are the stools watery? bloody? malodorous?"
"Is the diarrhea associated with abdominal pain? loss of appetite? nausea? vomiting?"

The acute onset of diarrhea after a meal suggests an acute infection or toxin. Watery stools are often associated with inflammatory processes of the small bowel and colon. Shigellosis is a disease of the colon that produces bloody diarrhea. Amebiasis is also associated with bloody diarrhea.

The patient with *chronic* diarrhea should be asked the following:

"How long have you had diarrhea?"
"Do you have periods of diarrhea alternating with constipation?"
"Are the stools watery? loose? floating? malodorous?"
"Have you noticed blood in the stools? mucus? undigested food?"
"What is the color of the stools?"
"How many bowel movements do you have a day?"
"Does the diarrhea occur after eating?"
"What happens when you fast? Do you still have diarrhea?"
"Is the diarrhea associated with abdominal pain? abdominal distention? nausea? vomiting?"

"Have you noticed that the diarrhea is worse at certain times of the day?"
"How is your appetite?"
"Has there been any change in your weight?"

The alternation of diarrhea and constipation is frequently seen in patients with colon cancer or diverticulitis. Loose bowel movements are common in diseases of the left colon, whereas watery movements are seen in severe inflammatory bowel disease and protein-losing enteropathies. Floating stools may result from malabsorption syndromes. Patients with ulcerative colitis commonly have stool mixed with blood and mucus. Any inflammatory process of the small bowel or colon can manifest with blood mixed with stool or undigested food. Irritable bowel syndrome classically produces more diarrhea in the morning.

Patients complaining of constipation should be asked these questions:

"How long have you been constipated?"
"How often do you have a bowel movement?"
"What is the size of your stools?"
"What is the color of your stools?"
"Is the stool ever mixed with blood? mucus?"
"Have you noticed periods of constipation alternating with periods of diarrhea?"
"Have you noticed a change in the caliber of the stool?"
"Do you have much gas?"
"How's your appetite?"
"Has there been any change in your weight?"

Change in the *caliber* of the stool is significant. "Pencil" diameter stools may result from an anal or a distal rectal carcinoma. A change in the color of stools is important. As will be discussed later, clay-colored stools indicate an absence of bile. This can be due to an obstruction to bile flow from the gallbladder or to decreased production of bile. Weight changes are important with the symptom of constipation. An increase in weight may indicate decreased metabolism seen in hypothyroidism; a decrease in weight may be associated with cancer of the colon.

Rectal Bleeding

Rectal bleeding may be manifested by bright red blood, blood mixed with stool, or black, tarry stools. Bright red blood per rectum (BRBPR), also known as *hematochezia,* can occur from colonic tumors, diverticular disease, or ulcerative colitis. Blood mixed with stool can be the result of ulcerative colitis, diverticular disease, tumors, or hemorrhoids. Ask the patient who describes rectal bleeding the following questions:

"How long have you noticed bright red blood in your stools?"
"Is the blood mixed with the stool?"
"Are there streaks of blood on the surface of the stool?"
"Have you noticed a change in your bowel habits?"
"Have you noticed a sensation in your rectum that you have to move your bowels but cannot?"

Tenesmus is the painful, continued, and ineffective straining at stool. It is caused by inflammation or tumor at the distal rectum or anus. Hemorrhoidal bleeding is a common cause of hematochezia and streaking of stool with blood.

Melena is a black, tarry stool that results from bleeding above the first section of the duodenum, with partial digestion of the hemoglobin. Inquire about the presence of melena. A useful way of questioning is to show the patient the black tubing on the stethoscope and ask, "Have your bowel movements ever been this color?" If asked directly whether the bowel movements have ever been black, the patient may answer in the affirmative, equating dark (normal) stools with black stools. Ask these questions of a patient who describes melena:

"Have you passed more than one black, tarry stool?" If so, *"When?"*
"How long have you been having black, tarry stools?"
"Have you noticed that you were lightheaded?"
"Have you had any nausea associated with these stools? any vomiting? diarrhea? abdominal pain? sweating?"

The answers to these questions can provide some information regarding the acuteness and the amount of the hemorrhage. Lightheadedness, nausea, and diaphoresis are seen with rapid gastrointestinal bleeding and hypotension.

The presence of *silver-colored stools* is rare but pathognomonic of acholic stools with melena, a condition resulting from cancer of the ampulla of Vater in the duodenum. The cancer produces biliary obstruction, and the cancerous fronds are sloughed, causing melena.

Jaundice

The presence of jaundice *(icterus)* must alert the examiner that there is either liver parenchymal disease or an obstruction to bile flow. The presence of icterus, or jaundice, results from a decreased excretion of conjugated bilirubin into the bile. This can result from intrahepatic biliary obstruction, known as *medical jaundice,* or from extrahepatic biliary obstruction, known as *surgical jaundice.* In any patient with icterus, the examiner should search for clues by asking the following questions:

"How long have you been jaundiced?"
"Did the jaundice develop rapidly?"
"Is the jaundice associated with abdominal pain? loss of appetite? nausea? vomiting? distaste for cigarettes?"
"Is the jaundice associated with chills? fever? itching? weight loss?"
"In the past year have you had any transfusions? tattooing? inoculations?"
"Do you use any 'recreational drugs'?" If so, *"Any intravenously?"*
"Do you eat raw shellfish? oysters?"
"Have you traveled abroad in the past year?" If so, *"Where?" "Did you drink any unclean water?"*
"Have you been jaundiced before?"
"Has your urine changed color since you noticed that you were jaundiced?"
"What is the color of your stools?"
"Do you have any friends or relations who are also jaundiced?"
"What type of work do you do?" "What other types of work have you done?"
"What are your hobbies?"

Viral hepatitis is associated with nausea, vomiting, a loss of appetite, and an aversion to smoking. Hepatitis A has a fecal-oral route of transmission and an incubation period of 2–6 weeks. It may be linked to ingestion of raw shellfish. Hepatitis B is blood-borne and has an incubation period of 1–6 months. Health professionals are at increased risk for hepatitis. Any contact with an individual with viral hepatitis places one at a higher risk of contracting viral hepatitis. Slowly developing jaundice that is accompanied by clay-colored stools and cola-colored urine is *obstructive jaundice,* either intra- or extrahepatic. Jaundice accompanied by fever and chills is considered *cholangitis* until proved otherwise. Cholangitis may result from stasis of bile in the bile duct that results from a gallstone or from cancer of the head of the pancreas. Determine whether chemicals are used in a patient's occupation or hobbies, because they may be related to the cause of the jaundice. Many industrial chemicals and drugs have been associated with liver disease. These agents may be responsible for a viral hepatitis–like illness, cholestasis, granulomas, or hepatic tumors. Occupational exposure to carbon tetrachloride and vinyl chloride is well known to cause liver disease. Ask questions related to alcohol abuse. These are described in Chapter 1, The Interviewer's Questions.

Abdominal Distention

Abdominal distention may be related to increased gas in the gastrointestinal tract or to the presence of ascites. Increased gas can result from malabsorption, irritable colon, or air swallowing *(aerophagia).* *Ascites* can be caused by a variety of causes, such as cirrhosis, congestive heart failure, portal hypertension, peritonitis, or neoplasia. To try to identify the cause of abdominal distention, ask these questions:

"How long have you noticed your abdomen to be distended?"
"Is the distention intermittent?"
"Is the distention related to eating?"

"Is the distention lessened by passing gas from above or below?"
"Is the distention associated with vomiting? loss of appetite? weight loss? change in your bowel habits? shortness of breath?"

Gaseous distention related to eating is intermittent and is relieved by the passage of flatus or belching. A patient with ascites has the insidious development of increased abdominal girth, noted through a progressive increase in belt size. Loss of appetite is often associated with cirrhosis and malignancy, although end-stage congestive heart failure may produce this symptom as well. Shortness of breath and ascites may be symptoms of congestive heart failure, but the shortness of breath may be the result of a decrease in pulmonary capacity owing to ascites from another cause. Questions related to alcoholic abuse are most appropriate and are outlined in Chapter 1.

Mass

An abdominal mass may be a neoplasm or a hernia. An abdominal *hernia* refers to a protrusion from the peritoneal cavity into which peritoneal contents are extruded. The contents may be omentum, intestine, or bladder wall. An abdominal hernia may be inguinal, femoral, umbilical, or internal, depending on its location. The most common complaint is swelling, which may or may not be painful. An inguinal hernia may manifest as a mass in the groin or scrotum. The major complications of a hernia are intestinal obstruction and intestinal strangulation from interference of blood supply. A hernia is termed *reducible* when it can be emptied of its contents by pressure or a change in posture.

A symptom of a pulsatile abdominal mass should alert the examiner to the possibility of an aortic aneurysm.

Pruritus

Pruritus, or itching, is a common symptom. Generalized itching may be a symptom of a diffuse skin disorder* or a manifestation of chronic renal or hepatic disease. Intense pruritus may be associated with lymphoma or Hodgkin's disease, as well as with malignancies of the gastrointestinal tract. In older individuals, pruritus may also be caused by dry skin alone. *Pruritus ani* is localized itching of the anal skin. It has many causes, including fistulae, fissures, psoriasis, parasites, poor hygiene, and diabetes.

Impact of Inflammatory Bowel Disease on the Patient

Inflammatory bowel disease constitutes a group of diseases of unknown cause. The symptoms produced depend on the location, extent, and acuteness of the inflammatory lesion(s). The common presenting features are fever, anorexia, weight loss, abdominal discomfort, diarrhea, rectal urgency, and rectal bleeding. It is a chronic, potentially disabling illness, often resulting in the need for multiple surgeries, in fistula formation, and in cancer.

Inflammatory bowel disease may lead to long absences from school or work, disruption of family life, malabsorption, malnutrition, and multiple hospitalizations. A patient can have 10–30 watery or bloody bowel movements each day. As a consequence, patients with inflammatory bowel disease have many psychological problems, particularly young adults. Sexual development may be delayed as a result of malnutrition. Social development is also retarded. The necessity of constantly having to remain near a bathroom inhibits patients' abilities to develop normal dating patterns. Many of these patients are socially immature, and social introversion is common. By necessity, they remain at home. Their lives revolve around their bowel habits.

In most cases, there is a positive correlation between the severity of the physical disease and the extent of emotional disturbance. *Dependency* is the most reported characteristic of patients with inflammatory bowel disease. Repressed rage, suppression of feelings, and anxieties are also common. It is reported that many patients have a

---

* For example, dermatitis herpetiformis, a blistering disease predominantly on the buttocks, shoulders, elbows, and knees.

constant desire to rid themselves of events in their lives. This characteristic can be acted out through the diarrhea. Another characteristic of these patients is to be *obsessive-compulsive*. The marked obsessive character becomes even more obvious when the patient is ill. It is typical for patients to worry incessantly about what is happening within their bowels. The patients are intelligent, often having read much literature, including medical textbooks, about their disease.

Denial is generally not a prominent symptom. In contrast, these patients concentrate obsessively on the details of their bowel habits.

Sexual problems are common. Interest and participation in sexual activity tend to be at a low level. Many of these individuals prefer to be fondled like a child and largely reject any genital contact. Patients are prone to regard sexual activity in anal terms, such as "dirty," "unclean," or "soiling." They are squeamish about body contact, odors, and secretions. The loss of libido and decreased sexual drive may be related to their fear of bowel action during intercourse, of perineal pain, or that sexual intercourse may in some way further damage the bowel.

The frequent hospitalizations cause anxiety and depression, which exacerbate the disease. The fear of cancer may be the basis of depression, which is a common response to the disease. It is well established that emotional factors are important in maintaining and prolonging an existing attack. Schoolwork deteriorates as young patients are forced to miss more and more school, further increasing their anxiety.

An often unappreciated major complication of inflammatory bowel disease is substance abuse. As a result of chronic pain, as many as 5% of patients with inflammatory bowel disease are physically addicted to oral narcotics. Many more are psychologically dependent on their pain medication.

Many patients with ulcerative colitis require an ileostomy. The fear of disfigurement, the loss of self-confidence, the potential lack of cleanliness, and the dread of unexpected spillage are common.

Time for listening and an interest in a patient's problem are important in gaining the patient's confidence. Listening may reveal and help unravel the emotional problems that may be the source of the exacerbation of the bowel disease. Talking to the patient may be more efficacious than anti-inflammatory agents or tranquilizers. Careful and thoughtful discussion of the illness strengthens the doctor-patient relationship and produces immeasurable therapeutic benefits.

Physical Examination

> The equipment necessary for the examination of the abdomen and rectum is a stethoscope, gloves, lubricant, tissues, and occult blood testing card and reagent.

The patient should be lying flat in bed, and the abdomen should be fully exposed from the sternum to the knees. The arms should be at the sides, and the legs flat. Frequently, patients tend to place their arms behind their head, which tightens the abdominal muscles and makes the examination more difficult. Placing a pillow beneath the knees often aids in relaxation. The examiner should be standing on the patient's right side. A sheet or towel is placed over the genitalia, as shown in Figure 15–4.

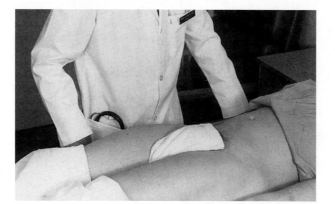

Figure 15–4

Technique for inspecting the abdomen.

If the patient has complained of abdominal pain, examine the area of pain *last*. If the examiner touches the area of maximal pain, the abdominal muscles will tighten, and the examination will be more difficult.

The physical examination of the abdomen includes the following:

- Inspection
- Auscultation
- Percussion
- Palpation
- Rectal examination
- Special techniques

Inspection

Evaluate General Appearance

The general appearance of the patient often furnishes valuable information as to the nature of the condition. Patients with renal or biliary *colic* writhe in bed. They squirm constantly and can find no comfortable position. In contrast, patients with *peritonitis* who have intense pain on movement characteristically remain still in bed because any slight motion worsens the pain. They may be lying in bed with their knees drawn up to help relax the abdominal muscles and reduce intra-abdominal pressure. Patients who are pale and sweating may be suffering from the initial *shock* of pancreatitis or a perforated gastric ulcer.

Determine Respiratory Rate

The respiratory rate is increased in patients with generalized peritonitis, intra-abdominal hemorrhage, or intestinal obstruction.

Inspect the Skin

Inspect the skin and sclera for jaundice. Whenever possible, the patient should be evaluated for jaundice in natural light, as incandescent light frequently masks the existence of icterus. Jaundice becomes apparent when the serum bilirubin level exceeds 2.5 mg/dL in adults or 6.0 mg/dL in neonates. Figure 15–5 shows a patient with jaundice. Notice the scleral icterus as well as the yellow discoloration of the skin. Hyperbilirubinemia can also result in intense generalized pruritus.

Inspect for *spider angiomas*. Spider angiomas have a high degree of sensitivity in patients with alcoholic cirrhosis but are nonspecific because they also occur in pregnancy and collagen vascular disorders. See Figure 6–60.

Figure 15–6 shows the leg of a patient with *pyoderma gangrenosum*. Notice the necrotic, undermined ulceration with pus. These tender ulcerations, commonly on the

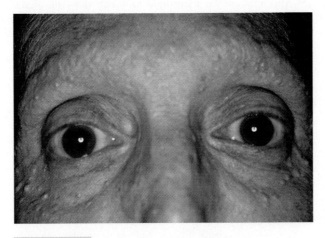

Figure 15–5

Jaundice.

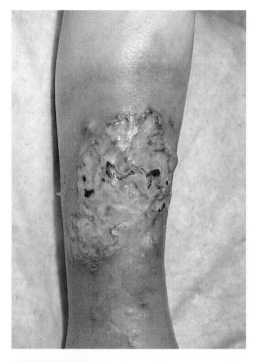

Figure 15–6

Pyoderma gangrenosum.

lower extremities, are associated with inflammatory bowel disease, especially ulcerative colitis. In general, the clinical course of pyoderma gangrenosum follows the course of the bowel disease. This condition is also seen in patients with rheumatoid arthritis, myeloid metaplasia, and chronic myelogenous leukemia.

Inspect the Hands

Is there muscle loss in the small muscles of the hands? This is associated with wasting.

The nails are examined for changes in the nail bed, especially an increase in the size of the lunula. The fingers of a patient with cirrhosis showing "half and half" nails are shown in Figure 15–7.

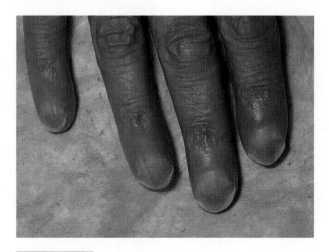

Figure 15–7

Lindsay's nails.

Inspect the Facies

Are the eyes sunken? Is temporal wasting present? These are signs of wasting and poor nutrition.

The skin around the mouth and oral mucosa may provide evidence of gastrointestinal disorders. Melanin deposition around and in the oral cavity, especially the buccal mucosa, suggests *Peutz-Jeghers syndrome.* Figure 10–10 shows the lips of a patient with the classic brown pigmentary changes of Peutz-Jeghers syndrome. This is an autosomal-dominant disorder characterized by generalized gastrointestinal, hamartomatous polyposis and mucocutaneous pigmentation. The benign polyps are most common in the jejunum and only rarely become malignant. The polyps, however, may bleed, cause intussusception, or cause obstruction. Telangiectasias of the lips and tongue are suggestive of *Osler-Weber-Rendu syndrome.* In this syndrome, multiple telangiectasias are present throughout the gastrointestinal tract. These may bleed insidiously, causing anemia. The classic oral lesions of a patient with Osler-Weber-Rendu syndrome are shown in Figure 15–8.

Hypercortisolism, or *Cushing's syndrome,* has a range of clinical manifestations. The most common are obesity, facial plethora, hirsutism, and hypertension. Obesity occurs in 90% of patients. Most patients with hypercortisolism characteristically have round, puffy, red faces called *moon facies.* They also have prominent fat deposits in the supraclavicular and retrocervical areas (buffalo hump). Figure 15–9 shows a patient with Cushing's syndrome and the typical moon facies.

Inspect the Abdomen

The contour of the abdomen should be assessed. A *scaphoid,* or concave, abdomen may be associated with cachexia; a *protuberant* abdomen may result from gaseous

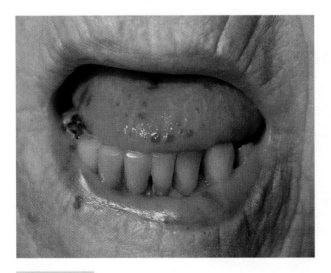

Figure 15–8

Osler-Rendu-Weber syndrome.

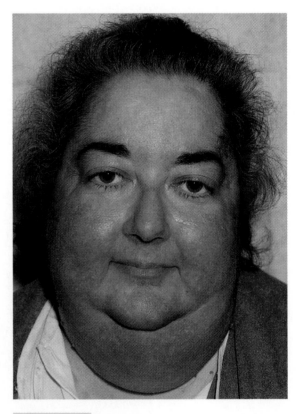

Figure 15–9

Cushing's syndrome.

distension of the intestines, ascites, organomegaly, or obesity. When a patient with ascites stands, the fluid sinks into the lower abdomen; when lying supine, the fluid bulges in the flanks. If a patient with ascites lies on a side, the fluid flows to the lower side. A patient with a protuberant abdomen as a result of carcinomatous ascites is shown in Figure 15–10.

The examiner should focus attention on the abdomen to adequately describe the presence of any asymmetry, distention, masses, or visible peristaltic waves. The examiner should then observe the abdomen from above, looking for the same signs. Inspection of the abdomen for striae and scars may provide valuable data. Silver striae are stretch marks consistent with weight loss. Pinkish-purple striae are classic signs of adrenocortical excess. Figure 15–11 shows the characteristic purplish striae in a patient with Cushing's disease.

Is the umbilicus everted? An everted umbilicus is often a sign of increased abdominal pressure, usually from ascites or a large mass. An umbilical hernia may also cause an umbilicus to become everted.

Are there ecchymoses on the abdomen or on the flanks? Massive ecchymoses may occur in these areas as a result of hemorrhagic pancreatitis or strangulated bowel. This is *Grey Turner's sign*.

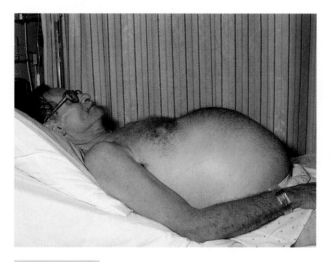

Figure 15–10

Ascites.

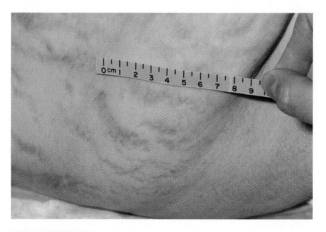

Figure 15–11

Abdominal striae.

Cullen's sign is a bluish discoloration of the umbilicus resulting from hemoperitoneum of any cause.

Recognition of classic surgical scars may be helpful. Figure 15–12 shows the locations of some common surgical scars.

Inspect for Hernias

The patient lying in bed should be asked to cough while the examiner inspects the inguinal, umbilical, and femoral areas. This maneuver, by increasing intra-abdominal pressure, may produce a sudden bulging in these areas, which may be related to a hernia. If the patient has had surgery, coughing may show a bulging along the abdominal scar from the previous incision. In addition, coughing may elicit pain localized to a specific area. This technique enables the examiner to identify the area of maximal tenderness and to perform most of the abdominal examination without too much

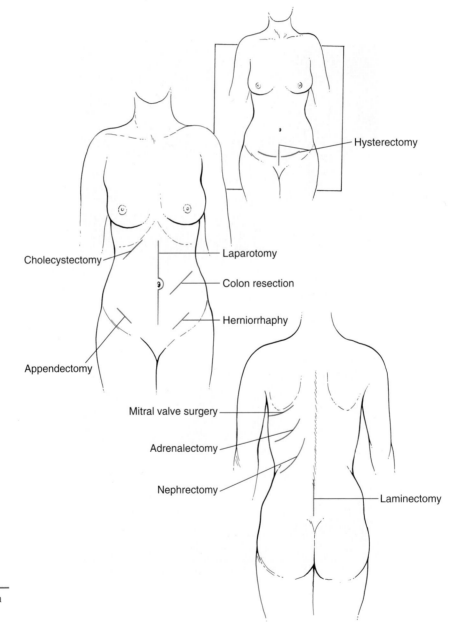

Figure 15–12

Locations of common surgical scars.

discomfort to the patient. Ascites secondary to metastatic breast carcinoma and an umbilical hernia are shown in Figure 15–13.

▤ Inspect the Superficial Veins

The venous pattern of the abdomen is usually barely perceptible. If visible in the normal individual, the drainage of the lower two thirds of the abdomen is downward. In the presence of vena caval obstruction, superficial veins may dilate, and the veins drain cephalad (toward the head). In patients with portal hypertension, the dilated veins appear to radiate from the umbilicus. This is due to backflow through the collateral veins within the falciform ligament, and this pattern is called *caput medusae*.

If the superficial veins are distended, evaluate the direction of drainage by the following technique. Place the tips of your index fingers on a vein that is oriented cephalad-caudad, not transverse, and compress it. Using continuous pressure, slide the index fingers apart for about 3–4 inches. Remove one finger and observe the refilling in the direction of flow. Repeat this procedure, but this time remove the other finger and observe the direction of flow. Figure 15–14 shows the abdomen of a patient with intrahepatic portal hypertension. Notice the engorged paraumbilical veins; the flow was away from the umbilicus toward the caval system.

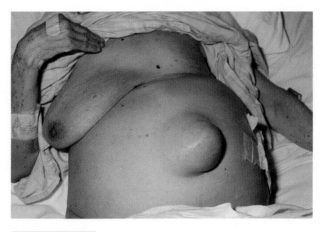

Figure 15–13

Ascites with umbilical hernia.

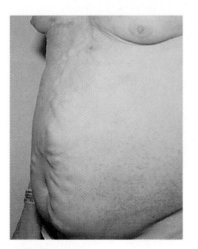

Figure 15–14

Abdominal venous pattern.

Auscultation

Auscultation of bowel sounds can provide information about the motion of air and liquid in the gastrointestinal tract. Many examiners perform auscultation of the abdomen before percussion or palpation, in contrast to the usual order. These examiners believe that percussion or palpation may change the intestinal motility; therefore, they believe that auscultation should be performed first to produce a more accurate assessment of the existing bowel sounds.

Evaluate Bowel Sounds

The patient is placed in a supine position. Auscultation of the abdomen is performed by placing the diaphragm of the stethoscope over the midabdomen, and the examiner listens for bowel sounds. This technique is shown in Figure 15–15.

Normal bowel sounds occur approximately every 5–10 seconds and have a high-pitched sound. If after 2 minutes no bowel sounds are heard, the statement "absent bowel sounds" may be made. The absence of bowel sounds suggests a paralytic ileus that is due to diffuse peritoneal irritation. There may be rushes of low-pitched rumbling sounds, termed *borborygmi,* which are associated with hyperperistalsis. These sounds are similar to the sound of the word "borborygmi" itself. They are common in early acute intestinal obstruction.

Rule Out Obstructed Viscus

A *succussion splash* may be detected in a distended abdomen as a result of the presence of gas and fluid in an obstructed organ. The examiner applies the stethoscope over the patient's abdomen while shaking the patient from side to side. The presence of a sloshing sound generally indicates distention of the stomach or colon. This technique is illustrated in Figure 15–16.

Rule Out Abdominal Bruits

Auscultation is also useful for determining the presence of bruits. Each quadrant should be evaluated for their presence. Bruits may result from stenosis of the renal artery or of the abdominal aorta. (See discussion of abdominal bruits in Chapter 13, The Peripheral Vascular System.)

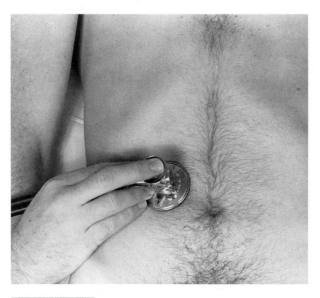

Figure 15–15

Technique for evaluating bowel sounds.

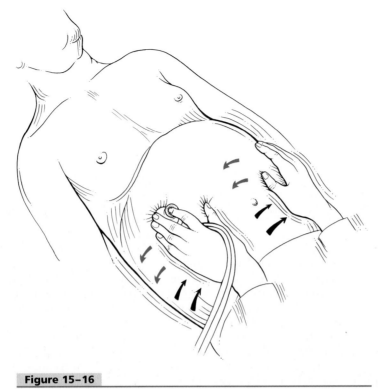

Figure 15–16

"Succussion splash" technique for assessing distention of abdominal viscera.

▩ Rule Out Peritoneal Rubs

A peritoneal friction rub, like a pleural or pericardial rub, is a sound that indicates inflammation. During respiratory motion, a friction rub may be heard in the right or left upper quadrants in the presence of hepatic or splenic disorder.

Percussion

Percussion is used to demonstrate the presence of gaseous distention and fluid or solid masses. In the normal examination, generally only the size and location of the liver and spleen can be determined. Some examiners prefer to palpate before percussion, especially if the patient complains of abdominal pain; either approach is correct. The technique of percussion is discussed in Chapter 11.

▩ Percuss the Abdomen

The patient lies supine. All four quadrants of the abdomen are evaluated by percussion. Tympany is the most common percussion note in the abdomen. This is due to the presence of gas within the stomach, small bowel, and colon. The suprapubic area when percussed may sound dull if the urinary bladder is distended or, in a woman, if the uterus is enlarged.

▩ Percuss the Liver

The upper border of the liver is percussed in the right midclavicular line, starting in the midchest. As the chest is percussed downward, the resonant note of the chest becomes dull as the liver is reached. As percussion continues still further, this dull note becomes tympanic because the percussion is now over the colon. The upper and lower borders of the liver should be no more than 10 cm apart. The technique is illustrated in Figure 15–17.

There are several problems with predicting liver size by percussion. If ascites is present, the examiner can only speculate about the correct size of the liver (or spleen). A more common cause of overestimating liver size (false-positive measurement) is some form of chronic obstructive lung disease. This makes percussion of the upper border of the liver difficult. Obesity can cause problems in both percussion and palpation. Distention of the colon may obscure the lower liver dullness. This may result in underestimating the size of the liver (false-negative measurement).

■ Percuss the Spleen

Although the size of the spleen is often difficult to determine, evaluation of the spleen should begin with percussion of splenic size. In normal individuals, the spleen lies hidden within the rib cage against the posterolateral wall of the abdominal cavity in *Traube's space*. Traube's space is defined by the sixth rib superiorly, the left anterior axillary line laterally, and the costal margin inferiorly. As the spleen enlarges, it remains close to the abdominal wall, and the tip moves downward and toward the midline. Because the early enlargement is in an anteroposterior direction, considerable enlargement may occur without its becoming palpable below the costal margin. Several investigators have felt that dullness to percussion in Traube's space—the loss of tympany from the air-filled colon and stomach by the enlarged spleen—is a useful sign for determining splenic enlargement.

Have the patient lie in the supine position. With the patient breathing normally, percuss in the lowest intercostal space in the left anterior axillary line. Normal percussion yields either a resonant or tympanic note. A positive test of splenomegaly is diagnosed when the percussion note is dull. Using ultrasonography as the standard (Barkun et al, 1989), splenic percussion has a sensitivity of 62% and a specificity of 72%. In leaner individuals who had not eaten in the previous 2 hours, the sensitivity was 78% and the specificity was 82%.

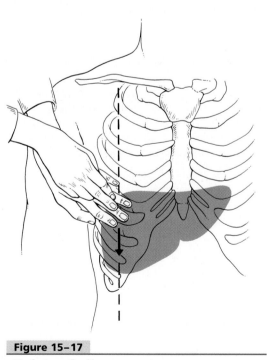

Figure 15–17

Technique for liver percussion.

■ Rule Out Ascites

On patients in whom ascites is thought to be present, a special percussion test for *shifting dullness* may be performed. While the patient is lying on the back, the examiner determines the borders of tympany and dullness. The area of tympany is present above the area of dullness. This is due to gas in the bowel that is floating on top of the ascites. The patient is then asked to turn on the side, and the examiner again determines the borders of the percussion notes. If ascites is present, dullness will "shift" to the more dependent position; the area around the umbilicus that was initially tympanic will become dull. Shifting dullness has a sensitivity of 83–88% and a specificity of 56%. The test for shifting dullness is illustrated in Figure 15–18.

An additional test for ascites is the presence of a *fluid wave*. Another examiner's hand or the patient's own hand is placed in the middle of the patient's abdomen. Indenting the abdominal wall will stop transmission of an impulse by the subcutaneous adipose tissue. The examiner then taps one flank while palpating the other side. Detection of a fluid wave suggests ascites. This technique is illustrated in Figure 15–19. The presence of a prominent fluid wave is the most specific of all physical diagnostic tests for ascites and has a specificity of 82–92%, based on several studies. A false-positive result may be obtained in obese individuals, and a false-negative result may be obtained when the ascites is small to moderate.

Another physical finding with ascites is the presence of *bulging flanks*. This occurs when the weight of free abdominal fluid is sufficient to push the flanks outward. It has a 93% sensitivity for detecting ascites and a 54% specificity (Simel et al, 1988).

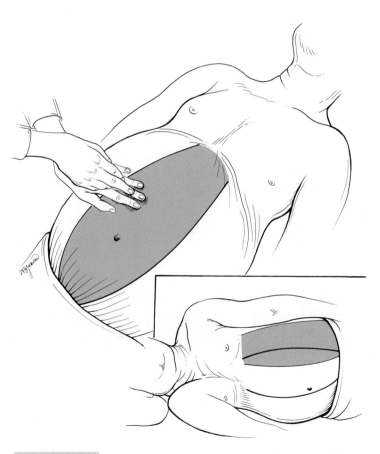

Figure 15–18

Technique for testing for shifting dullness. The colored areas represent the areas of tympany.

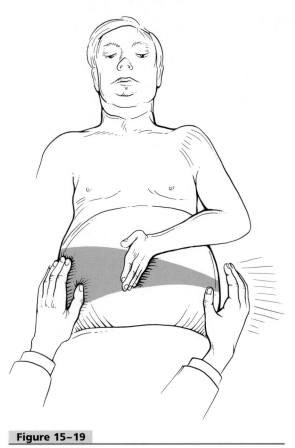

Figure 15–19

Technique for testing a fluid wave.

The most sensitive sign for ascites is the presence of shifting dullness, whereas the most specific sign is the presence of a prominent fluid wave. For an individual patient, the examiner must know the prevalence of disease or the pretest probability to apply sensitivity and specificity. Several studies have reviewed the operating characteristics of the physical examination tests for ascites. Their pooled sensitivity, specificity, and likelihood ratios for the presence of ascites are summarized in Table 15–4. The presence of a prominent fluid wave or shifting dullness increases the likelihood of the presence of ascites the most; the absence of bulging flanks, flank dullness, or shifting dullness decreases the likelihood.

Table 15–4   Characteristics of Physical Signs (Pooled Data) for Detection of Ascites*

Physical Sign	Sensitivity (%) Range	Specificity (%) Range	LR +	LR −
Bulging flanks	81 69–93	59 50–68	2.0	0.3
Flank dullness	84 80–94	59 47–71	2.0	0.3
Shifting dullness	86 64–90	72 63–81	2.7	0.3
Prominent fluid wave	62 47–77	90 84–96	6.0	0.4

* 95% confidence interval; data pooled from Cummings et al (1985), Simel et al (1988), Cattau et al (1982), and Williams and Simel (1992).

Simel et al (1988) reported that among the more common historical items perceived by patients, an increase in abdominal girth or recent weight gain increased the chance of ascites the most. The former has a positive likelihood ratio (LR+) of 4.16; the latter, an LR+ of 3.20. Conversely, the absence of the subjective increase in abdominal girth had a negative likelihood ratio (LR−) of 0.17; the absence of subjective ankle swelling carried an LR− of 0.10. Regarding the physical examination, the presence of a fluid wave or shifting dullness had the highest LR+ of 9.6 and 5.76, respectively. The absence of bulging flanks or edema made the presence of ascites least likely, with an LR− of 0.12 and 0.17, respectively.

Palpation

Abdominal palpation is commonly divided into the following:

- Light palpation
- Deep palpation
- Liver palpation
- Spleen palpation
- Kidney palpation

The patient is supine during palpation. Always begin palpation in an area of the abdomen that is farthest from the location of pain.

Light Palpation

Light palpation is used to detect tenderness and areas of muscular spasm or rigidity. The entire abdomen should be systematically palpated by using the flat part of the right hand or the pads of the fingers, *not* the fingertips. The fingers should be together, and sudden jabs are to be avoided. The hand should be lifted from area to area instead of sliding over the abdominal wall. Light palpation is demonstrated in Figure 15–20.

With patients who are ticklish, it may be useful to have them hold their hand over the examiner's hand, as shown in Figure 15–21.

During expiration, the rectus muscles usually relax and soften. If there is little change, *rigidity* is said to be present. Rigidity is involuntary spasm of the abdominal muscles and is indicative of peritoneal irritation. Rigidity may be *diffuse,* as in diffuse peritonitis, or *localized,* as over an inflamed appendix or gallbladder. In patients with generalized peritonitis, the abdomen is described as "board-like."

In patients who complain of abdominal pain, palpation should be performed gently. Lightly stroking the abdomen with a pin may reveal an area of increased sensation that is due to inflammation of the visceral or parietal peritoneum. This is *hyperesthesia.* The patient is asked to determine whether the pin feels sharper on one

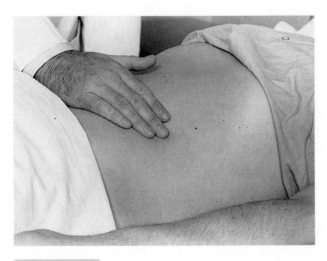

Figure 15–20

Technique for light palpation.

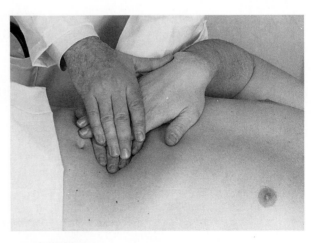

Figure 15–21

Technique used for ticklish patients. The patient's hand is sandwiched between the examiner's hands.

side of the abdomen than on the corresponding area on the other side. Although useful, the presence or absence of this finding must be considered in light of all other findings.

Deep Palpation

Deep palpation is used to determine organ size as well as the presence of abnormal abdominal masses. In deep palpation, the flat portion of the right hand is placed on the abdomen, and the left hand is placed over it. The fingertips of the left hand exert the pressure, while the right hand should appreciate any tactile stimulation. Pressure should be applied to the abdomen gently but steadily. The technique of deep palpation is shown in Figure 15–22.

During deep palpation, the patient should be instructed to breathe quietly through the mouth and to keep arms at the sides. Asking the patient to open the mouth when breathing seems to aid in generalized muscular relaxation. The palpating hands should be warm, because cold hands may produce voluntary muscular spasm called *guarding*. Engaging the patient in conversation often aids in relaxing the patient's abdominal musculature. Patients with well-developed rectus muscles should be instructed to flex their knees in order to relax the abdominal muscles. Any tender areas must be identified.

Rule Out Rebound Tenderness

In a patient with abdominal pain, it should be determined whether *rebound tenderness* is present. Rebound tenderness is a sign of peritoneal irritation and can be elicited by palpating deeply and *slowly* in an abdominal area away from the suspected area of local inflammation. The palpating hand is then quickly removed. The sensation of pain on the side of the inflammation that occurs on release of pressure is rebound tenderness. If generalized peritonitis is present, pain will be felt in the area of palpation. The patient should be asked, "Which hurts more, *now* (while pressing) or *now* (during release)?" This is a useful test, but because generalized pain will be elicited in the patient with peritonitis, the maneuver should be performed near the conclusion of the abdominal examination.

Liver Palpation

Palpation of the liver is performed by placing the examiner's left hand posteriorly between the patient's right twelfth rib and the iliac crest, lateral to the paraspinal muscles. The right hand is placed in the right upper quadrant parallel and lateral to the rectus muscles and below the area of liver dullness. The patient is instructed to take a deep breath as the examiner presses inward and upward with the right hand and pulls upward with the left hand. The liver edge may be felt to slip over the fingertips of the right hand as the patient breathes. Start as low as the pelvic brim and gradually work

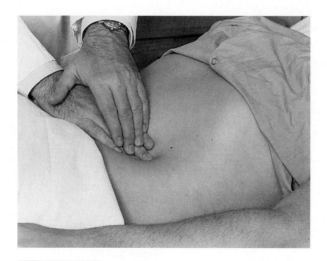

Figure 15–22

Technique for deep palpation.

upward. If the examination does not start low, a markedly enlarged liver edge will be missed. The technique of liver palpation is shown in Figure 15–23.

The normal liver edge has a firm, regular ridge, with a smooth surface. If the liver edge is not felt, repeat the maneuver after readjusting the right hand closer to the costal margin. Enlargement of the liver results from vascular congestion, hepatitis, neoplasm, or cirrhosis.

Another technique for liver palpation is the "hooking" method. The examiner stands near the patient's head and places both hands together below the right costal margin and the area of dullness. The examiner presses inward and upward and "hooks" around the liver edge while the patient inhales deeply. The technique of hooking the liver is shown in Figure 15–24.

Occasionally, the liver appears to be enlarged but the actual border is difficult to determine. The *scratch test* may be helpful in ascertaining the liver's edge. The bell of the stethoscope is held with the left hand and is placed below the right costal margin over the liver. While the examiner listens through the stethoscope, the right index finger "scratches" the abdominal wall at points in a semicircle equidistant from the stethoscope. As the finger scratches over the liver's edge, there will be a marked increase in the intensity of the sound. This technique is illustrated in Figure 15–25.

A palpable liver is not necessarily enlarged or diseased; however, a palpable liver does increase the possibility of hepatomegaly. A nonpalpable liver does not rule out hepatomegaly, but it does reduce the likelihood that an enlarged liver is present. The pooled LR+ for hepatomegaly, given a palpable liver, is 2.5; the LR− in the absence of a palpable liver for the presence of an enlarged liver detected by scintigraphic scanning is 0.45 (Naylor, 1994).

Rule Out Hepatic Tenderness

Hepatic tenderness is elicited by placing the palm of the left hand over the right upper quadrant and *gently* striking it with the ulnar surface of the fist of the right hand. Inflammatory processes involving the liver or gallbladder produce tenderness on fist palpation. Figure 15–26 shows this technique.

Occasionally during liver palpation, pain is elicited during inspiration, and the patient suddenly stops inspiratory efforts. This is called *Murphy's sign* and is suggestive of acute cholecystitis. Upon inspiration, the inflamed gallbladder descends against the palpating hand; pain is produced, and there is inspiratory arrest.

■ Spleen Palpation

Palpation of the spleen is more difficult than palpation of the liver. The patient lies on the back, with the examiner at the patient's right side. The examiner places the left

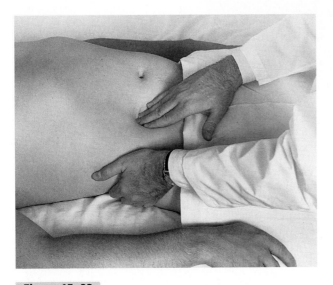

Figure 15–23

Technique for liver palpation.

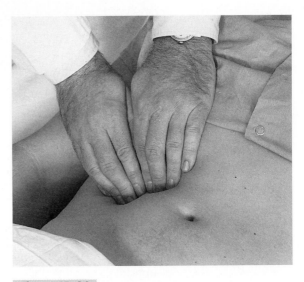

Figure 15–24

Technique for "hooking" the liver.

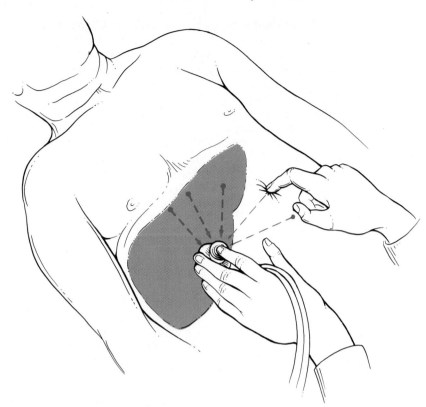

Figure 15–25

The scratch test for determining liver size.

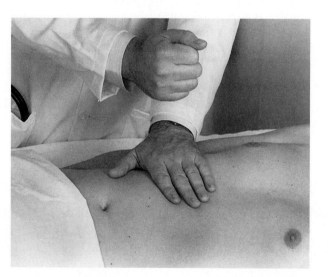

Figure 15–26

Liver tap technique for assessing liver tenderness.

hand over the patient's chest and elevates the patient's left rib cage. The right hand is placed flat below the left costal margin and presses inward and upward toward the anterior axillary line. The left hand exerts an anterior force to displace the spleen anteriorly. Figure 15–27 illustrates the positions of the hands for splenic palpation.

The patient is instructed to take a deep breath as the examiner presses inward with the right hand. The examiner should attempt to feel the tip of the spleen as it descends during inspiration. The tip of an enlarged spleen will lift the fingers of the right hand upward.

The examination of the spleen is repeated with the patient lying on the right side. This maneuver allows gravity to help bring the spleen anterior and downward into a

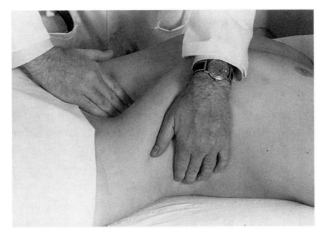

Figure 15–27

Technique for splenic palpation.

more favorable position for palpation. The examiner places the left hand on the patient's left costal margin while the right hand palpates in the left upper quadrant. The technique is shown in Figure 15–28.

Because the spleen enlarges diagonally in the abdomen from the left upper quadrant toward the umbilicus the right hand should always palpate near the umbilicus and gradually move toward the left upper quadrant. This is particularly important if the spleen is massively enlarged, because starting the palpation too high may cause the examiner to miss the splenic border.

The spleen is not palpable in normal conditions, but both techniques should be utilized to attempt to palpate it. Splenic enlargement (splenomegaly) may be due to hyperplasia, congestion, infection, or infiltration by tumor or myeloid elements. Massive splenomegaly in a patient with chronic myelocytic leukemia is shown in Figure 15–29.

▮ Kidney Palpation

More often than not, neither kidney can be palpated in the adult. The technique, however, is important to know.

Palpation of the right kidney is performed by deep palpation below the right costal margin. The examiner stands at the patient's right side and places the left hand behind the patient's right flank, between the costal margin and the iliac crest. The right hand is placed just below the costal margin with the tips of the fingers pointing to the examiner's left. The method of kidney palpation is shown in Figure 15–30.

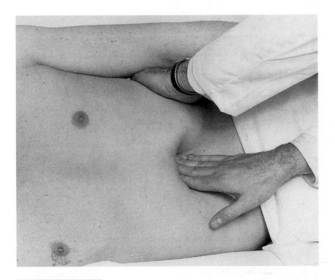

Figure 15–28

Another technique for splenic palpation.

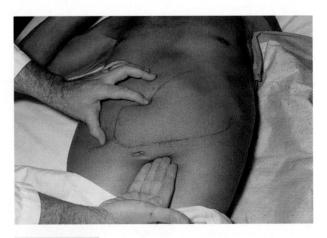

Figure 15–29

Splenomegaly. Note the splenic notch.

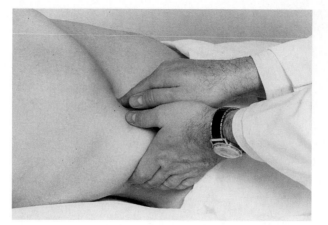

Figure 15–30

Technique for kidney palpation.

Very deep palpation may reveal the lower pole of the right kidney as it descends during inspiration. The lower pole may be felt as a smooth, rounded mass.

The same procedure is used for the left kidney except that the examiner is on the patient's left side. Because the left kidney is more superior than the right, the lower pole of a normal left kidney is rarely palpable. Occasionally, the spleen may be mistaken for an enlarged left kidney. The medial notch of the spleen is helpful in differentiating it from the kidney (see Fig. 15–29).

Rule Out Renal Tenderness

For this part of the examination, the patient should be seated. The examiner should make a fist and *gently* strike the area overlying the costovertebral angle on each side. Figure 15–31 shows the technique. Patients with pyelonephritis usually have extreme pain even on slight percussion in these areas. If pyelonephritis is suspected, only digital pressure should be used. As is described in Chapter 20, Putting the Examination Together, this portion of the abdominal examination is usually performed when the posterior chest is examined.

Rectal Examination

The routine abdominal examination concludes with the digital examination of the rectum. Because the anterior rectum has a peritoneal surface, the rectal examination may reveal tenderness if peritoneal inflammation is present.

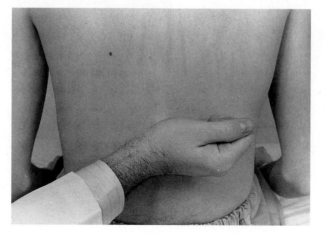

Figure 15–31

Assessing costovertebral angle tenderness.

The rectal examination for the male is discussed here; for the female, it is discussed in Chapter 17, Female Genitalia.

Patient Positioning

The examination of the rectum in the male may be performed with the patient lying on his back, lying on the left side, or standing, bent over the examination table. The modified lithotomy position (patient on his back with knees flexed) is used when the patient has difficulty standing or when a detailed examination of the anus is not required. The examiner passes the right hand under the patient's right thigh. The index finger in the patient's rectum is used in conjunction with the examiner's left hand, which is placed on the abdomen. This bimanual approach is useful and causes minimal disturbance of the sick patient.

The left lateral prone position, called *Sims' position,* is used commonly in patients who are weak and confined to bed. In this position, the right upper leg should be flexed while the left lower leg is semiextended. The modified lithotomy and left lateral prone positions are shown in Figure 15–32.

The standing position is the one most commonly used for men and allows for thorough inspection of the anus and palpation of the rectum. The patient is instructed to stand bent over, with shoulders and elbows supported on the bed or examination table. The examiner uses a gloved right hand to examine the anus and the tissue surrounding it while the left hand carefully spreads the buttocks. If infection is suspected, the examiner should wear gloves on both hands. The anal skin is inspected for signs of inflammation, excoriation, fissures, nodules, fistulae, scars, tumors, and hemorrhoids. Any abnormal areas should be palpated. The patient is asked to strain while the examiner inspects the anus for hemorrhoids or fissures. Figure 15–33 shows a patient with prolapsed internal hemorrhoids.

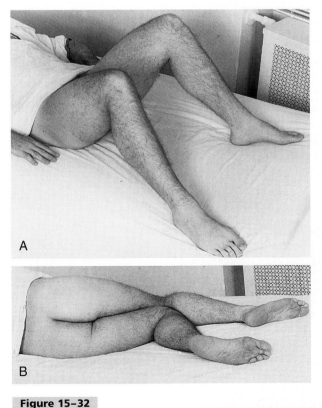

Figure 15–32

Positions for the rectal examination. *A,* Modified lithotomy position. *B,* Sims' position.

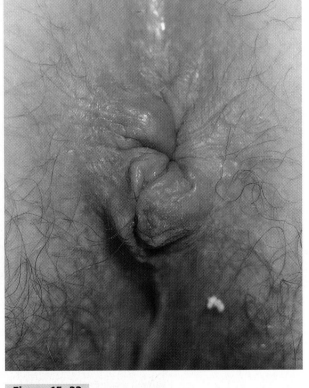

Figure 15–33

Prolapsed internal hemorrhoids.

The Technique

The patient is told that a rectal examination will now be performed. The examiner should tell the patient that a lubricant that will feel cool will be used, and this will be followed by the sensation of having to move the bowels; the patient should be assured that he will not do so.

The examiner lubricates the right gloved index finger and places the left hand on the patient's buttocks. As the left hand spreads the patient's buttocks, the examiner's right index finger is gently placed on the anal verge. The sphincter should be relaxed by gentle pressure with the palmar surface of the finger, as shown in Figure 15–34. Figure 15–35*A* illustrates the procedure.

The patient is instructed to take a deep breath, at which time the right index finger is inserted into the anal canal as the anal sphincter relaxes. The sphincter should close completely around the examining digit. The sphincter tone should be assessed. The finger should be inserted as far as possible into the rectum, although 10 cm is the probable limit of digital exploration. The left hand can now be moved to the patient's left buttock, while the right index finger examines the rectum. The examination is illustrated in Figure 15–35*B,* and the position of the hands is shown in Figure 15–36.

Palpate the Rectal Walls

The lateral, posterior, and anterior walls of the rectum are palpated. The lateral walls are felt by rotating the digit along the sides of the rectum. The ischial spines, coccyx, and lower sacrum can be felt easily. The walls are palpated for polyps, which may be sessile (attached by a base) or pedunculated (attached by a stalk). Any irregularities or undue tenderness should be noted. The only way to examine the entire circumference of the rectal wall fully is to turn your back to the patient, which will allow you to

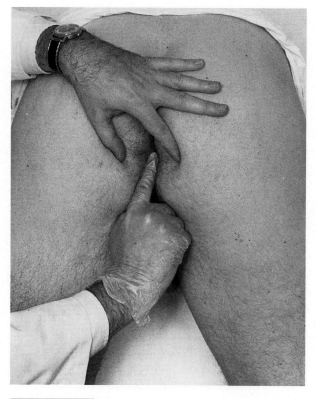

Figure 15–34

Technique of the rectal examination. The digit is inserted with the palm of the hand facing downward.

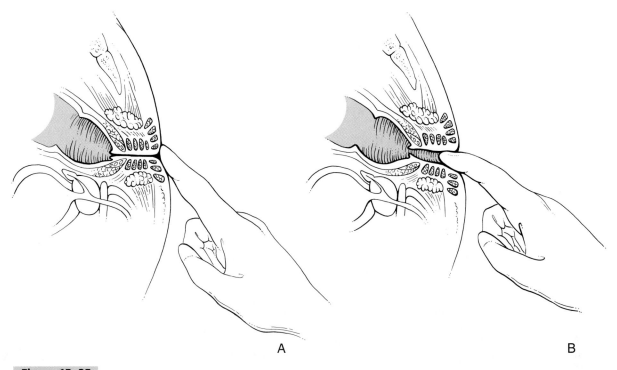

A   B

Figure 15-35

Illustration of the rectal examination. *A,* Sphincter is relaxed by gentle pressure with the palmar surface of the examiner's finger. *B,* With the examiner's left hand spreading the patient's buttocks, examination is carried out with the examiner's right index finger.

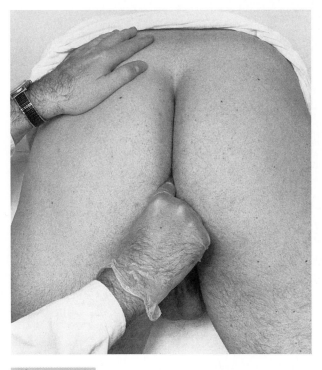

Figure 15-36

Technique for rectal examination. Note position of the examiner's left hand.

hyperpronate your hand. Unless you do so, you will be unable to examine the portion of the rectal wall between the 12 o'clock and 3 o'clock positions. A small lesion in this quadrant may go undetected.

Intraperitoneal metastases may be felt anterior to the rectum. These tumors are hard, and a shelf-like structure projects into the rectum as a result of infiltration of Douglas' pouch with neoplastic cells. This is *Blumer's shelf.*

■ Palpate the Prostate Gland

The prostate gland lies anterior to the wall of the rectum. The size, surface, consistency, sensitivity, and shape of the prostate gland should be assessed.

The prostate is a bilobed, heart-shaped structure approximately 4 cm in diameter. It is normally smooth and firm and has the consistency of a hard rubber ball. The apex of the heart shape points toward the anus. Identify the median sulcus and the lateral lobes. Note any masses, tenderness, and nodules. Only the lower apex portion of the gland is palpable. The superior margin is generally too high to reach. The examination of the prostate is illustrated in Figure 15–37. The size of the prostate in relation to the examiner's finger is shown in Figure 15–38.

A hard, irregular nodule produces asymmetry of the prostate gland and is suggestive of cancer. Carcinoma of the prostate frequently involves the posterior lobe, which can easily be identified during rectal examination. Carcinoma of the prostate is the second leading cause of death in men in the United States. In 1995, there were 35,000 deaths due to cancer of the prostate. Early detection is usually limited to detection of an abnormality on digital rectal examination.

Benign prostatic hypertrophy produces a symmetrically enlarged, soft gland that protrudes into the rectal lumen. This diffuse enlargement is common among men older than the age of 60 years. A boggy, fluctuant, or tender prostate may indicate acute prostatitis. The seminal vesicles lie superior to the prostate gland and are rarely felt, unless they are enlarged.

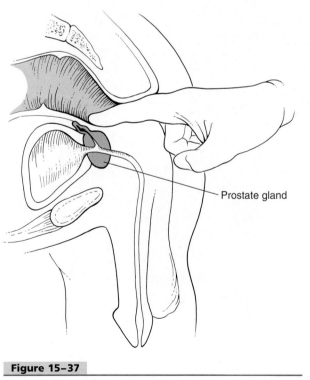

Prostate gland

Figure 15–37

Examination of the prostate.

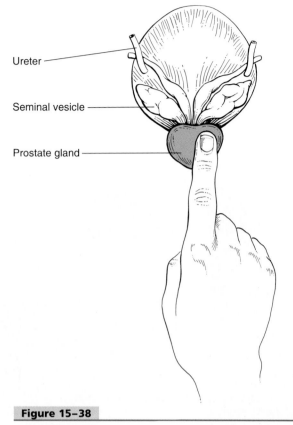

Ureter

Seminal vesicle

Prostate gland

Figure 15-38

Relationship of the size of the prostate gland to the examining finger.

The rectal examination is concluded by informing the patient that you are now going to withdraw your finger. Gently remove the examining finger, and give the patient tissues to wipe himself.

■ Test Stool for Occult Blood

The examining digit should be inspected. The color of the fecal material should be noted. The fecal material should be placed on the occult blood testing card and examined with the reagent.

The *guaiac* or *benzidine test* detects occult blood. If blood is present, a chemical reaction will result in a blue coloration on the card. The reaction is graded by the intensity of the blue color, from light blue (trace blood) to dark blue (4+ positive).

Although the examination for inguinal hernias is part of the abdominal examination, it is discussed in Chapter 16, Male Genitalia and Hernias.

Special Techniques

Intra-abdominal inflammation may involve the psoas muscle. A special test performed when there is suspicion of intra-abdominal inflammation is the *iliopsoas test*. The patient is asked to lie on the unaffected side and extend the other leg at the hip against the resistance of the examiner's hand. A *positive psoas sign* is abdominal pain with this maneuver. Irritation of the right psoas muscle by an acutely inflamed appendix produces a right psoas sign. This test is shown in Figure 15–39.

Another useful test for inflammation is the *obturator test*. While the patient is lying on the back, the examiner flexes the patient's thigh at the hip, with the patient's knees bent, and rotates the leg internally and externally at the hip. If there is an inflammatory process adjacent to the obturator muscle, pain is elicited. The obturator test is shown in Figure 15–40.

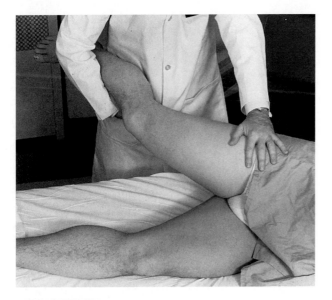

Figure 15–39

The iliopsoas test.

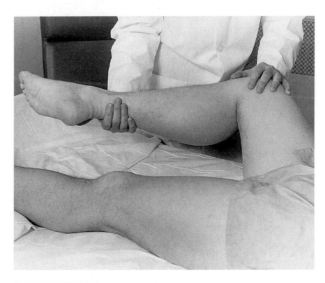

Figure 15–40

The obturator test.

Clinicopathologic Correlations

Table 15–2 lists the classic locations of pain referred from abdominal structures. Table 15–3 summarizes the maneuvers for ameliorating abdominal pain. Table 15–4 summarizes the sensitivities and specificities of the various maneuvers used to detect ascites. Table 15–5 is a comparison of the clinical manifestations of Crohn's disease and ulcerative colitis. Table 15–6 lists the clinical features of cancer of the stomach, pan-

Table 15–5   Clinical Comparison of Ulcerative Colitis and Crohn's Disease

	Ulcerative Colitis	Crohn's Disease
Diarrhea	Present	Present
Hematochezia	Common	Rare
Extraintestinal manifestations	Common	Common
Perirectal disease	Fissures	Fistulae Abscesses
Rectal disease	Present	Absent
Anal disease	Absent	Present

Table 15–6   Clinical Comparison of Cancer of the Stomach, Pancreas, and Colon

	Cancer of Stomach	Cancer of Pancreas	Cancer of Colon
Major Symptoms			
	Upper abdominal pain	Upper abdominal pain	Change in bowel habits
	Occult bleeding	Back pain	Gastrointestinal bleeding
	Weight loss	Weight loss	Lower abdominal pain
	Vomiting	Jaundice	
	Anorexia		
	Dysphagia		
Risk Factors			
	Adenomatous polyps	Smoking	Adenomatous polyps
	Pernicious anemia	Alcoholism (?)	Ulcerative colitis
	Family history		Familial polyposis
	Immigrants from Japan		Gardner's syndrome
			Villous adenomas

creas, and colon. Table 15–7 lists the variation of symptoms in right-sided and left-sided colon cancer and in rectal cancer. Table 15–8 compares the symptoms and signs of cirrhosis, which are numerous, as they relate to hepatocellular failure and portal hypertension.

Table 15–7   Variation of Symptoms of Cancer of the Right Colon, Left Colon, and Rectum

Symptom	Cancer of Right Colon	Cancer of Left Colon	Cancer of Rectum
Pain	Ill defined	Colicky*	Steady, gnawing
Obstruction	Infrequent	Common	Infrequent
Bleeding	Brick-red	Red mixed with stool	Bright red coating stool
Weakness†	Common	Infrequent	Infrequent

* Worse with ingestion of foods.
† Secondary to anemia.

Table 15–8   Signs and Symptoms of Cirrhosis

Hepatocellular Failure	Portal Hypertension
Spider angiomata	Ascites
Gynecomastia	Varices: esophageal
Palmar erythema	Hemorrhoids
Ascites	Caput medusae
Jaundice	Splenomegaly
Testicular atrophy	
Impotence	
Bleeding problems	
Changes in mental function	

Useful Vocabulary

Listed here are the specific roots that are important in order to understand the terminology related to abdominal disease.

Root	Pertaining to	Example	Definition
aer(o)-	air; gas	*aero*phagia	Air swallowing
celi(o)-	abdomen	*celi*ac	Pertaining to the abdomen
chol(e)-	bile	*chole*lith	Gallstone
cyst-	sac containing liquid	chole*cyst*itis	Inflammation of the gallbladder
enter(o)-	intestines	*enter*itis	Inflammation of the small intestines
gastr(o)-	stomach	*gastr*ectomy	Surgical removal of the stomach
lapar(o)-	loin; flank	*lapar*otomy	Surgical incision through the flank; generally, any abdominal incision
-phago-	eating	*phago*cyte	Any cell that ingests other cells or microorganisms
-tripsy	shock waves	litho*tripsy*	Noninvasive technique for breaking up stones by the use of shock waves

Writing Up the Physical Examination

Listed here are examples of the write-up for the examination of the abdomen.

- The abdomen is scaphoid without scars. Bowel sounds are present. The liver is felt 2 finger breadths below the right costal margin for a total span of 10 cm. Neither the spleen nor any masses are felt. The kidneys are not palpable. Rectal examination reveals normal sphincter tone. The prostate is soft, without any masses. The walls of the rectum are smooth, without masses. Testing of the stool for blood is negative. No costovertebral angle tenderness* is present.
- The abdomen has a scar in the right upper quadrant. Bowel sounds are absent. Marked tympany is present throughout the abdomen. Rigidity is present throughout. Marked tenderness is present in the abdomen, especially in the left lower quadrant. Examination of the rectum reveals tenderness in the same area. Stool guaiac is 4+ positive. The liver, spleen, and kidneys are not felt. No CVAT is present.
- The abdomen is obese. Bowel sounds are present. Percussion notes are normal. There is an area of significant pain in the right lower quadrant, immediately above the right midposition of the inguinal ligament. Rectal examination discloses severe pain in the same area. The obturator and straight leg raising signs are positive on the right. Stool guaiac is negative. Right CVAT is present. No organomegaly is felt.
- The abdomen is protuberant, with a midline well-healed scar. Bowel sounds are present. Shifting dullness and a fluid wave are present. A large mass 8 × 15 cm is felt in the right upper quadrant. Examination of the rectum is unremarkable except for a trace positive stool guaiac. There is no hepatosplenomegaly.
- The abdomen is scaphoid and soft, without guarding, rigidity, or tenderness. Bowel sounds are present. The liver measures 12 cm in span in the midclavicular line. The spleen tip is felt below the left costal margin. No masses are present. Rectal examination reveals a 2 cm hard nodule in the posterior lobe of the prostate, which is nontender. Stool guaiac is negative.

---

* Often abbreviated CVAT.

Bibliography

Barkun AN, Camus M, Green L, et al: The bedside assessment of splenic enlargement. Am J Med 91:512, 1991.

Barkun AN, Camus M, Meagher T, et al: Splenic enlargement and Traube's space: How useful is percussion? Am J Med 87:562, 1989.

Castell DO: The spleen percussion sign: A useful diagnostic technique. Ann Intern Med 67:1265, 1967.

Cattau EL Jr, Benjamin SB, Knoff TE, et al: The accuracy of the physical examination in the diagnosis of suspected ascites. JAMA 247:1164, 1982.

Cummings S, Papadakis M, Melnick J, et al: The predictive value of physical examination for ascites. West J Med 142:633, 1985.

Grover SA, Barkun AN, Sackett DL: Does this patient have splenomegaly? JAMA 270:2218, 1993.

Halpern S, Coel M, Ashburn W, et al: Correlation of liver and spleen size: Determinations by nuclear medicine studies and physical examination. Arch Intern Med 134:123, 1974.

Helzer JE, Chammas S, Norland CC, et al: A study of the association between Crohn's disease and psychiatric illness. Gastroenterology 86:324, 1984.

Latimer PR: Crohn's disease: A review of the psychological and social outcome. Psychol Med 8: 649, 1978.

Lindner AE: Emotional Factors in Gastrointestinal Illness. New York, American Elsevier, 1973.

McKegney FP, Gordon RO, Levine SM: A psychosomatic comparison of patients with ulcerative colitis and Crohn's disease. Psychosom Med 32:153, 1970.

Meidl EJ, Ende J: Evaluation of liver size by physical examination. J Gen Intern Med 8:635, 1993.

Mulvihill JJ: The frequency of hereditary large bowel cancer. In Ingall JRF, Mastromarino AJ (eds): Prevention of Hereditary Large Bowel Cancer. New York, Alan R Liss, 1983.

Naylor CD: Physical examination of the liver. JAMA 271:1859, 1994.

Simel DL, Halvorsen RA, Feussner JR: Quantitating bedside diagnosis: Clinical evaluation of ascites. J Gen Intern Med 3:423, 1988.

Williams JW, Simel DL: Does this patient have ascites? How to divine fluid in the abdomen. JAMA 267:2645, 1992.

CHAPTER 16

Male Genitalia and Hernias

If a man's urine is like the urine of an ass, like beer yeast, like wine yeast or varnish, that man is sick . . . and through a bronze tube in the penis pour oil and beer and licorice.

From the Sushruta Samhita
ca. 3000 BC

General Considerations

Since the beginning of recorded history, the external genitalia and the urologic system have been of special interest to people. Kidney stones and urologic surgery were well described in antiquity. One of the earliest reported kidney stones was found in a young boy who lived about 7000 BC.

Although *circumcision* has been considered as a measure of hygiene, there is much evidence that it was a ritualistic act. Circumcision is often depicted on the walls of temples dating from 3000 BC. In the Egyptian Book of the Dead, it is written, "The blood falls from the phallus of the Sun God as he starts to incise himself." The Hindus regarded the penis and testicles as a symbol of the center of life and sacrificed the prepuce as a special offering to the gods.

The Bible has many urologic references. In Genesis 17:7, Abraham makes a covenant with God for the Jews. He is told in Genesis 17:14, "And the uncircumcised male who is not circumcised in the flesh of his foreskin, that soul shall be cut off from his people; he hath broken My covenant." In Leviticus 12:3, the Jews were told, "And in the eighth day the flesh of his foreskin shall be circumcised." Leviticus 15:2–17 deals with discharges that render a man unclean.

The Bible, Hindu literature, and Egyptian papyruses described a disease now presumed to be gonorrhea. The Mesopotamian tablets described a variety of cures, such as: "If a man's penis on occasions of his pleasure hurts him, boil beer and milk and anoint him from the pubis." Avicenna's Canon of Medicine in 1000 AD was considered the authoritative text on medicine for centuries and described placing a louse in the penis to counteract a penile discharge.

Gonorrhea was probably first named by Galen in the 2nd century AD. Gonorrhea is the Greek translation of "a flow of offspring." Galen apparently thought that the purulent discharge was a leakage of semen. Many terms have been used to describe gonorrhea throughout the years. Perhaps the most common is *clap,* a name used for the past 400 years. It is thought that the term *clap* was derived from the red-light district in Paris, called "Le Clapier."

It is unclear when the scourge of *syphilis* began. There was much confusion between syphilis and gonorrhea. It was thought that gonorrhea was the first stage of syphilis. The cause of these diseases was also unknown. Many believed that syphilis was due to floods, eating disguised human meat, or poisoning of the water. It was not until 1500, when syphilis was pandemic in Europe, that the venereal origins of both diseases were understood. It is now believed that syphilis was introduced on the European continent in 1492 by the returning sailors who had been traveling with Columbus. After the invasion of Italy and the siege of Naples by France in 1495, syphilis became rampant throughout Europe. The *King's pox* and the *French pox* were the common terms used for syphilis.

Cancer of the genitourinary system is common. In the United States, it is estimated that prostatic cancer accounts for 19% of all cancers in men, and urinary tract cancers account for an additional 9%. Prostatic cancer accounts for 10% of all cancer deaths, whereas other genitourinary malignancies account for 5%. There were more than 97,000 new cases of prostatic cancer in 1994, making this diagnosis the second most common malignancy in men (lung cancer is the first). Approximately 95% of all prostatic cancers arise from the area of the gland that can be readily detected by rectal examination.

Although testicular cancer accounts for only 1% of all cancers in men, testicular carcinoma represents the most common cancer in men in the 15–35 year old age group. Approximately 90% of all testicular tumors manifest as an asymptomatic testicular mass. Once these tumors are detected and treatment is begun, the cure rate can approach 90%. The most important prognostic factors have been shown to be early detection by routine physical examination and self-examination. All men should be instructed in testicular self-examination.

Structure and Physiology

Cross-sectional and frontal views of the male genitalia are shown in Figure 16–1.

The *penis* is composed of three elongated, distensible structures: two paired *corpora cavernosa* and a single *corpus spongiosum.* The urethra runs through the corpus spongiosum. The penis has two surfaces, dorsal and ventral (urethral), and consists of the root, the shaft, and the head. The shaft is composed of erectile tissue, which when engorged with blood produces a firm erection necessary for sexual intercourse. The corpora cavernosa also contain smooth muscle that contract rhythmically during ejaculation.

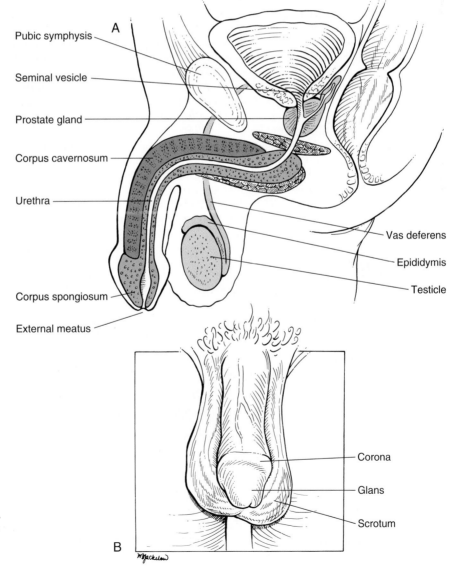

Figure 16–1

Diagrams of male genitalia. *A,* Cross section. *B,* Frontal view.

On the dorsal aspect in the midline of the penis runs the dorsal vein with an artery and nerve on either side. The distal end of the corpus spongiosum expands to form the head, or *glans penis.* The glans penis covers the end of the corpora cavernosa. The glans has a prominent margin on its dorsal aspect, the *corona.* A slit-like opening on the tip of the glans is the *external meatus* of the urethra.

The skin of the penis is smooth, thin, and hairless. At the distal end of the penis, a free fold of skin called the *prepuce* (foreskin) covers the glans. Mucus secretion and sloughed epithelial cells called *smegma* collect between the prepuce and the glans, providing a lubricant during sexual intercourse. The prepuce can be retracted to expose the glans as far as the corona. During circumcision, the prepuce is removed.

The root of the penis lies deep to the scrotum, in the perineum. At the root, the corpora cavernosa diverge from each other. Each corpus cavernosum is enveloped in a dense, fibroelastic covering called the *tunica albuginea,* and these tunicae fuse to form the median septum of the penis. A cross section through the penis is shown in Figure 16–2.

The blood supply to the penis is from the internal pudendal artery, from which the dorsal and deep arteries of the corpora cavernosa are derived. The veins drain into the dorsal vein of the penis. In the flaccid state, the venous channels and arteriovenous anastomoses are widely patent, whereas the arteries are partially constricted. In the erect state, the arteriovenous channels are closed, and the arteries are widely opened. Muscular pillars are present in the walls of the arteries, veins, and arteriovenous anastomoses, which aid in occluding the lumens. The physiology of erection is illustrated in Figure 16–3.

The *urethra* extends from the internal urinary meatus of the bladder to the external meatus of the penis. The urethra can be divided into three portions: the prostatic (posterior) portion, the membranous portion, and the cavernous (anterior) portion. The short posterior portion passes through the prostate gland. The common ejaculatory duct as well as several prostatic ducts enters at the distal end of this portion. The external urethral sphincter surrounds the membranous urethra, and on either side lie Cowper's bulbourethral glands. The anterior urethra is the longest and passes through the corpus spongiosum. The ducts of Cowper's glands enter the anterior urethra near its proximal end.

The *scrotum* is the pouch containing the testes, which is suspended externally from the perineum. It is divided into halves by the interscrotal septum, one testis lying on each side. The wall of the scrotum contains involuntary smooth muscle and voluntary striated muscle. A major role of the scrotum is temperature regulation of the testes. The testes are maintained about 2°C lower than the peritoneal cavity, a condition necessary for spermatogenesis. The size of the scrotum is variable according to the individual and his response to ambient temperature. During exposure to cold temperatures, the scrotum is contracted and very rugated. In a warm environment, the scrotum becomes pendulous and smoother.

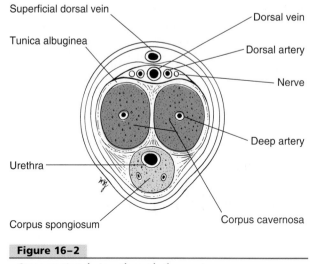

Figure 16–2

Cross-sectional view through the penis.

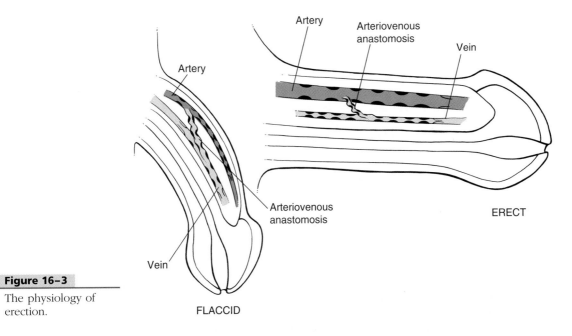

Figure 16–3

The physiology of erection.

The *testes,* or *testicles,* are ovoid, smooth, and approximately 3.5–5 cm in length. The left testicle commonly lies lower than the right. The testes are covered with a tough fibrous coat called the *tunica albuginea testis.* Each testicle has a long axis directed slightly anteriorly and upward and contains long, microscopic, convoluted seminiferous tubules that produce sperm. The tubules end in the *epididymis,* which is comma-shaped and located on the posterior border of the testis. It consists of a head that is swollen and overhangs the upper pole of the testicle. The inferior portion or tail of the epididymis continues into the *vas deferens.* The testicular artery enters the testicle in its posterior midportion. The veins draining the testicle form a dense network called the *pampiniform plexus,* which drains into the testicular vein. The right testicular vein drains directly into the inferior vena cava, whereas the left drains into the left renal vein. The lymphatic drainage of the testes is to the pre-aortic and precaval nodes, not to the inguinal nodes. This is important to recognize, because the testes are embryologically intra-abdominal organs, and neoplasms and inflammations of the testis produce adenopathy of these nodal chains. In general, inguinal adenopathy is rare.

The relationship of the testicle and epididymis is shown in Figure 16–4.

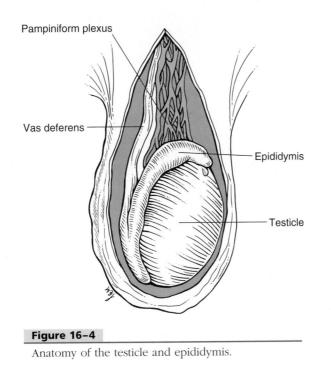

Figure 16–4

Anatomy of the testicle and epididymis.

The vas deferens is a cord-like structure, easily felt in the scrotum. The vas deferens, testicular arteries, and veins form the *spermatic cord,* which enters the inguinal canal. The vas deferens passes through the internal ring and, after a convoluted course, reaches the fundus of the bladder. It passes between the rectum and the bladder and approaches the vas deferens of the opposite side near the seminal vesicles. Near the base of the prostate, the vas deferens joins with the duct of the corresponding seminal vesicle to form the *ejaculatory duct,* which passes through the prostate gland to enter the posterior urethra.

The *prostate gland* is about the size of two almonds, or approximately 3.5 cm long by 3 cm wide. Traversing through the gland in the midline is the posterior urethra. On either side is an ejaculatory duct. The prostate is commonly divided into five lobes. The posterior lobe is clinically important, because carcinoma frequently affects this lobe. In the presence of cancer, the midline groove between the two lateral lobes may be obliterated. The middle and lateral lobes are above the ejaculatory ducts and are typically involved with benign hypertrophy. The anterior lobe is of little clinical importance.

The male genitalia showing the sources and direction of seminal fluid flow are illustrated in Figure 16–5.

The descent of the testes is important to review at this time. In the normal full-term male, both testes are in the scrotum at birth. The testes descend to this position just before birth. About the 12th week of gestation, the *gubernaculum* develops in the inguinal fold and grows through the body wall to an area that will ultimately lie in the scrotum. This tract marks the location of the future inguinal canal. A dimple called the *processus vaginalis* forms in the peritoneum and follows the course of the gubernaculum. By the 7th month of gestation, the processus vaginalis has reached the aponeurosis of the external oblique muscle. Each testis then begins its descent from the abdominal cavity through the internal ring to lie in the abdominal wall. During the 8th month, the testes descend along the inguinal canal; at birth, they are in the scrotum. At birth,

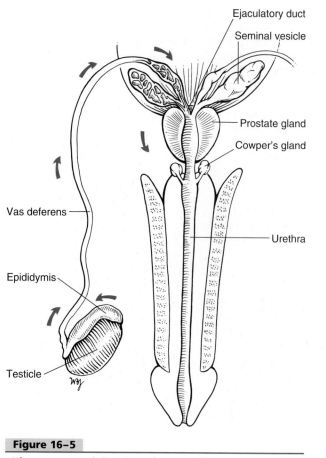

Figure 16–5

The sources and direction of seminal flow.

the gubernaculum is barely distinguishable, and the processus vaginalis becomes obliterated within the spermatic cord. In about 5% of male infants, there is imperfect descent of the testis *(cryptorchidism)*. The descent of the testes is illustrated in Figure 16–6.

The genital development stages for boys are illustrated in Figure 22–23 (and discussed in Chapter 22, The Pediatric Patient).

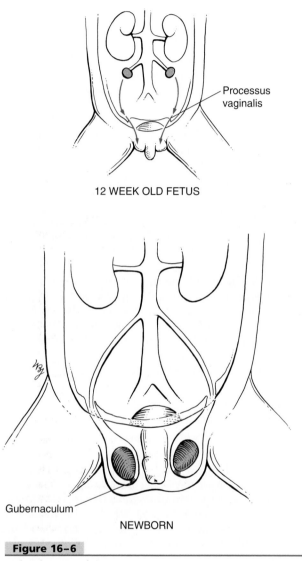

12 WEEK OLD FETUS

NEWBORN

Figure 16–6

The descent of the testes.

Review of Specific Symptoms

The most common symptoms of male genitourinary disease are as follows:

- Pain
- Dysuria
- Changes in urine flow
- Red urine
- Penile discharge
- Penile lesions
- Scrotal enlargement
- Groin mass or swelling
- Impotence
- Infertility

Pain

Sudden distention of the ureter, renal pelvis, or bladder may cause flank pain. Any patient with flank pain should be asked the following questions:

"When did the pain begin?"
"Where did the pain begin?" "Can you point to the area?"
"Do you feel the pain in any other area of your body?"
"Did the pain start suddenly?"
"Have you ever had this type of pain before?"
"Is the pain constant?"
"What seems to make the pain worse? less?"
"Has the color of your urine changed?"
"Is the pain associated with nausea? vomiting? abdominal distention? fever? chills? burning on urination?"

Gradual enlargement of an organ is usually painless. An aching pain in the costovertebral angle may be related to sudden distention of the renal capsule, which results from acute pyelonephritis or obstructive hydronephrosis. The spasmodic, colicky pain from upper ureteral dilatation may cause referred pain to the testis on the same side. Lower ureteral dilatation may cause pain referred to the scrotum. The pain of ureteral distention is severe, and the patient is restless and uncomfortable in any position. Bladder distention causes lower abdominal fullness and suprapubic pain, with an intense desire to urinate. Pain in the groin may result from pathologic processes in the spermatic cord, testicle, or prostate gland; from lymphadenitis of any cause; from hernia; from herpes zoster; or from a disorder that is neurologic in origin.

Testicular pain can result from nearly any disease of the testis or epididymis. Such diseases include epididymitis, orchitis, hydrocele, spermatic cord torsion, and tumor. Referred pain from the ipsilateral ureter must always be considered. *Priapism* is a painful, persistent erection of the penis that is not a result of sexual excitation. The sustained erection results from thrombosis of the corpora cavernosa. This occurs in patients with sickle cell anemia or leukemia. The exact mechanism is unknown but appears to result from a blockage of venous drainage from the penis, while the arteries remain patent. Chronic priapism often results in organic impotence.

Dysuria

Pain on urination, called *dysuria,* is frequently described as "burning." Dysuria is evidence of inflammation of the lower urinary tract. The patient may describe discomfort in the penis or in the suprapubic area. Dysuria also implies difficulty in urination. This may result from external meatal stenosis or from a urethral stricture. Painful urination is usually associated with urinary frequency and urgency. When the patient describes pain or difficulty in urination, ask the following questions:

"How long have you noticed burning on urination?"
"How often do you urinate each day?"
"How does your urination feel different?"
"Is your urine clear?"
"Does the urine smell bad?"
"Do you have a discharge from your penis?"
"Does the urine seem to have gas bubbles in it?"
"Have you noticed any solid particles in your urine?"
"Have you noticed pus in your urine?"

Pneumaturia is the passage of air in the urine producing what the patient describes as "bubbles of gas in the urine." The air or gas is emitted usually at the end of urination. Normally, there is no gas in the urinary tract. The symptom of pneumaturia indicates the introduction of air by instrumentation, a fistula to the bowel, or a urinary tract infection by gas-forming bacteria, such as *Escherichia coli* or clostridia.

Fecaluria is the presence of fecal material in the urine and is rare. The passage of feculent-smelling material results from either an intestinovesicular fistula or a urethrorectal fistula. These fistulae occur as a consequence of ulceration from the bowel to the urinary tract. Diverticulitis, carcinoma, and Crohn's disease are frequent causes.

Pus in the urine, or *pyuria,* is the body's response to inflammation of the urinary tract. Bacteria is the most common cause of inflammation resulting in pyuria, although pyuria is also seen in patients with neoplasms and kidney stones. Cystitis and prostatitis are common causes of pyuria.

Changes in Urine Flow

Changes in urine flow include frequency and incontinence. Urinary *frequency* is the most common symptom of the genitourologic system. Frequency is defined as passing urine more often than normal. *Nocturia* is urinary frequency at night. There are several causes of frequency: decreased bladder size, bladder wall irritation, and increased urine volume. If an obstructed bladder cannot be completely emptied at each voiding, its effective capacity is diminished. The following questions, in addition to the ones pertaining to dysuria, should be asked to help define the problem:

> *"Do you find that you must wake up at night to urinate?"*
> *"Can you estimate the amount of urine passed each time you urinate?"*
> *"Do you have sudden urges to urinate?"*
> *"Have you found that despite an urge to urinate you cannot start the stream?"*
> *"Has there been a change in the caliber of the stream?"*
> *"Have you found that you must wait longer for the stream to start?"*
> *"Do you have the sensation that after urination has stopped you still have the urge to urinate?"*
> *"Do you have to strain at the end of urination?"*
> *"Have you been drinking more fluids recently?"*

Prostatic hypertrophy is the most common cause in men of reduced usable bladder capacity. Most bladder diseases, such as cystitis, cause frequency that is due to irritation of the bladder mucosa. *Polyuria,* or voiding large amounts of urine, is usually accompanied by excessive thirst, *polydipsia.* Diabetes mellitus and diabetes insipidus are common causes of polydipsia.

Urinary *incontinence* is the inability of the patient to retain his urine voluntarily. The urge to urinate may be so intense that incontinence may result. In addition to the questions regarding dysuria and frequency, ask the following:

> *"Do you involuntarily lose small amounts of urine?"*
> *"Do you lose your urine constantly?"*
> *"Do you lose your urine when lifting heavy objects? laughing? coughing? bending over?"*
> *"Do you have to press on your abdomen to urinate?"*

In patients who have chronically distended bladders, as in patients with prostatic hypertrophy, there is always a large amount of residual urine. The pressure within the bladder is constantly elevated. A slight increase in intra-abdominal pressure raises the intravesicular pressure sufficiently to overcome bladder neck resistance, and urine escapes. Leakage may be steady or intermittent. This type of incontinence is *overflow* incontinence. *Stress* incontinence is leakage that occurs only when the patient strains. The primary defect is a loss of muscular support in the urethrovesicular region. Residual urine is insignificant. Any increase in intra-abdominal pressure causes leakage. This type of incontinence is more common in women and is further discussed in Chapter 17, Female Genitalia.

Polyuria is the symptom of increased amounts of urination, frequently greater than 2–3 liters per day. The normal daily urine output varies from 1 to 2 liters. The most important diseases to differentiate are diabetes mellitus, diabetes insipidus, and psychological diabetes insipidus. Ask the following questions:

> *"How long have you been passing large amounts of urine?"*
> *"Was the onset sudden?"*
> *"How often do you have to urinate at night?"*

"Is there any variability in the urine flow from day to day?"
"Do you have an excessive thirst?"
"Do you prefer water or other fluids?"
"What happens if you don't drink? Will you still have to urinate?"
"How is your appetite?"
"Do you have any visual problems? headaches?"
"Are you aware of any emotional problems?"

Patients with diabetes mellitus have a high osmotic load and have polyuria. Increased appetite is also common. Diabetes insipidus is due to a vasopressin deficiency related to a lesion in the hypothalamus or pituitary gland. In these patients, the urine cannot become concentrated despite a rise in plasma osmolality. Patients with psychogenic diabetes insipidus, which is more common, have polyuria related to compulsive drinking of water. It is seen in patients with psychological problems. The abrupt onset of polyuria is seen in psychogenic diabetes insipidus. These patients also have no preference for the type of fluid they drink. In contrast, patients with true diabetes insipidus prefer water. Because true diabetes insipidus is related to intracranial lesions, it is not surprising that these individuals suffer from headaches and visual disturbances, especially visual field abnormalities.

Red Urine

Red urine often indicates *hematuria,* or blood in the urine. There are many causes of red urine, and it should not be automatically assumed that red urine indicates bleeding. Vegetable dyes, drugs such as pyridium, and excessive ingestion of beets can cause red urine. When it is determined that the urine is red as a result of the presence of blood, the hematuria is termed *gross hematuria.* Hematuria may be the first symptom of serious disease of the urinary tract. Ask the following questions of any patient with the symptom of red urine:

"How long have you noticed red urine?"
"Have you had red urine previously?"
"Have you noticed that the urine starts red and then clears? starts clear and then turns red? is red throughout?"
"Have you noticed clots of blood in the urine?"
"Have you done any severely strenuous physical activity recently, such as prolonged hiking, running, or marching?"
"Did you have an upper respiratory infection or a sore throat a few weeks ago?"
"Is the red urine associated with flank pain? abdominal pain? burning on urination? fever? weight loss?"
"Are you aware of any bleeding problems?"
"Are you taking any medications?"
"Do you eat beets often?"

Individuals who participate in strenuous activities may traumatize blood cells as these cells travel through the small vessels on the feet. A condition called *march hemoglobinuria* may result, causing intravascular hemolysis and hemoglobinuria. The temporal relationship of blood in the urine is an important factor. Blood only at the beginning, or *initial* hematuria, usually has a source in the urethra. Blood only at the end of urination, *terminal* hematuria, indicates a disorder at the bladder neck or at the posterior urethra. Blood evenly distributed throughout urination is *total* hematuria and implies disease above the prostate gland or a massive hemorrhage at any level. Blood staining of undergarments without blood in the urine indicates pathologic processes in the external urethral meatus. Weight loss and hematuria are seen in renal cell carcinoma. Red urine that has occurred 10–14 days after an upper respiratory infection may indicate acute glomerulonephritis.

Penile Discharge

Discharge from the penis is a continuous or intermittent flow of fluid from the urethra. Ask the patient whether he has ever had a discharge and, if he has, whether it was bloody or purulent. Bloody penile discharges are associated with ulcerations, neoplasms, or urethritis. Purulent discharges are thick and yellowish-green and may be associated with gonococcal urethritis or chronic prostatitis. Determine when the discharge was first noted. Figure 16–7 shows a purulent penile discharge in a male with gonococcal urethritis. Gonorrhea is caused by *Neisseria gonorrhoeae*. After exposure, approximately 25% of males and more than 50% of females will contract the disease. In males, the acute symptoms of dysuria and a purulent urethral discharge begin 2–10 days after exposure. In females, a vaginal discharge and dysuria develop days to weeks after exposure; however, up to 50% of women may be asymptomatic.

Tactful direct questioning of any history of or exposure to sexually transmitted diseases is essential. The interviewer should determine the patient's sexual orientation and the type of sexual exposure—oral, vaginal, or anal—as this information will help determine the types of bacteriologic cultures necessary. It is appropriate to ask whether the patient has more than one sexual partner and whether the partner or partners have any known illnesses. The sexual history questions suggested in Chapter 1, The Interviewer's Questions, may be helpful.

Penile Lesions

A history of lesions on the penis should alert the examiner to the possibility of venereal disease. Ask the patient whether he has had gonorrhea, syphilis, herpes, trichomoniasis, or other venereal disease.

Scrotal Enlargement

It is not uncommon for a male to complain of enlargement of his scrotum, but it is often difficult for him to determine which anatomic structures in the scrotum are enlarged. Ask these questions:

"When did you first notice the enlargement?"
"Is it painful?"
"Have you sustained any injury to your groin?"
"Does the enlargement change in size?"
"Have you ever had it before?"

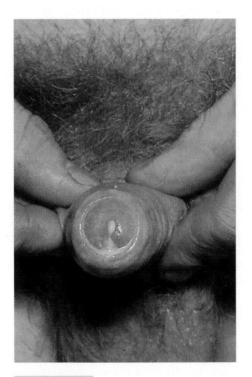

Figure 16–7

Purulent penile discharge.

"Have you ever had a hernia?"
"Have you had any problems with fertility?"

Swellings in the scrotum can be related to testicular or epididymal enlargement, a hernia, a varicocele, a spermatocele, or a hydrocele. Testicular enlargement can result from inflammation or tumor. Most of the time, enlargement is unilateral. Painful scrotal enlargements can result from acute inflammation of the epididymis or testis, torsion of the spermatic cord, or a strangulated hernia. Varicoceles are often a cause of decreased fertility.

Groin Mass or Swelling

If a patient describes a mass in the groin, ask the following questions:

"When did you first notice it?"
"Is the mass painful?"
"Does it change in size with different positions?"
"Have you had any venereal disease?"

The most common cause of swelling in the groin is a hernia. Hernias are reduced in size after the patient has been lying down. Adenopathy from any infection of the external genitalia may produce inguinal swelling. Carcinoma of the testis produces inguinal node enlargement only if the scrotal skin is involved.

Impotence

Erectile impotence frequently provides an insight into emotional problems of the patient. A delicate approach to the patient must be taken. It is necessary to use tact and appropriate language that will be understood by the patient. Explaining that impotence is a common problem often sets the tone. Deep-seated problems require careful questioning. Sometimes the interviewer will discover latent homosexuality. Guilt and taboos during early life may leave a lasting impression on sexual performance. Key and direct questions are important. It is appropriate to ask the following:

"Do you have early morning erections or nighttime emissions?"
"Do any individuals other than your partner arouse you?"
"Are you able to masturbate to an erection or climax?"

An affirmative answer to any of these questions will allow the interviewer to be reassured that the impotence is psychological in origin. Allowing the patient to discuss his problems may serve to vent some of his anxieties. The patient's confidence must be secured by guaranteeing confidentiality. The interviewer must resolve his or her own sexual anxieties in order to have a confident and straightforward discussion. An open dialogue about the anxieties surrounding sexual intercourse may be productive. The interviewer must be careful not to impose his or her own moral standards on the patient. Improving communication between partners is helpful.

Infertility

Infertility is the inability to conceive or to cause pregnancy. Infertility is a common problem found in as many as 10% of all marriages. A couple is said to be infertile when after 1 year of normal intercourse without the use of contraceptives pregnancy does not occur. It has been estimated that almost 30% of all infertility is due to a male factor. Any patient with the history of infertility should be questioned regarding a history of mumps, testicular injury, venereal disease, exposure to x-rays, or any urologic surgical procedure. Determine frequency of sexual intercourse and difficulty in achieving or maintaining an erection. Take a careful history of general work habits, alcohol consumption, and sleeping habits.

Impact of Impotence on the Male

Impotence may be described as the inability of a male to achieve or maintain an erection sufficient to accomplish coitus. Impotence may be either erectile or ejaculatory. This inability may also be partial or complete. Males may complain of difficulty in achieving or maintaining an erection or of premature ejaculations. The prevalence of some degree of impotence ranges from 20 to 30% of the married population. As the male ages, there is a natural loss of both libido and potency. In general, this does not occur before the age of 50 years. Some men remain sexually vigorous well into old age. If a patient suffering from impotence has occasional erections or can achieve orgasm during masturbation, he may have a primary emotional problem. In almost 90% of patients complaining of impotence, the inadequacy is found to be caused by emotional rather than anatomic factors.

Hearing about a friend's sexual activities, especially if they are exaggerated, will deflate a patient's ego and heighten his sense of inadequacy. The cultural environment of the patient must set the standard for adequacy. It is almost impossible to compare the cultural patterns of Occidentals with those of Orientals. In 1948, Kinsey and his group obtained factual data on Anglo-American sexual patterns. The frequency of sexual intercourse varied from one to four times per week. The period of maximum sexual activity was from the ages 20 to 30 years. It was shown that there were marked variations among individuals as well as among socioeconomic groups. The lower the socioeconomic group, the more frequent were the sexual encounters.

Boredom, anxiety, peer pressure, aging, deterioration of the stereotypical male role, and female "aggressiveness" are factors contributing to psychogenic impotence. Diabetes mellitus is one of the more common causes of organic impotence. Patients with multiple sclerosis, spinal cord tumors, degenerative diseases of the spinal cord, and local injury suffer from a gradual loss of potency. Certain medications can cause impotence: beta-blockers, carbonic anhydrase inhibitors, and antihypertensive agents, for example.

Guilt, anxiety, and hypochondriasis are common in the male with psychogenic impotence. Frigidity in a woman may make the male feel further insecure in his own marital adjustment, worsening his impotence. The self-image of the male may be low. It is common for the male with marginal difficulties to worry incessantly about his next attempt. His fear of failure generates enormous anxiety, which reinforces his inadequacy, and a vicious circle is begun. Each failure worsens the next attempt. If the act of coitus is not satisfactory to the patient or his partner, embarrassment and guilt develop.

Some males may be able to maintain an erection but have difficulty in ejaculation. They may become physically exhausted and may have to stop intercourse before ejaculation. The ejaculatory ducts may become so inflamed or even ulcerated that if ejaculation does occur, blood is present in the semen. This produces further anxiety and emotional upset that aggravate the situation.

Regardless of the cause, impotence has vast implications. The male may feel emasculated with an inferiority complex. Anger and depression are common. If the patient's impotence is associated with an anatomic defect, there may be additional changes in his self-image related to the physical disease state. If sexual problems are not resolved, the patient may develop personality changes. His fear of losing his sexual partner interferes with his work. Sleep and rest are disturbed. If sexual maladjustment continues, neurotic complaints may ensue. Without proper guidance, the man may become completely impotent, and suicidal tendencies can develop.

Severe psychiatric disturbances must be treated by a trained psychiatrist or sexual therapist. Success depends to a great extent on the ability of the clinician and the patient's sexual partner to inspire confidence in the patient.

Physical Examination

The only equipment necessary for the examination of the male genitalia is latex gloves.

Many students are concerned about the possibility that a patient will have an erection during the examination. Although possible, it is rare for a male to become sexually excited, because he will usually be nervous in these circumstances. If the examination is performed in an objective manner, it should not be a source of stimulation to the patient.

Although the wearing of protective gloves may decrease the examiner's sensitivity, disposable latex gloves should be worn.

Examination of the male genitalia is performed with the patient first lying and then standing. This postural change is important, because hernias or scrotal masses may not be apparent in the lying position.

The examination of the male genitalia consists of the following:

- Inspection and palpation with the patient lying
- Inspection and palpation with the patient standing
- Hernia examination

Inspection and Palpation with the Patient Lying

■ Inspect the Skin and Hair

While the patient is lying, the skin in the groin should be inspected for the presence of a superficial fungal infection, excoriations, and other rashes. Excoriations may indicate a scabies infection.

Observe the distribution of hair. Inspect the pubic hair for the presence of crab lice or nits (egg cases) attached to the hair. Are there any burrows of scabies present? See Figure 6–67.

■ Inspect the Penis and Scrotum

In the examination of the penis and scrotum, note the following:

- Whether the male is circumcised
- The size of the penis and scrotum
- Any lesions on the penis and penile edema

Figure 16–8 shows ectopic sebaceous glands on the shaft of the penis. The glands appear as pinhead-sized, whitish-yellow papules. These are commonly seen in normal men on the corona, the inner foreskin, and on the shaft of the penis. Their appearance is very similar to Fordyce's spots of the oral mucosa. Ectopic sebaceous glands may be found also in normal women on the labia minora and labia majora.

Figure 16–9 shows the penis of a patient with the chancre of primary syphilis. Although the typical syphilitic chancre is described as nontender, approximately 30% of

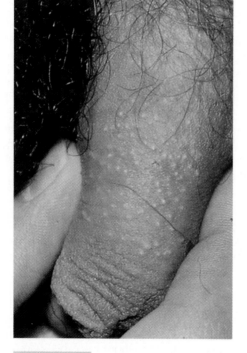

Figure 16–8

Ectopic sebaceous glands on the penis.

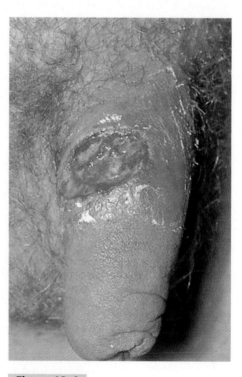

Figure 16–9

Primary syphilis.

patients with primary syphilis describe some pain or tenderness. Usually only a single lesion is present. The edge of the chancre is usually indurated. Moderate, nontender, inguinal adenopathy was present in this patient.

Figure 16–10 shows the penis of a patient with chancroid. In contrast to the chancre of syphilis, the ulceration of chancroid is extremely painful. The ulcer has a purulent, grayish surface that becomes granulating. Characteristically, the base of the ulcer and its vicinity are not infiltrated. There is also usually moderate, tender adenopathy associated with the genital lesions. Another important difference between the ulceration of chancroid and the chancre of syphilis is the frequent presence of multiple lesions in the former. This patient had a similar lesion on the other side of his penis.

Are there any papules on the penis or scrotum? Figure 16–11 shows genital papules in a patient with scabies.

The scrotum is inspected for any sores or rashes. Pinpoint, dark red, slightly raised, telangiectatic lesions on the scrotum are common in individuals older than the age of 50 years. They are *angiokeratomas* and are benign. *Fabry's disease,* which is a rare, sex-linked inborn error of glycosphingolipid metabolism, is characterized by pain, fever, and diffuse angiokeratomas in a "bathing suit" distribution, especially around the umbilicus and scrotum. The scrotum of an 18 year old patient with Fabry's disease and multiple angiokeratomas is shown in Figure 16–12.

The patient in Figure 16–13 has acquired immunodeficiency syndrome (AIDS) and Kaposi's sarcoma. Notice the marked penile and scrotal edema as well as the lesions of Kaposi's sarcoma on his thighs and scrotum.

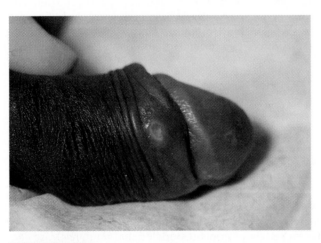

Figure 16–10

Chancroid.

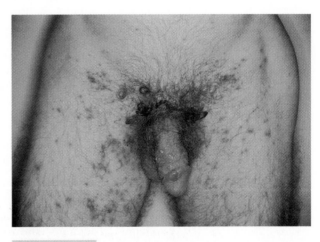

Figure 16–11

Scabies in the groin and on the penis.

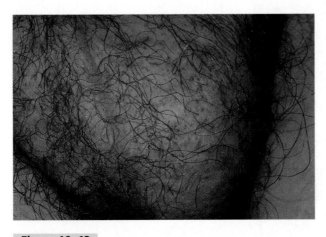

Figure 16–12

Angiokeratomas in a patient with Fabry's disease.

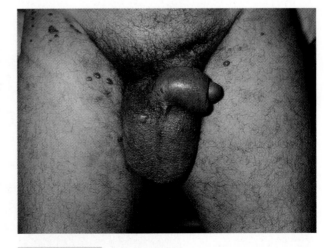

Figure 16–13

Kaposi's sarcoma and AIDS-related edema.

The examiner elevates the patient's scrotum to inspect the perineum carefully for any inflammation, ulceration, warts, abscesses, or other lesions.

▧ Palpate the Inguinal Nodes

By rolling the fingers along the inguinal ligament, the examiner may assess the presence of inguinal adenopathy. Commonly, small (0.5 cm), freely mobile lymph nodes are present in this area. Because the lymphatics from the perineum, legs, and feet drain into this area, it is not surprising that small lymph nodes are frequently encountered.

▧ Inspect for Groin Mass

Ask the patient to cough or strain while you inspect the groin. A sudden bulge may indicate an inguinal or femoral hernia.

Inspection and Palpation with the Patient Standing

The patient is asked to stand while the examiner assumes a seated position in front of him.

▧ Inspect the Penis

If the patient is not circumcised, the foreskin should be retracted. Some examiners prefer the patient to retract it himself, whereas others would rather determine the tightness of the foreskin. The cheesy, white material under the foreskin is smegma and is normal.

Phimosis is present when the foreskin cannot be retracted and prevents adequate examination of the glans. Because the glans also cannot be cleaned, smegma builds up, leading to possible inflammation of the glans and prepuce, *balanoposthitis.* Inflammation of the glans penis alone is *balanitis.* This chronic irritation may be a causative factor in cancer of the penis.

The glans is inspected for ulcers, warts, nodules, scars, and signs of inflammation. Figure 16–14 shows a patient with the characteristic rash of *genital lichen planus.* Notice the white reticulate pattern over the violaceous lesions.

▧ Inspect the External Meatus

The examiner should note the position of the external urethral meatus. It should be central on the glans. The meatus is evaluated by the examiner placing hands on either side of the glans penis and opening the meatus. The technique for examining the meatus is shown in Figure 16–15.

The meatus should be observed for any discharge, warts, and stenosis. Venereal warts, *condylomata acuminata,* may be found near the meatus, on the glans, in the perineum, at the anus, and on the shaft of the penis. Condylomata acuminata are the characteristic lesions of human papillomavirus infection. Typically, these papules have

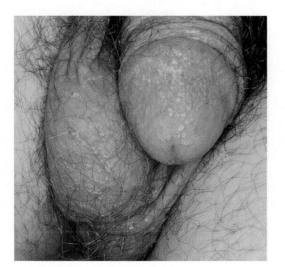

Figure 16–14

Genital lichen planus.

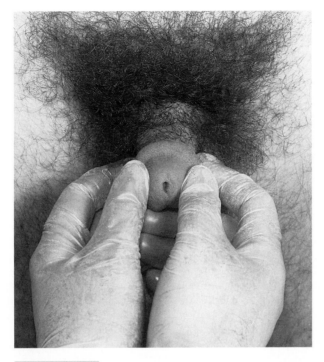

Figure 16–15

Technique for inspecting the external urethral meatus.

a verrucous surface resembling cauliflower. They are highly contagious, with transmission occurring in 30–60% of patients after a single exposure. Figure 16–16 shows meatal condylomata acuminata.

Occasionally, the urethral meatus opens on the ventral surface of the penis; this condition is *hypospadias*. A less common condition is *epispadias,* in which the meatus is located on the dorsal surface of the penis.

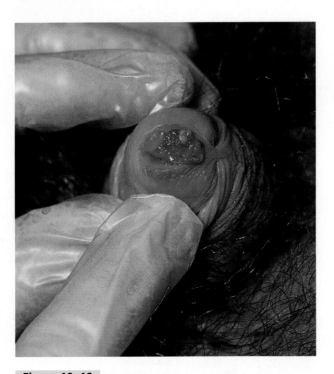

Figure 16–16

Condylomata acuminata.

Palpate the Penis

Palpate the shaft from the glans to the base of the penis. The presence of scars, ulcers, nodules, induration, and signs of inflammation must be noted. Palpation of the corpora cavernosa is performed by holding the penis between the fingers of both hands and using the index fingers to note any induration. Figure 16–17 illustrates the method of palpation of the penis.

The presence of nontender induration or fibrotic areas under the skin of the shaft suggests *Peyronie's disease*. Patients with this condition may also complain of penile deviation on erection. The erect penis shows a deviation in the long axis, making sexual intercourse difficult or impossible. The patient or his partner may also complain of pain. The site of predilection is the dorsal aspect of the penis, especially in the middle or proximal third. Figure 16–18 shows a patient with Peyronie's disease.

Palpate the Urethra

The urethra should be palpated from the external meatus through the corpus spongiosum to its base. To palpate the base of the urethra, the examiner elevates the penis with the left hand while the right index finger invaginates the scrotum in the midline and palpates deep to the base of the corpus spongiosum. The pad of the right index finger should palpate the entire corpus spongiosum from the meatus to its base. This technique is shown in Figure 16–19. If a discharge is present, "milking the urethra" may allow a drop to be placed on a glass slide for microscopic evaluation.

The foreskin, if retracted, should be replaced. *Paraphimosis* is a condition in which the foreskin can be retracted but cannot be replaced and becomes caught behind the corona.

Inspect the Scrotum

The scrotum is now reevaluated while the patient is standing. Observe the contour and contents of the scrotum. Two testicles should be present. Normally the left testicle is lower than the right. The presence of any fullness not seen while the patient was lying should be noted.

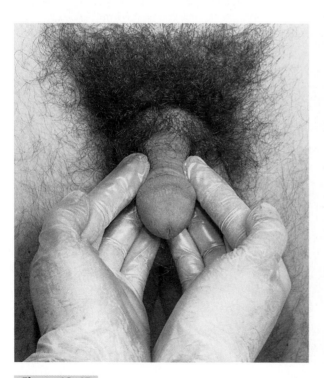

Figure 16–17

Technique for palpation of the penis.

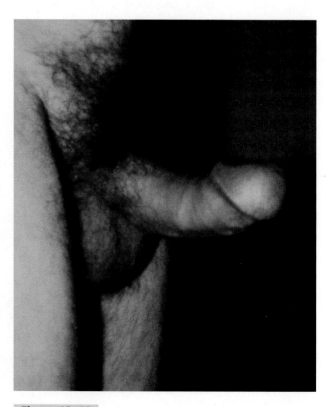

Figure 16–18

Peyronie's disease.

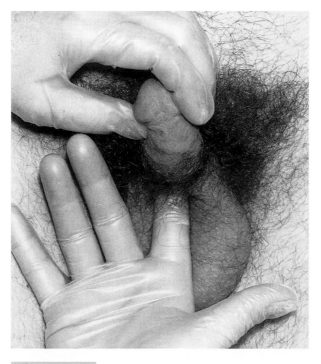

Figure 16–19

Technique for palpation of the base of the urethra.

Palpate the Testes

Each testis is palpated separately. Use both hands to grasp the testicle gently. While the left hand holds the superior and inferior poles of the testicle, the right hand palpates the anterior and posterior surfaces. The technique for palpation of the testicle is shown in Figure 16–20.

Note the size, shape, and consistency of each testicle. No tenderness or nodularity should be present. Normal testicles have a firm, rubbery consistency. The size and consistency of one testicle is compared with those of the other. Does one testicle feel

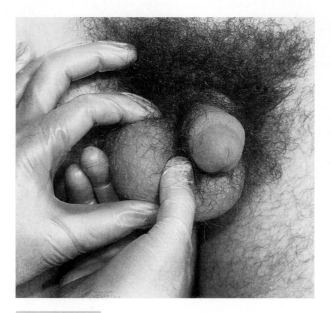

Figure 16–20

Technique for palpation of the testicle.

heavier than the other? If a mass is present, can the examining finger get above the mass within the scrotum? Because inguinal hernias arise from the abdominal cavity, the examining finger will be unable to get above such a mass. In contrast, the examining finger can frequently get above a mass that arises from within the scrotum.

Palpate the Epididymis and Vas Deferens

Next, locate and palpate the epididymis on the posterior aspect of the testicle. The head and tail should be carefully palpated for tenderness, nodularity, or masses.

The spermatic cord is palpated from the epididymis up to the external abdominal ring. The patient is asked to elevate his penis gently. If the penis is elevated too much, the scrotal skin will be reduced, and the examination will be more difficult. The examiner should hold the scrotum in the midline by placing both thumbs in front of and both index fingers on the perineal side of the scrotum. Using both hands, the examiner should simultaneously palpate both spermatic cords between the thumbs and index fingers as the fingers are pulled laterally over the scrotal surface. The most prominent structures in the spermatic cord are the vasa deferens. The vasa are felt as firm cords about 2–4 mm in diameter and feel like partially cooked spaghetti. The sizes are compared, and tenderness or beading is noted. Absence of the vas deferens on one side is often associated with absence of the kidney on the same side. The technique of spermatic cord palpation is shown in Figure 16–21.

A common enlargement of the spermatic cord that is due to a dilatation of the pampiniform plexus is a *varicocele*. These varicosities are usually on the left side, and the impression on palpation has been likened to that of feeling a bag of worms. Because the varicocele is gravity-dependent, it is usually visible only while the patient is standing or straining. The patient is asked to turn his head and cough while the spermatic cords are held between the fingers as indicated previously. A sudden pulsation, especially on the left side, confirms the diagnosis of a varicocele. Although the diagnosis is usually made from palpation, large varicoceles may be discovered on mere inspection, as can be seen in the patient in Figure 16–22.

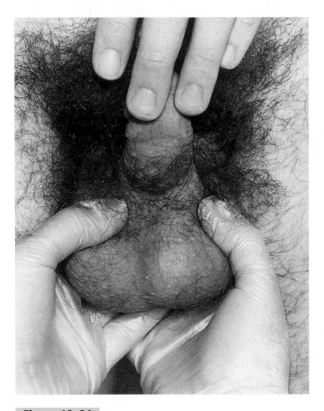

Figure 16–21

Technique for palpation of the spermatic cord.

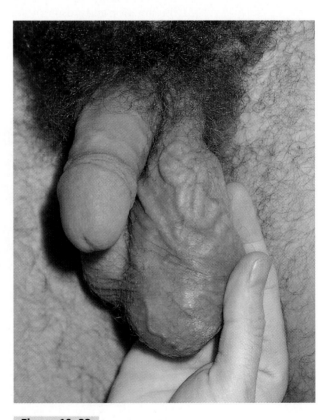

Figure 16–22

Varicocele.

■ **Transilluminate Scrotal Masses**

If a scrotal mass is detected, transillumination is necessary. In a darkened room, a light source is applied to the side of scrotal enlargement. Vascular structures, tumors, blood, a hernia, and a normal testicle do not transilluminate. The transmission of the light as a red glow indicates a serous fluid–containing cavity, such as a *hydrocele* or a *spermatocele*. A hydrocele is an abnormal collection of clear fluid in the tunica vaginalis. The testicle is contained within this cystic mass, preventing actual palpation of the testis itself. By transillumination, it may even be possible to view the relationship of the normal-sized testicle within the hydrocele. A spermatocele is a pea-sized, nontender, mass that contains spermatozoa usually attached to the upper pole of the epididymis. A hydrocele, seen only as massive scrotal enlargement, is shown in Figure 16–23. Transillumination of a hydrocele in another patient is shown in Figure 16–24. An illustration of a hydrocele is shown in Figure 16–25.

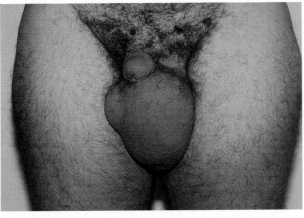

Figure 16–23

Hydrocele.

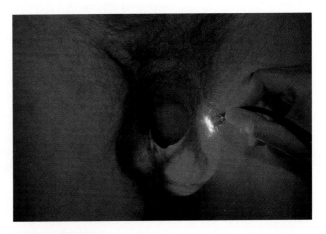

Figure 16–24

Transilluminated hydrocele.

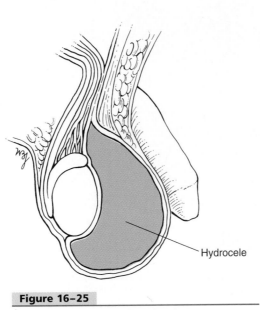

Figure 16–25

Cross section of a hydrocele, showing its anatomy.

Hernia Examination

■ **Inspect Inguinal and Femoral Areas**

Although hernias may be defined as any protrusion of a viscus, or part of it, through a normal or abnormal opening, 90% of all hernias are located in the inguinal area. Commonly, a hernial impulse is better seen than felt.

Instruct the patient to turn his head to the side and to cough or strain. Inspect the inguinal and femoral areas for any sudden swelling during coughing, which may indicate a hernia. If a sudden bulge is seen, ask the patient to cough again, and compare the impulse with that of the other side. If the patient complains of pain while coughing, determine the location of the pain, and reevaluate the area.

■ **Palpate for Inguinal Hernias**

Palpation for inguinal hernias is performed by the examiner placing the right index finger in the patient's scrotum above the left testis and invaginating the scrotal skin. There should be sufficient scrotal skin to reach the external inguinal ring. The finger should be placed with the nail facing outward and the pad of the finger inward. This is shown in Figure 16–26. The examiner's left hand may be placed on the patient's right hip for better support.

The examiner's right index finger should follow the spermatic cord laterally into the inguinal canal parallel to the inguinal ligament and upward toward the external inguinal ring, which is superior and lateral to the pubic tubercle. The external ring may be dilated and allow the finger to enter. The correct position of the right hand is shown in Figure 16–27 and is illustrated in Figure 16–28.

With the index finger placed either against the external ring or in the inguinal canal, ask the patient to turn his head to the side and to cough or strain down. Should a hernia be present, a sudden impulse against either the tip or the pad of the examining finger will be felt. If a hernia is present, have the patient lie down, and observe whether it can be reduced by gentle, sustained pressure on the mass. If the hernia

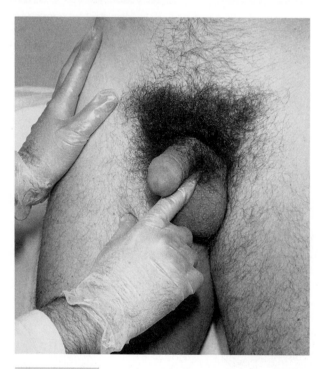

Figure 16–26

Technique for examination for inguinal hernias. Notice that the examiner's right index finger is directed inward, and the examiner's left hand is placed on the patient's hip for support and better patient contact.

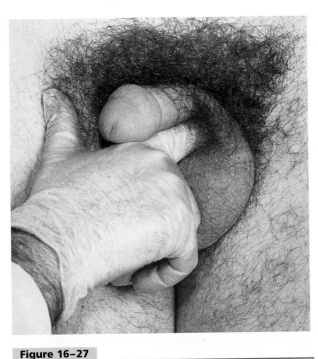

Figure 16–27

Technique for palpation of inguinal hernias.

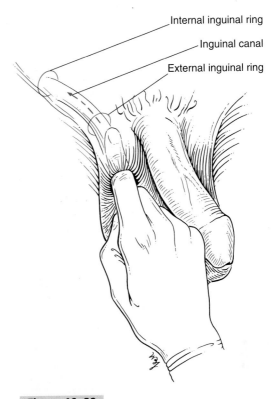

Internal inguinal ring

Inguinal canal

External inguinal ring

Figure 16–28

Position of examining finger in the inguinal canal.

examination is performed with adequate scrotal skin and is done *slowly,* it is painless. The characteristics of hernias are discussed in the next section.

After the left side is evaluated, the procedure is repeated by using the right index finger to examine the right side. Some examiners prefer to use the right index finger for examining the patient's right side and the left index finger for the patient's left side. Try both techniques to see which one is more comfortable for you.

If a large scrotal mass that does not transilluminate is present, an indirect inguinal hernia may be present in the scrotum. Auscultation of the mass may be performed to determine whether bowel sounds are present in the scrotum, a sign useful in diagnosing an indirect inguinal hernia.

Examination of the prostate was discussed in Chapter 15, The Abdomen. If the rectal examination has not yet been performed, this is the appropriate time to examine the rectum and prostate.

Clinicopathologic Correlations

Gross hematuria that is usually painless is often the first indication of a urinary tract tumor, commonly located in the bladder. Table 16–1 lists the common causes of gross hematuria in different age groups and by sex.

Scrotal disorders are relatively common. In a man with scrotal swelling, a careful history and a thorough physical examination often provide enough information for a correct diagnosis. Intrascrotal masses are common findings on physical examination. Although most masses are benign, testicular cancer is the leading solid malignancy in men younger than the age of 35 years. Testicular carcinoma is diagnosed annually in more than 3000 men.

Some of the important considerations in the history include the patient's age, time of onset of symptoms (if any), associated problems (e.g., fever, weight loss, dysuria), past medical history, and sexual history.

Intrascrotal masses may be categorized as acute and nonacute, intra- and extratesticular, and neoplastic and non-neoplastic.

Table 16–1	Causes of Hematuria by Age and Sex	
Age (yr)	Male	Female
Younger than 20	Congenital urinary tract anomaly Acute glomerulonephritis Acute urinary tract infection	
20–40	Acute urinary tract infection Kidney stone Bladder tumor	
40–60	Bladder tumor Kidney stone Acute urinary tract infection	Acute urinary tract infection Kidney stone Bladder tumor
Older than 60	Prostatic disorder Bladder tumor Acute urinary tract infection	Bladder tumor Acute urinary tract infection

The most common pathologic disorders in the category of *acute, non-neoplastic lesions* include testicular torsion, epididymitis, and trauma. Testicular torsion is a surgical emergency in which a twisting of the testis leads to venous obstruction, edema, and eventual arterial obstruction. The prompt recognition (within 10–12 hours) of this condition enables physicians to salvage the testis in 70–90% of cases. Torsion is most commonly seen in adolescents from 12 to 18 years of age. Patients complain of acute, unilateral testicular pain that is often accompanied by nausea and vomiting. On physical examination, the testis is enlarged and is extremely sensitive. It may be retracted and is often lying in a horizontal position.

Epididymitis is the most common cause of acute scrotal swelling. It accounts for more than 600,000 visits to physicians annually in the United States. It occurs in young, sexually active men and in older adults with associated genitourinary problems. Patients usually complain of recent onset of testicular pain that is associated with fever, dysuria, and scrotal swelling. On examination, the epididymis is tender and indurated; the testis may also be enlarged and tender. This variant of epididymitis is epididymoorchitis.

Trauma is the third major cause of acute scrotal swelling. Trauma may produce a scrotal and/or testicular hematoma. An important fact to keep in mind is that 10–15% of patients with testicular tumors seek medical attention after trauma.

The most common types of intrascrotal pathologic conditions are the *nonacute, non-neoplastic lesions*. These include hydrocele, spermatocele, and varicocele. A hydrocele (see Fig. 16–23) is a collection of fluid within layers of the tunica vaginalis. It manifests as a painless swelling of the scrotum. A hydrocele may be congenital, acquired, or idiopathic. Acquired hydroceles may result from trauma, infection, renal transplantation, and neoplasm. Idiopathic hydroceles are the most common; patients may have no symptoms or may complain of a dull ache or scrotal heaviness. In general, hydroceles are anterior to the testis. They are smooth-walled and will transilluminate. Figure 16–24 shows a transilluminated hydrocele.

Spermatoceles are cystic collections of fluid in the epididymis. They are frequently found on routine physical examination, because they usually produce no symptoms. Because they are fluid-filled, they can often be transilluminated.

A varicocele is a common intrascrotal mass resulting from abnormal dilatation of the veins of the pampiniform plexus. A man with a varicocele is generally asymptomatic but may have a history of infertility or of a sensation of heaviness in the scrotum. The varicocele can best be visualized on examination by observing the patient in a standing position. A mass resembling a bag of worms may be seen and felt superior to the testis. These varicosities typically enlarge during Valsalva's maneuver and are reduced when the patient lies down. Varicoceles are found predominantly on the left side. A right-sided varicocele suggests some obstruction of the inferior vena cava, whereas an acute left-sided varicocele may indicate a left-sided hypernephroma or other left renal tumor. Figure 16–22 shows a patient with a varicocele. Notice the markedly dilated veins in the scrotum.

Most patients with *testicular neoplasms* are asymptomatic, but some patients may seek medical attention because of acute pain related to trauma, hemorrhage, hydrocele, and epididymitis. Other men may present with weight loss, fever, abdominal pain, lower extremity edema, or bone pain resulting from advanced metastatic disease. A history of cryptorchidism is important because of a high association of this condition with testicular malignancies. The most common finding on physical examination is a nodule or a painless swelling of one testicle. Extratesticular tumors are uncommon and are generally benign.

Table 16–2 provides a differential diagnosis of common scrotal swellings.

Sexually transmitted diseases are common. Of every 100 outpatient visits to a venereal disease clinic, 25% of men have gonorrhea, 25% have nongonococcal urethritis, 4% have venereal warts, 3.5% have herpes, 1.7% have syphilis, and 0.1% have chancroid. The incidence of both gonococcal and nongonococcal urethritis has increased dramatically during the last two decades. On college campuses, 85% of urethritis is nongonococcal in origin.

Genital lesions of venereal diseases may be ulcerative or nonulcerative. The incidence of genital lesions has changed greatly throughout the years. At one time, chancroid was common, and herpes was rare; today, herpes is common, and chancroid is rare. Figure 16–29 shows the vesicular stage of a herpetic infection. Anal ulcerative lesions are being seen more commonly, particularly in the population of men with homosexual behavior.

Table 16–2	**Differential Diagnosis of Common Scrotal Swellings**			
Diagnosis	Usual Age (yr)	Transillumination	Scrotal Erythema	Pain
Epididymitis	Any	No	Yes	Severe, increasing severity
Torsion of testis	<20	No	Yes	Severe, sudden
Testis tumor	15–35	No	No	Minimal or absent
Hydrocele (see Fig. 16–23)	Any	Yes (see Fig. 16–24)	No	None
Spermatocele	Any	Yes	No	None
Hernia (see Figs. 16–34 and 16–35)	Any	No	No	None to moderate*
Varicocele (see Fig. 16–22)	>15	No	No	None

* Unless incarcerated, at which time pain may be severe.

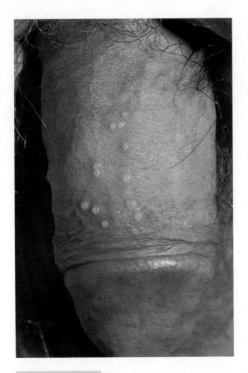

Figure 16–29

Herpes simplex.

Molluscum contagiosum is a common, usually self-limited, cutaneous eruption affecting the skin and mucous membranes. It is often seen in the pediatric population and is caused by a large DNA poxvirus. Adults can acquire infection through sexual contact. The characteristic lesions are flesh-colored papules that range in size from pinpoint to 1 cm in diameter. The central depression is the most important diagnostic sign. The painful lesions may occur anywhere on the body; on the face and trunk in children, and around the genitals of adults. Any adult with this disease must be screened for other sexually transmitted diseases. The lesions, as the name indicates, are highly infectious. As the lesions develop, there may be a surrounding patch of eczema. In the AIDS patient, the lesions become widespread, attaining sizes up to 1–2 cm in diameter. Figure 16–30 shows the classic, umbilicated lesions of molluscum contagiosum. Figure 16–31 shows a patient with lesions of molluscum contagiosum of the penis. Table 16–3 lists a differential diagnosis of genital papular lesions.

The primary lesion of *syphilis* is the chancre (see Fig. 16–9), which occurs from 10 days to 3 weeks after infection at the site of the inoculation. The chancre is a painless ulcer with an indurated edge. It usually heals spontaneously within a month. If the patient is not treated for syphilis, the disease may evolve to the secondary stage. This occurs about 2 months after the appearance of the chancre. The patient may present with a widespread nonpruritic, maculopapular rash over the genitalia, trunk, palms, and soles. There is a tendency for cropping of the lesions. The healed chancre may still be evident. There is also generalized lymphadenopathy. In the genital and perianal areas, the papules may coalesce and erode. These large, moist, painful papules, which appear as if they were "pasted" on the skin, are called *condylomata lata*. They are covered with an exudate and are teeming with active spirochetes. If untreated, the patient may recover but may have a relapse of the eruption within 2 years. After this period, there is a long latent period during which time the disease may progress to cardiovascular syphilis, or neurosyphilis, a condition known as tertiary syphilis.

The skin lesions of syphilis are important to recognize. Figure 16–32 shows the typical skin lesions of secondary syphilis on the feet. Figure 16–33 shows condylomata

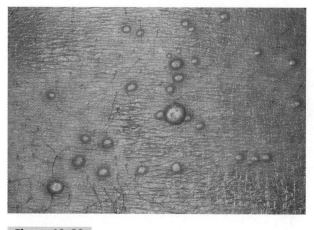

Figure 16–30

Umbilicated lesions of molluscum contagiosum.

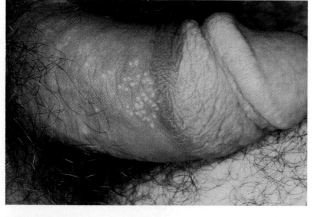

Figure 16–31

Lesions of molluscum contagiosum of the penis.

Table 16–3   Differential Diagnosis of Genital Papules

Condition	Appearance	Pain	Lymphadenopathy
Herpes	Multiple, ulcers, vesicles	Painful	Present
Condylomata lata (see Fig. 16–33)	Multiple, moist, flat, round	Painful	Present
Condylomata acuminata (see Fig. 16–16)	Multiple, verrucous	Absent	Absent
Molluscum contagiosum	1–5 mm umbilicated papules, often in clusters; caseous material expressible from center	Painful	Rarely

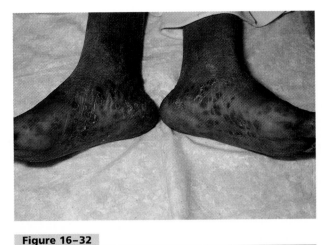

Figure 16–32

Secondary syphilis.

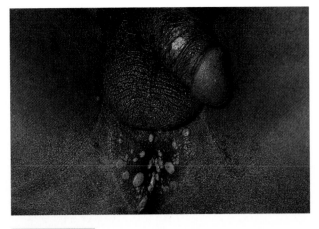

Figure 16–33

Condylomata lata. Notice the healing primary chancre on the penis.

lata in the perineum of the same patient. The healing chancre of primary syphilis is also seen on the penis of this patient.

Hernias are common. The major types of external hernias are the indirect and direct inguinal, and the femoral hernias. Figure 16–34 shows a patient with a massive left indirect inguinal hernia. Figure 16–35 shows a patient with a small right direct inguinal hernia. Figure 16–36 illustrates and lists the major differences in the differential diagnosis of hernias.

Useful Vocabulary

Listed here are the specific roots that are important in order to understand the terminology related to urologic disease.

Root	Pertaining to	Example	Definition
andr-	man	*andr*ogen	Substance possessing masculinizing properties
cyst(o)-	urinary bladder	*cysto*tomy	Incision of the urinary bladder
litho-	stone	*litho*tomy	Incision of an organ for the removal of a stone
nephro-	kidney	*nephro*pathy	Disease of the kidneys
orchi(o)-	testes	*orchi*tis	Inflammation of the testis
pyel(o)-	pelvis of kidney	*pyelo*gram	X-ray film of the kidney and ureter
ureter(o)-	ureter	*uretero*lith	A stone lodged or formed in the ureter
urethr(o)-	urethra	*urethro*plasty	Plastic surgery of the urethra
vas(o)-	vas deferens	*vas*ectomy	Excision of the vas deferens

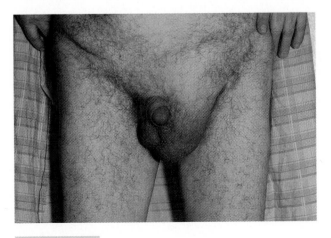

Figure 16–34

Left indirect inguinal hernia.

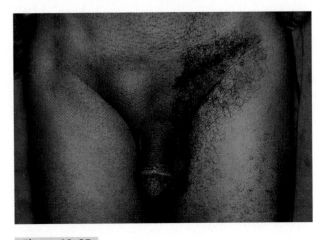

Figure 16–35

Right direct inguinal hernia.

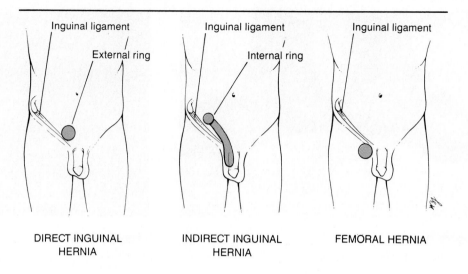

Feature	Direct Inguinal*	Indirect Inguinal†	Femoral
Occurence	Middle-aged and elderly men	All ages	Least common: more frequently found in women
Bilaterality	55%	30%	Rarely
Origin of swelling	Above inguinal ligament. Directly behind and through external ring.	Above inguinal ligament. Hernial sac enters inguinal canal at internal ring and exists at external ring.	Below inguinal ligament
Scrotal involvement	Rarely	Commonly	Never
Impulse location	At side of finger in inguinal canal	At tip of finger in inguinal canal	Not felt by finger in inguinal canal; mass below canal

Figure 16–36

Differential diagnosis of hernias.

*See Figure 16–35.
†See Figure 16–34.

Writing Up the Physical Examination

Listed here are examples of the write-up for the examination of the male genitalia.

- The penis is circumcised. Both testes are in the scrotum and are within normal limits. There are no abnormal scrotal masses. No inguinal hernias are present. No inguinal adenopathy is present.
- The penis is uncircumcised. The foreskin is easily retracted. The left hemiscrotum is markedly enlarged by a painless mass, which transilluminates. The left testicle cannot be palpated. The right testicle is within normal limits. No inguinal hernias are present. A small 2 × 2 soft, nonfixed, nontender lymph node is present in the right inguinal area.
- The penis is circumcised. There is a 1–2 cm verrucous mass at the external meatus. A thick, yellow, purulent urethral discharge, which can be milked from the urethra, is seen at the meatus. The scrotal contents are within normal limits. No inguinal hernias are present.
- The penis is uncircumcised. The foreskin is tight, although it can be retracted by the patient. A large amount of smegma is present behind the corona. There is a large mass of nontender, dilated veins present in the left hemiscrotum seen and felt when the patient stands. An impulse is felt in the left spermatic cord upon coughing. No inguinal hernias are present.
- The penis is circumcised. The left testicle is soft and measures 2 × 3 cm. The right testicle appears normal. The scrotal contents are within normal limits. The hernia examination on the left side reveals a prominent impulse when the patient coughs. This impulse is felt at the tip of the examiner's finger.
- The penis is circumcised. There is a 1 cm painless ulcer with a clean, nonpurulent base at the corona. The ulcer is indurated and has a smooth, regular, sharply defined border. Painless, firm, movable inguinal lymphadenopathy is present bilaterally. The testes are normal, as are the other scrotal contents. No inguinal hernias are present.

Bibliography

Blandy J: Lecture Notes on Urology, 4th ed. Oxford, Blackwell Scientific, 1989.

Bullock N, Sibley G, Whitaker R: Essential Urology. Edinburgh, Churchill Livingstone, 1989.

Chisholm GD, Fair WF (eds): Scientific Foundations of Urology, 3rd ed. Oxford, Heinemann Medical Books, 1990.

Herman JR: Urology: A View Through the Retrospectroscope. Hagerstown, MD, Harper & Row, 1973.

Kinsey AC, Pomeroy WB, Martin CE: Sexual Behavior in the Human Male. Philadelphia, W.B. Saunders, 1948.

McConnell EA, Zimmermann MF: Care of Patients with Urologic Problems. Philadelphia, J.B. Lippincott, 1983.

Murphy LJT: The History of Urology. Springfield, IL, Charles C Thomas, 1972.

Tanagho EA, McAninch JW: Smith's General Urology. East Norwalk, CT, Appleton & Lange, 1988.

CHAPTER 17

Female Genitalia

In young girls, as I said, and in women past childbearing, it [the uterus] is without blood, and about the size of a bean. In a marriageable virgin it has the magnitude and form of a pear. In women who have borne children, and are still fruitful, it equals in bulk a small gourd or a goose's egg; at the same time, together with the breasts, it swells and softens, becomes more fleshy, and is heat increased. . . .

William Harvey
1578–1657

General Considerations

Gynecology and obstetrics had their beginnings with the origin of the human race. From a statistical analysis of worldwide populations in 1982, more than 4.7 million live births have occurred each year: over 12,000 each day, over 600 each hour, and over 10 every minute. Almost 98% of all live-born infants survive. The 1982 population is expected to double by the year 2010.

Records of obstetrics and gynecology date back to the time of Hippocrates in 400 BC. He was probably the first physician to describe midwifery, menstruation, sterility, symptoms of pregnancy, and puerperal (the period after labor) infections. Most of the early gynecologic history stems from Soranus in the 2nd century AD. His works included chapters on anatomy, menstruation, fertility, signs of pregnancy, labor, care of the infant, dysmenorrhea (painful menstruation), uterine hemorrhage, and even the use of vaginal specula.

William Harvey, the "father" of the theory of blood circulation, was also responsible for a monumental treatise on obstetrics. This work, published in 1651, included a detailed assessment of uterine changes throughout life.

The 18th century saw a further understanding of pregnancy, labor, and fertility. However, it was not until the 19th century that diseases of the female genitalia were better understood. As recently as 1872, Noeggerath published his investigations on gonorrhea, which ultimately changed the opinion of the medical world about the significance of this disorder. He was the first to suggest that "latent gonorrhea" was associated with sterility in women. Although the first cesarean section was described in 1596 by Mercurio, the development of the current technique of Max Sänger was described as recently as 1882.

Since the middle 1960s, deaths from cancer of the uterus and cervix in the United States have declined by 57%. Cancer of the uterus and cervix now accounts for 13% of all cancers and 5% of all cancer deaths in women. In 1994, there were more than 10,000 deaths from cancer of the cervix and uterus. The decline in mortality from cervical cancer is largely attributed to early detection by physical examination. Of the many risk factors that have been evaluated, the age at first sexual intercourse and the fact of multiple sexual partners seem to be the ones most often associated with an increased risk of cervical cancer.

Although ovarian carcinoma accounts for only 4% of all cancers in women, more than 5% of cancer deaths in women is due to ovarian cancer. In 1994, the American Cancer Society recorded 13,000 deaths from ovarian cancer. Among the gynecologic malignancies, cancer of the ovary accounts for nearly 50% of all deaths that are due to cancer. The carefully performed pelvic examination has been shown to be the cornerstone of diagnosis of ovarian cancer.

Structure and Physiology

The external female genitalia are shown in Figure 17–1. The *vulva* consists of the mons veneris, the labia majora, the libia minora, the clitoris, the vestibule and its glands, the urethral meatus, and the vaginal introitus. The *mons veneris* is a rounded

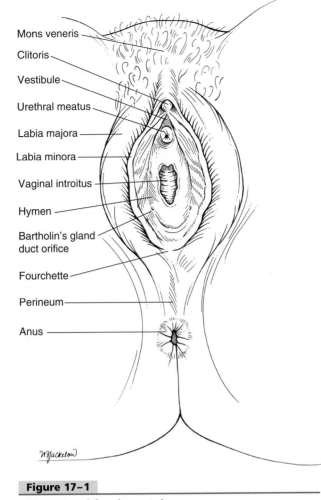

Mons veneris

Clitoris

Vestibule

Urethral meatus

Labia majora

Labia minora

Vaginal introitus

Hymen

Bartholin's gland
duct orifice

Fourchette

Perineum

Anus

Figure 17–1

The external female genitalia.

prominence of fat tissue overlying the pubic symphysis. The *labia majora* are two wide skin folds that form the lateral boundaries of the vulva. They meet anteriorly at the mons veneris to form the anterior commissure. The labia majora and the mons veneris have hair follicles and sebaceous glands. The labia majora correspond to the scrotum in the male. The *labia minora* are two narrow, pigmented skin folds lying between the labia majora and enclose the *vestibule,* which is the area lying between the labia minora. Anteriorly, the two labia minora form the prepuce of the *clitoris.* The clitoris, analogous to the penis, consists of erectile tissue and a rich supply of nerve endings. It has a glans and two corpora cavernosa. The external *urethral meatus* is located in the anterior portion of the vestibule below the clitoris. Paraurethral glands, or *Skene's glands,* are small glands that open lateral to the urethra. Secretion of sebaceous glands in this area protects the vulnerable tissues against urine.

The major vestibular glands are known as *Bartholin's glands,* or vulvovaginal glands. These pea-sized glands correspond to the Cowper's glands in the male. Each Bartholin's gland lies posterolaterally to the vaginal orifice. During sexual intercourse, a watery fluid is secreted that serves as a vaginal lubricant.

Inferiorly, the labia minora unite at the posterior commissure to form the *fourchette.* The *perineum* is the area between the fourchette and the anus.

The *hymen* is a circular fold of tissue that partially occludes the *vaginal introitus.* There are marked variations in its size as well as the number of openings in it. The vaginal introitus is the border between the external and internal genitalia and is located in the lower portion of the vestibule.

The blood supply to the external genitalia and perineum is predominantly from the internal pudendal arteries. The lymphatic drainage is into the superficial and deep inguinal nodes.

The internal genitalia are shown in Figure 17–2. The *vagina* is a muscularly walled, hollow canal that passes upward and slightly backward, at a right angle to the uterus. The vagina lies between the urinary bladder anteriorly and the rectum posteriorly. The vaginal walls are thrown into transverse rugae, or folds. The lower portion of the cervix projects into the upper portion of the vagina and divides it into four fornices. The anterior fornix is shallow and is just posterior to the bladder. The posterior fornix is deep and is just anterior to the rectovaginal pouch, known as the *cul-de-sac (pouch) of Douglas,* and the pelvic viscera lie immediately above this pouch. The lateral fornices contain the broad ligaments. The fallopian tubes and ovaries may be palpated in the lateral fornices. The superficial cells of the vagina contain glycogen, which is acted upon by the normal vaginal flora to produce lactic acid. This is in part responsible for the resistance of the vagina to infection.

The arterial supply to the vagina is derived from the internal iliac, uterine, and middle hemorrhoidal arteries. The lymphatic channels of the lower third of the vagina drain into the inguinal nodes. The lymphatic channels of the upper two thirds enter the hypogastric and sacral nodes.

The *uterus* is a hollow muscular organ with a small central cavity. The lower end is the *cervix;* the upper portion is the *fundus.* The size of the uterus is different during various stages of life. At birth, the uterus is only 3–4 cm long. The adult uterus is 7–8 cm long and 3.5 cm wide, with an average wall thickness of 2–3 cm. The growth of the uterus and the relationship of the size of the fundus to the size of the cervix are shown in Figure 17–3.

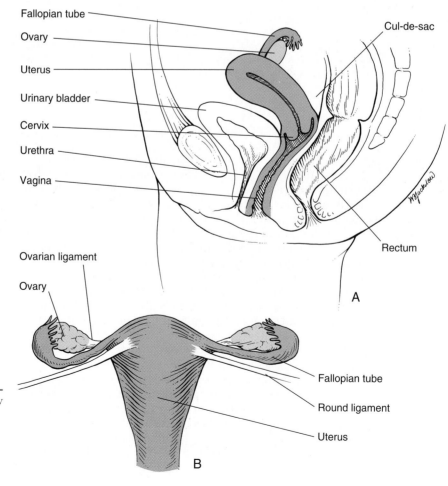

Figure 17–2

A, Cross-sectional view of the internal female genitalia. *B,* Frontal view of uterus, fallopian tubes, and ovaries.

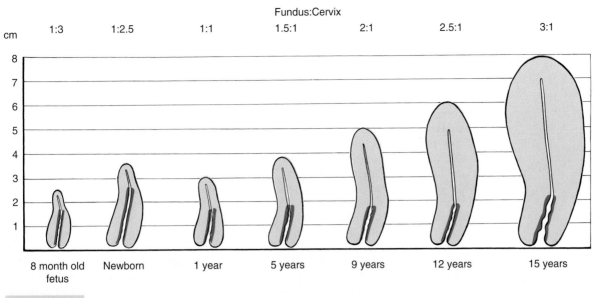

Fundus:Cervix

Figure 17–3

The growth of the uterus and changes in the fundus : cervix ratio with development. The darker red area represents the length of the cervix.

The triangular uterine cavity is 6–7 cm in length and is bounded by the *internal cervical os* inferiorly and the entrances of the fallopian tubes superiorly. Normally, the long axis of the uterus is bent forward on the long axis of the vagina. This is *anteversion.* The fundus is also bent slightly forward on the cervix. This is *anteflexion.*

The uterus is freely mobile and is located centrally in the pelvic cavity. It is supported by the broad and uterosacral ligaments as well as by the pelvic floor. The peritoneum covers the fundus anteriorly down to the level of the internal cervical os. Posteriorly, the peritoneum covers the uterus down to the pouch of Douglas. The function of the uterus is childbearing. A detailed anatomic representation of the uterus is shown in Figure 17–4.

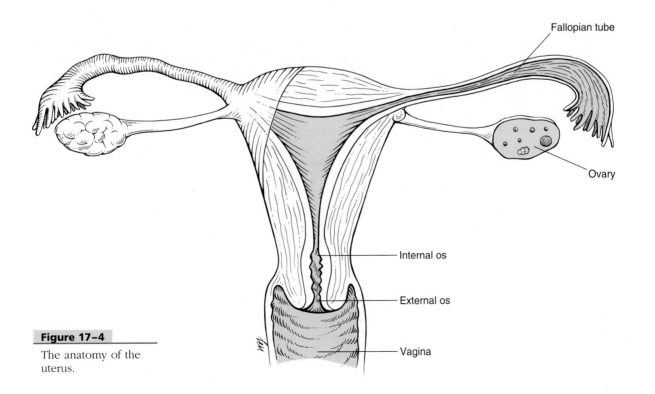

Figure 17–4

The anatomy of the uterus.

The cervix is the vaginal portion of the uterus. The greater portion of the cervix has no peritoneal covering. The cervical canal extends from the *external cervical os* to the internal cervical os, where it continues into the cavity of the fundus. The external cervical os in women who have not given birth vaginally is small and circular. In women who have had vaginal deliveries, the external cervical os is linear or oval.

With increasing levels of estrogens, the external cervical os begins to dilate, and cervical mucus secretion becomes clear and watery. With high levels of estrogens, cervical mucus, when placed between two glass slides that are then pulled apart, can be stretched 15–20 cm before breaking. This property of cervical mucus to be drawn into a fine thread is termed *spinnbarkeit.* When cervical mucus is allowed to dry on a glass slide and is examined under low power of a light microscope, a *fern pattern* made up of salt crystals may be seen. Spinnbarkeit and ferning reach a maximum at the midpoint of the menstrual cycle. Sperm can more easily penetrate mucus with these characteristics.

The blood supply to the uterus comes from the uterine and ovarian arteries. The lymphatics of the fundus enter into the lumbar nodes.

The *fallopian tubes,* or *oviducts,* enter the fundus at its superior aspect. They are small muscular tubes that extend outward into the broad ligament toward the pelvic wall. The other end of the oviduct opens into the peritoneal cavity near the ovary. These endings are surrounded by fringed-shaped projects called *fimbriae.* The primary function of the fallopian tube is to provide a conduit for and convey the egg from the corresponding ovary to the uterus, a trip that takes several days. Sperm traverse the oviduct in the opposite direction, and it is usually in the oviduct that fertilization takes place.

The *ovaries* are almond-shaped structures about 3–4 cm long and are attached to the broad ligament. The primary functions of the ovary are oogenesis and hormone production.

The ovaries, fallopian tubes, and supporting ligaments are termed the *adnexa.*

The female reproductive system is under the influence of the hypothalamus, whose releasing factors control the secretion of the anterior pituitary gonadotropic hormones: *follicle-stimulating hormone* and *luteinizing hormone.* In response to these hormones, the ovarian graafian follicle secretes estrogens and discharges its ovum. After ovulation, the ovarian follicle is termed the *corpus luteum,* which secrets estrogens and progesterone. With the secretion of progesterone, the basal body temperature rises. This is a reliable sign of ovulation. Under the influence of the ovarian hormones, the uterus and breasts undergo the characteristic changes of the menstrual cycle.

If pregnancy does not occur, the corpus luteum regresses, and the level of ovarian hormones begins to fall. At this time, before menstruation, many women have symptoms of weakness, depression, and irritability. Breast tenderness is also common. These symptoms are termed *premenstrual syndrome.* About 5 days after the fall in the level of the hormones, the menstrual period begins. Menstruation throughout the 5 day period measures about 50–150 mL, only half of which is blood; the remainder is mucus. Because menstrual blood does not contain fibrin, it does not clot. When the menstrual flow is heavy, as it is on days 1–2, "clots" may be described. These clots are not fibrin clots but are combinations of red cells, glycoproteins, and mucoid substances that are believed to form in the vagina rather than in the uterine cavity.

Some of the hormone-dependent changes related to the menstrual cycle are shown in Figure 17–5.

About 1.5 years before puberty, gonadotropins are measurable in the urine. The ovaries enter a period of rapid growth at ages 8–9 years, which marks the onset of puberty. Secretion of estrogens begins to increase rapidly at about the age of 11 years. Concomitantly with estrogen production, the sexual organs begin to mature. During puberty, the secondary sex characteristics begin to develop. The breasts enlarge, hair develops on the pubis, the vulva enlarges, the labia minora become pigmented, and the body contour changes. Puberty lasts for approximately 4–5 years. The first menstrual cycle, called *menarche,* occurs at the end of puberty at about 12.5 years of age. There is, however, a wide variation in the age at menarche. The cycles continue approximately every 28 days, with a flow lasting 3–5 days. The first day of the period is taken to be the first day of the cycle. It is rare for a woman to be absolutely regular, and cycles of 25–34 days are considered normal.

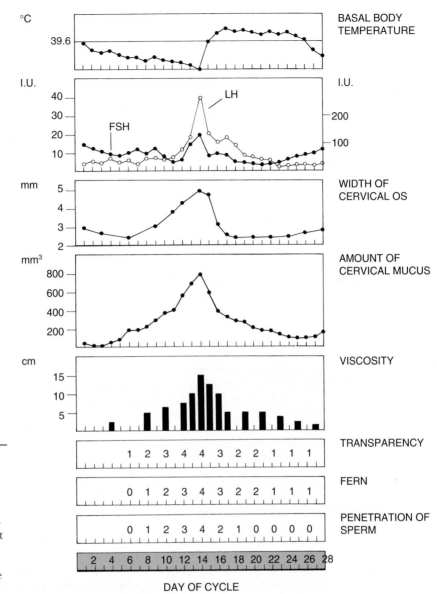

Figure 17-5

Physiologic changes associated with the menstrual cycle. The numbers 0 to 4 indicate an increasing characteristic of cervical mucus. Notice that ferning, transparency, and the ability for sperm penetration are maximal at midcycle.

At the time of menarche, the menstrual cycle is usually anovulatory* and irregular. After 1–2 years, ovulation begins. After stabilization of the menses, ovulation occurs about midcycle in a woman with a regular cycle.

Menopause marks the ends of menstruation. Menopause is defined as the last uterine bleeding induced by ovarian function. It usually occurs between 45 and 55 years of age. Ovulation and corpus luteum formation no longer occur, and the ovaries decrease in size. The period after menopause is termed *postmenopausal*.

Review of Specific Symptoms

The most common symptoms of female genitourinary disease are as follows:

- Abnormal vaginal bleeding
- Dysmenorrhea

---

* Not accompanied by the release of an ovum from the ovary.

- Masses or lesions
- Vaginal discharge
- Vaginal itching
- Abdominal pain
- Dyspareunia
- Changes in hair distribution
- Changes in urinary pattern
- Infertility

Abnormal Vaginal Bleeding

Ask these questions of any woman with abnormal vaginal bleeding:

"How long have you noticed the vaginal bleeding?"
"What types of contraceptives do you use?"
"How often are your periods?"
"What is the duration of your menstrual flow?"
"How many tampons or napkins do you use on each day of your flow?"
"Are there any clots of blood?"
"When was your last period?"
"Have you noticed bleeding between your periods?"
"Do you have abdominal pain during your periods?"
"Do you have hot flashes? cold sweats?"
"Do you have children?" If so, *"When was your last one born?"*
"Do you think you might be pregnant?"
"Are you under any unusual emotional stress?"
"Have you noticed an intolerance to cold? heat?"
"Have you noticed a change in your vision?"
"Have you had any headaches? nausea? change in hair pattern? milk discharge from your nipples?"
"What is your diet like?"

Abnormal bleeding, also known as *dysfunctional uterine bleeding,* includes amenorrhea, menorrhagia, metrorrhagia, and postmenopausal bleeding. *Amenorrhea* is the cessation or nonappearance of menstruation. Before puberty, amenorrhea is physiologic, as it is during pregnancy and after menopause. In primary amenorrhea, menstruation has never occurred; in secondary amenorrhea, menstruation has occurred but has ceased, as in pregnancy. Long-distance joggers, anorectics, or any woman with abnormally low body fat may have secondary amenorrhea. Diseases of the hypothalamus, pituitary gland, ovary, uterus, and thyroid gland are associated with amenorrhea. Galactorrhea, or milk discharge from the nipples, is commonly seen in many individuals with pituitary tumors. Chronic disease is also frequently associated with secondary amenorrhea.

Menorrhagia is excessive bleeding at the time of the menstrual cycle. The flow may be increased, the duration may be increased, or both. The number of pads or tampons a patient uses each day of the cycle will help to quantify the flow. Menorrhagia in some cases may be associated with blood disorders such as leukemia, inherited clotting abnormalities, and decreased platelet states. Uterine fibroids are a leading cause of menorrhagia. Menorrhagia secondary to fibroids is related to the large surface area of the endometrium from which bleeding occurs.

Metrorrhagia is uterine bleeding of normal amount at irregular noncyclic intervals. Foreign bodies such as intrauterine devices as well as ovarian and uterine tumors can cause metrorrhagia. Often there is increased bleeding between cycles as well as heavier periods; this is termed *menometrorrhagia.*

Postmenopausal bleeding occurs after 6–8 months of amenorrhea after menopause. Any postmenopausal bleeding must be investigated. Uterine fibroids or tumors of the cervix, uterus, or ovary may be responsible.

Dysmenorrhea

Dysmenorrhea, or painful menstruation, is a common symptom. It is often difficult to define as abnormal, because many healthy women have some degree of menstrual discomfort. In most women, these mild cramps subside soon after the commencement of the menstrual flow. There are two types of dysmenorrhea: primary and secondary. Primary dysmenorrhea is far more common. It begins shortly after menarche, is associated with colicky uterine contractions, and occurs with every period. Childbirth frequently alleviates this state permanently. Secondary dysmenorrhea is caused by acquired disorders within the uterine cavity (such as intrauterine devices, polyps, or fibroids), obstruction to flow (e.g., cervical stenosis), or disorders of the pelvic peritoneum.* It usually occurs after several years of painless periods. Regardless of its cause, dysmenorrhea is described as intermittent, crampy pain accompanying the menstrual flow. The pain is felt in the lower abdomen and back, sometimes radiating down the legs. In severe cases, fainting, nausea, or vomiting may occur.

Masses or Lesions

Masses or lesions of the external genitalia are common. They may be related to veneral diseases, tumors, or infections. Ask these questions of any woman with a lesion on the genitalia:

"When did you first notice the mass (lesion)?"
"Is it painful?"
"Has it changed since you first noticed it?"
"Have you ever had it before?"
"Have you been exposed to anyone with venereal disease?"

Syphilis may result in a chancre on the labia. Often unnoticed, it is a small, painless nodule or ulcer with a sharply demarcated border. Small, acutely painful ulcers may be chancroid or genital herpes. A patient with an abscess of Bartholin's gland may present with an extremely tender mass in the vulva. Benign tumors, such as venereal warts (condylomata acuminata), and malignant conditions present as a mass on the external genitalia.

Some patients complain of a sensation of fullness or mass in the pelvis as a result of pelvic relaxation. *Pelvic relaxation* applies to the descent or protrusion of the vaginal walls or uterus through the vaginal introitus. This is caused by a weakening of the pelvic supports. The anterior vaginal wall can descend, producing a *cystocele* that triggers urinary symptoms such as frequency and stress incontinence. The posterior vaginal wall can descend, producing a *rectocele,* which triggers bowel symptoms such as constipation, tenesmus, or incontinence. The uterus can also descend, which results in uterine prolapse. In its most severe state, the uterus may lie outside the vulva with complete vaginal inversion, a condition known as *procidentia.* The consequences of pelvic relaxation are discussed further in the Clinicopathologic Correlations section in this chapter.

Vaginal Discharge

Vaginal discharges, also known as *leukorrhea,* are common. Is there an associated foul odor? Although a whitish discharge is often normally present, a fetid discharge often indicates a pathologic problem. The most common pathologic odor is a foul, fishy odor related to the volatilization of amines that are produced by anaerobic metabolism. Is itching also present? Women with moniliasis (candidiasis) complain of a white, dry discharge that looks like cottage cheese with intense pruritus. Has the woman taken any medications, such as antibiotics, recently? Antibiotics change the normal vaginal flora, and an overgrowth of *Candida* may result. Table 17–1 summarizes the important characteristics of vaginal discharge.

---

* Endometriosis or pelvic inflammatory disease, for example. Endometriosis is the presence of endometrial tissue outside the uterus and is a cause of chronic pelvic pain.

Table 17–1 **Characteristics of Common Vaginal Discharges**

Feature	Physiologic Discharge	Nonspecific Vaginitis	Trichomonas	Candida	Gonococcal
Color	White	Gray	Grayish-yellow	White	Greenish-yellow
Fishy odor	Absent	Present	Present	Absent	Absent
Consistency	Nonhomogeneous	Homogeneous	Purulent, often with bubbles	Cottage cheese–like	Mucopurulent
Present	Dependent	Adherent to walls	Often pooled in fornix	Adherent to walls	Adherent to walls
Discharge at introitus	Rare	Common	Common	Common	Common
Vulva	Normal	Normal	Edematous	Erythematous	Erythematous
Vaginal mucosa	Normal	Normal	Usually normal	Erythematous	Normal
Cervix	Normal	Normal	May show red spots	Patches of discharge	Pus in os

Vaginal Itching

Vaginal itching is associated with monilial infections, glycosuria,* vulvar leukoplakia, and any condition that predisposes a woman to vulvar irritation. Pruritus may also be a symptom of psychosomatic disease.

Abdominal Pain

Ask the following questions in addition to those indicated in Chapter 15, The Abdomen, of any woman with abdominal pain:

> *"When was your last period?"*
> *"Have you ever had any type of venereal disease?"*
> *"Is the pain related to your menstrual cycle?"* If so, *"At what time in your cycle does it occur?"*
> *"Do you experience burning when you urinate?"*

Abdominal pain may be acute or chronic. Is the patient pregnant? Acute abdominal pain may be a complication of pregnancy. Spontaneous abortion, uterine perforation, and ectopic tubal pregnancy all are life-threatening situations. Acute inflammation by gonococci of the fallopian tubes and ovary, *salpingo-oophoritis,* can produce intense lower abdominal pain. Acute lower abdominal pain localized to one side that occurs at the time of ovulation is termed *mittelschmerz.* This pain is related to a small amount of intraperitoneal bleeding at the time of ovum release. Urinary tract infection may also cause acute pain. Patients with urinary tract infections usually have associated urinary symptoms of burning or frequency.

Chronic abdominal pain may result from ectopic endometrial tissue, chronic pelvic inflammatory disease of the fallopian tubes and ovaries, and pelvic muscle relaxation with protrusion of the bladder, rectum, or uterus.

Dyspareunia

Dyspareunia is pain during or after sexual intercourse. Dyspareunia may be physiologic or psychogenic. Infections of the vulva, introitus, vagina, cervix, uterus, fallopian tubes, and ovaries have been associated with dyspareunia. Tumors of the rectovaginal septum, uterus, and ovaries have been described in patients who have experienced painful sexual intercourse. Dyspareunia is often present in the absence of a disorder. A history of painful pelvic examinations and fears about pregnancy are common in these pa-

---

* High levels of glucose in the urine, as in diabetes.

tients. Women may have "penetration anxiety" until they are assured that their vagina can be penetrated by a penis. In these individuals, such anxiety may lead to *vaginismus,* a condition of severe pelvic pain and spasm when the labia are merely touched. In other women, dyspareunia may develop during times of stress or emotional conflicts. The examiner can obtain valuable information by asking, "What else is going on in your life now?" Dryness of the vagina and labia may cause irritation that can result in dyspareunia.

Changes in Hair Distribution

Hair loss or change in hair distribution may occur during certain states of hormonal imbalance. *Hirsutism* is an excessive growth of hair on the upper lip, face, ear lobes, upper pubic triangle, trunk, or limbs. *Virilization* is extensive hirsutism associated with receding temporal hair, a deepening of the voice, and clitoral enlargement. Increased androgen production by the adrenal glands or ovaries may be responsible for these phenomena. Tumors of the ovary are usually associated with amenorrhea, rapidly developing hirsutism, and virilization. Polycystic ovarian disease is associated with menstrual irregularities, infertility, obesity, and hirsutism. It is important to determine whether the patient is taking any medications. A drug used to treat hypertension, minoxidil, has been found to have the unexpected side effect of causing diffuse hair growth on the face.

Hair loss, or *alopecia,* is a distressing problem. Many drugs may have a profound effect on hair growth. The interviewer must inquire whether the patient has taken any chemotherapeutic agents or has been exposed to radiation. Different areas of the head seem to respond differently to androgens. The top and front of the scalp respond to increased androgen production by hair loss, whereas the face responds with increased hair growth. Has the patient been dieting? Because hair has a high metabolic rate, crash diets and infectious diseases reduce the nutrients available for hair growth. Secondary alopecia may result.

Changes in Urinary Pattern

Changes in the patterns of urination are common. Chapter 16, Male Genitalia and Hernias, reviews many of the symptoms of changes in the urinary pattern. These symptoms may occur in women as well.

Stress incontinence is incontinence of urine on straining or coughing. Stress incontinence is more common among women than among men. The female urinary bladder and urethra are maintained in position by several muscular and facial supports. It has been postulated that estrogens may, at least in part, be responsible for a weakening of the pelvic support. With aging, the support of the bladder neck, the length of the urethra, and the competence of the pelvic floor are weakened. Repeated vaginal deliveries, strenuous exercise, and chronic coughing increase the chance for stress incontinence. Ask a patient these questions:

> *"Do you lose your urine on straining? coughing? lifting? laughing?"*
> *"Do you lose your urine constantly?"*
> *"Do you lose small amounts of urine?"*
> *"Are you aware of a full bladder?"*
> *"Do you have to press on your abdomen to void?"*
> *"Are you aware of any weakness in your limbs?"*
> *"Have you ever had a loss of vision?"*
> *"Do you have diabetes?"*

Patients with pure stress incontinence describe urine loss without urgency that occurs during any activity that momentarily increases intra-abdominal pressure. Although stress incontinence is common among women, it is important to rule out other types of incontinence, such as neurologic, overflow, and psychogenic. *Neurologic incontinence* may result from cerebral dysfunction, spinal cord disease, and peripheral nerve lesions. Multiple sclerosis is a chronic relapsing neurologic disorder causing urinary incontinence. Most individuals suffer from an episode of temporary visual loss as an early symptom. *Overflow incontinence* occurs when the pressure in the bladder exceeds the urethral pressure in the absence of bladder contraction. This may occur in patients with diabetes and an atonic bladder. In *psychogenic incontinence,* individuals have been known to urinate in bed at night to "warm" themselves or during the daytime in group settings to bring attention to themselves.

Infertility

Infertility may result from failure to ovulate, called *anovulation,* or from inadequate function of the corpus luteum. Both of these conditions can occur in women with cyclic menstrual bleeding. Therefore, having a period does not indicate fertility. The woman with the symptom of infertility should be asked these questions:

> *"Do you have regular menstrual periods?"*
> *"Have you kept a charge of your basal body temperature?"*
> *"Have you ever had venereal disease?"*
> *"Have you been tested for thyroid disease?"*
> *"Have you taken any medications to promote fertility?"*

Charting basal body temperatures is a reliable method for detecting ovulation. Gonococcal disease in a woman may lead to salpingo-oophoritis, with scarring of the fallopian tubes and infertility. Hypothyroidism is well known to be responsible for infertility.

General Suggestions

Even in the absence of specific symptoms, all women, regardless of age, should be asked several important questions. The answers to the following questions will provide a complete gynecologic, obstetric, and reproductive history. The first group of questions is related to the *gynecologic history* and menstrual cycle:

> *"At what age did you start to menstruate?"*
> *"How often do your periods occur?"*
> *"Are they regular?"*
> *"For how many days do you have menstrual flow?"*
> *"How many pads or tampons do you use each day of your flow?"*
> *"During your menstrual cycle, do you experience any breast tenderness or breast pain? bloating? swelling? headache? edema?"*
> *"When was your last menstrual period?"*

The *catamenia* refers to the menstrual history and summarizes the age at menarche, the cycle length, and the duration of flow. If a woman reached menarche at age 12 years and has had regular periods every 29 days lasting for 5 days, the catamenia can be summarized as CAT 12 × 29 × 5. The date of the last menstrual period can be abbreviated as LMP: December 3, 1997.

Any recurrent, midcyclic symptom associated with the menstrual period, such as breast tenderness, bloating, and so forth, is termed *molimen.* The presence of molimen correlates with ovulation, although not all women experience molimen when ovulation occurs. Therefore, molimen is a specific but nonsensitive sign of ovulation.

The next group of questions is related to the *obstetric history:*

> *"Have you ever been pregnant?"*
> *"How many full-term pregnancies have you had?"*
> *"Have you had any children born prematurely?"*
> *"Have you ever had a miscarriage or an elective abortion?"*
> *"Were any of your children stillborn?"*
> *"How many living children do you have?"*
> *"How were your children delivered (vaginally, cesarean)?"*
> *"What were the birth weights of your children?"*

The obstetric history includes the number of pregnancies, known as *gravidity,* and the number of deliveries, known as *parity.* If a woman has had three full-term infants (born at 37 weeks or more of gestation), two premature infants (born at less than 37 weeks of gestation), one miscarriage (or abortion), and four living children, her obstetric history can be summarized as *para 3–2–1–4.* An easy way to remember this four digit parity code is with the mnemonic *Florida Power And Light,* the abbreviation of which stands for *f*ull term, *p*remature, *a*bortions (miscarriages), *l*iving. The woman in this example is *gravida 6.*

When asking a woman about the date of her last menstrual period, never assume that menopause has occurred. Even a 62 year old woman should be asked when her last menstrual period occurred. Allow the patient to say that she has not had a period in, for example, 12 years.

A careful sexual history is important. Chapter 1, The Interviewer's Questions, provides several ways of broaching the topic. The interviewer might start by asking, "Are you satisfied with your sex life?" It is important for the examiner to determine the marital status of the patient. Is the patient married? How many times? How long? Are there other sexual partners? If the patient is not married, is she currently having sexual relationship(s)? What type of birth control is being used?

Determine whether the patient's mother was given diethylstilbestrol (DES)* during her pregnancy.

Use words that will be understood by the patient. It may be necessary to use such terms as "lips" to refer to the labia or "privates" to refer to the genitalia.

Impact of Infertility on the Female

The problem of infertility is not new. From ancient times, cultures have practiced fertility rites to ensure the continuation of their people. Many societies considered a woman's worth in terms of her ability to have children. The "barren woman" was frequently banished.

The average time taken for a woman to conceive is 4–5 months. The American Fertility Society defines infertility as the inability to conceive "after one year of regular coitus without contraception." During this period, more than 80% of women conceive. After 3 years of regular sexual intercourse, 98% of women become pregnant.

It has been estimated that approximately one of every six couples in the United States has some problem with fertility. Infertility should be considered a problem of both men and women. It was previously thought that infertility was *functional* (no demonstrable organ disorder) in 30–50% of all cases, but it is now recognized that more than 90% of infertile couples have a pathologic cause. However, only about 50% of these couples achieve pregnancy. Fifty percent of infertility is related to a female problem,† 30% to a male problem,‡ and 20% to a combined problem.

Infertility is one of the several important developmental crises of adult life. The impact of infertility on a woman can be severe. The influence of the higher nervous system on ovulation is well known but only partially understood. When the woman is told that she is infertile, she may be shocked and distressed about the loss of an important function of her body. This psychological injury lasts for variable amounts of time. Often the woman feels defective or inadequate. This extends to her interactions with others, in addition to her sexual function. Her attitude toward her job may change; her work productivity may decline. There is a significant decrease in sexual desire. Depression, the loss of libido, and the concern whether conception will ever occur contribute to making sex a less pleasurable activity, and all decrease the possibility of normal ovulation. A period of mourning and frustration usually occurs.

Often the woman becomes preoccupied with her menstrual periods. When will the next one come? Is she pregnant? Did she have any symptoms of ovulation? When the next menstrual cycle occurs, the woman suffers further grief.

The infertile woman may fear that her partner will resent her, and she may feel alienated from him. She may experience jealousy and resentment toward friends or relations who have children. Her infertility lowers her self-esteem and may make her feel that she is unfit to be a parent.

---

* DES was given to many pregnant women from 1940 to 1975 for a variety of reasons, such as a threatened abortion and premature labor. Vaginal involvement by adenosis often developed in the exposed daughters. Carcinoma of the vagina or cervix, as well as cervical incompetence, has also been occasionally reported in the offspring.

† In general, fallopian tubal patency or ovulation problems.

‡ Vas deferens obstruction, varicocele, chromosomal defects, testicular infection, autoimmune states, and decreased sperm count are the most important.

Regardless of the cause of infertility, the treatment must work to lessen the psychological side effects. Both partners must be encouraged to communicate. Education regarding the physical problem is important throughout the medical work-up. Communication between the partners and the physician is paramount. The patient needs to be protected from her own insecurities while given empathy and compassion.

In some women, psychogenic factors may be the sole cause of infertility. Such factors may act at various phases in the reproductive process. These women may have an immature personality and fear the responsibilities of motherhood. They use their infertility as a defense mechanism. In other cases, emotional conflicts may lead to somatic symptoms and signs. Vaginismus is the most common psychosomatic disorder causing infertility. In this condition, the introitus may become so constricted that it inhibits the penis from entering. Vaginismus protects the patient from conception. Many of these women view sexual intercourse as exploitative and degrading. Intercourse is feared because it is painful. These patients do well with psychotherapy that allows them to express their fears about intercourse, genitalia, and childbearing.

Physical Examination

The equipment necessary for the examination of the female genitalia and rectum is vaginal speculum, lubricant, cervical scrapers, cotton-tipped applicators, gloves, glass slides, occult blood testing card and reagent, culture media (as appropriate), fixative, tissues, and a light source.

General Considerations

Unlike most other parts of the physical examination, the pelvic examination is often viewed with apprehension by the patient. This is frequently related to a previous bad experience. An examination performed slowly and gently with adequate explanations goes a long way in developing a good doctor-patient relationship. Communication is the key to a successful pelvic examination. The examiner should talk to the patient and tell her exactly what is going to be done. Eye contact is also necessary to decrease the patient's anxiety. A relaxed patient will provide a more accurate and less traumatic examination.

If the examiner is a male, he should examine the patient's genitalia in the presence of a female attendant. The woman attendant is important for assistance as well as for medicolegal considerations. Although not required by law, the presence of a female attendant is important, especially when the patient appears overly upset or seductive. At times, the patient may request that a family member be present. The examiner should grant such a request if no other attendant is available.

Throughout the world, certain patient positions are preferred for facilitating the pelvic examination. These include the woman's lying on her back on an examining table, lying in bed on her left side, lying on her back in bed with her legs abducted, and sitting upright in a chair with legs abducted. In the United States, the woman usually lies on her back on an examination table with her feet in heel rests. This position is uncomfortable and demeaning.

Preparation for the Examination

The patient should be instructed to empty her bladder and bowels before the examination. The patient is assisted onto an examination table with her buttocks placed near its edge. The heel rests of the table are extended, and the patient is instructed to place her heels in them. If possible, some cloth should be placed over the rests. Alternately, the patient can be given plastic foam booties to protect her feet from cold metal heel rests. Shortening the heel rest brackets will help the woman bend her knees in order to lower the position of the cervix. The older patient with osteoarthritis may require the heel rests to be longer, because there may be limitation of hip and knee motion. Offer the patient a mirror that she can use to observe the examination.

The head of the examination table should be elevated so that eye contact between the physician and the patient will occur. A sheet is usually draped over the lower abdomen and knees of the patient. Some patients prefer not to have the sheet used. The patient should be asked for her preference.

The knees are drawn up sufficiently to relax the abdominal muscles as the thighs are abducted. Ask the patient to let her legs fall to the sides or to drop her knees to each side. Never tell a patient to "spread her legs."

Gloves should be worn for the examination of the female genitalia. The examiner should be seated on a stool between the legs of the patient. Good lighting, including a light source directed into the vagina, is essential.

The examination of the female genitalia consists of the following:

- Inspection and palpation of external genitalia
- Examination with speculum
- Bimanual palpation
- Rectovaginal palpation

Inspection and Palpation of External Genitalia

Inspect the External Genitalia and Hair

To make the woman more comfortable during inspection of the external genitalia, it is often useful to touch the patient. Tell the patient that you are going to touch her leg. Use the *back* of your hand to touch the inside of the patient's thigh.

The external genitalia should be inspected carefully. The mons veneris is inspected for lesions and swelling. The hair is inspected for its pattern and for pubic lice and nits. The skin of the vulva is inspected for redness, excoriation, masses, leukoplakia, and pigmentation. Lesions should be palpated for tenderness. *Kraurosis vulvae* is a condition in which the skin of the vulva shows a uniform reddened, smooth, shiny, almost transparent appearance. Although most common in the postmenopausal woman, it may be seen in patients of all ages. White patches of hyperkeratosis, *leukoplakia vulvae,* frequently appear on the labia and perineum. The principal importance of this lesion is that it commonly precedes carcinoma. Leukoplakia is less common than kraurosis vulvae. Figure 17–6 shows an ulcerated lesion of squamous cell carcinoma of the vulva.

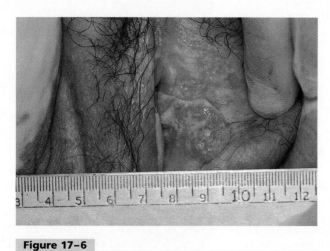

Figure 17–6

Vulvar carcinoma.

Inspect the Labia

Tell the patient that you are now going to spread the labia. With your right hand, the labia majora and minora are spread apart between the right thumb and index fingers, as shown in Figure 17–7. The vaginal introitus is inspected.

Inflammatory lesions, ulceration, discharge, scarring, warts, trauma, swelling, atrophic changes, and masses are noted. Figure 17–8 shows condylomata acuminata of the labia.

Inspect the Clitoris

The clitoris is inspected for size and lesions. The clitoris is normally 3–4 mm in size.

Inspect the Urethral Meatus

Is pus or inflammation present? If pus is present, determine its source. Dip a cotton-tipped applicator into the discharge, and spread the sample on a microscope slide for later evaluation.

Inspect the Area of Bartholin's Glands

Tell the patient that you are going to palpate the glands of the labia. Palpate the area of the right gland (at 7–8 o'clock positions) by grasping the posterior portion of the right labia between the right index finger in the vagina and the right thumb on the outside, as shown in Figure 17–9. Is any tenderness, swelling, or pus present? Normally, Bartholin's glands can be neither seen nor felt. Use the left hand to examine the area of the left gland (at 4–5 o'clock positions).

Figure 17–10 shows a patient with an abscess in the left Bartholin's gland.

Inspect the Perineum

The perineum and anus are inspected for masses, scars, fissures, and fistulae. Is the perineal skin reddened? The anus should be inspected for hemorrhoids, irritation, and fissures.

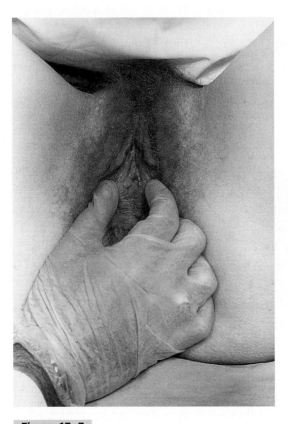

Figure 17–7

Technique for inspecting the labia.

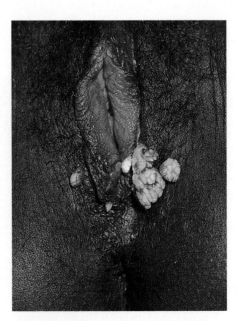

Figure 17–8

Condylomata acuminata.

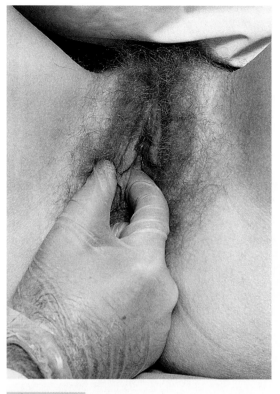

Figure 17-9

Technique for palpation of Bartholin's glands.

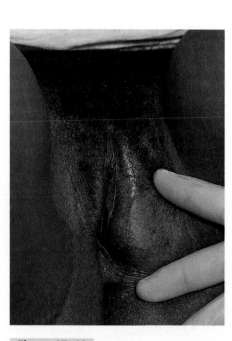

Figure 17-10

Bartholin's gland abscess.

▪ Test for Pelvic Relaxation

With the labia spread widely, the patient is asked to bear down or cough. If vaginal relaxation is present, ballooning of the anterior or posterior walls may be seen. Bulging of the anterior wall is associated with a cystocele; bulging of the posterior wall indicates a rectocele. If stress incontinence is present, the coughing or bearing down may trigger a spurt of urine from the urethra.

Examination with Speculum

▪ The Preparation

The speculum examination inspects the vagina and cervix. There are several types of specula. The metal *Cusco,* or *bivalve,* speculum is the most popular. This speculum consists of two blades or bills that are introduced closed into the vagina and are then opened by squeezing the handle mechanism. The vaginal walls are held apart by the bills, and adequate visualization of the vagina and cervix is achieved. There are basically two types of bivalve specula: the Graves and the Pedersen. The *Graves* speculum is the more common one and is used for most adult women. The bills are wider and are curved on the sides. The *Pedersen* speculum has narrower, flat bills and is used for women with a small introitus. The plastic, disposable bivalve speculum is becoming more commonly used. A disadvantage to its use is a loud click that is made as the lower bill is disengaged during removal from the vagina. If a plastic speculum is used, the patient should be informed that this sound will occur. Check the bills to make sure that there are no rough edges.

Before using the speculum in a patient, practice opening and closing it. If the patient has never had a speculum examination, show the speculum to her. You should warm the speculum with warm water and then touch it to the back of your hand to determine that the temperature is suitable. Jelly lubricant should not be used because it may interfere with cervical cytologic determination and gonococcal cultures. Tell the patient that you are now going to perform the speculum part of the internal examination.

■ The Technique

While the examiner uses the left index and middle fingers to separate the labia and firmly depress the perineum, the closed speculum, held by the examiner's right hand, is introduced at an oblique angle *slowly* into the introitus over the examiner's left fingers. This procedure is shown in Figures 17–11 and 17–12 and is illustrated in Figure 17–13. Do not introduce the speculum vertically, because injury to the urethra or meatus may occur.

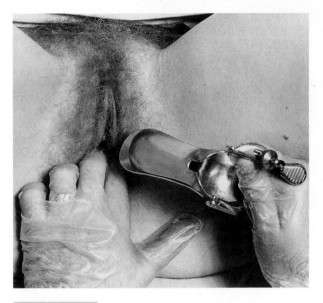

Figure 17–11

Technique for insertion of the vaginal speculum. Note the examiner's fingers pressing downward on the perineum.

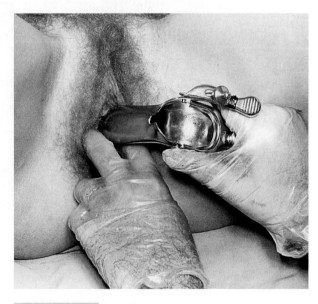

Figure 17–12

Technique for insertion of the vaginal speculum. Note that the speculum rides over the examiner's fingers, avoiding contact with the external urethral meatus and clitoris.

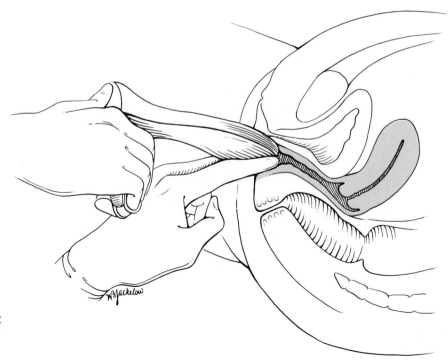

Figure 17–13

Cross-sectional view of the speculum examination.

Inspect the Cervix

The speculum is introduced as far into the vagina as possible. When it is inserted completely, the speculum is rotated to the transverse position, with the handle now pointing downward, and is opened *slowly*. With the bills open, the vaginal walls and cervix can be visualized. The cervix should rest within the bills of the speculum. This is shown in Figure 17–14 and illustrated in Figure 17–15. To keep the speculum open,

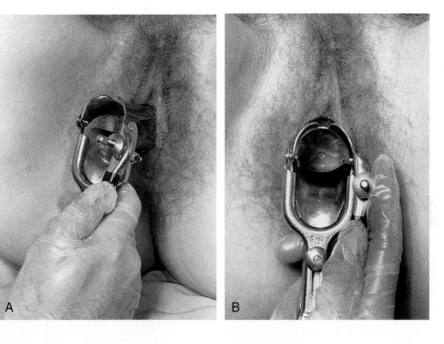

Figure 17–14

Technique for inspecting the cervix. *A,* The opening of the speculum bills after the speculum has been fully inserted and rotated to the transverse position. *B,* The internal view of the cervix when the speculum is correctly inserted.

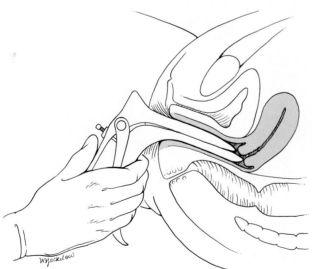

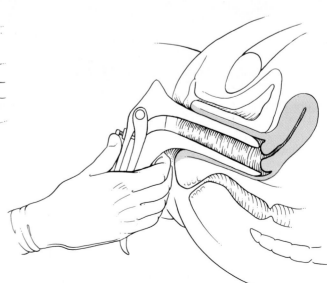

Figure 17–15

Cross-sectional view illustrating the position of the speculum during inspection of the cervix.

the set screw can be tightened. If the cervix is not immediately seen, gently turn the bills in various directions to expose the cervix. The most common reason for not visualizing the cervix is failure to insert the speculum far enough before opening it.

If a discharge is obscuring any part of the vaginal walls or cervix, the discharge should be removed with a cotton-tipped applicator and spread onto a glass microscope slide.

Inspect the cervix for discharge, erythema, erosion, ulceration, leukoplakia, and mass. What is the shape of the external cervical os? What is the color of the cervix? A bluish discoloration may be an indication of pregnancy or a large tumor.

A normal cervix is seen in Figure 17–16. Notice that the external cervical os is linear, which is characteristic of a cervix of a woman who has had a vaginal delivery.

Pap Smear

A Pap* smear is obtained with a wooden Ayres' cervical scraper inserted through the speculum, as shown in Figure 17–17. The longer end of the scraper is inserted into the external cervical os (Fig. 17–18). The scraper is then rotated 360° while scraping off cells from the external cervical os. Other specimens are taken with a cotton-tipped applicator from the posterior and lateral vaginal fornices and from the endocervix. The specimens are smeared separately onto glass slides and are fixed either by dropping

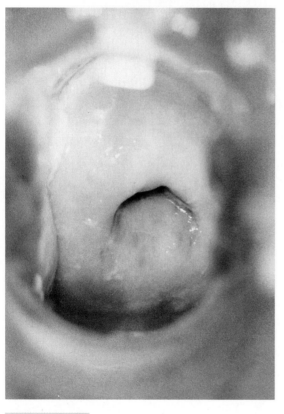

Figure 17–16

A normal cervix. Note the linear external cervical os, which is commonly seen in women who have had vaginal deliveries. The external cervical os in a nulliparous woman is perfectly round.

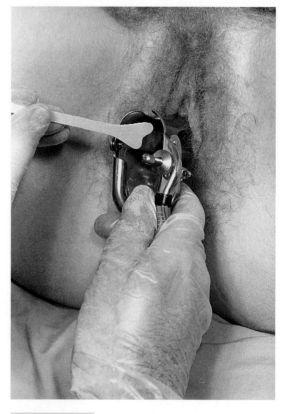

Figure 17–17

Technique for obtaining a smear for the Pap test.

---

*Pap is the abbreviated name for George N. Papanicolaou, the physician who developed this screening technique. The properly performed test can accurately lead to the diagnosis of cervical carcinoma in 98% of cases and can detect 80% of cases of endometrial carcinoma.

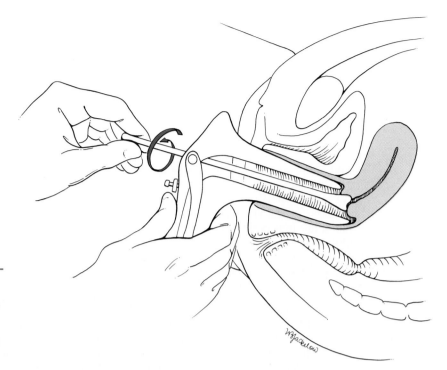

Figure 17–18

Technique for obtaining a smear for the Pap test. Note that the longer end of the wooden spatula is placed in the cervical os.

them in a solution of equal parts of 95% methyl alcohol and ether or by spraying them with a rapidly drying fixative, such as Spraycyte. Because the Pap smear may cause the cervix to bleed slightly, advise the patient that she may have a little spotting, which is normal. Any significant bleeding, however, should be evaluated.

Inspect the Vaginal Walls

The patient is told that the speculum will now be removed. The set screw is released with the examiner's right index finger, and the speculum is rotated back to the original oblique position. As the speculum is slowly withdrawn and closed, the vaginal walls are inspected for masses, lacerations, leukoplakia, and ulcerations. The walls should be smooth and nontender. A moderate amount of colorless or white mucus is usually present.

Bimanual Palpation

The bimanual examination is used for palpation of the uterus and adnexa. Lower the head of the examination table to 15° or to flat, depending on the patient's preference. In this examination, the examiner's hands are placed in the patient's vagina and on the abdomen, and the pelvic structures are palpated between the hands. The choice of which hand to use vaginally is a matter of preference. In general, the right hand is inserted into the vagina, and the left hand palpates the abdomen.

The Technique

The physician should be positioned between the patient's legs. If the right hand is to be used vaginally, the examiner places the right foot on a small footrest or stool. A suitable jelly lubricant is held in the left hand, and a small amount is dropped from the tube onto the examiner's gloved right index and middle fingers. The examiner should not touch the tube of lubricant to the gloves because the lubricant will become contaminated. The patient is told that the internal examination will now begin.

As the bimanual examination is being performed, the examiner should observe the patient's face. Her expression will quickly reveal whether the examination is painful. The examiner should tell the woman that he or she is again going to touch her leg as the examination begins. The back of the examiner's left hand should touch the inside of the patient's right thigh. The labia are spread, and the examiner's lubricated right index and middle fingers are introduced vertically into the vagina. A downward pressure toward the perineum is applied. The right fourth and fifth fingers are flexed into the palm of the hand. The right thumb is extended. The area around the clitoris should not be touched. The examiner may now rest the right elbow on his or her right knee so that undue pressure is not placed on the patient.

The correct positions of the physician, assistant, and patient are shown in Figure 17–19.

The vaginal walls are palpated for nodules, scarring, and induration.

Once inserted into the vagina, the examiner's right hand is rotated 90° clockwise so that the palm is facing upward. Some physicians prefer not to rotate the vaginal hand because this may decrease the depth of penetration. The left hand is now placed on the abdomen approximately one third of the way to the umbilicus from the pubic symphysis. The wrist of the abdominal hand should not be flexed or supinated. The right (vaginal) hand pushes the pelvic organs up out of the pelvis and stabilizes them while they are palpated by the left (abdominal) hand. It is the abdominal, not the vaginal, hand that performs the palpation. The technique for the bimanual examination is shown in Figure 17–20 and is illustrated in Figure 17–21.

■ Palpate the Cervix and Uterine Body

The cervix is palpated. What is its consistency (soft, firm, nodular, friable)?

Tell the patient that she will now feel you move her cervix and uterus, but this should not be painful. The cervix can usually be moved 2–4 cm in any direction. The cervix is pushed backward and upward toward the abdominal hand as the abdominal hand pushes downward. Any restriction of motion or the development of pain on movement should be noted. Pushing the cervix up and back tends to tip an anteverted, anteflexed uterus forward into a position that is more easily palpated. The uterus should then be felt between the two hands. Describe its *position, size, shape, consistency, mobility,* and *tenderness.* Determine whether the uterus is anteverted or retroverted, enlarged, firm, and mobile. Are any irregularities felt? Is there any tenderness when the uterus is moved?

Palpation by the bimanual technique is possible only if the uterus is anteverted and anteflexed, which is the most common uterine position. A retroverted uterus is directed toward the spine and is not easily felt by bimanual palpation.

■ Palpate the Adnexa

After the uterus has been evaluated, the right and left adnexa are palpated. If the patient has complained of pain on one side, start the examination on the other side. The right hand should move to the left lateral fornix while the left (abdominal) hand moves to the patient's left lower quadrant. The vaginal fingers lift the adnexa toward

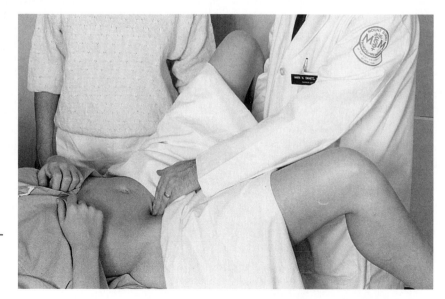

Figure 17–19

The positions of the examiner, assistant, and patient for the bimanual examination.

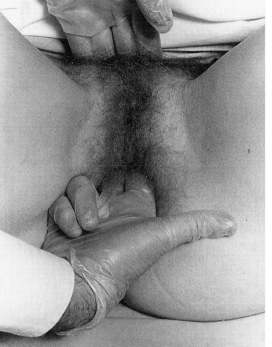

Figure 17–20

Technique for the bimanual examination.

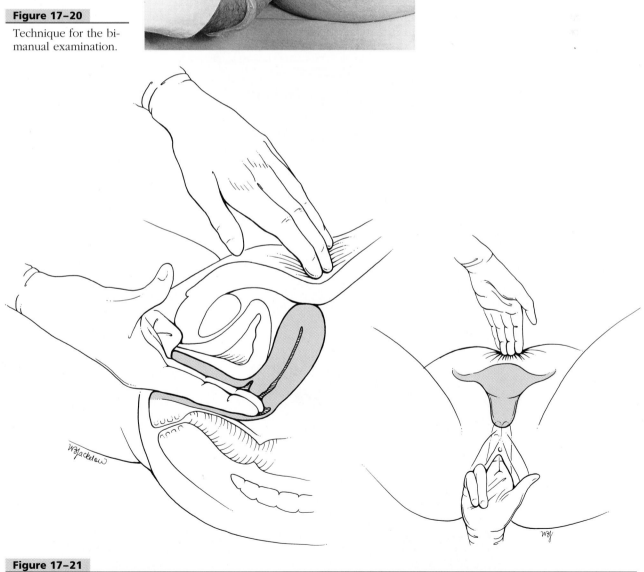

Figure 17–21

The bimanual examination. Cross-sectional view through the pelvic organs. Position of the uterus between the examining hands. Note the position of the right thumb, held away from the clitoris.

the abdominal hand, which attempts to palpate the adnexal structures. This is illustrated in Figure 17–22.

The adnexa should be explored for masses. Describe the *size, shape, consistency,* and *mobility,* as well as any *tenderness,* of the structures in the adnexa. The normal

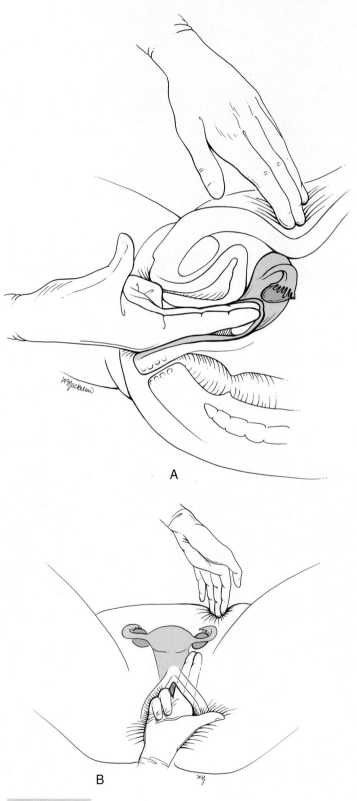

A

B

Figure 17–22

Technique for palpating the left adnexa. *A,* Cross-sectional view through the pelvic organs. *B,* Position of the ovary and fallopian tube between the examining hands.

ovary is sensitive to pressure when squeezed. After the left side is examined, the right adnexa are palpated by moving the right (vaginal) hand to the right lateral fornix and the left (abdominal) hand to the right lower quadrant of the patient.

In many women, the adnexal structures cannot be palpated. In thin women, the ovaries are frequently palpable. Adnexal tenderness or enlargement is relatively specific for a pathologic state.

After completion of the examination of the adnexa, the examining vaginal fingers move to the posterior fornix to palpate the uterosacral ligaments and the pouch of Douglas. Marked tenderness and nodularity suggest endometriosis.

If the patient has borne children, the examiner should have no difficulty in using the right index and middle fingers in the vagina for bimanual palpation. If the introitus is small, the examiner should introduce the right middle finger first and gently push downward toward the anus. By stretching the introitus, the right index finger can then be introduced with little discomfort. If the patient is a virgin, only the right middle finger should be used.

Rectovaginal Palpation

▓ Palpate the Rectovaginal Septum

Tell the patient that you will now examine the vagina and rectum. The rectovaginal examination allows for better evaluation of the posterior portion of the pelvis and the cul-de-sac than does the bimanual examination alone. You can often get 1–2 cm higher into the pelvis by the rectovaginal examination. Remove your hand from the vagina, and change your glove. Lubricate the gloved index and middle fingers. Inspect the anus. Insert the index finger back into the vagina while the middle finger is introduced into the anus. Explain to the patient that this technique will make her feel as if she has to defecate but will not do so. The examining right index finger is positioned as far up the posterior surface of the vagina as possible. This technique is shown in Figure 17–23 and is illustrated in Figure 17–24.

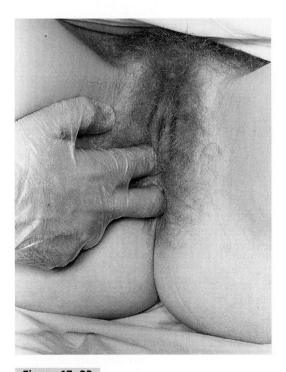

Figure 17–23

Technique for performing the rectovaginal examination.

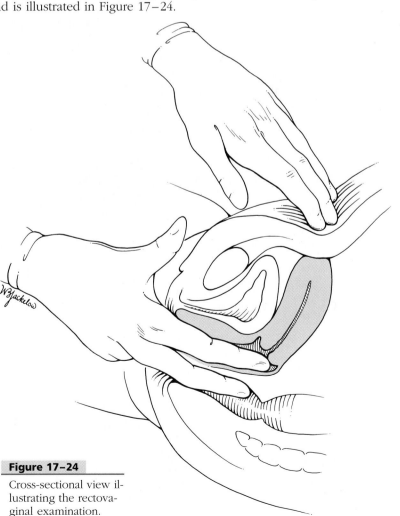

Figure 17–24

Cross-sectional view illustrating the rectovaginal examination.

The rectovaginal septum is palpated. Is it thickened or tender? Are nodules or masses present? The right middle finger should feel for tenderness, masses, or irregularities in the rectum.

The patient is told that the internal examination is completed and that you are about to remove your hand. When you withdraw your fingers, inspect them for discharge or blood. Offer the woman tissues to wipe off any excess lubricant.

▨ Test Stool for Occult Blood

Any fecal material on the middle (rectal) finger should be tested with the occult blood testing card and reagent.

Ask the woman to move back on the examination table, remove her legs from the heel rests, and then sit up slowly. Remove your gloves, and wash your hands. This concludes the examination of the female genitalia.

Clinicopathologic Correlations

Figure 17–25 shows several of the common uterine positions.

Pelvic relaxation is a common problem. The consequences include cystocele, rectocele, and uterine prolapse. Figure 17–26 illustrates these sequelae of relaxation of the pelvic floor.

A summary of dysfunctional uterine bleeding is illustrated in Figure 17–27.

Vaginitis is an inflammation of the vagina and vulva that is marked by pain, itching, and vaginal discharge. Normal vaginal discharge originates in mucous secre-

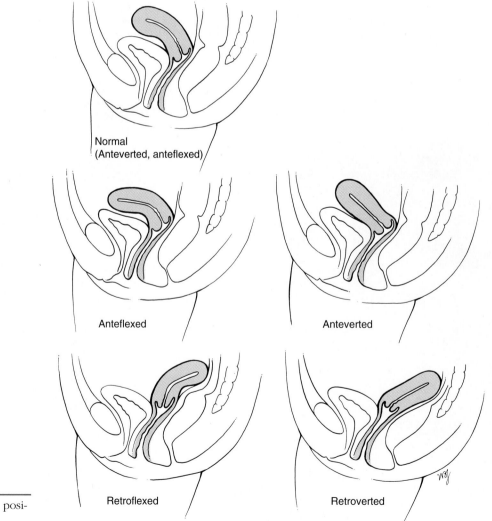

Figure 17–25

Common uterine positions.

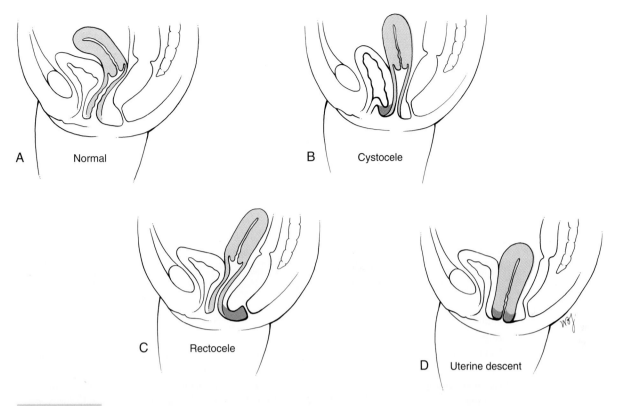

Figure 17–26

Sequelae of pelvic floor relaxation. *A,* Normal anatomy, *B,* A cystocele, which is protrusion of the wall of the urinary bladder through the vagina. *C,* A rectocele, which is a protrusion of the rectal wall through the vagina. *D,* Uterine descent, which is a protrusion of the uterus through the vagina.

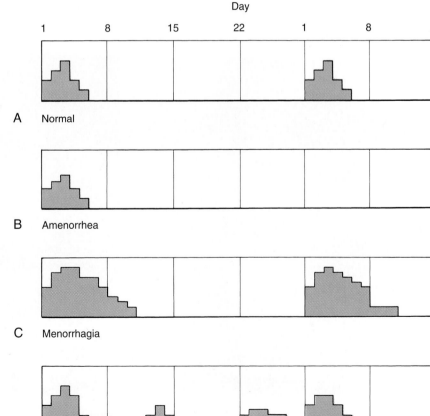

Figure 17–27

Types of dysfunctional uterine bleeding. *A,* Normal 28 day cycle. Note that menstrual flow occurs on day 1 and lasts for approximately 5 days. *B,* Amenorrhea. After a menstrual flow of 5 days, the period does not recur. *C,* Menorrhagia. Note that the flow occurs at 28 day intervals, but the amount of flow is heavier, and its duration is longer than normal. *D,* Metrorrhagia. In this condition, flow is regular, but there is bleeding between the normal menstrual flow cycles.

tions from the cervix and vagina as well as in exfoliated vaginal cells. A normal vaginal discharge is thin and transparent and has little odor. When the normal bacterial flora in the vagina is disturbed, one or more organisms can multiply out of their normal proportions. This change in the normal flora may also make the vagina more susceptible to other invading organisms. The rapid growth of organisms produces an excess of waste products that irritate tissues, cause burning and itching, and produce a discharge with an unpleasant odor. The discharges caused by different organisms have different appearances.

Table 17–1 lists the characteristics of common vaginal discharges. Table 17–2 summarizes the clinical features of genital ulcerations. Figure 17–28 shows the vesicular stage of herpes simplex infection. Figure 17–29 shows a chancre in a woman with primary syphilis.

Table 17–2   Clinical Features of Genital Ulcerations

Feature	Genital Herpes*	Primary Syphilis†	Chancroid
Incubation period	3–5 days	9–90 days	1–5 days
Number of ulcers	Multiple	Single	Multiple
Appearance at onset	Vesicle	Papule	Papule/pustule
Later appearance	Small, grouped	Round, indurated	Irregular, ragged
Ulcer pain	Present	Absent	Present
Inguinal adenopathy	Present, tender	Present, painless	Present, painful
Healing	Within 2 weeks	Slowly for weeks	Slowly for weeks
Recurrence (even if not infected)	Common	Rare	Common

* See Figure 17–28.
† See Figure 17–29.

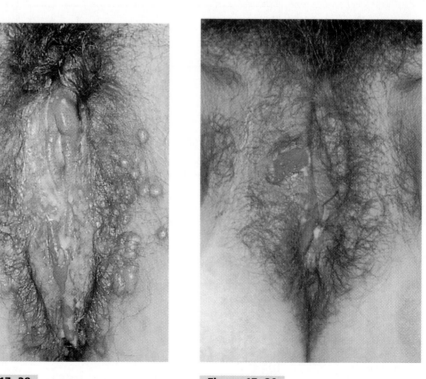

Figure 17–28

Herpes simplex infection.

Figure 17–29

Chancre.

Useful Vocabulary

Listed here are the specific roots that are important in order to understand the terminology related to diseases of the female genitalia.

Root	Pertaining to	Example	Definition
amni(o)-	amnion	*amnio*rrhexis	Rupture of the amnion
colp(o)-	vagina	*colpo*scopy	Examination of vagina (and cervix)
-cyesis	pregnancy	pseudo*cyesis*	False pregnancy
gyn(e)-	woman	*gyne*cology	Branch of medicine that deals with treating diseases of the genital tract in women
hyster(o)-	uterus	*hyster*ectomy	Surgical removal of the uterus
metro-	uterus	*metro*rrhagia	Uterine bleeding
oophor(o)-	ovary	*oophoro*tomy	Incision of an ovary
ov-	egg	*ov*ulation	The discharge of an egg from the ovary
salping(o)-	fallopian tube	*salping*itis	Inflammation of the fallopian tube

Writing Up the Physical Examination

Listed here are examples of the write-up for the examination of the female genitalia.

- Examination of the vulva is within normal limits. No lesions are present. The cervix appears pink, smooth, and nulliparous. There is no discharge from the external cervical os. The vaginal walls appear normal. Bimanual palpation reveals an anteverted, anteflexed uterus without masses or tenderness. The adnexa are unremarkable. Rectovaginal examination reveals a thin rectovaginal membrane without tenderness. Stool guaiac is negative.

- Examination of the vulva reveals groups of tense vesicles and scattered erosions that are covered with exudate. The cervix is pink and multiparous. No cervical lesions are present. No discharge is present. The vagina is within normal limits. The uterus is anteverted and anteflexed. A 6 × 6 cm mass is felt with the uterus. The ovaries and tubes are unremarkable. Rectovaginal examination is within normal limits.

- The vulva appears within normal limits without masses or lesions. The cervix has an erosion with a thick, white, cottage cheese–like discharge in the vagina. The discharge is adherent to the vaginal walls. The uterus is retroverted and cannot be adequately examined. A walnut-sized mass is felt in the left adnexa. It appears rubbery and is freely mobile. The rectovaginal examination is normal. Stool guaiac is negative.

- The vulva is normal. Upon straining, a rectocele becomes apparent. The vagina is normal. The cervix is smooth, pink, and multiparous. The uterus is anteverted and anteflexed and is not enlarged. The adnexa are difficult to assess because of obesity of the patient. No tenderness is present.

Bibliography

Magee J: The pelvic examination: A view from the other end of the table. Ann Intern Med 83:563, 1975.

Mazor MD, Simons HF (eds): Infertility: Medical, Emotional and Social Considerations. New York, Human Sciences Press, 1984.

Peckham BM, Shapiro SS: Signs and Symptoms in Gynecology. Philadelphia, J.B. Lippincott, 1983.

Priest RG: Psychological Disorders in Obstetrics and Gynaecology. London, Butterworth, 1985.

CHAPTER 18

The Musculoskeletal System

The hand of the Lord was upon me . . . and set me down in the midst of the valley which was full of bones . . . behold, there were very many in the open valley; and, lo, they were very dry. . . . Thus saith the Lord God unto these bones: Behold, I will cause breath to enter into you, and ye shall live. And I will lay sinews upon you, and will bring up flesh upon you, and cover with skin, and put breath in you, and ye shall live . . . there was a noise, and behold a commotion, and the bones came together, bone to bone . . . and skin covered them . . . and the breath came into them, and they lived, and stood up upon their feet. . . .

Ezekiel XXXVII: 1–10

General Considerations

Diseases of the musculoskeletal system rank first among disease conditions that alter the quality of life. This is related to limitation of activity, disability, and impairment. In the United States, one of every seven persons suffers from some sort of musculoskeletal disorder, the cost of which exceeds 60 billion dollars annually. This includes lost earnings and medical expenses.

Diseases of the musculoskeletal system are divided into two categories: *systemic* and *local*. Patients with a systemic disease, such as rheumatoid arthritis, systemic lupus erythematosus, or polymyositis, may appear chronically ill, with generalized weakness, pain, and episodic stiffness of their joints. Patients with a local disease are basically healthy individuals who suffer restriction of motion and pain from a single area. Included in this group of patients are those suffering from back pain, tennis elbow, arthritis, or bursitis. Despite the fact that these patients may have only local symptoms, their disability can greatly limit their work capacity, and the disease can have severe impact.

Diseases of the musculoskeletal system rank first in cost to workers' compensation insurance carriers. Nearly 100,000 workers receive disability payments annually, with a total cost to the carriers of more than 200 billion dollars annually.

It has been estimated that musculoskeletal-related problems rank second (after cardiovascular disorders) in the number of visits to internists and rank third in the number of surgical procedures in hospitals.*

Although not primarily fatal disorders, musculoskeletal conditions affect the quality of life. Studies have indicated that backache is experienced by more than 80% of all Americans at some time in their lives. Patients with backache for longer than 6 months constitute a large portion of permanently disabled individuals. More than 50% of these patients never return to work. More than 25 million Americans suffer from arthritis that requires medical attention. Arthritis ranks second to cardiac disease as a cause of limitation of activity.

In the United States, at least 10% of the population experiences a bone fracture, dislocation, or sprain annually. Each year, more than 1.2 million fractures are sustained by women over the age of 50 years. There are more than 200,000 hip fractures annually, and these are associated with prolonged disability. Osteoporosis† is the most common musculoskeletal disorder in the world and is second only to arthritis as a leading cause of morbidity in the geriatric population. Postmenopausal osteoporosis and age-related osteoporosis increase the risk of fractures in the older population. There are more than 40 million women in the United States older than the age of 50 years, and more than 50% of them have evidence of spinal osteoporosis. Almost 90% of women older than the age of 75 years have significant radiographic evidence of osteoporosis.

The high prevalence of musculoskeletal disease in the elderly requiring assistance has a significant impact on the American economy. The cost for nursing home care for

---

* Gynecologic surgery is first, followed by abdominal surgery.
† *Osteoporosis* is a state of decreased density of normal mineralized bone.

patients with musculoskeletal disease is almost 75 billion dollars. More than 10 million individuals in the United States have some form of inflammatory arthritis, the most prevalent being rheumatoid arthritis. It is estimated that more than 7 million of these patients have this form of arthritis. Although trauma to the spinal cord that produces paraplegia or quadriplegia is rare, the average total lifetime cost per patient exceeds $150,000.

Musculoskeletal problems have their most significant financial effect on the aged population. More than 1 billion dollars is spent annually by Medicare for hospitalizations of patients with these conditions. This represents 20% of all Medicare payments.

Structure and Physiology

The principal functions of the musculoskeletal system are to provide support and protection of the body and to bring about movement of the extremities for locomotion and for the performance of tasks.

The parts of the musculoskeletal system are composed of variable forms of dense connective tissue, which include the following:

- Bone
- Skeletal muscle
- Ligaments and tendons
- Cartilage

Bone is composed of an organic matrix that consists of collagen fibers embedded in a cementing gel made up of calcium and phosphate. Bone is an actively changing tissue constantly undergoing *remodeling* while reappropriating its mineral stores and matrix according to mechanical stresses. Normal bone is composed of collagen fibers aligned parallel to the tension stresses to which the bone is exposed. The long bones in the adult are composed of tubes of *cortical,* or compact, bone surrounding a medullary cavity of *cancellous,* or spongy, bone. Cortical bone exists in areas where support is necessary, whereas cancellous bone is found in areas where hematopoiesis and bone formation occur. In cortical bone, the bone cells, or *osteocytes,* are enclosed in lacunae, which are spaces in the sheets of bone tissue called *lamellae.* Several lamellae are arranged concentrically around a vascular channel and are termed a *haversian canal.* In cancellous bone, the lamellae are not arranged in haversian systems but are organized into a spongy network called *trabeculae.* These trabeculae align along lines of stress.

The ends of the long bones, called *epiphyses,* are expanded near the articular surfaces and are composed of spongy bone. The shaft of the long bone, the *diaphysis,* is covered with a layer of *periosteum.* The inner cavity of the long bone is lined with *endosteum* and is filled with marrow.

For a period of time, a layer of cartilage exists between the diaphysis and the epiphysis. This cartilage is known as the *growth plate* or *epiphyseal plate.* The purpose of the growth plate is to determine the longitudinal growth of the bone. The parts of a long bone are illustrated in Figure 18–1.

Cells in the periosteum can develop into *osteoblasts,* which lay down new bone, or into *osteoclasts,* which resorb bone. Trauma, infection, and tumors stimulate the development of osteoblasts. Osteoblasts secrete the matrix that is refashioned into lamellae and is arranged to meet the mechanical stresses to which the bone is subjected.

A pathologic process that interferes with the normal architecture of bone will tend to weaken it. Paget's disease is a disease of bone in which there is a disruption of the normal architecture. Patients with this condition are extremely susceptible to pathologic fractures.

Skeletal muscle is an organ, the contraction of which produces movement.

Ligaments attach bone to bone, and *tendons* attach muscle to bone. Both are dense connective tissues that offer great resistance to a pulling force.

Cartilage is a type of connective tissue with great resilience. It plays an important role in joint function and in determining bone length.

The basic functional unit of the musculoskeletal system is the *joint.* A joint is a union of two or more bones. There are several types of joints in the body. They include joints that are:

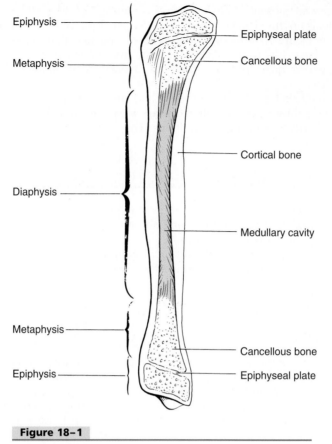

Epiphysis ——————
Epiphyseal plate
Metaphysis ——————
Cancellous bone

Diaphysis ——————

Cortical bone

Medullary cavity

Metaphysis ——————
Cancellous bone
Epiphysis ——————
Epiphyseal plate

Figure 18–1

Anatomy of a long bone.

- Immovable
- Slightly movable
- Movable

Immovable joints are joints fixed as a result of fibrous tissue banding. Examples of this type of joint are the sutures of the skull. *Slightly movable joints* are termed *symphyses*. In this type of joint, fibrocartilage joins the articulating bones. The pubic symphysis is an example of a slightly movable joint. The most common type of joint is the *movable joint*. The body has many different types of movable joints, also known as *synovial joints*. In synovial joints, the bone structures come in contact with each other and are covered with hyaline articular cartilage. A capsule surrounds the joint by attaching to the bones on either side of the joint. Within the capsule is a small amount of synovial fluid, which plays a role in joint lubrication and nourishment of the articular cartilage. Synovial joints are classified according to the type of movement their structure permits. The classifications include the following:

- Hinge joint
- Pivot joint
- Condyloid joint
- Saddle joint
- Ball-and-socket joint
- Plane joint

A *hinge joint* permits movement in only one axis, namely flexion or extension. The axis is transverse. An example of a hinge joint is the elbow. A *pivot joint* permits rotation in one axis. The axis is longitudinal along the shaft of the bone. One bone moves around a central axis without any displacement from that axis. An example of a pivot joint is the proximal radioulnar joint. A *condyloid joint* permits movement in two axes. The articular surfaces are oval and have been described as an "egg-in-spoon joint." One axis is the long diameter of the oval, and the other axis is the short diameter of the oval. The wrist joint is an example of a condyloid joint. A *saddle joint* is also a biaxial joint. The articular surfaces are saddle-shaped, with the movements similar to those of the condyloid joint. The carpometacarpal joint of the thumb is an example of the saddle joint. The *ball-and-socket joint* is an example of a polyaxial joint; motion is possible in many axes. In a ball-and-socket joint, the articular surfaces are reciprocal segments of a sphere. The hip and shoulder joints are examples of ball-and-socket joints. A *plane joint* is also a polyaxial joint. In the plane joint, the articular surfaces are flat, and one bone merely rides over the other in many directions. The patellofemoral joint is an example of a plane joint. These different types of movable joints are shown in Figure 18–2 according to the movement permitted.

The stability of a joint depends on the following:

- The shape of the articular surfaces
- The ligaments
- The associated muscles

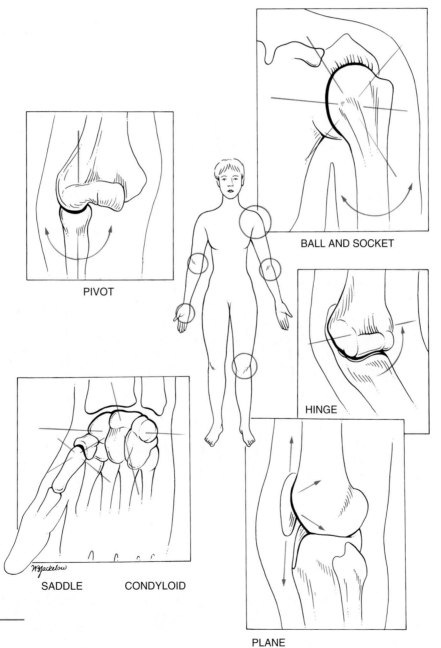

PIVOT

BALL AND SOCKET

HINGE

SADDLE   CONDYLOID

PLANE

Figure 18–2

Types of movable joints.

There are certain anatomic terms that refer to positions with which the reader must be familiar (Table 18–1). The *median plane* bisects the body into a right and left half. A plane parallel to the median plane is a *sagittal plane.* The terms *medial* and *lateral* are used in reference to the sagittal plane. A position closer to the median plane is medial; farther from the median plane is lateral. In the upper limb, *ulnar* is often substituted for medial, and *radial* is used to denote lateral. In the lower limb, *tibial* is used to denote medial, and *peroneal* or *fibular* is substituted for lateral.

The anatomic terms are illustrated in Figure 18–3.

The front of the body is the *anterior,* or *ventral,* surface, and the back of the body is the *posterior,* or *dorsal,* side. The *palmar,* or *volar,* aspect of the hand is the anterior

Table 18–1	Anatomic Terms for the Upper and Lower Limb		
	Limb	Medial	Lateral
	Upper	Ulnar	Radial
	Lower	Tibial	Peroneal
			Fibular

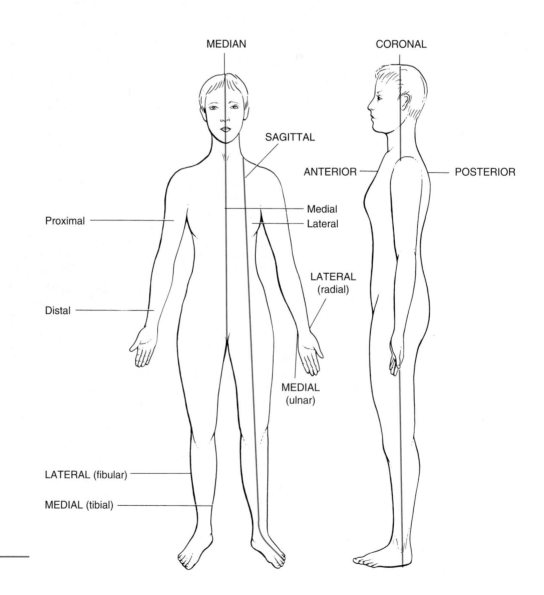

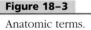

Figure 18–3

Anatomic terms.

surface. The dorsal aspect of the foot faces upward, and the *plantar* aspect is the sole. *Proximal* refers to the part of an extremity that is closest to its root; *distal* refers to the part farthest from the root.

The most important terms relating to deformities of the bone structure are *valgus* and *varus*. In a valgus deformity, the distal portion of the bone is displaced away from the midline, and angulation is toward the midline. In a varus deformity, the distal portion of the extremity is displaced toward the midline, and angulation is away from the midline. The name of the deformity is determined by the joint involved. An example of a valgus deformity of the knees is called knock-knee, termed *genu valgum*. An example of a varus deformity of the knee is known as bowleg, termed *genu varum*.

In the evaluation of a joint, assess the *range of motion*. Each joint has a characteristic range of motion that can be measured passively and actively. *Passive* range of motion is the motion elicited by the examiner as a result of the examiner's moving the patient's body. *Active* range of motion is the motion that the patient performs as a result of moving the musculature. The passive range of motion usually equals the active range of motion except in paralysis of muscles or in ruptured tendons. The range of motion of individual joints is discussed later in this chapter. Joint motion is measured in degrees of a circle, with the joint at the center. If a limb is extended with the bones in a straight line, the joint is at *zero position*. The zero position is the neutral position of the joint. As the joint is flexed, the angle increases. The concept of range of motion is illustrated in Figure 18–4.

The six basic types of joint motion are as follows:

- Flexion and extension
- Dorsiflexion and plantar flexion
- Adduction and abduction
- Inversion and eversion
- Internal and external rotation
- Pronation and supination

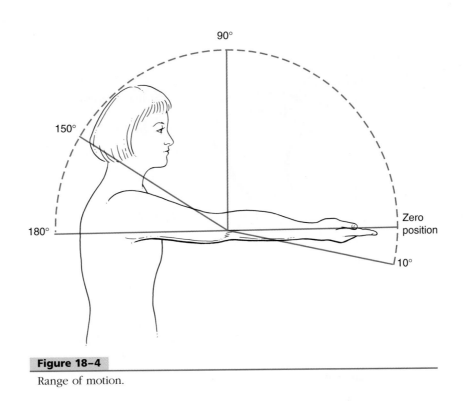

Figure 18-4

Range of motion.

The definitions of these motions and the joints at which the motions are seen are summarized in Table 18–2.

The anatomy of the *shoulder joint* is illustrated in Figure 18–5. The joint movements at the shoulder are abduction and adduction, flexion and extension, and internal and external rotation. These motions are illustrated in Figure 18–6.

Table 18–2	Joint Motion	
Motion	**Definition**	**Example**
Flexion	Motion away from the zero position	Most joints
Extension	Return motion to the zero position*	Most joints
Dorsiflexion	Movement in the direction of the dorsal surface	Ankle, toes, wrist, fingers
Plantar (or palmar) flexion	Movement in the direction of the plantar (or palmar) surface	Ankle, toes (wrist, fingers)
Adduction	Movement toward the midline†	Shoulder, hip, metacarpophalangeal, metatarsophalangeal joints
Abduction	Movement away from the midline	Shoulder, hip, metacarpophalangeal, metatarsophalangeal joints
Inversion	Turning of the plantar surface of the foot inward	Subtalar and midtarsal joints of the foot
Eversion	Turning of the plantar surface of the foot outward	Subtalar and midtarsal joints of the foot
Internal rotation	Turning of the anterior surface of a limb inward	Shoulder, hip
External rotation	Turning of the anterior surface of a limb outward	Shoulder, hip
Pronation	Rotation so that the palmar surface of the hand is directed downward	Elbow, wrist
Supination	Rotation so that the palmar surface of the hand is directed upward	Elbow, wrist

* If motion goes beyond the zero position, *hyperextension* is said to be present.
† In the hand or foot, the midline is a line drawn through the middle finger or middle toe, respectively.

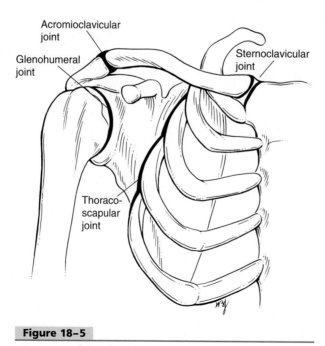

Figure 18–5

Anatomy of the shoulder joint.

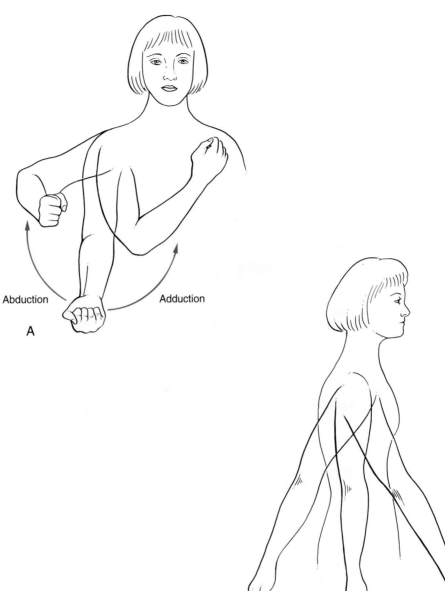

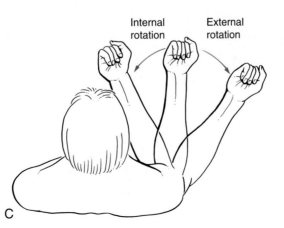

Figure 18–6

Range of motion at the shoulder. *A,* Abduction and adduction. *B,* Flexion and extension. *C,* Internal and external rotation.

The anatomy of the *elbow joint* is shown in Figure 18–7. The joint movements at the elbow are flexion and extension and supination and pronation. These motions are illustrated in Figure 18–8.

The anatomy of the *wrist* and *fingers* is illustrated in Figure 18–9. The joint movements at the wrist are dorsiflexion (or extension) and palmar flexion and supination and pronation. These motions are illustrated in Figure 18–10. The joint movements

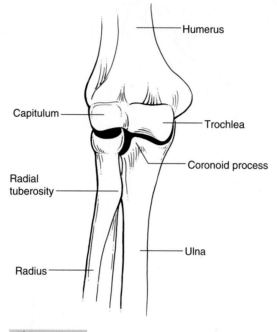

Figure 18–7

Anatomy of the elbow joint.

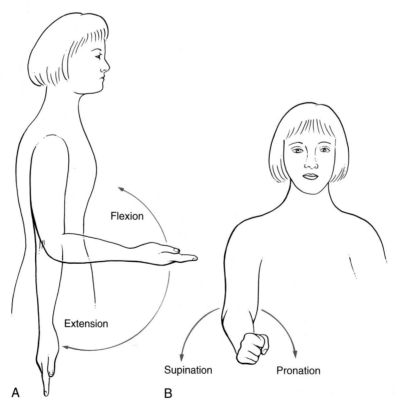

Figure 18–8

Range of motion at the elbow joint. *A,* Flexion and extension. *B,* Supination and pronation.

A   B

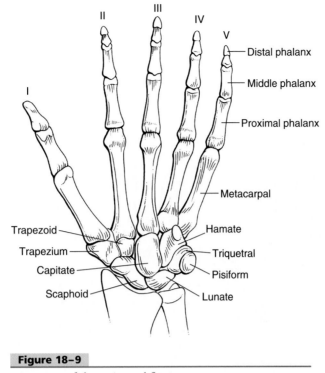

II   III   IV   V

Distal phalanx

Middle phalanx

Proximal phalanx

I

Metacarpal

Trapezoid   Hamate

Trapezium   Triquetral

Capitate   Pisiform

Scaphoid   Lunate

Figure 18-9

Anatomy of the wrist and fingers.

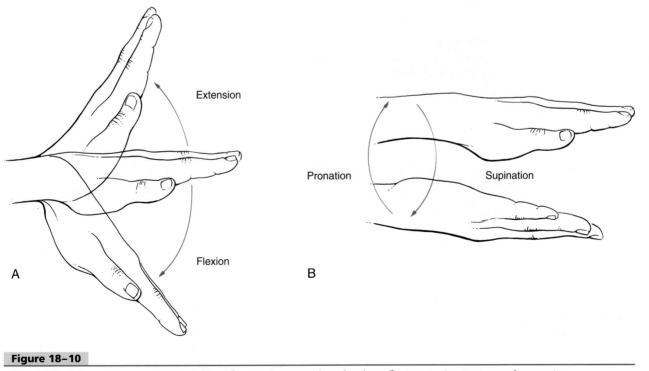

Extension

Pronation   Supination

Flexion

A   B

Figure 18-10

Range of motion at the wrist joint. *A,* Dorsiflexion (extension) and palmar flexion. *B,* Supination and pronation.

at the fingers are abduction and adduction and flexion. These motions are illustrated in Figure 18–11.

The joint movements of the *thumb* are flexion and extension and opposition. These motions are illustrated in Figure 18–12.

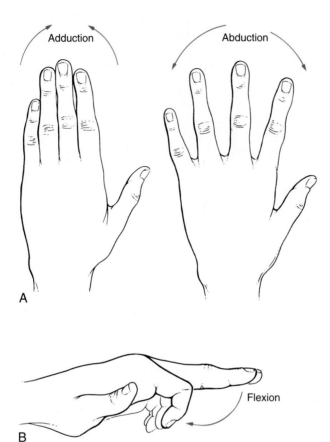

Figure 18–11

Range of motion at the finger joints. *A,* Abduction and adduction. *B,* Flexion.

Figure 18–12

Range of motion of the thumb. *A,* Flexion and extension. *B,* Opposition.

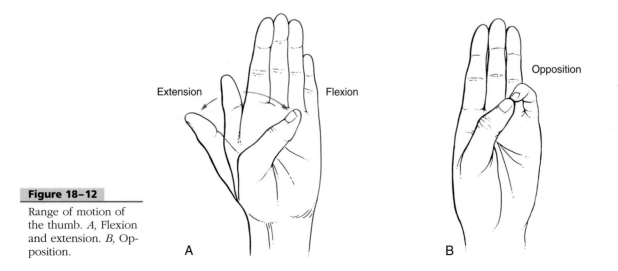

The anatomy of the *hip* is illustrated in Figure 18–13. The joint movements at the hip are flexion and extension, abduction and adduction, and internal and external rotation. These motions are illustrated in Figure 18–14.

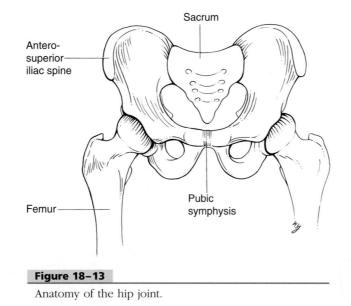

Figure 18–13

Anatomy of the hip joint.

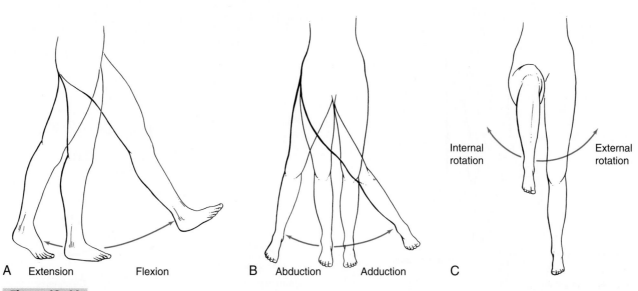

Figure 18–14

Range of motion at the hip joint. *A,* Flexion and extension. *B,* Abduction and adduction. *C,* Internal and external rotation.

The anatomy of the *knee* is shown in Figure 18–15. The joint movements at the knee are flexion and hyperextension. These motions are illustrated in Figure 18–16.

The anatomy of the *ankle* and *foot* is illustrated in Figure 18–17. The joint movements at the ankle are dorsiflexion and plantar flexion and eversion and inversion. These motions are illustrated in Figure 18–18.

The anatomy of the *cervical spine* is shown in Figure 18–19. The joint movements of the neck are flexion and extension, rotation, and lateral flexion. These motions are illustrated in Figure 18–20.

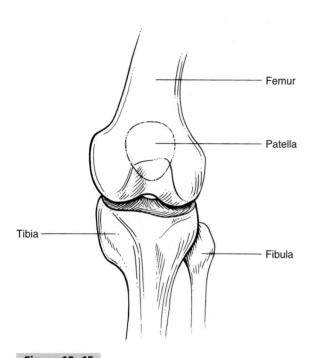

Figure 18–15

Anatomy of the knee joint.

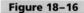

Figure 18–16

Range of motion at the knee joint: flexion and hyperextension.

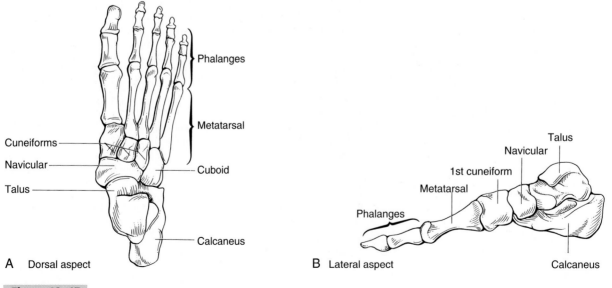

A   Dorsal aspect

B   Lateral aspect

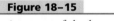

Figure 18–17

Anatomy of the ankle and foot joints. *A,* View from above. *B,* Medial view.

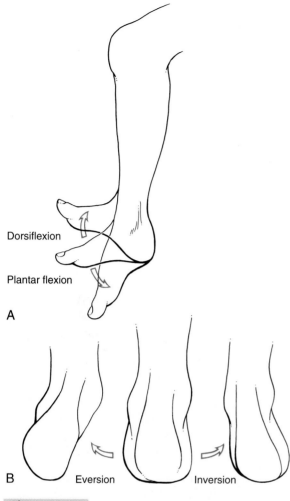

Dorsiflexion

Plantar flexion

A

B Eversion Inversion

Figure 18–18

Range of motion at the ankle and foot joints. *A,* Dorsiflexion and plantar flexion. *B,* Eversion and inversion.

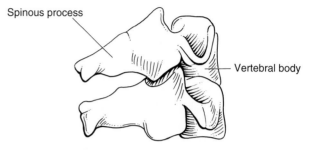

Spinous process

Vertebral body

Figure 18–19

Anatomy of the cervical spine.

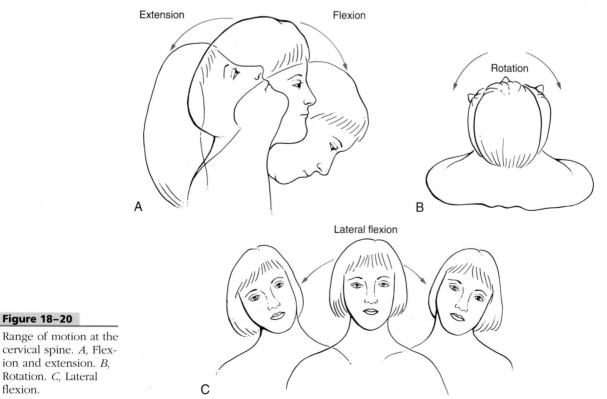

Extension

Flexion

A

Rotation

B

Lateral flexion

C

Figure 18–20

Range of motion at the cervical spine. *A,* Flexion and extension. *B,* Rotation. *C,* Lateral flexion.

The anatomy of the *lumbar spine* is illustrated in Figure 18–21. The joint movements of the lumbar spine are flexion and extension, rotation, and lateral extension. These motions are illustrated in Figure 18–22.

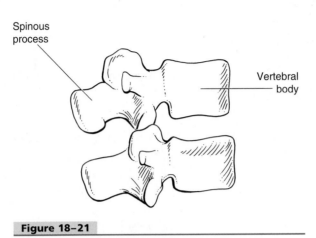

Figure 18–21

Anatomy of the lumbar spine.

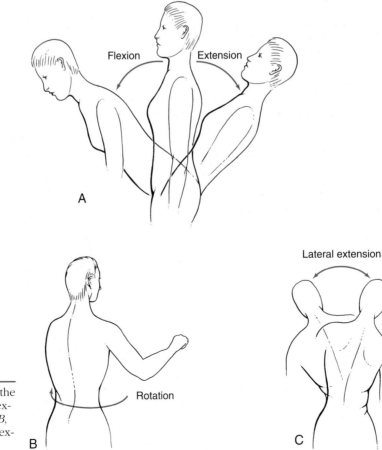

Figure 18–22

Range of motion at the lumbar spine. *A,* Flexion and extension. *B,* Rotation. *C,* Lateral extension.

Review of Specific Symptoms

The most common symptoms of musculoskeletal disease are as follows:

- Pain
- Weakness
- Deformity
- Limitation of movement
- Stiffness
- Joint clicking

The location, character, and onset of each of these symtpoms must be ascertained. It is important for the interviewer to determine the time course of any of these symptoms.

Pain

Pain can result from disorders of the bone, muscle, or joint. Ask the following questions:

"When did you first become aware of the pain?"
"Where do you feel the pain? Point to the most painful spot with one finger."
"Did the pain occur suddenly?"
"Does the pain occur daily?"
"During which part of the 24 hour day is your pain worse: morning? afternoon? evening?"
"Did a recent illness precede the pain?"
"What makes the pain worse?"
"What do you do to relieve the pain?"
"Is the pain relieved by rest?"
"What kind of medications have you taken to relieve the pain?"
"Have you noticed that the pain changes according to the weather?"
"Do you have any difficulty in putting on your shoes or coat?"
"Does the pain ever awaken you from sleep?"
"Does the pain shoot to another part of your body?"
"Have you noticed that the pain moves from one joint to another?"
"Has there been any injury, overuse, or strain?"
"Have you noticed any swelling?"
"Are other bones, muscles, or joints involved?"
"Have you had a recent sore throat?"

Bone pain may occur with or without trauma. It is typically described as "deep," "dull," "boring," or "intense." The pain may be so intense that the patient is unable to sleep. Typically, bone pain is not related to movement unless a fracture is present. Pain from a fractured bone is often described as "sharp." Muscle pain is frequently described as "crampy." It may last briefly or last longer. Muscle pain in the lower extremity on walking, described in Chapter 13, The Peripheral Vascular System, suggests ischemia of the calf or hip muscles. Muscle pain associated with weakness is suspicious for a primary muscular disorder. Joint pain is felt around or in the joint. In some conditions, the joint may be exquisitely tender. Movement usually worsens the pain, except with rheumatoid arthritis, in which movement often reduces the pain. Pain of several years' duration rules out an acute septic process and usually malignancy. Chronic infection that is due to tuberculosis or fungal infections may smoulder for years before pain is present. The severity of the pain may often be assessed by the interval between the onset of the pain and the time the patient sought medical attention.

The time of day when the pain is worse may be helpful in diagnosing the disorder. The pain of many rheumatic disorders tends to be accentuated in the morning, particularly on arising. Tendinitis worsens during the early morning hours and eases off by midday. Osteoarthritis worsens as the day progresses.

Sudden onset of pain in a metatarsophalangeal joint should raise suspicion of gout. Entrapment syndromes are apt to radiate pain distally. Severe pain may awaken any patient from sleep. Rheumatoid arthritis and tendinitis often cause early awakening because of pain, particularly when the patient is lying on the affected limb.

Acute rheumatic fever, leukemia, gonococcal arthritis, sarcoidosis, and juvenile rheumatoid arthritis are commonly associated with *migratory polyarthritis,* in which one joint is affected, the disease subsides, and then another joint becomes involved.

Viral illnesses are commonly associated with muscle aches and pains. A recent history of a sore throat, with joint pains occurring 10–14 days later, is suspicious for rheumatic fever. If rest does not relieve the pain, serious musculoskeletal disease may be present. The interviewer should keep in mind the possibility of *referred pain.* Pain from a hip disorder is frequently referred to the knee, especially in a child.

Weakness

Muscular weakness should always be differentiated from fatigue. Ascertain which functions the patient is unable to perform as a result of "weakness." Is the weakness related to proximal or distal muscle groups? *Proximal weakness* is usually a myopathy; *distal weakness* is usually a neuropathy. The patient with the symptom of muscular weakness should be asked these questions:

"Do you have difficulty in combing your hair?"
"Do you have difficulty in lifting objects?"
"Have you noticed any problem with holding a pen or pencil?"
"Do you have difficulty in turning doorknobs?"
"Do you have trouble standing up after sitting in a chair?"
"Do you find that, as the day goes on, there is a change in the weakness?" If so,
    "Does the weakness worsen or improve?"
"Have you noticed any decrease in your muscle size?"
"Are the weak muscles stiff?"
"Do you have trouble with double vision? swallowing? chewing?"

The patient with proximal weakness of the lower extremity has difficulty in walking and in crossing the knees. A proximal weakness of the upper extremity is manifested by difficulty in brushing hair or lifting objects. Patients with polymyalgia rheumatica have proximal muscle weakness. This condition is discussed in Chapter 23, The Geriatric Patient. A distal weakness of the upper extremity is manifested by difficulty in turning doorknobs or buttoning a shirt or blouse. Patients with myasthenia gravis have generalized weakness and have difficulty due to diplopia and in swallowing and chewing.

Deformity

Deformity may be the result of a congenital malformation or an acquired condition. In any patient with a deformity, it is important to determine the following:

"When was the deformity first noticed?"
"Did the deformity occur suddenly?"
"Did the deformity occur as a result of trauma?"
"Has there been any change in the deformity with time?"

Limitation of Motion

Limitation of motion may result from changes in the articular cartilage, scarring of the joint capsule, or muscle contractures. Determine the types of motion that the patient can no longer perform easily, such as combing the hair, putting on shoes, or buttoning a shirt or blouse.

Stiffness

Stiffness is a common symptom of musculoskeletal disease. For example, a patient with arthritis of the hip may have difficulty in crossing the legs to tie shoes. Ask the patient whether the stiffness is worse at any particular time of the day. Patients with rheumatoid arthritis tend to experience stiffness after periods of joint rest. These patients typically describe morning stiffness, which may take several hours to improve.

Joint Clicking

Joint clicking is commonly associated with specific movements in the presence of dislocations of the humerus, displacement of the biceps tendon from its groove, degenerative joint disease, damaged knee meniscus, and temporomandibular joint problems.

Impact of Musculoskeletal Disease on the Patient

Musculoskeletal diseases have an enormous impact on the life of patients and their families. The perturbation of a patient's personal life and restriction of activities as a result of disability are frequently more catastrophic than the muscle or joint pain itself.

Diseases of the musculoskeletal system range from minor aches and pains to severe crippling disorders, often associated with premature death. Rheumatoid arthritis is a crippling disorder striking many patients in the prime of life. In addition to having the joint pain and reduction of activity, patients with rheumatoid arthritis fear the possibility of being crippled for the rest of their lives. Greater dependence on others occurs as the disease progresses. The disability alters patients' self-image and self-esteem. The altered body image may be devastating; patients often become withdrawn.

The physical limitations of musculoskeletal disease, especially when accompanied by joint or muscle pain, threaten the integrity of patients in their social world. Marital and familial ties may suffer as patients become further debilitated and withdrawn. Because of the disability, patients may have to change occupations, which causes further anxiety and depression. The loss of status and financial adjustments may further jeopardize the marital situation. The fear of loss of independence is extremely common. Patients are forced to make more demands but recognize that this may only worsen their relationships with others.

Rehabilitation is important for the physical and psychological improvement of the patient. The patient is the key contributor to this rehabilitative process. Motivation may be provided first by those caring for the patient, but it is the patient's own attitude that determines whether the rehabilitation process will be successful. The motivation of the patient to tackle the disability depends on many factors, which include self-image as well as psychological, social, and financial resources. It is incumbent on the clinician to gain the patient's confidence to help overcome the disability.

Physical Examination

No special equipment is necessary for the examination of the musculoskeletal system.

The purpose of the internist's musculoskeletal examination is as a screening examination to indicate or exclude functional impairment of the musculoskeletal system. The examination should take only a few minutes and should be part of the routine examination of all patients. If an abnormality is noted or if the patient has specific symptoms referable to a particular joint, a more detailed examination of that area is indicated. The detailed description of the examination of specific joints follows the discussion of the screening examination.

The Screening Examination

The screening examination should pay specific attention to the following:

- Inspection
- Palpation
- Passive and active range of motion
- Muscle strength
- Integrated function

General Principles

During inspection, asymmetry should be assessed. Nodules, wasting, masses, or deformities may be responsible for the absence of symmetry. Are there any signs of inflammation? *Swelling, warmth, redness,* and *tenderness* suggest inflammation. To determine a difference in temperature, use the back of your hand to compare one side with the other.

Palpation may reveal areas of tenderness or discontinuity of a bone. Is *crepitus* present? Crepitus is a palpable crunching sensation often felt in the presence of roughened articular cartilages.

The *assessment of range of motion* of specific joints is next. Keep in mind that inflamed or arthritic joints may be painful. Move these joints *slowly.*

Muscle function and *integrated function* are usually evaluated during the neurologic examination, and these topics are discussed in Chapter 19, The Nervous System.

Evaluate Gait

The first part of the screening examination consists of inspection of gait and posture. To determine any eccentricity of gait, ask the patient to disrobe down to underwear and walk barefoot. Have the patient walk away from you, then back to you on tiptoes, away from you on the heels, and finally back to you in tandem gait. If there is difficulty in gait, modification of these maneuvers must be performed.

Observe the rate, rhythm, and arm motion employed in walking. Does the patient have a staggering gait? Are the feet lifted high and slapped downward firmly? Does the patient walk with an extended leg that is swung laterally during walking? Are the steps short and shuffling? A complete discussion of gait abnormalities is in Chapter 19. Figure 19–59 illustrates the more common types of gait abnormalities.

Evaluate the Spine

Attention should then be forcused on the spine to detect any abnormal spinal curvatures. Have the patient stand erect, and stand at the patient's side to inspect the profile of the patient's spine. Are the cervical, thoracic, and lumbar curves normal?

Move to inspect the patient's back. What is the level of the iliac crests? A difference may result from a leg length inequality, scoliosis, or flexion deformity of the hip. An imaginary line drawn from the posterior occipital tuberosity should fall over the intergluteal cleft. Any lateral curvature is abnormal. Figure 18–23 illustrates this point.

Ask the patient to bend forward, flexing at the trunk as far as possible with the knees extended. Note the smoothness of this action. This position is best for determining whether a scoliosis is present. As the patient bends forward, the lumbar concavity should flatten. A persistence of the concavity may indicate an arthritic condition of the spine called ankylosing spondylitis.

Ask the patient to bend to each side from the waist and then bend backward from the waist to test *extension of the spine,* as shown in Figure 18–24A.

To test *rotation of the lumbar spine,* sit on a stool behind the patient and stabilize the patient's hips by placing your hands on them. Ask the patient to rotate the shoulders one way and then reverse, as shown in Figure 18–24B.

Evaluate Strength of the Lower Extremities

To assess the function of all major joints of the lower extremities, stand in front of the patient. Have the patient squat, with knees and hips fully flexed. Assist the patient by holding the hand to secure balance. This is shown in Figure 18–25. Ask the patient to stand. Observing the manner in which the patient squats and then stands provides an excellent impression of the muscle strength and joint action of the lower extremities.

In addition, assessment of specific muscle groups can be performed and can be integrated into the arthrometric examination. Muscle strength can be graded according to the scale described in Chapter 19.

Measure the dorsiflexors and plantarflexors. With the patient seated, have the patient dorsiflex and plantarflex the foot against resistance. This can also be accomplished by asking the patient to walk toward and away from the examiner on the heels and then on the toes. Injury to the common peroneal nerve will cause weakness of the anterior muscle group with a diminished capacity to dorsiflex the foot. Injury to the Achilles tendon or to the gastrosoleus complex will impair plantarflexion.

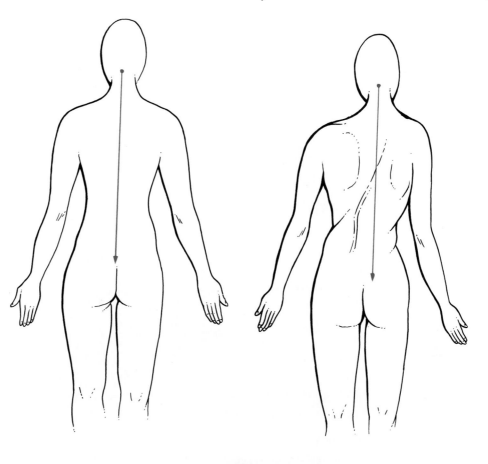

Figure 18–23

Technique of evaluating patient for "straightness" of the spine. The lateral deviation of the spine may be related to a herniated disc or to spasm of the paravertebral muscles. This functional deviation is often termed a *list*. True scoliosis may be due to an actual deformity of the spine. In many cases, the spine may twist in the opposite direction, so that a plumb line may actually be in the center.

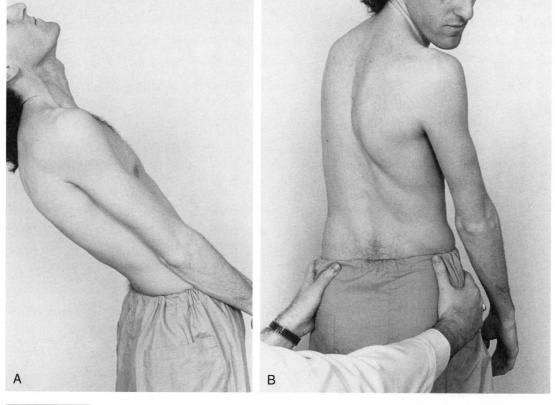

Figure 18–24

Technique for evaluating motion of the lumbar spine. *A,* Test for extension of the spine. *B,* Test for rotation of the spine.

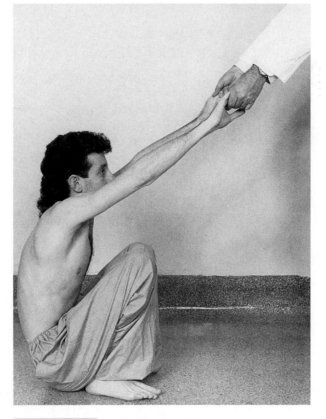

Figure 18–25

Technique for evaluating strength of the lower extremities.

Measure invertors and evertors. With the patient seated, have the patient invert and then evert the foot against resistance.

Measure the quadraceps and hamstrings. With the patient seated, have the patient extend and then flex the knee against resistance.

Measure the hip flexors and extensors. With the patient seated, have the patient raise the knee off the examination table against the examiner's downward opposing force. Hip extensors can be assessed by asking the patient to rise from a seated position unassisted. Human immunodeficiency virus–related myopathy affects proximal muscle groups first, and patients may initially complain of difficulty rising from a chair or ascending stairs.

Evaluate Neck Flexion

The patient is instructed to sit, and the range of motion of the neck is assessed. The patient is asked to put chin on chest, with the mouth closed, as shown in Figure 18–26. This tests full flexion of the neck.

Evaluate Neck Extension

To test full extension of the neck, place your hand between the occiput and the spinous process of C7. Instruct the patient to trap your hand by extending the neck. This is shown in Figure 18–27.

Evaluate Neck Rotation

Rotation of the neck is determined by asking the patient to rotate the neck to one side and touching chin to shoulder. This is shown in Figure 18–28. The examination is then repeated on the other side.

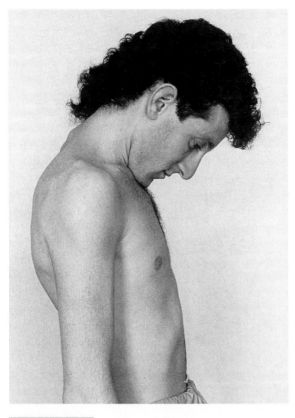

Figure 18–26

Technique for testing flexion of the neck.

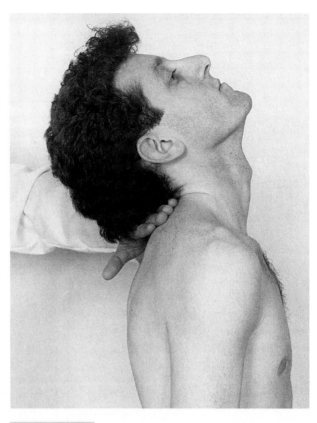

Figure 18–27

Technique for testing extension of the neck.

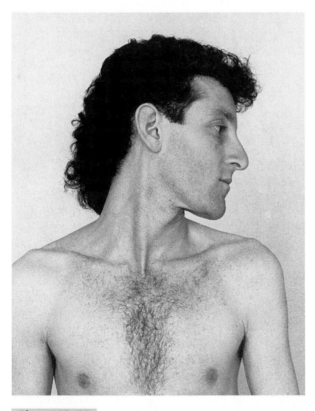

Figure 18–28

Technique for testing rotation of the neck.

▨ Evaluate Intrinsic Muscles of the Hand

The patient is instructed to stretch out the arms, with the fingers spread. The examiner attempts to compress the fingers together against resistance, as shown in Figure 18–29. This tests the intrinsic muscles of the hands.

▨ Evaluate External Rotation of the Arm

To test the functional range of rotation of the humerus as well as the *shoulder, acromioclavicular,* and *sternoclavicular joints,* instruct the patient to abduct the arms fully and place palms together above the head. The arms should touch the patient's ears with the head and cervical spine in the vertical position. This is shown in Figure 18–30.

▨ Evaluate Internal Rotation of the Arm

The patient is then asked to place hands on back between the scapulae. The hands should normally reach the level of the inferior angle of the scapulae. This is shown in Figure 18–31. This maneuver tests internal rotation of the humerus and the range of motion at the elbow.

▨ Evaluate Strength of the Upper Extremities

The final test of the screening examination assesses the power of the major groups of muscles in the upper extremity. The patient is asked to grasp the index and middle fingers of the examiner in each hand. The patient is instructed to resist upward, downward, lateral, and medial movement by the examiner. This position is shown in Figure 18–32.

This completes the basic musculoskeletal screening examination. The remainder of this chapter describes the symptoms and examination of specific joints.

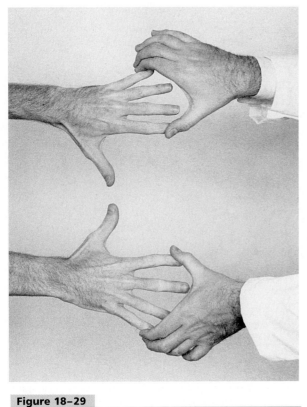

Figure 18–29

Technique for testing the intrinsic muscles of the hand.

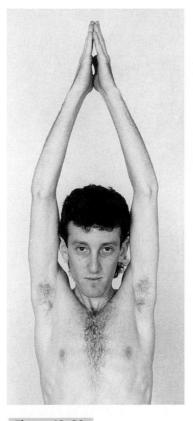

Figure 18–30

Technique for testing external rotation of the arm.

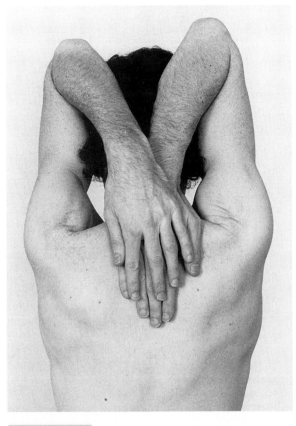

Figure 18–31

Technique for testing internal rotation of the arm.

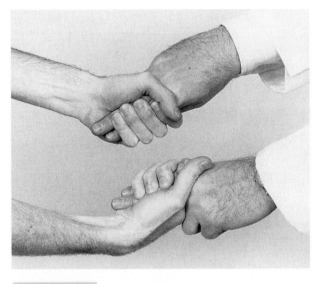

Figure 18–32

Technique for assessing strength in the upper extremities.

Examinations of Specific Joints

Any area must be inspected for evidence of swelling, atrophy, redness, and deformity, as well as palpated for swelling, muscle spasm, and local painful areas. The range of motion is assessed both actively and passively.

■ Temporomandibular Joint

Symptoms

The patient with temporomandibular joint problems may complain of unilateral or bilateral jaw pain. The pain is worse in the morning and after chewing or eating. The patient may also complain of "clicking" of the jaw.

Examination

To examine this joint, the examiner should place his or her index fingers in front of the tragus and instruct the patient to open and close the jaw slowly. The examiner should observe the smoothness of the range of motion and note any tenderness. This is illustrated in Figure 18–33.

■ The Shoulder

Symptoms

Although shoulder pain may be related to a primary shoulder disorder, *always* consider the possibility that shoulder pain is referred from either the chest or the abdomen. Coronary artery disease, pulmonary tumors, and gallbladder disease are commonly associated with referred pain to the shoulder.

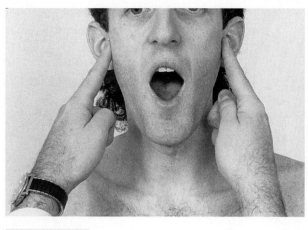

Figure 18–33

Technique for evaluating the temporomandibular joint.

Pain is the main symptom of shoulder disorders. Inflammation of the *supraspinatus muscle* causes pain that is usually worse at night or when the patient lies on the affected shoulder. The pain often radiates down the arm as far as the elbow. The pain is commonly referred to the lower part of the deltoid area and is characteristically aggravated by combing the hair, putting on a coat, or reaching into the back pocket. Diffuse tenderness of the shoulder associated with pain on moving the humerus posteriorly is associated with disorders of teres minor, infraspinatus, and subscapularis muscles. In this case, the pain usually does not radiate into the arm and is generally absent when the arm is dependent.

The movements of the shoulder occur at the *glenohumeral, thoracoscapular, acromioclavicular,* and *sternoclavicular joints.* The glenohumeral joint is a ball-and-socket joint. In contrast to the hip joint, which is also a ball-and-socket joint, in the glenohumeral joints the humerus sits into the very shallow glenoid socket. Therefore, the function of the joint depends on the muscles surrounding the socket for stability. These muscles and their tendons form the *rotator cuff* of the shoulder. For this reason, many shoulder problems are muscular, not bone- or joint-related, in origin.

Examination

Inspect the shoulder for deformity, wasting, and asymmetry. The shoulder should be palpated for local areas of tenderness. The range of motion for abduction, adduction, external and internal rotation, and flexion is evaluated and compared with that of the other side. Any pain is noted.

Special tests are required to determine specific diagnoses. The impingement syndrome, tears of the rotator cuff, and bicipital tendinitis are common. The examinations for these conditions are described in this section.

The *impingement syndrome,* also known as *rotator cuff tendinitis,* is usually secondary to sports trauma. Irritation of the avascular portion of the supraspinatus tendon progresses to an inflammatory response termed *tendinitis.* This inflammatory response later involves the biceps tendon, subacromial bursa, and acromioclavicular joint. With continued trauma, rotator cuff tears and calcification may occur. The most reliable test for the impingement syndrome is the reproduction of pain induced by the examiner forcibly flexing the patient's arm with the elbow extended against resistance.

Sudden onset of shoulder pain in the deltoid area within 6–10 hours after trauma suggests a *rotator cuff tear* or *rupture.* Extreme tenderness over the greater tuberosity of the humerus and pain and restricted motion at the glenohumeral joint are usually present. Active abduction of the glenohumeral joint is markedly reduced. When the examiner attempts to abduct the arm, pain and a characteristic *shoulder shrug* result.

Generalized tenderness anteriorly over the long head of the biceps associated with pain, especially at night, should raise suspicion of *bicipital tendinitis.* In this condition, there is normal abduction and forward flexion. The hallmark of bicipital tendinitis is the reproduction of anterior shoulder pain during resistance to forearm supination. The patient is asked to place the arm at the side with the elbow flexed 90°. The patient is instructed to supinate the arm against the resistance by the examiner. If there is pain in the triceps area with resisted extension of the elbow, *tricipital tendinitis* may be present.

The Elbow

The most common symptom of elbow disorders is well-localized elbow pain.

Symptoms

Although it is a simple hinge joint, the elbow is the most complicated joint of the upper extremity. The distal end of the humerus articulates with the proximal ulna and radius. Flexion and extension of the elbow are effected through the humeroulnar portion of the joint. The radius plays little role in this action: its role is primarily in pronation and supination of the forearm. The ulnar nerve lies in a vulnerable position as it passes around the medial epicondyle of the humerus.

Examination

Palpate the elbow for swelling, masses, tenderness, and nodules.

Test flexion and extension.

To test for pronation and supination, the elbows should be flexed at 90° and placed firmly on a table. The patient is asked to rotate the forearm and wrist down (pronation), as shown in Figure 18–34*A*, and up (supination), as shown in Figure 18–34*B*. Any limitation of motion or pain is noted.

Tennis elbow, also known as *lateral epicondylitis,* is a common condition characterized by pain in the region of the lateral epicondyle of the humerus. The pain radiates down the extensor surface of the forearm. Patients with tennis elbow often experience pain when attempting to open a door or when lifting a glass. To test for tennis elbow, the examiner should flex the elbow and fully pronate the hand. Pain over the lateral epicondyle while extending the elbow is diagnostic of tennis elbow. Another test involves having the patient clench the fist, dorsiflex the wrist, and extend the elbow. Pain will be elicited by trying to force the dorsiflexed hand into palmar flexion.

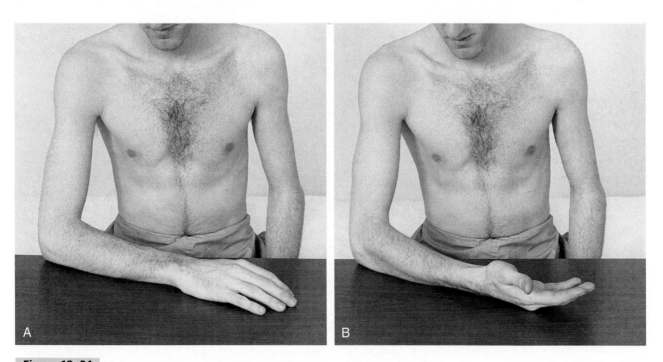

Figure 18–34

Technique for evaluating pronation and supination at the elbow. *A,* Pronation. *B,* Supination.

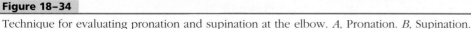

The Wrist

Symptoms

The symptoms of wrist disorders include pain in the wrist or hand, numbness or tingling in the wrist or fingers, loss of movement and stiffness, and deformities. It should be remembered that pain in the hand may be referred from the neck or elbow.

The wrist is composed of the articulation of the distal end of the radius with the proximal row of the carpal bones. The stability of the wrist is due to the banding of these bones together by strong ligaments. The distal ulna does not articulate with any of the carpal bones. On the volar aspect of the wrist, the carpal bones are connected by the carpal ligament. The passage under this ligament is the *carpal tunnel,* through which the median nerve and all the flexors of the wrist pass. Entrapment of the nerve, known as the *carpal tunnel syndrome,* produces symptoms of numbness and tingling.

Examination

Palpate the patient's wrist joint between your thumb and index fingers, noting tenderness, swelling, or redness (Figure 18–35).

The range of motion of dorsiflexion and palmar flexion is noted. With the forearms fixed, the degree of supination and pronation is evaluated. Is ulnar or radial deviation present?

When the diagnosis of carpal tunnel syndrome is suspected, a sharp tap or pressure directly over the median nerve may reproduce the paresthesias of the carpal tunnel syndrome, called *Tinel's sign.* Another useful test is for the examiner to stretch the median nerve by extending the patient's elbow and dorsiflexing the wrist. The development of pain or paresthesias suggests the diagnosis. A third test entails the patient's holding both wrists in a fully palmar-fixed position for 2 minutes. The development or exacerbation of paresthesias is suggestive of the carpal tunnel syndrome.

The Hand

Symptoms

Pain and swelling of joints are the most important symptoms of disorders of the hand.

Examination

Palpate the patient's metacarpophalangeal joints and note swelling, redness, or tenderness, as shown in Figure 18–36. Palpate the medial and lateral aspects of the proximal and distal interphalangeal joints between your thumb and index fingers, as shown in Figure 18–37. Again, note swelling, redness, or tenderness.

The range of motion of the fingers includes the movements at the distal interphalangeal joint, the proximal interphalangeal joint, and the metacarpophalangeal joints of the fingers and the thumb.

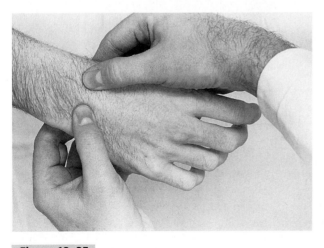

Figure 18–35

Technique for palpation of the wrist joint.

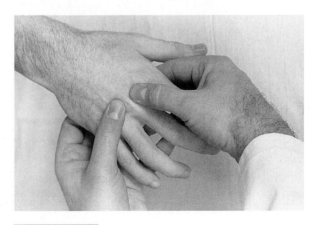

Figure 18–36

Technique for palpation of the metacarpophalangeal joints.

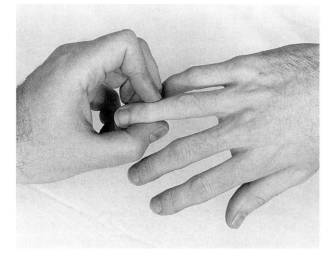

Figure 18–37

Technique for palpation of the interphalangeal joints.

Ask the patient to make a fist with the thumb across the knuckles and then extend and spread the fingers. The normal fingers should flex to the distal palmar crease. The thumb should oppose to the distal metacarpal head. Each finger should extend to the zero position in relation to its metacarpal.

Tenosynovitis of the thumb abductors and extensors is known as *de Quervain's disease*. The patient complains of weakness of grip and of pain at the base of the thumb that is aggravated by certain movements of the wrist. To confirm the diagnosis, ask the patient to flex the thumb and close the fingers over it. You should now attempt to move the hand into ulnar deviation. Excruciating pain will accompany this maneuver if de Quervain's tenosynovitis is present.

■ The Spine

Symptoms

The most common symptom of disorders of the spine is pain. Pain from the thoracic spine often radiates around the trunk along the lines of the intercostal nerves. Pain from the upper lumbar spine may be felt in the front of the thighs and knees. Pain originating in the lower lumbar spine can be felt in the coccyx, hips, and buttocks as well as shooting down the back of the legs to the heels and feet. The pain is often intensified by movement. Patients with a herniated vertebral disc may complain of pain that is exacerbated by sneezing or coughing. Determine whether there is associated numbness or tingling in the lower extremity, which is related to nerve root lesions.

Examination

The cervical spine may be examined with the patient seated. You should inspect the cervical spine from the front, back, and sides for deformity and unusual posture. Test range of motion of the cervical spine. Palpate the paravertebral muscles for tenderness and spasm.

The thoracolumbar spine is examined with the patient standing in front of you. Inspect the spine for deformity or swelling. Inspect the spine from the side for abnormal curvature. Test range of motions. Palpate the paravertebral muscles for tenderness. Percuss each spinous process for tenderness.

The range of motions tested for the spine is composed of forward flexion, extension, lateral flexion, and rotation.

The presence of a *cervical rib* may cause coldness, discoloration, and trophic changes as a result of ischemia to an upper extremity. To test for a cervical rib, palpate the radial pulse. Move the arm through its range of motions. Obliteration of the pulse by this maneuver is suggestive of a cervical rib. Ask the patient to turn the head toward the affected side and take a deep breath while you are palpating the radial pulse on the same side. Obliteration of the pulse by this maneuver is also suggestive of a cervical rib. Often, auscultation over the subclavian artery will reveal a bruit suggestive of mechanical obstruction by a cervical rib. Repeat any of these tests on the opposite side. Cervical ribs are rarely bilateral.

Pain from entrapment of the sciatic nerve is called *sciatica*. Patients with sciatica describe pain, burning, or aching in the buttocks radiating down the posterior thigh to the posterolateral aspect of the calf. Pain is worsened by sneezing, laughing, or straining at stool. One of the tests for sciatica is the straight leg raising test. The patient is asked to lie supine while the examiner flexes the extended leg to the trunk at the hip. The presence of pain is a positive test. The patient is asked to plantarflex and dorsiflex the foot. This stretches the sciatic nerve even more. If sciatica is present, this test will reproduce pain in the leg. The test is illustrated in Figure 18–38.

Another test for sciatica is the sitting knee extension test. The patient sits off the side of the bed and flexes the neck, placing chin on chest. The examiner fixes the thigh on the bed with one hand while the other hand extends the leg. If sciatica is present pain will be reproduced as the leg is extended. This test is demonstrated in Figure 18–39.

The Hip

Symptoms

The main symptoms of hip disease are pain, stiffness, deformity, and a limp. Hip pain may be localized to the groin or may radiate down the medial aspect of the thigh. Stiffness may be related to periods of immobility. An early symptom of hip disease is difficulty in putting on a shoe. This requires external rotation of the hip, which is the first motion to be lost with degenerative disease of the hip. This is followed by loss of abduction and adduction; finally, hip flexion is the last movement to be lost.

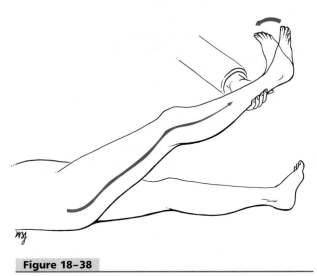

Figure 18–38

The straight leg raising test.

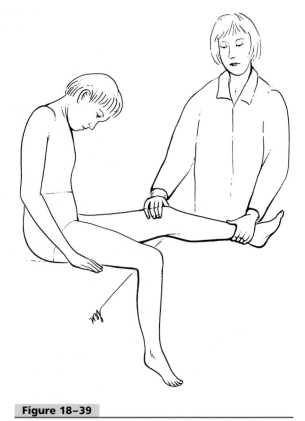

Figure 18–39

The sitting knee extension test.

Examination

The examination of the hip is performed with the patient standing and lying on the back.

Inspection of the hips and gait have already been described. The *Trendelenburg test* indicates a disorder between the pelvis and the femur. The patient is asked to stand on the "good" leg, as illustrated in Figure 18–40*A*. The examiner should note that the pelvis on the opposite side elevates, demonstrating that the gluteal medius is working efficiently. When the patient is asked to stand on the "bad" leg, as shown in Figure 18–40*B*, the pelvis on the opposite side will fall. This is termed a positive Trendelenburg test.

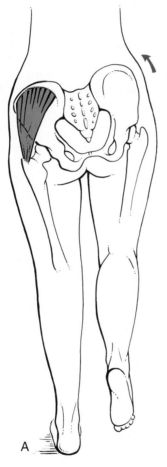
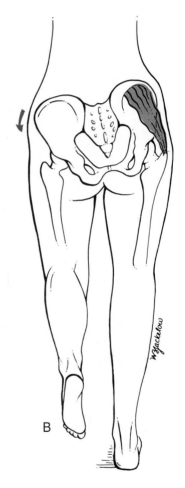

Figure 18–40

The Trendelenburg test. *A,* Position of the hips when standing on the normal left leg. Note hip elevates as a result of contraction of the left hip musculature. *B,* Position of the hips when standing on the abnormal right leg. Note that the left hip falls as a result of lack of adequate contraction of the right hip muscles.

Ask the patient to lie on the back. The hip is acutely flexed on the abdomen to flatten the lumbar spine. A flexion of the opposite thigh suggests a flexion deformity of that hip. Figure 18–41 illustrates the technique.

Leg length measurements are useful in evaluating hip disorders. The distance between the anterosuperior iliac spine to the tip of the medial malleolus is measured on each side and compared. A difference in leg length may be caused by hip joint disorders.

As indicated, loss of rotation of the hip is an early finding in hip disease. To test this movement, ask the patient to lie on the back. You should flex the hip and knee to 90° and rotate the ankle inward for external rotation, as illustrated in Figure 18–42A, and outward for internal rotation, as shown in Figure 18–42B. Restriction of this motion is a sensitive sign of degenerative hip disease.

■ The Knee

Symptoms

Although the knee is the largest joint in the body, it is not the strongest. The knee is a hinge joint between the femur and the tibia and permits flexion and extension. When flexed, a small degree of lateral motion is also normal. As with the shoulder, the knee depends on the strong muscles and ligaments around the joint for its stability.

Pain, swelling, joint instability, and limited movement are the main symptoms of knee disorders. Knee pain is exacerbated by movement and may be referred to the calf or thigh. Swelling of the knee indicates a synovial effusion or bleeding into the joint, also known as *hemarthrosis*. Knee trauma may result in hemarthrosis and limitation of joint motion. *Locking* of the knee results from small pieces of broken cartilage lodged between the femur and the tibia, blocking full extension of the joint.

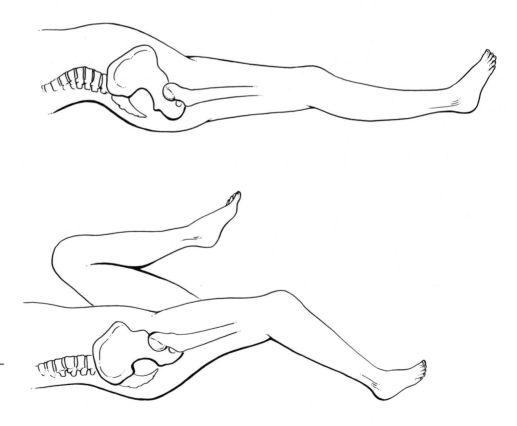

Figure 18–41

Evaluation for a flexion deformity of the hip.

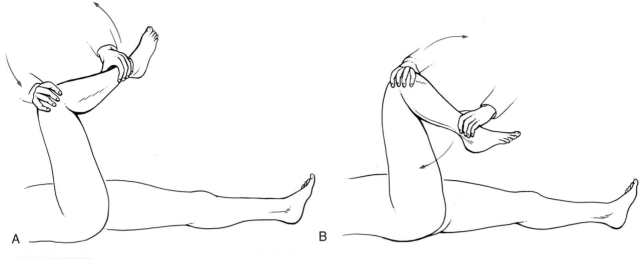

Testing the range of motion at the hip. The examiner flexes the patient's hip and knee to 90° and rotates the ankle inward for external rotation *(A)* and outward for internal rotation *(B)*.

Examination

The examination of the knee is performed with the patient standing and lying on the back.

While the patient is standing, any varus or valgus deformity should be noted. Is there wasting of the quadriceps muscle? Is there swelling of the knee? An early sign of knee joint swelling is the loss of the slight depressions on the lateral sides of the patella. You should inspect for swelling in the popliteal fossa. A *Baker cyst* in the popliteal fossa may be responsible for a swelling in the popliteal fossa, causing calf pain.

The patient is then asked to lie on the back. The contours of the knee are evaluated. The patella is palpated in extension for tenderness. By stressing the patella against the femoral condyles, pain may be elicited. This occurs in osteoarthritis.

Testing for *knee joint effusion* is performed by pressing the fluid out of the suprapatellar pouch down behind the patella. Start about 15 cm above the superior margin of the patella and slide your index finger and thumb firmly downward along the sides of the femur, milking the fluid into the space between the patella and the femur. While you maintain pressure on the lateral margins of the patella, tap on the patella with the other hand. This technique is termed *ballottement*. In the presence of an effusion, a palpable tap will be felt, and the transmitted impulse will be felt by the fingers on either side of the patella. This technique is shown in Figure 18–43.

To palpate the *collateral ligaments,* the patient's foot should be resting on the bed, with the knee flexed at 90°. Grasp the patient's leg and, using your thumbs, try to elicit tenderness over the patellar tendon beneath the femoral epicondyles. A *medial collateral ligament* rupture is illustrated in Figure 18–44.

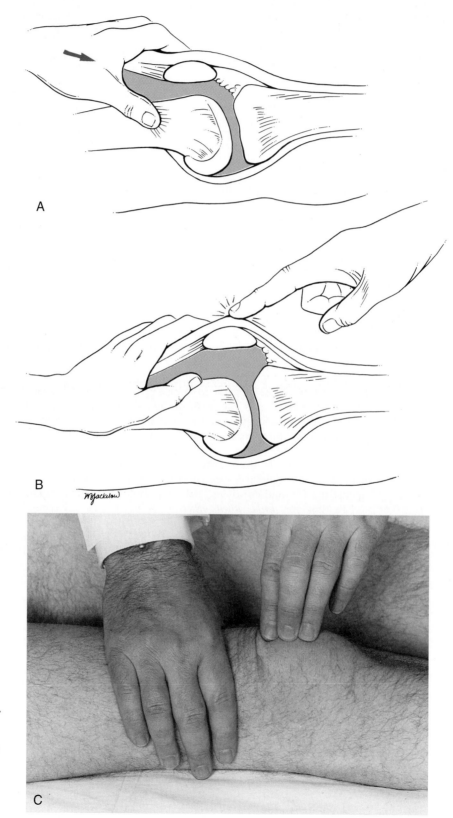

Figure 18–43

Technique for testing for a knee joint effusion. *A,* Position of the hand for pushing fluid out of the bursae. *B,* and *C,* Position for tapping the patella.

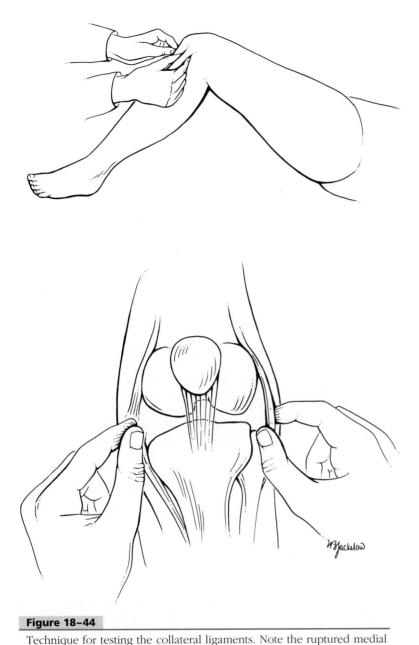

Figure 18–44

Technique for testing the collateral ligaments. Note the ruptured medial collateral ligament in the lower illustration.

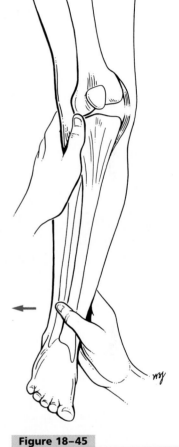

Figure 18–45

Another technique for testing the collateral ligaments.

Another test for collateral ligament rupture is performed by placing the left hand on the lateral aspect of the patient's knee at the level of the joint. The knee is flexed about 25°, and the lower leg is pushed outward by the examiner's right hand, using the left hand as a fulcrum. This maneuver attempts to "open up" the medial side of the knee joint. The finding should be compared with that of the other side. Abnormal lateral motion is seen in rupture of the medial collateral ligament, as illustrated in Figure 18–45. The maneuver may be used to test for rupture of the lateral collateral ligament by reversing the positions.

The drawer test is used to test for rupture of the *cruciate ligaments*. The patient is instructed to flex the knee to 90°. The examiner should sit close to the foot to steady it. The examiner then grasps the leg just below the knee with both hands and jerks the tibia forward, as illustrated in Figure 18–46. Abnormal forward mobility of 2 cm or more suggests rupture of the anterior cruciate ligament. This maneuver may be used to test the posterior cruciate ligament by flexing the knee to 90°, steadying the foot, and attempting to jerk the leg backward. Abnormal backward motion of 2 cm or more indicates rupture of the posterior cruciate ligament.

The Ankle and Foot

Symptoms

The ankle is a hinge joint between the lower end of the tibia and the talus.

Although symptoms in the ankle and foot usually have a local cause, they can also be secondary to systemic disorders. Symptoms may include pain, swelling, and deformities.

The patient's only complaint may be shoe wear. In normal sole wear, the sole is fairly evenly worn. The lateral sides may show maximal wear. Patients with flat feet wear down their soles on the medial side extending to the tip of the shoe. The outer portion of the heel is also worn out early. Scuff marks are usually present on the medial sides of the shoes. Patients with unusually high arches have excessive wear under the metatarsal head area. There is also excessive wear on the backs of the heels.

Examination

The examination of the ankle and foot is performed with the patient standing and then sitting.

Ask the patient to stand. Inspect the ankles and feet for swellings and deformities. Compare one foot with the other with regard to symmetry. Describe abnormalities of the longitudinal arch. A *cavus foot* has an abnormally high arch. In *flat foot,* the longitudinal arch is flatter than normal. Common foot abnormalities are illustrated in Figure 18–47.

Ask the patient to sit with the feet dangling off the side of the bed. Palpate the medial and lateral malleoli. Palpate the Achilles tendon. Are any nodules present? Is tenderness present?

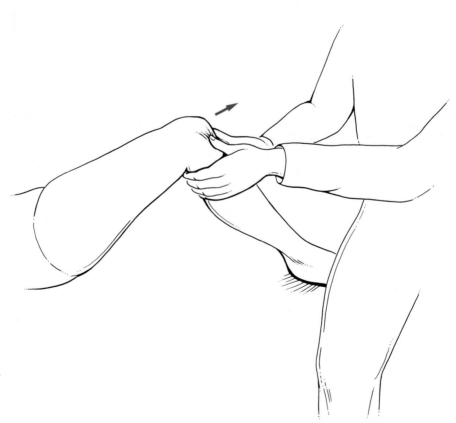

Figure 18–46

Technique for testing the cruciate ligaments: the drawer test.

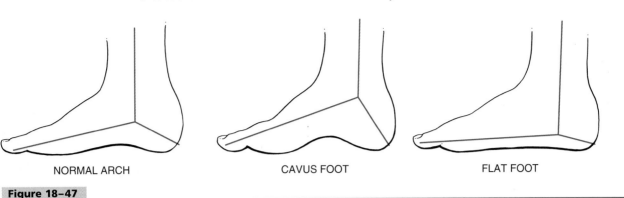

NORMAL ARCH   CAVUS FOOT   FLAT FOOT

Figure 18–47

Common foot abnormalities.

Test the range of motion at the ankle, which includes dorsiflexion and plantar flexion. The range of motion necessary for normal gait is 10° dorsiflexion and 20° plantar flexion. Ankle joint dorsiflexion with the knee flexed should approach 15°.

If dorsiflexion at the ankle joint is less than 10°, measurement should again be taken with the knee flexed. If dorsiflexion is less than 10° in both positions, limitation of motion is usually due to an osseous block at the ankle. If dorsiflexion increases with knee flexion, a tight gastrosoleus complex is probably responsible.

Test the range of motion at the subtalar joint, which includes eversion and inversion. With the patient lying prone on the examination table, hold the patient's leg in one hand, and move the heel with the other hand into inversion and eversion. Measure the excursion of the heel with respect to the bisection of the lower one third of the leg. This technique is shown in Figure 18–48. The average range of motion of the subtalar joint is 20° of inversion and 10° of eversion.

Test the range of motion at the midtarsal joint, which includes eversion and inversion. With the patient in the prone position, stabilize the heel with one hand, and

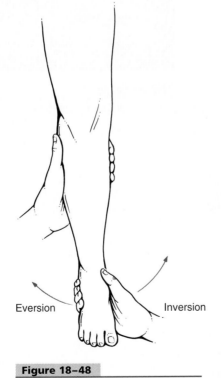

Eversion   Inversion

Figure 18–48

Evaluating the range of motion at the subtalar joint.

rotate the forefoot into inversion and eversion. Measure excursion of the plane of the metatarsal heads with respect to the bisection of the heel. This is shown in Figure 18–49.

The movements of the metatarsophalangeal joints are tested individually. Palpate the head of each metatarsal and the base of each proximal phalanx as well as the groove between them. Is tenderness or joint effusion present?

Describe abnormalities of the joints, including hallux abductovalgus (*bunion*) deformities and flexion contractions of the lower digits (*hammer toes*). Figure 18–50 shows a patient with hallux abductovalgus deformity, flexion contractures of the interphalangeal joints, and bowstringing of the extensor tendons. This is a typical presentation in the geriatric age group. Note the hyperkeratotic lesion over the right bunion from shoe pressure.

Measure the range of motion of the first metatarsophalangeal joint. Dorsiflexion of the hallux is measured against the bisection of the first metatarsal. The normal dorsal range of motion is 65–75°. Limitation of motion of this joint is termed *hallux limitus* and is most commonly due to osteoarthritis.

Bunion deformities can be a source of undue pressure in the diabetic patient, leading to ulceration and infection. A diabetic patient with a large pressure ulceration over the medial eminence of the first metatarsophalangeal joint from shoe irritation is shown in Figure 18–51.

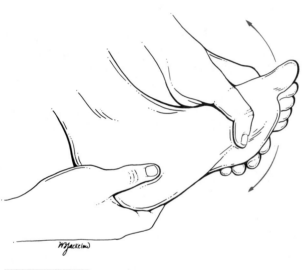

Figure 18–49

Evaluating the range of motion at the midtarsal joint.

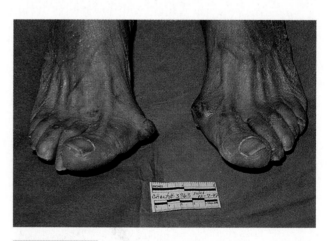

Figure 18–50

Bunion deformity and hammer toes.

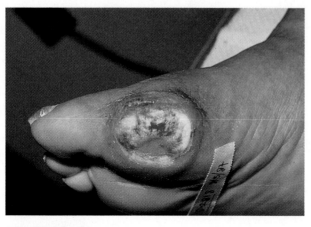

Figure 18–51

Hallux abductovalgus deformity and ulceration.

Figure 18–52 shows a patient with chronic tophaceous gout with ulceration over the distal interphalangeal joint of the fourth toe. Note the bunion deformity and underlapping hallux. An acute attack of gout commonly presents with severe pain, swelling, and inflammation in the first metatarsophalangeal joint, a condition termed *podagra*. A patient with acute gout and podagra is shown in Figure 18–53. Notice the erythema of the left hallux and the generalized swelling of the left foot.

Examine the lesser metatarsophalangeal joints. Grasp the metatarsophalangeal joints between your thumb and index fingers and attempt to compress the forefoot. Pain elicited by this maneuver is often an early sign of *rheumatoid arthritis*. This test is shown in Figure 18–54.

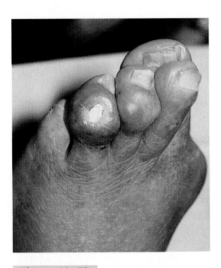

Figure 18–52

Gout of the lesser metatarsophalangeal joints.

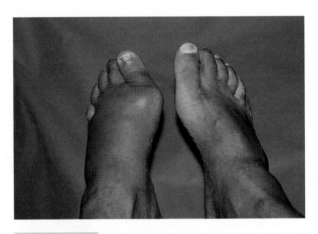

Figure 18–53

Acute gout and podagra.

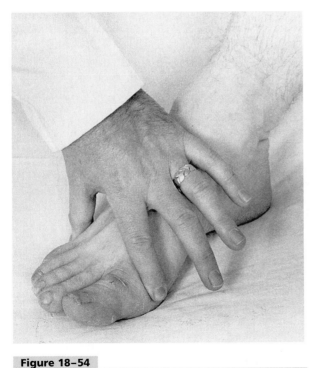

Figure 18–54

Technique for evaluating the metatarsophalangeal joints.

Clinicopathologic Correlations

Rheumatoid arthritis is a common musculoskeletal disorder and is the most destructive and disabling of the principal joint diseases. It is a condition of chronic inflammation of joints and of many other organs. However, the joints display the most marked destructive changes. The most characteristic changes are in the hands. In the early stages of the disease, there is swelling of the proximal interphalangeal, the metacarpophalangeal, and the wrist joints. As the disease progresses, there is bone erosion, which produces the classic signs of the disease. The most characteristic deformity of the fingers is ulnar deviation at the metacarpophalangeal joints. The two main deformities of the interphalangeal joints are:

- The swan-neck deformity
- The boutonnière deformity

The *swan-neck deformity,* which results from shortening of the interosseous muscles, produces flexion of the metacarpophalangeal joints, hyperextension of the proximal interphalangeal joints, and flexion of the distal interphalangeal joints. The *boutonnière deformity* is a flexion deformity of the proximal interphalangeal joints with hyperextension of the distal interphalangeal joints. Figure 18–55 shows the hands of a woman with rheumatoid arthritis. Note the marked ulnar deviation of the metacarpophalangeal joints. Figure 18–56 shows another example of a characteristic swan-neck deformity.

Osteoarthritis, or degenerative joint disease, is also common. In most cases, the inflammatory response is minimal compared with that of rheumatoid arthritis. The form of osteoarthritis depends on the joints involved. One of the joints more frequently involved is the distal interphalangeal joint. Progressive enlargement of these joints is termed *Heberden's nodes.* As the disease progresses, the proximal interphalangeal joints may become involved. The name often given to involvement of these joints is *Bouchard's nodes.* Figure 18–57 shows the hands of a woman with osteoarthritis.

Gout is a metabolic disease characterized by high levels of uric acid, recurrent attacks of acute arthritis, and deposition of urate crystals in and around the joints. The initial presentation is frequently acute pain in the first metatarsophalangeal joint, often waking the patient from sleep. Even at rest, the pain is severe, but the slightest movement of the joint is agonizing. Within a few hours, the joint becomes swollen, shiny, and red. The higher the level of uric acid, the more likely the patient is to develop *tophi,* which are subcutaneous and periarticular deposits of urate crystals. The commonly involved sites are over the first metatarsophalangeal joint, the finger, the ear, the elbow, and the Achilles tendon. Figure 18–58 shows the arms of a patient with chronic tophaceous gout who has large tophi on her elbows as well as smaller tophi on her hands. Tophi frequently develop over the distal interphalangeal joints of the

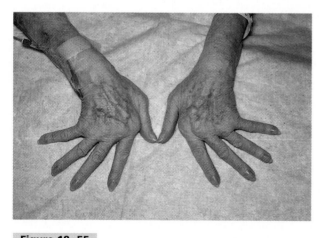

Figure 18–55

Rheumatoid arthritis. Note the marked ulnar deviation of the wrists.

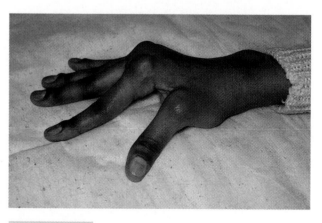

Figure 18–56

Rheumatoid arthritis. Note the swan-neck deformity.

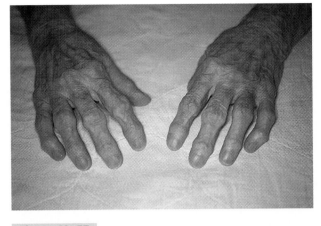

Figure 18–57

Osteoarthritis. Note Heberden's and Bouchard's nodes.

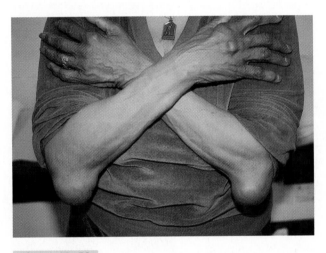

Figure 18–58

Gout. Note tophi on the elbows and hands.

fingers and in the olecranon and prepatellar bursae. Figure 18–59 shows the hands of a patient with tophi on her fingers.

Approximately 7% of patients with psoriasis develop joint disease. The most common form of *psoriatic arthritis* (70%) is asymmetric arthritis involving only two or three joints at a time. *Arthritis mutilans* is the most deforming type of psoriatic arthritis. In

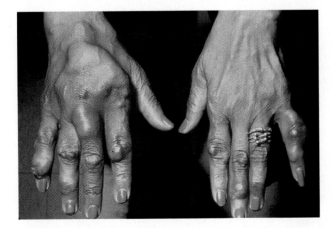

Figure 18–59

Tophi on fingers.

the most severe cases, there is osteolysis of the phalangeal and metacarpal joints, resulting in "telescoping of the digits," also known as the "opera-glass" deformity. The hands of a patient with this deforming form of psoriatic arthritis is shown in Figure 18–60.

Figure 18–61 shows a patient with psoriasis of the feet. Note the hyperkeratosis on an erythematous base.

Tuberous sclerosis is a dominantly inherited hamartomatous disorder characterized by mental retardation, seizures, eye lesions, and skin lesions. The classic triad of symptoms is mental retardation, seizures, and adenoma sebaceum. *Adenoma sebaceum* occurs near the nasolabial folds and over the cheeks. These lesions are facial angio-fibromas. Other common skin lesions are periungual and subungual fibromas. Figure 18–62 shows a patient with tuberous sclerosis and periungual fibromas.

Lesions of Kaposi's sarcoma are frequently seen on the feet. Figure 18–63 shows the foot of a patient who presented with this lesion between his fourth and fifth toes. A

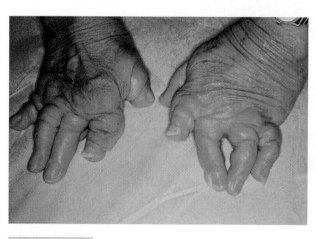

Figure 18–60

Psoriatic arthritis.

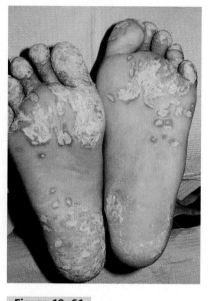

Figure 18–61

Psoriasis of the feet.

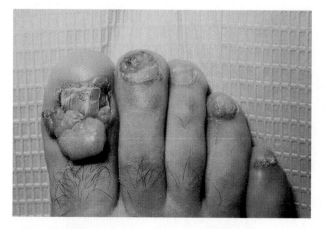

Figure 18–62

Tuberous sclerosis and periungual fibromas.

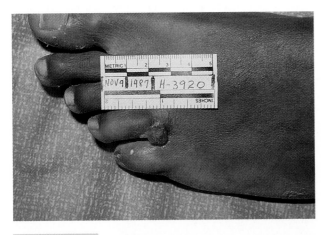

Figure 18–63

Kaposi's sarcoma between toes.

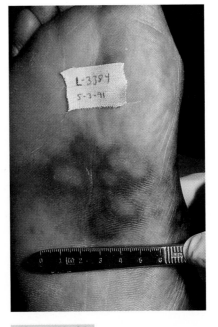

Figure 18–64

Kaposi's sarcoma on the plantar arch.

biopsy of the lesion confirmed the diagnosis of Kaposi's sarcoma. This was this patient's first manifestation of the acquired immunodeficiency syndrome. Figure 18–64 shows the plantar arch of another patient who presented with painful nodules. A biopsy confirmed the diagnosis of Kaposi's sarcoma.

Another common podiatric complaint is an exostosis at the metatarsocuneiform joint, which produces a painful dorsal lesion. Figure 18–65*A* shows a patient with this type of problem; Figure 18–65*B* is an x-ray film of the foot showing the bony abnormality.

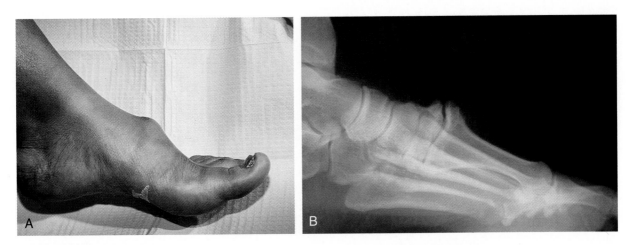

Figure 18–65

A, Exostosis at the metatarsocuneiform joint; *B*, X-ray film of the metatarsocuneiform joint.

Figure 18–66 shows a patient with a severe paronychia with exuberant granulation tissue. Such lesions must be differentiated from amelanotic melanomas.

Although *squamous cell carcinomas* are usually in sun-exposed areas, the patient shown in Figure 18–67 has such a lesion on the plantar aspect of the foot. A callus is also present under the head of the first metatarsal.

It is common for diabetics, with their decreased sensitivity in their feet, to present with a foreign body in their toe or foot. Figure 18–68 shows the right foot of a diabetic patient and a foreign body protruding from the tip of the third toe. This patient had dropped a needle in the carpet and some time later stepped on the needle, which penetrated the toe. Only after noticing it did the patient seek medical attention.

Scleroderma, or progressive systemic sclerosis, is a chronic multisystem disease manifested by thickening of the skin and varying degrees of organ involvement. There is a broad spectrum of disease manifestations of scleroderma, ranging from limited skin lesions associated with *c*alcinosis, *R*aynaud's phenomenon, *e*sophageal motility problems, *s*clerodactyly, and *t*elangiectasia (CREST variant) to full encasement of the body by diffuse sclerosis. Calcification of the soft tissues can produce a stony-hard tissue and

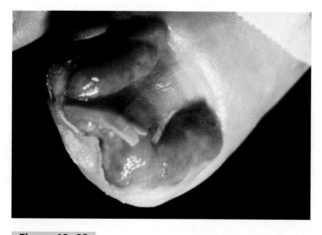

Figure 18–66

Paronychia with extensive granulation.

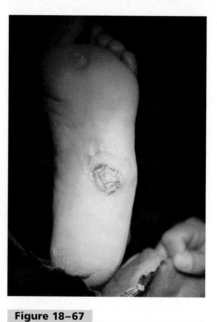

Figure 18–67

Squamous cell carcinoma on the plantar surface.

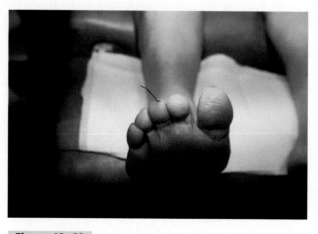

Figure 18–68

Foreign body in toe of diabetic patient.

can range from a small area to massive calcium deposits. Figure 18–69*A* shows a patient with the CREST syndrome with Raynaud's phenomenon and calcinosis cutis. Note the telangiectasias of the finger tips. Figure 18–69*B* shows the same patient with calcinosis cutis of the heel. Commonly, the distal finger pad assumes a tapered appearance with a tuft of scarred tissue between the fingertip and the nailbed. Ulceration can also occur that can lead to osteomyelitis. Figure 18–70 shows the plantar view of the hallux in the same patient with CREST syndrome; note the characteristic tapering of the digit and pterygium inversus (growth of soft tissue along the ventral aspect of the nail plate).

Figure 18–71 shows a subungual presentation of *malignant melanoma* of the hallux. Determine the cause of all subungual pigmented lesions.

Pain in the heel and pain in the first metatarsophalangeal joints are common complaints, most often caused by mechanical factors. However, pain can be secondary

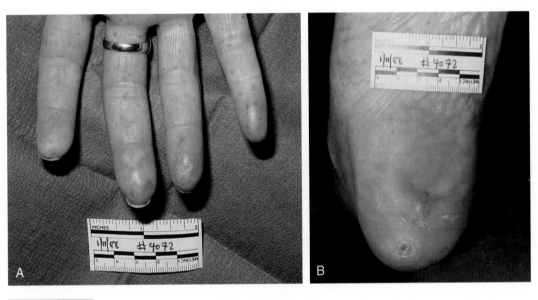

Figure 18–69

CREST syndrome. *A,* Telangiectasias of the finger tips. *B,* Calcinosis cutis of heel.

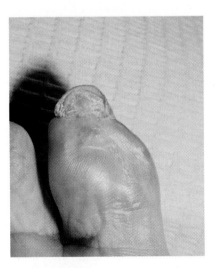

Figure 18–70

CREST syndrome with tapered digit and pterygium inversus.

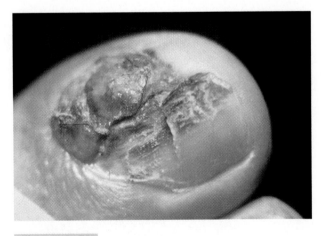

Figure 18–71

Subungual presentation of a malignant melanoma.

to several other causes. Table 18–3 lists the most common disorders associated with heel pain; Table 18–4 lists disorders associated with first metatarsophalangeal joint pain.

Table 18–5 summarizes the clinical features that differentiate rheumatoid arthritis from osteoarthritis. Table 18–6 summarizes some of the features of diseases affecting the hands and wrists. Table 18–7 outlines the clinical features that differentiate common musculoskeletal disorders affecting the elbow. Table 18–8 lists the clinical features that differentiate significant diseases affecting the knee. Table 18–9 lists the clinical features differentiating diseases of the foot. Table 18–10 summarizes the normal joint ranges of motion.

Table 18–3   Disorders Causing Heel Pain

Plantar calcaneal spur (enthesopathy)
Plantar fasciitis
Inferior calcaneal bursitis
Atrophy of plantar fat pad
Rheumatoid arthritis
Ankylosing spondylitis
Reiter's syndrome
Gout
Fracture
Neoplasm
Foreign body
Nerve entrapment

Table 18–4   Disorders Causing Pain in the First Metatarsophalangeal Joint

Osteoarthritis
Bursitis/capsulitis
Fracture
Sesamoiditis
Gout
Rheumatoid arthritis
Reiter's syndrome
Septic arthritis

Table 18–5   Clinical Features Differentiating Rheumatoid Arthritis from Osteoarthritis

Clinical Feature	Rheumatoid Arthritis*	Osteoarthritis†
Patient's age (yr)	3–80	Older than 45
Morning stiffness	More than 1 hr	Less than 1 hr
Disability	Often great	Variable
Joint distribution		
Distal interphalangeal joint	Rare	Very common
Proximal interphalangeal joint	Very common	Common
Metacarpophalangeal joint	Very common	Absent
Wrist	Very common	Absent
Soft-tissue swelling	Very common	Rare
Interosseous muscle wasting	Very common	Rare
Swan-necking	Common	Rare
Ulnar deviation	Common	Absent

* See Figures 18–55 and 18–56.
† See Figure 18–57.

Table 18-6   Clinical Features Differentiating Diseases Affecting the Hands and Wrists

Clinical Feature	Rheumatoid Arthritis	Psoriatic Arthritis*	Acute Gout¶	Osteoarthritis	Carpal Tunnel Syndrome
Age (yr)	3–80	10–60	30–80	50–80	40–80
Sex	F	M	M	F	M, F
Pain onset	Gradual	Gradual	Abrupt	Gradual	Gradual
Stiffness	Very common	Common	Absent	Common	Absent
Swelling	Common	Common	Common	Common	Common
Redness	Absent	Uncommon	Common	Uncommon	Absent
Deformity	Flexion of PIP and MCP; swan-neck,† boutonnière; ulnar deviation‡	Frequent DIP, PIP, and MCP involvement; "sausage"-shaped digits§	None in acute stage; resembles RA if deposits occur in tendon sheaths in chronic gout	Flexion and lateral deviation of DIP and PIP‖	Thenar muscle atrophy

* Needlepoint pitting of the nails is often associated with psoriatic arthritis. See Figures 6–12 and 6–13.
† See Figure 18–56.
‡ See Figure 18–55.
§ See Figure 18–60.
¶ See Figure 18–53.
‖ See Figure 18–57.
   Abbreviations: PIP = proximal interphalangeal joint; MCP = metacarpophalangeal joint; DIP = distal interphalangeal joint; RA = rheumatoid arthritis.

Table 18-7   Clinical Features Differentiating Diseases Affecting the Elbow

Clinical Feature	Rheumatoid Arthritis	Psoriatic Arthritis	Acute Gout*	Osteoarthritis	Tennis Elbow
Age (yr)	3–80	10–60	30–80	50–80	20–60
Sex	F	M	M	F	M, F
Pain onset	Gradual	Gradual	Abrupt	Gradual	Gradual
Stiffness	Very common	Common	Absent	Common	Occasional
Swelling	Common	Common	Common	Common	Absent
Redness	Absent	Uncommon	Common	Absent	Absent
Deformity	Flexion contractures, usually bilaterally	Flexion contractures, usually bilaterally	Flexion contractures only in chronic state	Flexion contractures	None

* See Figure 18–58, which shows a patient with chronic tophaceous gout and painless tophi on the elbows.

Table 18-8   Clinical Features Differentiating Diseases Affecting the Knee

Clinical Feature	Rheumatoid Arthritis	Psoriatic Arthritis	Acute Gout	Osteoarthritis	Torn Meniscus
Age (yr)	3–80	10–60	30–80	50–80	20–60
Sex	F	M	M	F	M
Pain onset	Gradual	Gradual	Abrupt	Gradual	Abrupt
Stiffness	Very common	Common	Absent	Common	Occasional
Swelling	Common	Common	Common	Common	Common
Redness	Absent	Uncommon	Common	Absent	Absent
Deformity	Flexion contractures	Flexion contractures	Flexion contractures only in chronic state	Flexion contractures	None

Table 18–9　Clinical Feature Differentiating Diseases Affecting the Foot

Clinical Feature	Rheumatoid Arthritis	Psoriatic Arthritis	Acute Gout	Osteoarthritis	Reiter's Syndrome
Age (yr)	3–80	10–60	30–80	50–80	10–80 (peak 30s)
Sex	F	M	M	F	M
Pain Onset	Gradual	Gradual	Abrupt	Gradual	Gradual
Stiffness	Very common	Common	Common	Common	Common
Swelling	Common	Common	Very common	Uncommon	Common
Redness	Uncommon	Uncommon	Very common	Uncommon	Common
Joint Predilection and Deformity	Abductovalgus deformity of MTP*	Fusiform swelling of DIP*	First MTP (may also have hallux abductovalgus deformity)	Hallux abductovalgus deformity	Ankle, heel, toes ("sausage" swelling of digits)

Abbreviations: MTP = metatarsophalangeal joint; DIP = distal interphalangeal joint.

Table 18–10　Joint Ranges of Motion

Joint	Flexion	Extension	Lateral Bending	Rotation
Cervical Spine	45°	55°	40°	70°
Thoracic and lumbar spine	75°	30°	35°	30°
			Abduction	Adduction
Shoulder	180°	50°	180°	50°
			Pronation	Supination
Elbow	150°	180°	80°	80°
			Radial Motion	Ulnar Motion
Wrist	80°	70°	20°	55°
MCP*	90°	20°		
Hip	90° with knee extended	30° with knee extended	40°	45°
	120° with knee flexed		Abduction	Adduction
			45°	30°
Knee	135°	0–10°		
Ankle	50°	15°		
			Inversion	Eversion
Subtalar			20°	10°
First MTP*	40°	65–75°		

Abbreviations: MCP = metacarpophalangeal joint; MTP = metatarsophalangeal joint.

Useful Vocabulary

Listed here are the specific roots that are important in order to understand the terminology related to musculoskeletal diseases.

Root	Pertaining to	Example	Definition
ankyl(o)-	stiff	*ankylo*sis	Immobile or stiff joint
arthr(o)-	joint	*arthro*gram	An x-ray of a joint
chir(o)-	hand	*chiro*spasm	Writer's cramp
dactyl(o)-	finger or toe	*dactylo*spasm	Cramping of a digit
myo-	muscle	*myo*pathy	Disease of muscle
oste(o)-	bone	*osteo*malacia	A condition marked by softening of the bones
pod-	foot	*pod*iatrist	Specialist in conditions of the foot
scolio-	twisted	*scolio*sis	Lateral deviation of the spine
spondyl(o)-	vertebrae	*spondyl*itis	Inflammation of vertebrae
teno-	tendon	*teno*tomy	Surgical cutting of a tendon

Writing Up the Physical Examination

Listed here are examples of the write-up for the examination of the musculoskeletal system.

- All the joints have a full range of motion. No deformities, tenderness, or abnormalities are detected.
- There is marked ulnar deviation of both hands associated with a flexion deformity of all the proximal interphalangeal joints and hyperextension of all the distal interphalangeal joints. Marked tenderness of both wrists is present.
- There is abnormal forward mobility of the knee. There is 3–4 cm of motion detected.
- The left first metatarsophalangeal joint is markedly erythematous and painful. The joint is shiny and edematous.
- No joint deformities are noted. There is marked reduction of hip internal and external rotation. No pain is produced by these movements. Pain is produced by abduction of the right shoulder against resistance. The range of right shoulder abduction is reduced. The range of motion of the hands, wrists, spine, knees, and ankles is normal.

Bibliography

Birnbaum JS: The Musculoskeletal Manual. Orlando, FL, Grune & Stratton, 1986.

Cooper BS, Rice DP: The economic cost of illness revisited. Soc Secur Bull 39:21, 1976.

D'Ambrosia RD: Musculoskeletal Disorders: Regional Examination and Differential Diagnosis. Philadelphia, J.B. Lippincott, 1986.

Dieppe PA, Bacon PA, Bamji AN, et al: Atlas of Clinical Rheumatology. Philadelphia, Lea & Febiger, 1986.

Gartland JJ: Fundamentals of Orthopaedics, 4th ed. Philadelphia, W.B. Saunders, 1987.

Kelsey JL, Pastides H, Bisbee GE Jr: Musculo-Skeletal Disorders: Their Frequency of Occurrence and Their Impact on the Population of the United States. New York, Prodist, 1978.

Kosinski MA, Stewart D: Nail changes associated with systemic disease and vascular insufficiency. Clin Podiatr Med Surg 6:295, 1989.

CHAPTER 19

The Nervous System

As the debility increases and the influence of the will over the muscles fades, the tremulous agitation becomes more vehement. It now seldom leaves him for a moment; but even when exhausted nature seizes a small portion of sleep, the motion becomes so violent as not only to shake the bed-hangings, but even the floor and sashes of the room. The chin is now almost immovably bent down upon the sternum. The slops with which he is attempted to be fed, with the saliva, are continually trickling from the mouth. The power of articulation is lost. The urine and faeces are passed involuntarily; and at the last, constant sleepiness, with slight delirium, and other marks of extreme exhaustion, announce the wished-for release.

James Parkinson
1755–1824

General Considerations

By the 2nd century AD, Galen had already described the cerebral ventricles, 7 of the 12 cranial nerves, and the cerebral convolutions. There was, however, little further interest in the anatomy and physiology of the neurologic system until the 16th century. In 1543 Vesalius illustrated the basal ganglia, and in 1552 Eustachius described the cerebellar peduncles and the pons.

The 17th century saw the descriptions and illustrations by Willis of the cerebral circulation, the "striate body," and the internal capsule. Bartholin and others felt that the function of the cerebral cortex was to protect the blood vessels, whereas other investigators felt that the cerebrum possessed higher functions. Pourfour du Petit stressed that the cortex was responsible for motor activity. This concept lay dormant until the end of the 19th century.

Careful anatomic descriptions of the tracts, nuclei, and gyri were described in the writings of the scientists of the 18th and early 19th centuries. Reil and Burdach provided names for the many gross anatomic structures that had been illustrated by others in the previous centuries. Reil has been credited with the naming of the insula, the capsule, the uncinate and cingular fasculi, and the tapetum. The uncus, lenticular nucleus, pulvinar, and gyrus cinguli were named by Burdach. During this same period, Soemmering, Vicq d'Azyr, Gall, Gratiolet, and Rolando made many detailed illustrations of the cerebral convolutional patterns.

The early 19th century saw the beginnings of the descriptions of several disease states. In 1817 James Parkinson wrote an essay describing the "shaking palsy" that now bears his name. In 1829 Charles Bell wrote:

> The next instance was in a man wounded by the horn of an ox. The point entered under the angle of the jaw and came out before the ear. . . . He remains now a singular proof of the effects of the loss of function in the muscles of the face by this nerve being divided. The forehead of the corresponding side is without motion, the eyelids remain open, the nostril has no motion in breathing, and the mouth is drawn to the opposite side.

This is the classic description of facial nerve (seventh cranial nerve) palsy, also known as Bell's palsy.

In the mid-19th century, an interest in microscopic neuroanatomy developed. Purkinje, Schwann, and Helmholtz were a few of the many neuroanatomists who contributed valuable information about the intricacies of the nervous system. However, not until the late 19th century were specific staining techniques developed by Golgi, Marchi, and Nissl, which led the way to our current understanding of neuronal disease. The nerve cell had finally been discovered.

The 20th century saw further progress in the description of the cerebral cortex, anterior commissure, thalamus, and hypothalamus. A major advance came from the work of Cajal in 1904. His histologic exploration clarified the complexities of the neuron. Not until 1925 were the hypophysio-hypothalamic connections described, and even to this day, the function of the hypothalamus is not fully understood.

It has been suggested that more than 40% of patients who present to the internist have symptoms referable to neurologic disease. The internist must have the ability to identify the early signs and symptoms of neurologic disease to initiate the appropriate therapy. All too often, subtle signs and symptoms may be ignored, and a diagnosis is not made until advanced disability is apparent.

The internist holds an important position, because the patient with a neurologic problem will usually seek help from that specialist first. A thorough knowledge of the basic neuroanatomy and physiology is the cornerstone of neurologic diagnosis.

Structure and Physiology

The brain, which is enclosed in the cranium and surrounded by the meninges, is the center of the nervous system. The brain can be divided into paired cerebral hemispheres, basal ganglia, diencephalon (thalamus and hypothalamus), brain stem, and cerebellum.

The two *cerebral hemispheres* make up the largest portion of the brain. Each hemisphere may be subdivided into four major lobes named for the cranial bones that overlie them: frontal, parietal, occipital, and temporal. The fissures and sulci divide the cerebral surface. A deep midline, longitudinal fissure separates the two hemispheres. The convolutions, or *gyri,* lie between the sulci. A lateral view of the left cerebral hemisphere is shown in Figure 19–1. Figure 19–2 shows a medial view of the right cerebral hemisphere. A basal view of the cerebral hemispheres is shown in Figure 19–3.

The cerebrum is responsible for motor, sensory, associative, and higher mental functions. The primary *motor cortex* is located in the precentral gyrus. Neurons in this area control voluntary movements of the skeletal muscle on the opposite side of the body. An irritative lesion in this area may cause seizures or changes in consciousness. Destructive lesions in this area can produce contralateral flaccid paresis or paralysis.

The primary *sensory cortex* is located in the postcentral gyrus. Irritative lesions in this area may produce paresthesias ("numbness" or "pins and needles" sensations) on the opposite side. Destructive lesions produce an impairment in cutaneous sensation on the opposite side.

The primary *visual cortex* is located in the occipital lobe along the calcarine fissure, which divides the cuneus from the lingual gyri. Irritative lesions in this area produce visual symptoms such as flashes of light or rainbows. Destructive lesions cause an homonymous hemianopsia on the contralateral side. Central macular vision is spared.

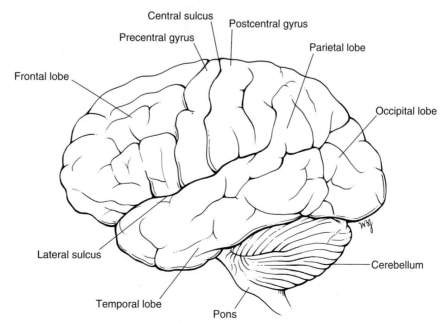

Figure 19–1

Lateral view of the left cerebral hemisphere.

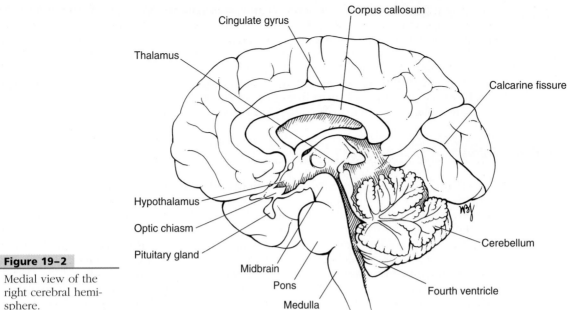

Medial view of the right cerebral hemisphere.

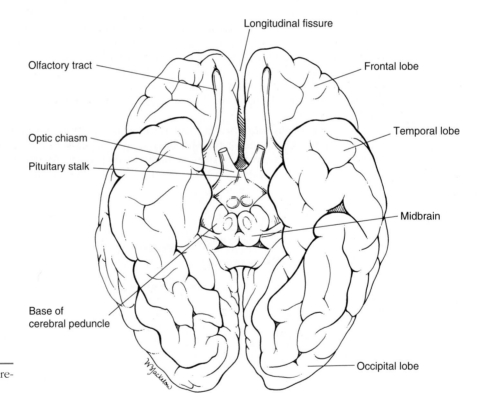

Basal view of the cerebral hemispheres.

The primary *auditory* cortex is located in the temporal lobe along the transverse temporal gyrus. Irritative lesions in this area produce a buzzing or ringing in the ears. Destructive lesions rarely produce deafness.

The *basal ganglia* are situated deep within the cerebral hemispheres. The structures constituting the basal ganglia include the caudate and lenticular nuclei as well as the amygdala. The amygdala is part of the limbic system concerned with emotion. All other components are important structures in the extrapyramidal system, which is concerned with modulating voluntary body movements, postural changes, and autonomic integration. The basal ganglia are especially involved with fine movements of the extremities. Disturbances of the basal ganglia can result in tremors and rigid movements.

The *thalamus* is a large nuclear mass located on each side of the third ventricle. The thalamus is the chief sensory and motor integrating mechanism of the neuraxis. All sensory impulses, except olfactory ones, and the major output from systems that modulate and modify motor function (i.e., cerebellum and corpus striatum) terminate in the thalamus, from which they are projected to specific areas of the cerebral cortex. The thalamus is concerned with certain emotional connotations that accompany most sensory experiences. The thalamus can influence visceral and somatic effectors serving primarily affective reactions, through its connections with the hypothalamus and striatum. Through its control of the electrical excitability of the cerebral cortex, the thalamus plays a dominant role in the maintenance and regulation of the state of consciousness, alertness, and attention. The thalamus may be the critical structure for the perception of pain and thermal sense, which remain after complete destruction of the primary sensory cortex. Thermal sense endows sensation with discriminative faculties and is not concerned with the recognition of crude sensory modalities.

The *hypothalamus* is located below the thalamus. It includes the optic chiasm and the neurohypophysis. The hypothalamus is responsible for many regulatory mechanisms, such as temperature regulation; neuroendocrine control of catecholamines, thyroid-stimulating hormone, adrenocorticotropic hormone, follicle-stimulating and luteinizing hormones, prolactin, and growth hormones; thirst; appetite; water balance; and sexual behavior.

The brain stem consists of the midbrain, pons, and medulla. Figure 19–4 shows the external anatomy of the brain stem. The brain stem is responsible for relaying all messages between the upper and lower levels of the central nervous system. Cranial nerves III to XII also arise from the brain stem. The brain stem contains the reticular formation, a network that provides for constant muscle stimulation to counteract the force of gravity. In addition to its antigravity effects, this area of the brain is essential for the control of consciousness. The neurons in the recticular activating system are capable of waking and arousing the entire brain.

The *midbrain* contains the superior and inferior colliculi, the cerebral peduncles, and the motor nuclei of the trochlear and oculomotor nerves. The superior colliculi are associated with the visual system, and the inferior colliculi are associated with the

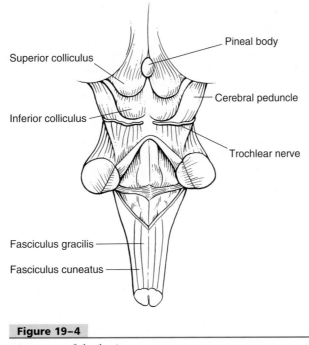

Figure 19–4

Anatomy of the brain stem.

auditory system. The cerebral peduncles converge from the inferior aspect of the cerebral hemispheres and enter the pons. A destructive lesion of the superior colliculi causes paralysis of upward gaze. Destructive lesions of the cranial nerve nuclei produce the classic paralysis of the affected nerve. A destructive lesion of the cerebral peduncle gives rise to spastic paralysis on the other side of the body. Destruction of still other tracts in the midbrain results in rigidity and involuntary movements.

The *pons* lies ventral to the cerebellum and rostral to the medulla. The abducens, facial, and acoustic (and vestibular) nuclei are found within the pons, and their nerves exit through a groove that divides the pons from the medulla. The motor and sensory nuclei of the trigeminal nerve are also located in the pons. At this level, the corticospinal tracts (also known as the pyramidal tracts) have not yet crossed, and a lesion at this level will produce loss of voluntary movement on the opposite side. Destructive lesions of the pons may produce a variety of clinical syndromes, such as the following:

- Contralateral hemiplegia with ipsilateral trigeminal hemiplegia (paralysis of the jaw muscles and loss of sensation over the same side of the face)
- Contralateral hemiplegia with ipsilateral facial palsy (Bell's palsy)
- Contralateral hemiplegia with ipsilateral facial palsy and ipsilateral abducens palsy (paralysis of the lateral rectus muscle on the same side of the face)
- Contralateral hemiplegia with ipsilateral abducens palsy
- Quadriplegia and nystagmus

The *medulla* is the portion of the brain stem between the pons and the spinal cord. The nuclei of the hypoglossal, vagus, glossopharyngeal, and spinal accessory nerves are located within the medulla. It is within the medulla that the majority of fibers in the corticospinal tracts cross to the opposite side. Destructive lesions in the medulla produce symptoms that are referable to the tracts interrupted by the lesion. Some clinical syndromes are as follows:

- Contralateral hemiplegia with ipsilateral hypoglossal palsy*
- Ipsilateral vagal palsy† with contralateral loss of pain and temperature sense
- Ipsilateral vagal palsy with ipsilateral spinal accessory palsy‡
- Ipsilateral vagal palsy with ipsilateral hypoglossal palsy
- Ipsilateral vagal palsy, ipsilateral spinal accessory palsy, and ipsilateral hypoglossal palsy

There are many more clinical syndromes, which are beyond the scope of this text. The reader is advised to review the neuroanatomy further in order to understand the complexities of these neurologic syndromes.

The *cerebellum* is located in the posterior fossa of the skull and is composed of a small midline vermis and two large lateral hemispheres. The cerebellum acts to keep the individual oriented in space and to halt or check motions. The cerebellum is also responsible for the fine movements of the hands. Essentially, the cerebellum coordinates and refines the action of muscle groups to produce steady and precise movements. Destructive lesions of the cerebellum cause swaying, staggering, intention tremors,§ and inability to change movements rapidly.

The blood supply to the brain is 80% through the internal carotid arteries and 20% through the vertebral basilar arteries. Each internal carotid artery terminates as the anterior cerebral and middle cerebral arteries. The posterior cerebral artery arises from the basilar artery, which joins with the posterior communicating artery, a branch of the internal carotid artery. The two anterior cerebral arteries are joined by the anterior communicating artery. This vascular network forms the circle of Willis, located at the base of the brain. This is illustrated in Figure 19–5.

Continuous with the medulla is the *spinal cord,* a cylindrical mass of neuronal tissue measuring 40–50 cm in length in the adult. Its distal end attaches to the first

---

* Paralysis of the tongue muscles on the same side of the lesion. The tongue deviates to the side of the lesion when the patient is asked to stick out the tongue.
† Paralysis of the soft palate and difficulty in speaking, termed *dysarthria.*
‡ Paralysis of the sternocleidomastoid and/or trapezius muscles. This results in the inability to turn the head to the side opposite the lesion and to shrug the shoulder.
§ Tremors that result when the individual moves the hands to do something but that may not be present at rest.

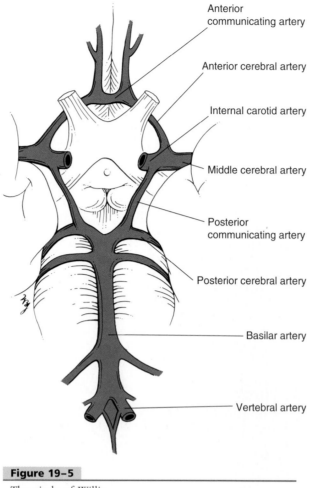

Figure 19–5

The circle of Willis.

segment of the coccyx. The spinal cord is divided into two symmetric halves by the anterior median fissure and the posterior median sulcus. Each half contains white and gray matter, which can be further subdivided. This is illustrated in Figure 19–6.

In the center of the spinal cord is the *gray matter*. The anterior gray matter, the *anterior horn,* is the motor portion of the spinal cord and contains multipolar cells of origin of the *anterior roots* of the peripheral nerves. The *lateral horn* (sympathetic

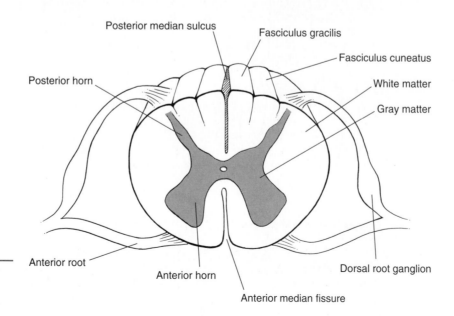

Figure 19–6

Cross-sectional view through the spinal cord.

preganglionic neurons) is found at T1–L2 spinal levels. The posterior gray matter, the *posterior horn,* is the receptor portion of the spinal cord.

The *white matter* of the spinal cord consists of tracts that serve to link segments of the spinal cord and to connect it to the brain. There are three main columns (funiculi). Between the anterior median fissure and the anterolateral sulcus is the *anterior white column,* which contains the descending fibers of the *ventral corticospinal tract* and the ascending fibers of the *ventral spinothalamic tract.* The ventral corticospinal tract is involved with voluntary motion, and the ventral spinothalamic tract carries light touch.

The *lateral white column* is located between the anterolateral and posterolateral sulci and contains the descending fibers of the *lateral corticospinal tract* and the

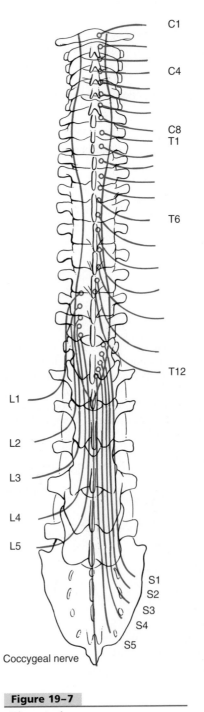

Figure 19–7

The spinal nerves.

ascending *spinocerebellar* and *lateral spinothalamic tracts.* The lateral corticospinal tract is responsible for voluntary movement; the spinocerebellar tracts carry reflex proprioception; the lateral spinothalamic tract carries pain and temperature sensation.

The *posterior white column* is located between the posterolateral and posterior median sulcus. The most important fibers in this column are the ascending fibers of the *fasciculus gracilis* and the *fasciculus cuneatus.* These tracts carry vibration sense, passive motion, joint position, and two-point discrimination.

There are 31 pairs of spinal nerves, each having a ventral (motor) and dorsal (sensory) root. The ventral root consists of *efferent* nerve fibers, which originate in the anterior and lateral (T1–T2 only) gray matter and travel to the peripheral nerve and muscle. This is the motor root. The dorsal root consists of *afferent* nerve fibers, whose cell bodies are in the *dorsal root ganglion.* This is the sensory root.

The spinal nerves are grouped into 8 cervical (C1–C8), 12 thoracic (T1–T12), 5 lumbar (L1–L5), 5 sacral (S1–S5), and 1 coccygeal nerve. These nerves are shown in Figure 19–7.

A *spinal reflex* involves an afferent neuron and an efferent neuron at the same level in the spinal cord. The basis for this reflex arc is an intact sensory limb, functional synapses in the spinal cord, an intact motor limb, and a muscle capable of responding. The afferent and the efferent limbs travel together in the same spinal nerve. When a stretched muscle is suddenly stretched farther, the afferent sensory limb sends impulses through its spinal nerve that travel to the dorsal root of that nerve. After synapsing in the gray matter of the spinal cord, the impulse is transmitted to the ventral nerve root. These impulses are then conducted through the ventral root to the neuromuscular junction, where a brisk contraction of the muscle completes the reflex arc. Figure 19–8 illustrates a reflex spinal arc.

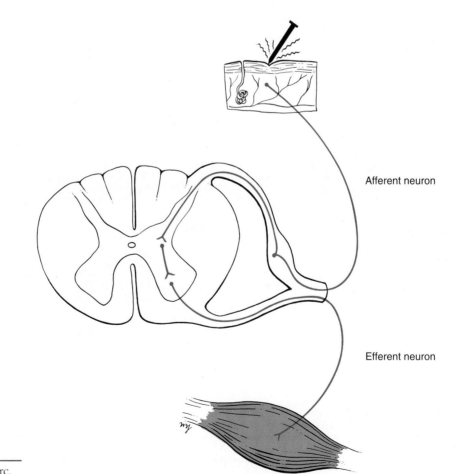

Afferent neuron

Efferent neuron

Figure 19–8

The reflex spinal arc.

The afferent sensory limb is important not only in the reflex arc but also in the conscious appreciation of sensation. Nerve fibers carrying pain and temperature sensation enter the spinal cord and cross to the other side within one or two spinal segments. They ascend in the contralateral *lateral spinothalamic tract,* travel through the brain stem and the thalamus, and end in the postcentral gyrus of the parietal lobe, as illustrated in Figure 19–9A. Fibers carrying *proprioceptive* sensation from muscles, joints, and tendons enter the dorsal root and participate in the reflex arc. Other fibers carrying proprioceptive sensation pass directly into the *posterior columns* and ascend in the fasciculi gracilis and cuneatus to their ipsilateral nuclei, cross in the medial lemniscus, synapse in the thalamus, and end in the postcentral gyrus of the parietal lobe. Still other proprioceptive fibers ascend crossed and uncrossed in the spinocerebellar tracts to the cerebellum. These additional pathways are illustrated in Figure 19–9B.

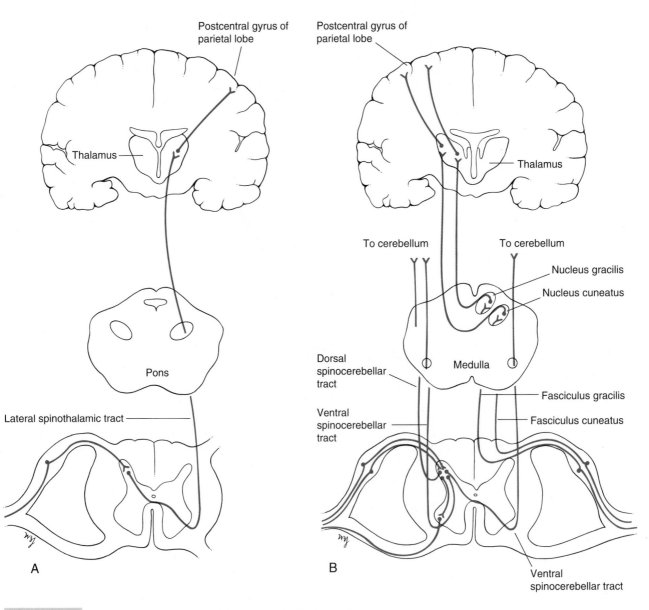

Figure 19–9

The conscious appreciation of sensation. *A,* Nerve pathways for pain and temperature sensation through the lateral spinothalamic tracts. *B,* Pathways of the fibers carrying proprioceptive sensation through the posterior columns and in the spinocerebellar tracts.

Review of Specific Symptoms

The most common symptoms of neurologic disease are as follows:

- Headache
- Loss of consciousness
- "Dizziness"
- Ataxia
- Changes in consciousness
- Visual disturbances
- Dysphasia
- Brain failure
- Cerebral vascular accidents
- Gait disturbances
- Tremor
- "Numbness"
- "Weakness"
- Pain

Headache

Headache is the most common neurologic symptom. It has been estimated that more than 35 million individuals in the United States suffer from recurrent headaches. Most of these patients have headaches that are related to migraine, muscle contraction, or tension. A headache pattern that is unchanged and has been present for several years is unlikely to be related to the present illness of the patient. Several points must be clarified in any patient complaining of a recent change in the frequency or severity of the headaches. Ask the following questions:

"How long have you been having headaches?"
"When did you notice a change in the pattern or severity of your headaches?"
"How has the pattern of your headaches changed?"
"How often do your headaches occur?"
"How long does each headache last?"
"Which part of your head aches?"
"Describe what the headache feels like."
"How quickly does the headache reach its maximum?"
"When you get the headaches, do you have any other symptoms?"
"Are you aware of anything that produces the headaches?"
"Are there any warning signs?"
"Does anything make the headaches worse?"
"What makes the headaches better?"

Patients complaining of a *sudden* onset of headache generally have more serious illnesses than patients with headaches of chronic duration. A continuous headache can be related to muscle spasm, whereas a *recurrent* headache may be migraine or cluster. A *throbbing* headache often has a vascular cause. Certain headaches are associated with visual phenomena, nausea, or vomiting. In patients with increased intracranial pressure, any maneuver that increases the pressure, such as coughing or bending, may worsen the headache.

Migraine is a biphasic type of headache associated with a prodromal phase, called the *aura,* followed by the headache phase. During the aura, one or more physiologic events may occur. These include transient autonomic, visual, motor, or sensory phenomena. Common visual symptoms are photophobia, blurred vision, and scotomata. As the aura fades, the headache begins. It is usually unilateral, often described as pulsating, and lasts for hours to days. Migraine headaches are often triggered by stress, anxiety, the use of birth control pills, and hormonal changes. Many patients experience migraine headaches after a period of excitement. Other important triggers are hunger and the ingestion of certain foods such as chocolate, cheese, cured meats, and highly spiced foods. There is often a family history of migraine.

Cluster headaches are associated with oculosympathetic disturbances. The patient is frequently a middle-aged man complaining of recurrent episodes of pain centered around the eye lasting for up to 1 hour. Classically, cluster headaches awaken the patient from sleep on successive nights for 2–4 weeks. There is ipsilateral miosis, ptosis, conjunctival edema, tearing, and nasal stuffiness during the headache. It is thought that alcohol may precipitate such attacks.

Headache may be the result of referred pain from sinus infections, ocular disease, and dental disease. Systemic conditions such as viral infections, chronic obstructive pulmonary disease, and poisoning may produce headaches. Determine whether the patient is taking any medications that may be producing the head pain. (See Table 19–2, in the Clinicopathologic Correlations section, which provides an approach to the patient with the symptom of headache.)

Loss of Consciousness

Loss of consciousness—syncope—may result from cardiovascular or neurologic causes. The cardiovascular causes are discussed in Chapter 12, The Heart, and Chapter 13, The Peripheral Vascular System. The term *blackout* is commonly used but may mean different conditions to the patient and interviewer. Any patient who uses this term should be asked to clarify its meaning. The term *to blackout* or *to fall out* is often used by the patient to indicate an actual loss of consciousness, dimming of vision, or a decreased awareness of the environment without an actual loss of consciousness.

A useful way to clarify the symptom of loss of consciousness is to ask the patient, "Have you ever lost consciousness, fainted, or felt that you were not aware of your surroundings?" If the patient answers in the affirmative, identify the cause of the loss of consciousness. Ask the following questions:

> *"Can you describe the attack to me? I want you to describe every event as it occurred until you lost consciousness."*
> *"Did anyone witness the attack?"**
> *"Were there any symptoms that preceded the attack?"*
> *"Were you told that there were body movements?"*
> *"I would like you to describe everything you remember after the attack until you felt completely normal."*
> *"Was there a period of sleepiness that followed?"* If so, *"For how long did this period last?"*
> *"How did you feel after the attack? Were you confused?"*
> *"Did you notice afterward that you had urinated or had a bowel movement during the attack?"*

Epileptic seizures, or fits, may produce a loss of consciousness and are caused by the sudden, excessive disorderly discharge of neurons. The first step in approaching the symptom of "seizure" is to identify its type. If the discharge is *focal,* the clinical seizure reflects the effect of the excessive discharge in that area of the body. For example, if the discharge is located in the inferior precentral gyrus, involved with hand and arm motion, the seizure will result in involuntary motion of the hand and arm. A *generalized* seizure results from a discharge in the subcortical structures, such as the thalamocortical radiations. These have widespread bilateral cortical connections. There are three main types of generalized seizures:

- Petit mal
- Grand mal
- Myoclonic

A *petit mal* seizure is characterized by a sudden attack of unconsciousness lasting only about 10 seconds, usually without any warning. During the petit mal seizure, the patient appears to be staring or daydreaming. There is no associated falling or involuntary limb motion. The patient rapidly returns to normal activity without being aware of the attack. These seizures are most common in children from the ages of 5 to 15 years. Occasionally they may persist into adulthood.

A *grand mal* seizure is a generalized major motor convulsion. Patients lose consciousness, and many fall rigidly to the floor. In 50% of patients with grand mal

---

* Obtain a history from an observer, if possible.

seizures, there is an aura of giddiness, involuntary twitching, change in mood, confusion, or epigastric discomfort as the seizure begins. Some patients may cry out initially. During this *tonic* phase, there is an increase in muscle tone, resulting in a rigid, flexed posture and then a rigid, extended posture. The patient may become apneic and cyanotic. The eyes may open and stare or may be deviated to one side. The *clonic* phase follows with involuntary movements of the body. These are often associated with salivation, eye rolling, and incontinence. Biting the tongue is common. After the clonic phase, the individual passes into a phase of resembling sleep from which she or he cannot be easily awakened. *Postictally,* or after the seizure, the patient may be confused and often falls into a deep sleep that lasts for hours. Accompanying muscle pain and headache are common.

A *myoclonic* seizure is a minor motor seizure characterized by sudden muscle contractions of the face and upper extremities. The eyelids and forearms are commonly affected. There is no detectable loss of consciousness.

Febrile convulsions are common in children from the ages of 6 months to 6 years and are similar to grand mal seizures. When a child has a high fever, a seizure lasting less than 10 minutes may occur. The younger the child at the time of the first febrile seizure, the greater the likelihood that a seizure will recur.

"Dizziness"

Dizziness is a term used frequently by the patient and should be avoided by the interviewer. Dizziness may be the patient's description of vertigo, ataxia, or lightheadedness. Any time the patient uses the term dizziness, it must be clarified by additional questioning, because different pathophysiologic mechanisms may be responsible. The interviewer needs to differentiate vertigo from ataxia. If the patient complains of "dizziness," it is important to ask these questions:

> *"Would you describe the dizziness as a funny spinning sensation in your head?"*
> *"Did the room spin, or did it feel as if you were spinning?"*
> *"Were you unsteady while walking?"*

Vertigo is partially discussed in Chapter 9, The Ear and Nose. Froehling et al (1994) reviewed the pathophysiology of vertigo and nystagmus as well as how to elicit the symptoms and signs of vertigo. Vertigo is the hallucination of movement. Acute vertigo may be associated with nausea, vomiting, perspiration, and a sense of anxiety. Ask patients whether they have the sensation that objects are moving around them or that they are spinning or moving. In addition to the questions in Chapter 9, ask the following questions:

> *"During the attack, did you experience any nausea or vomiting?"*
> *"Have you noticed any problem with hearing or ringing in your ears?"*
> *"Have you ever been given an antibiotic called gentamicin?"*

Ménière's disease can result in protracted attacks of severe vertigo associated with vomiting. Patients with Ménière's disease often have the associated symptoms of tinnitus and a hearing loss. During the attacks, the patient is unsteady, with horizontal nystagmus directed away from the affected ear. Certain drugs (such as gentamicin) are associated with changes in the labyrinth of the ear and cause vertigo and deafness.

Ataxia

Disruption of the vestibulo-ocular-cerebellar control mechanism produces ataxia. Ataxia is persistent unsteadiness while upright. Any patient complaining of dizziness must be evaluated for abnormal function of the vestibular, visual, proprioceptive, and cerebellar systems. Equilibrium requires the integration of sensory input and motor output acting primarily at a reflex level for the maintenance of balance. The ears and eyes and their central connections in the brain stem and the cerebellum are intimately involved in balance. Any patient with ataxia should be asked:

> *"Are you unsteady when you walk?"*
> *"Have you noticed that the dizziness is worse when your eyes are open or closed?"*
> *"What does your diet consist of? What did you eat yesterday?"*
> *"Have you ever had syphilis?"*

Abnormal proprioceptive input from the lower extremities can cause ataxia. Severe posterior column damage from syphilis, vitamin B_{12} deficiency, or multiple sclerosis may produce a "sensory" ataxia resulting in a wide-based, high-stepping gait. The gait is worsened by having the patient close the eyes and is improved by having the patient observe the feet. Vitamin B_{12} deficiency may result from pernicious anemia or from inadequate intake, although poor nutrition is a rare cause. "Motor" ataxia results from an abnormality in the cerebellum and central vestibular pathways. It is characterized by wide-based, irregular placement of the feet and poor placement of the center of gravity, with a lurching to either side.

Changes in Consciousness

Changes in consciousness may be related to changes in attention span, perception, or arousal, or a combination. In *confusional states,* the patient has the ability to receive information normally, but the processing is disturbed. In *delirium,* the individual perceives the information abnormally. Any patient, or member of the patient's family, who indicates that a change in consciousness has occurred should be asked the following:

"Has the change occurred suddenly?"
"Have there been other symptoms associated with the change of consciousness?"
"Do you use any medications? depressants? insulin? alcohol? recreational drugs?"
"Is there a history of psychiatric illness?"
"Is there a history of kidney disease? liver disease? thyroid disease?"
"Have you ever had an injury to your head?"

Many factors may produce changes in consciousness. The acuteness of the change in consciousness is often helpful in making a diagnosis. Hemiparesis, paresthesia, hemianopsia, garbled speech, and arm and leg weakness are common associated symptoms of supratentorial lesions. Brain stem lesions are often associated with changes in consciousness and with nystagmus, vomiting, double vision, nausea, and yawning. Drugs of any type are associated with acute changes in consciousness. A history of earlier psychiatric illness is important. Toxic and metabolic changes are frequently associated with changes in consciousness. Liver or kidney failure, myxedema, and diabetic ketoacidosis are common causes of metabolic abnormalities. A history of head trauma may result in a subdural hematoma and produce a gradual change in consciousness.

Visual Disturbances

Visual disturbances are common neurologic presenting symptoms. The most important symptoms are acute visual loss, chronic visual loss, and double vision. Ask any patient complaining of visual disturbances the following questions:

"How long have you noticed these visual changes?"
"Is the visual loss associated with pain?"
"Did it occur suddenly?"
"Do you have a history of glaucoma?"
"Have you ever been told that you have or had a thyroid problem?"
"Do you have diabetes?"

Acute painless visual loss is caused by either a vascular accident or a retinal detachment. Acute narrow-angle glaucoma may also be responsible for transient loss of vision associated with intense ocular pain. Painless loss of vision over a longer period is seen with compression of the optic nerve or tract or radiation. Glaucoma is often the cause of chronic, insidious, painless loss of vision. Episodes of migraine may produce transient episodes of visual loss before the development of the headache. *Amaurosis fugax* is transient visual loss lasting up to 3 minutes and is a feature of internal carotid artery disease.

Diplopia is discussed in Chapter 8, The Eye. Ocular motor palsies, thyroid abnormalities, myasthenia gravis, and brain stem lesions are well-known causes of diplopia. Ocular motor palsies are seen in trauma, multiple sclerosis, myasthenia gravis, aneurysms of the circle of Willis, diabetes, and tumors. Ask the following questions of any patient complaining of diplopia:

"Are you diabetic?"
"In which field of gaze do you have double vision?"
"Did the double vision occur suddenly?"
"Was there any pain associated with the double vision?"
"Has there been any injury to the head or eye?"
"Have you ever been told that your blood pressure has been elevated?"
"Does the double vision get worse when you are tired?"
"Have you been exposed to the AIDS (acquired immunodeficiency syndrome) virus?"

When a cranial nerve is affected, resulting in an extraocular muscle palsy, a patient may complain of diplopia in one field of gaze when the affected eye is unable to move conjugately with the other. Ocular palsies involve the 3rd, 4th, and 6th cranial nerves. A complete 3rd nerve palsy causes ptosis, mydriasis, and the loss of all extraocular movements except abduction. Trauma, multiple sclerosis, tumors, and aneurysms are the most frequent causes. Aneurysms of the posterior communicating artery can involve the 3rd nerve as this nerve passes near the artery on its way to the cavernous sinus. Cavernous sinus thrombosis, not infrequently seen in patients suffering from AIDS, may also produce a complete 3rd nerve palsy. Pupil-sparing 3rd nerve, trochlear nerve, and abducens nerve palsies are seen in diabetics and in patients with longstanding hypertension. Patients with myasthenia gravis often have diplopia in the later part of the day as the muscles tire and weaken.

Dysphasia

Speech abnormalities, or dysphasia, may be either nonfluent (expressive) or fluent (receptive). In *expressive aphasia,* the speech pattern is hesitant and labored, with poor articulation. The patient has no problem with comprehension. When asked to say, "No ifs, ands, or buts," the patient has great difficulty. In *receptive aphasia,* the speech is rapid and appears fluent but is full of syntax errors, with the omission of many words. Handwriting changes are nonspecific but indicate an impairment of neuromuscular control. Ask the following questions:

"Have you noticed any recent change in your speech pattern, such as slurring of your words?"
"Do you have trouble understanding things that are said to you?"
"Have you had any difficulty in finding the right word in conversation?"
"Has your handwriting changed recently?"

Brain Failure

An important symptom of neurologic disease is failing memory. The term *brain failure* replaces *dementia.* Brain failure can be defined as the progressive impairment of orientation, memory, judgment, and other aspects of intellectual function. Brain failure is a symptom rather than a specific disease entity. The most important cause of brain failure is *Alzheimer's disease.* Other causes include Parkinson's disease, vascular disorders, metabolic disorders, drugs, tumors, vitamin B_{12} deficiency, and normal pressure hydrocephalus. It is common for patients with early brain failure to recognize an increasing failure to comprehend written material. Ask the patient, friends, and family the following:

"Have you noticed any change in your memory lately?"
"Do you have difficulty in reading or understanding what you have read?"
"What was the patient's personality like a few years ago?"
"When was the last time the patient seemed normal?"
"What does the patient's diet consist of?" "Does he or she eat well?"
"Can the patient live alone?"

Cerebral Vascular Accidents

Strokes, or cerebral vascular accidents, are common. Most are thromboembolic (80%), but some are hemorrhagic (20%). Thirty percent of patients with a stroke die within the first month. Most patients with strokes have paresis of at least one limb. *Transient ischemic attacks* (TIAs) are short episodes manifested by focal neurologic dysfunction.

They generally last only a few minutes, after which complete recovery occurs. The importance of TIAs is that in 30% of patients, a stroke occurs within 4–5 years.

Gait Disturbances

Gait disturbances may occur for a variety of reasons. Gait may be changed by local pain in the foot, pain in a joint, claudication of the hip or leg, bone disease, vestibular problems, and extrapyramidal disorders. Interruption of the corticospinal tracts in the cerebrum following a stroke produces a spastic weakness in the contralateral leg. The foot is dragged, and the whole leg appears stiff and extended. Lesions in the spinal cord may produce a spastic paralysis affecting both legs. The gait is slow and stiff, with small steps. Patients suffering from Parkinson's disease walk stooped over, with short, quick, shuffling steps. Any patient with a gait disturbance should be asked the following:

> *"Do you have pain in your leg or hip when you walk?"*
> *"Do you have a history of diabetes?"*
> *"Have you ever had syphilis?"*
> *"What do you eat?" "Tell me everything you ate yesterday."*

Patients with vascular occlusive disease of the hip or leg may experience pain while walking and may alter their gait. Diabetes, syphilis, and pernicious anemia may produce a sensory loss, and each condition may result in gait abnormalities.

Tremor

A tremor is a rhythmic motion of the distal parts of the limbs or head. A physiologic tremor has an oscillation of 10–12 cycles per second and is more obvious after exercise. A pathologic tremor is slower. *Parkinson's disease* is the most frequently encountered extrapyramidal movement disorder. In this condition, the tremor is present at rest and is decreased with action. It has a frequency of 3–6 cycles per second and is worsened by anxiety. An intention, or *ataxic,* tremor is slow (at 2–4 cycles per second) and worsens on attempted movement. Multiple sclerosis is one of the many causes of an intention tremor. Metabolic problems from liver or kidney failure are frequently responsible. Withdrawal from alcohol or from caffeine is often a precipitating factor. Any patient with the symptom of a tremor should be asked these questions:

> *"Does the tremor worsen when you try to do something?"*
> *"Is there a history of thyroid disease?"*
> *"Have you been told of any problems with your liver or kidneys?"*
> *"What is your daily consumption of alcoholic beverages?"*
> *"How much coffee or tea do you drink?"*
> *"How much chocolate do you eat?"*

Chorea is involuntary jerky motions of the face and limbs. A common cause is *Huntington's disease,* in which chorea is accompanied by brain failure. The patients frequently present with personality changes and symptoms of brain failure.

"Numbness"

Numbness is another term used by patients to indicate a variety of problems. "Numbness" can be used by patients to describe "pins and needles" sensations, coolness, pain, and clumsiness. The interviewer should be careful to clarify the meaning. The examiner must be careful during the physical examination to palpate the distal pulses in any patient complaining of numbness, because arterial insufficiency is a possible cause.

"Weakness"

"Weakness" may be a symptom of the motor system. A patient with a *proximal arm* motor weakness complains of difficulty in brushing hair, shaving, or reaching up to shelves. A patient with *distal arm* weakness complains of difficulty in putting a button through a buttonhole, using keys, or writing with a pen or pencil. *Proximal leg* weakness is characterized by difficulty in climbing stairs or getting into bed or the bathtub. Foot drop is a classic sign of *distal leg* motor weakness. Chapter 18, The Musculoskeletal System, reviews some of the important questions relating to weakness.

Pain

Pain is an infrequent symptom of neurologic disease, but it does deserve mention. *Trigeminal neuralgia,* also known as *tic douloureux,* is the occurrence of severe, jabbing pain lasting only seconds in the distribution of the maxillary or mandibular divisions of the trigeminal nerve (Fig. 19–10). It is frequently provoked by motion, touch, eating, or exposure to cold temperatures. Another cause of facial pain is the cluster headache, already discussed. *Herpes zoster* infection of a sensory nerve root, also known as *shingles,* manifests with intense pain along the distribution of that nerve root. Three to 4 days later, the classic linear, vesicular skin eruption develops along the distribution of the nerve. Figure 6–53 shows the classic dermatologic manifestations of herpes zoster infection of spinal nerve T3.

Sciatica is intense pain shooting down the leg in the distribution of the sciatic nerve. In this condition, there is an impingement of portions of the sciatic nerve by the vertebrae. Arthritis of the lumbosacral spine is frequently the cause.

Sometimes the paresthesias associated with demyelinating diseases are so intense, the patient may describe them as pain.

Impact of Chronic Neurologic Disease on the Patient

The ramifications of chronic neurologic disease on the patient and the family are enormous. All family members experience emotional pain while observing the progressive clinical changes. The family bears an immense personal burden in assisting the patient to cope with disability.

One example of a progressive neurologic condition is Alzheimer's disease. A devastating chronic disorder of unknown cause, Alzheimer's disease is the most common diffuse brain degeneration causing brain failure. This condition is characterized by progressive and widespread brain degeneration with a hopeless prognosis.

Memory problems and impairment of intellectual function are the main symptoms of Alzheimer's disease. Depression is common. Patients may have significant cognitive impairment, ruining their ability to negotiate in their environment. They may forget

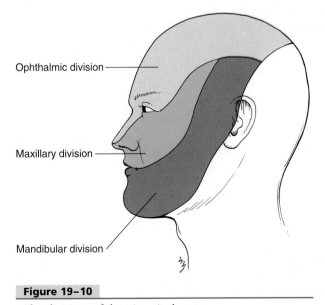

Figure 19–10

The divisions of the trigeminal nerve.

where they live. They might forget to turn off a gas burner on the stove or to put out a cigarette. They may wander aimlessly through the streets.

Patients represent a clinical spectrum from awareness of the disability to a vegetative state. Many patients lose touch with reality. During an interview with such a patient, it may become clear that even the ability to describe the patient's own medical history has been lost.

Early in the course of the disease, patients may use a number of circumlocutions, substituting words when they cannot find the more appropriate ones. Another early change is the disorientation to time and place. Visual hallucinations are common. Sexual disinterest is almost universal. Motor behavior diminishes progressively as impairment of consciousness increases. An important characteristic is the development of bizarre thoughts and fantasies that come to dominate consciousness. Delusions are common, especially delusions of persecution.

In the early stages of the disease, when patients are still aware of their environment but have experienced the symptoms of memory loss, mild depression, anxiety, and irritability are common. As the disease progresses, apathy is the dominant feature. Patients may actually appear indifferent and emotionally withdrawn. In others in whom there is increased motor activity, anxiety and fear are common. In these individuals, terror and panic attacks are not uncommon. Hostility and paranoia develop rapidly. Regression and sudden displays of highly charged emotion are the responses to their frequent hallucinations.

In the milder cases, depression, hypochondriasis, and phobic features abound. Hysterical conversion reactions, such as hysterical blindness, may occur. Social interaction is lost, and the patient may suddenly explode with anger, anxiety, or tears. As the disease progresses, suicidal attempts are common. Emotional lability is often extreme, with periods of laughter followed by crying. With progressive disease, dullness of affect and a lack of an emotional response occur as gross neurologic disability develops. In the terminal stages, patients with Alzheimer's disease may show severe body wasting with profound brain failure.

Physical Examination

The equipment necessary for the neurologic examination is safety pins, cotton-tipped applicators, 128 Hz tuning fork, gauze pads, familiar objects (coins, keys), and a reflex hammer.

The neurologic examination consists of assessment of the following:

- Mental status
- Cranial nerves
- Motor function
- Reflexes
- Sensory function
- Cerebellar function

Mental Status

During the interview, the examiner has already gained much insight into the mental status of the patient. The interviewer may have already been able to assess the patient's remote memory, affect, and judgment. The formal mental status portion of the neurologic examination is introduced by the examiner saying to the patient, "I would like to ask you a few routine questions. Some of them you will find very easy. Others will be more difficult. Do the best you can."

The mental status examination consists of evaluation of the following:

- Level of consciousness
- Speech
- Orientation
- Knowledge of current events
- Judgment

- Abstraction
- Vocabulary
- Emotional responses
- Memory
- Calculation ability
- Object recognition
- Praxis

Assess Level of Consciousness

The level of consciousness can be assessed as soon as you introduce yourself to the patient. Is the patient awake? Alert? Is the patient's sensorium clouded by exogenous or endogenous insults? Does the patient appear confused? If the patient does not respond to your introduction, hold the patient's hand and softly say, "Hello, Mr./Ms. _____, can you hear me? If you hear me, squeeze my hand." If there is no response, try gently shaking the patient. If there is still no response and the patient appears obtunded, squeezing the nipple or applying pressure with your thumb to the bony ridge under the eyebrow is a painful maneuver that may rouse the patient. If these maneuvers fail to awaken the patient, the patient is in *coma*. Patients who are in coma are completely unconscious and cannot be roused even by painful stimuli. If either painful stimulus is used, be careful not to pinch the skin or bruise the patient. If friends or relatives are present, make sure to indicate to them what you are doing.

Evaluate Speech

If the patient is awake and alert, you will have already observed the speech. The patient should now be asked to recite short phrases such as "no ifs, ands, or buts." Is dysarthria, dysphonia, dysphasia, or aphasia present? *Dysarthria* is difficulty in articulation. In general, lesions of the tongue and palate are responsible for dysarthria. *Dysphonia* is difficulty in phonation. The result is an alteration in the volume and the tone of voice. Lesions of the palate and vocal cords are often responsible. *Dysphasia* is difficulty with comprehension or with speech as a result of cerebral dysfunction. Patients with a total loss of speech have *aphasia*. Different areas of the brain are responsible for the different types of aphasia. A motor, expressive, nonfluent aphasia is present when patients know what they want to say but have motor impairment and cannot articulate properly. They understand written and verbal commands but cannot repeat them. A frontal lobe lesion is often the cause. A sensory, receptive, fluent aphasia is present when the patient articulates spontaneously but uses words inappropriately. The patient has difficulty in understanding written and verbal commands and cannot repeat them. A temporoparietal lesion is frequently the cause.

Evaluate Orientation

The patient's orientation to person, place, and time must be established. Orientation refers to the person's awareness of self in relation to other persons, places, and time. Disorientation occurs in association with impairment of memory and attention span. The patient should be asked these questions:

"What is today's date?"
"What is the day of the week?"
"What is the name of this hospital (or building)?"

Evaluate Knowledge of Current Events

A knowledge of current events can be assessed by asking the patient to name the last four presidents of the United States. Asking the patient the name of the mayor or governor is also useful. If the patient is not American or is unfamiliar with American affairs, asking the patient about more general current events may be more useful. The ability to name current events requires an intact orientation, intact recent memory, and the ability to think abstractly.

Assess Judgment

Evaluation of judgment is performed by asking the patient to interpret a simple problem. Ask the patient the following:

> *"What would you do if you noticed an addressed envelope with an uncanceled stamp on it on the street near a mailbox?"*
> *"What would you do if you were in a crowded movie theatre and a fire started?"*

A correct response to the first question would be to pick up the letter and mail it. An example of an incorrect response might be, "I'd throw it in the trash." Judgment requires higher cerebral function.

Assess Abstraction

Abstraction is a higher cerebral function that requires comprehension and judgment. Proverbs are commonly used to test abstract reasoning. The patient should be asked to interpret the following:

> *"People who live in glass houses shouldn't throw stones."*
> *"A rolling stone gathers no moss."*

A patient with an abnormality in abstract reasoning might interpret the first quote by using a *concrete* interpretation such as, "The glass will break if you throw a stone through it." A concrete interpretation of the second proverb might be, "Moss only grows under rocks that don't move and not under a rolling stone." Concrete responses are common in patients with mental retardation or with brain failure. Schizophrenic patients often answer with concrete interpretations, but bizarre assessments are also common. Be careful in assessing abstraction in patients who are not fluent in English.

Another method of testing abstract reasoning is to ask the patient how a pair of items are similar or dissimilar. You might ask, "What is similar about a dog and a cat?" "What is similar about a church and a synagogue?" or "What is dissimilar about an apple and a chicken?"

Assess Vocabulary

Vocabulary is often difficult to assess. It is based on many factors, which include the patient's education, background, work, environment, and cerebral function. It is, however, an important parameter in assessing intellectual capacity. Patients who are mentally retarded have a limited vocabulary, whereas those with mild brain failure have a well-preserved vocabulary. Patients should be asked to define words or use them in sentences. Any words can be used, but they should be asked with increasing levels of difficulty. The examiner may wish to consider these words in the following order:

> Car
> Ability
> Dominant
> Voluntary
> Telescope
> Reticent
> Enigma

Assess Emotional Responses

Although emotional response has probably already been informally observed, inquire specifically whether the patient has noticed any sudden mood changes. It is appropriate for the examiner to ask, "How are your spirits?" During the interview, the interviewer has already noticed the patient's *affect*. Affect is the emotional response to an event. The response may be *appropriate, abnormal,* or *flat*. An appropriate response to a loved one's death may be to cry. An inappropriate response is to laugh. A flat response shows little emotional response. Patients with bilateral cerebral damage lose control of their emotions.

Assess Memory

To test memory, have the patient recall the recent and the remote past. *Recent* memory is easily tested by presenting three words to the patient and asking for them to be repeated 5 minutes later. For example, tell the patient, "Repeat these words after me and remember them. I will ask for them later: necklace, thirty-two, barn." Continue with the mental status examination. Five minutes later, ask the patient, "What were those words I asked you to remember?"

A simpler test of memory is to have the patient recall as many elements in a category as possible. Ask the patient:

"Name as many flowers as you can."
"Name as many occupations as you can."
"Name as many tools as you can."

An abnormality in recent memory may be related to a lesion in the temporal lobe.

To test the *remote past* memory, ask the patient about well-known events in the past. Don't ask about events that you cannot verify.

Assess Calculation Ability

The ability to calculate depends on the integrity of the dominant cerebral hemisphere as well as on the patient's intelligence. Ask the patient to perform simple arithmetic problems, such as subtracting 7 from 100, then 7 from the result, then 7 from the result, and so forth. This is the *serial sevens* test. If there is difficulty with serial sevens, ask the patient to add or subtract several numbers, such as "How much is 5 plus 7? How much is 12 plus 9? How much is 27 minus 9?"

Assess Object Recognition

Object recognition is termed *gnosia*. *Agnosia* is the failure to recognize a sensory stimulus despite normal primary sensation. Show the patient a series of well-known objects, such as coins, pens, eyeglasses, or pieces of clothing, and ask the person to name them. If the patient has normal vision and fails to recognize the object, *visual agnosia* is present. *Tactile agnosia* is the inability to recognize an object by palpation in the absence of a sensory deficit. This occurs with a lesion in the nondominant parietal lobe. *Autotopagnosia* is the term used to describe the inability to recognize a patient's own body part, such as the hand or leg.

Assess Integration of Motor Activity

Praxis is the ability to perform a motor activity. *Apraxia* is the inability to perform a voluntary movement in the absence of deficits in motor strength, sensation, or coordination. *Dyspraxia* is the decreased ability to perform the activity. The patient hears and understands the command but cannot integrate the motor activities that will complete the action. Ask a patient to pour water from the bedside pitcher into a glass and drink the water. A patient with dyspraxia may either drink the water from the pitcher or may drink from the empty glass. A deep frontal lobe lesion is frequently responsible for this disorder.

Another type of apraxia is *constructional apraxia*. In this condition, the patient has an inability to construct or draw simple designs. The examiner draws a shape and asks the patient to copy it. Alternatively, the patient can be asked to draw the face of a clock. Patients with constructional apraxia often have a lesion in the posterior portion of the parietal lobe.

Cranial Nerves

The examination of the cranial nerves should be carried out in an orderly fashion. Several of the cranial nerves have already been evaluated. Table 19–1 lists the cranial nerves, their functions, and the clinical findings when a lesion exists.

▧ Cranial Nerve I: Olfactory

The olfactory nerve supplies nerve endings to the superior nasal concha and upper one third of the nasal septum. The olfactory nerve is not routinely tested. However, any patient in whom a frontal lobe disorder is suspected should be evaluated.

Test Olfaction

The patient is asked to close the eyes and one nostril as the examiner brings a test substance close to the patient's other nostril. The patient is instructed to sniff the test substance. The substance must be volatile and nonirritating, such as cloves, vanilla bean, freshly ground coffee, or lavender. The use of an irritating agent such as alcohol will involve cranial nerve V as well as cranial nerve I, and the test will be inaccurately performed.

Table 19–1 **Cranial Nerves**

Cranial Nerve	Function	Clinical Findings with Lesion
I: Olfactory	Smell	Anosmia
II: Optic	Vision	Amaurosis
III: Oculomotor	Eye movements; pupillary constriction; accommodation	Diplopia; ptosis; mydriasis; loss of accommodation
IV: Trochlear	Eye movements	Diplopia
V: Trigeminal	General sensation of face, scalp, and teeth; chewing movements	"Numbness" of face; weakness of jaw muscles
VI: Abducens	Eye movements	Diplopia
VII: Facial	Taste; general sensation of palate and external ear; lacrimal gland and submandibular and sublingual gland secretion; facial expression	Loss of taste on anterior two thirds of tongue; dry mouth; loss of lacrimation; paralysis of facial muscles
VIII: Vestibulocochlear	Hearing; equilibrium	Deafness; tinnitus; vertigo; nystagmus
IX: Glossopharyngeal	Taste; general sensation of pharynx and ear; elevates palate; parotid gland secretion	Loss of taste on posterior one third of tongue; anesthesia of pharynx; partially dry mouth
X: Vagus	Taste: general sensation of pharynx, larynx, and ear; swallowing; phonation; parasympathetic to heart and abdominal viscera	Dysphagia; hoarseness; palatal paralysis
XI: Spinal accessory	Phonation; head, neck, and shoulder movements	Hoarseness; weakness of head, neck, and shoulder muscles
XII: Hypoglossal	Tongue movements	Weakness and wasting of tongue

Each nostril is tested separately. The examiner asks the patient to identify the test material. A unilateral loss of smell, known as unilateral *anosmia,* is more important than the bilateral loss, because it indicates a lesion affecting the olfactory nerve or tract on that side.

Cranial Nerve II: Optic

The optic nerve ends in the retina. The examinations for visual acuity as well as the ophthalmoscopic examination are discussed in Chapter 8.

Cranial Nerve III: Oculomotor

The oculomotor nerve supplies the medial, superior, and inferior rectus muscles and the inferior oblique muscle, which control most eye movements. The third nerve also innervates the intrinsic muscles, controlling pupillary constriction and accommodation.

Extraocular muscle movements are discussed in Chapter 8. A patient with an oculomotor palsy is shown in Figure 8–55. The pupillary light reflex depends on the function of cranial nerves II and III. This reflex is discussed in Chapter 8. Visual fields are part of the eye examination and the neurologic examination. The technique for visual field testing is discussed in Chapter 8.

Cranial Nerve IV: Trochlear

The trochlear nerve is responsible for the movement of the superior oblique muscle. Extraocular muscle movements are discussed in Chapter 8.

Cranial Nerve V: Trigeminal

The trigeminal nerve is responsible for supplying sensation to the face, the nasal and buccal mucosa, and the teeth. The motor division supplies the muscles of mastication. The three major subdivisions of the trigeminal nerve are the ophthalmic, the maxillary, and the mandibular. These divisions are shown in Figure 19–10.

The *ophthalmic division* supplies sensation to the frontal sinuses, the conjunctiva, the cornea, the upper lid, the bridge of the nose, the forehead, and the scalp as far as the vertex of the skull. The *maxillary division* supplies sensation to the cheek, the maxillary sinus, the lateral aspects of the nose, the upper teeth, the nasal pharynx, the hard palate, and the uvula. The *mandibular division* supplies sensation to the chin, the lower jaw, the anterior two thirds of the tongue, the lower teeth, the gums and floor of the mouth, and the buccal mucosa of the cheek. The motor division supplies the muscles of mastication and the tensor tympani.

The examination of the trigeminal nerve consists of the following:

- Testing the corneal reflex
- Testing the sensory function
- Testing the motor function

Test Corneal Reflex

The corneal reflex depends on the function of cranial nerves V and VII. To evaluate the corneal reflex, the examiner uses a cotton-tipped applicator, the tip of which has been pulled into a thin strand about ½ inch in length. The examiner then stabilizes the patient's head by placing a hand on the patient's eyebrow and head. The patient is asked to look to the right side as the cotton tip is brought in from the left side to touch the left cornea gently. This is shown in Figure 19–11. A prompt bilateral reflex closure of the lids is the normal response. The examination is repeated on the other side by reversing the directions.

The responses on the two sides are compared. The sensory limb of the corneal reflex is the ophthalmic division of the trigeminal nerve; the motor limb is conducted through the facial nerve.

In performing the corneal reflex, touch the cornea and not the eyelashes or conjunctiva, which will give an inaccurate result.

Test Sensory Function

The sensory function of the trigeminal nerve is tested by asking the patient to close the eyes and to respond when a touch is felt. A piece of gauze is applied to one side of the forehead and then to the corresponding position on the other side. This test is then performed on the cheeks, and then on the jaw, testing all three subdivisions of the nerve. The patient is also asked if one side feels the same as or different than the other side. The examination is shown in Figure 19–12.

The procedure is repeated with the use of a sharp pin, alternating between the sides.

Test Motor Function

The motor function of the trigeminal nerve is tested by having the patient bite down or clench the teeth while the masseter and temporalis muscles are palpated bilaterally.

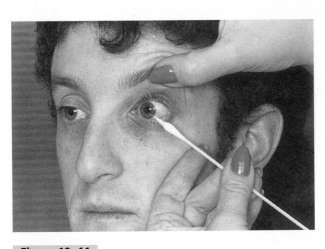

Figure 19–11

Technique for evaluating the corneal reflex.

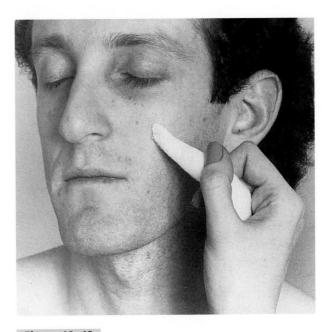

Figure 19–12

Technique for testing the sensory function of the trigeminal nerve.

This is shown in Figure 19–13. Unilateral weakness will cause the jaw to deviate toward the side of the lesion.

Cranial Nerve VI: Abducens

The abducens nerve is responsible for movement of the lateral rectus muscle. Extraocular muscle movements are discussed in Chapter 8.

Cranial Nerve VII: Facial

The facial nerve innervates the facial muscles and supplies taste to the anterior two thirds of the tongue. A small component also supplies general sensation to the external ear. The facial nerve also carries parasympathetic motor fibers to the salivary glands and chorda tympani. Testing for abnormalities of taste is generally not performed by an internist.

Test Motor Function

The patient is asked to bare the teeth while the examiner observes for asymmetry. The patient is asked to puff out the cheeks against resistance and then to wrinkle the forehead. It is helpful if the examiner actually demonstrates these maneuvers for the patient. These maneuvers are shown in Figure 19–14.

The patient is then asked to close the eyes tightly while the examiner tries to open them. The patient is told to close the eyes as tightly as possible. The examiner can say, "Don't let me open them." This procedure is demonstrated in Figure 19–15*A*. Each eye is examined separately, and the strengths are compared. Normally the examiner should not be able to open the patient's eyes. Look at the patient in Figure 19–15*B*. Notice the marked weakness of the left orbicularis oculi muscle as a result of a stroke involving the facial nucleus.

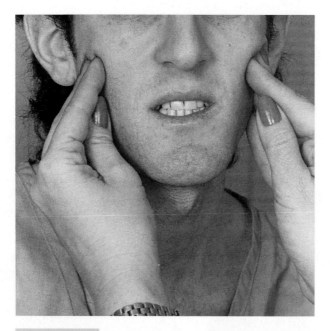

Figure 19–13

Technique for testing the motor function of the trigeminal nerve.

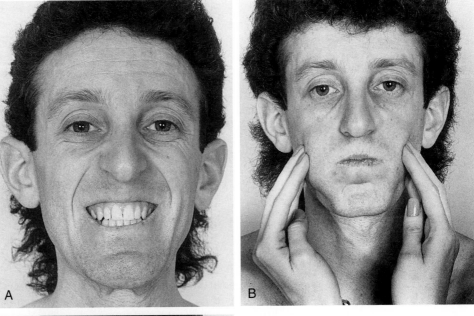

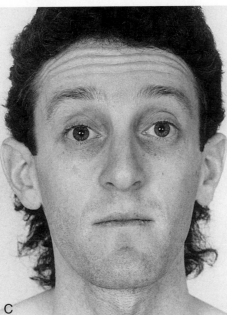

Figure 19–14

Testing the facial nerve. *A* and *B*, Tests for the lower division. *C*, Test for the upper division.

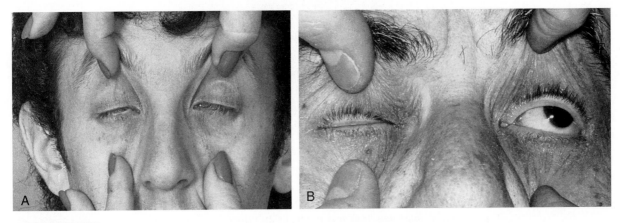

Figure 19–15

Testing the strength of eyelid closure. *A*, Normal response. Note that the eyelids cannot be opened by the examiner. *B*, Test in a patient with a stroke that involved the facial nerve nucleus. Note the loss in strength of the muscle around the left eye.

The innervations of the facial nerve are shown in Figure 19–16. There are two types of facial weakness. Upper motor neuron lesions such as a stroke involving the corticobulbar pathways will produce contralateral weakness of the lower face, with normal function of the upper face. The patient will still be able to wrinkle the forehead. This is related to the bilateral innervation of the upper face by the corticobulbar fibers. The lower face has only unilateral innervation from contralateral cortical centers. This type of upper motor neuron lesion is illustrated by lesion A in Figure 19–16. The second type of facial weakness will produce total involvement of the ipsilateral facial muscles, with no area being spared. This may result from lesions of the nerve as it exits from the skull or from involvement of the facial nucleus in the pons, as shown by lesion B in Figure 19–16.

Look at the patient in Figure 19–17. When he was asked to smile, the right side of his face was drawn to the left. This patient has a right facial palsy, also known as a right Bell's palsy. Further maneuvers revealed that the entire right side of his face was involved as a result of a lesion affecting the right facial nucleus.

Cranial Nerve VIII: Vestibulocochlear

The vestibulocochlear nerve is responsible for hearing, balance, and an awareness of position. Auditory testing is discussed in Chapter 9. Tests for the vestibular function of cranial nerve VIII are generally not performed.

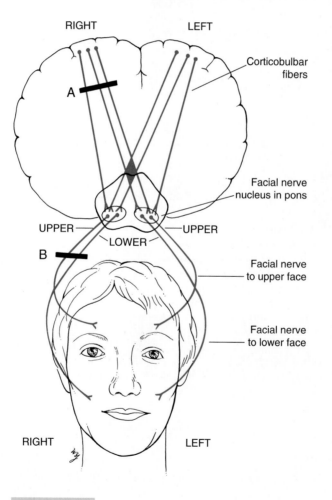

Figure 19–16

Types of facial weakness. Lesion *A* produces an upper motor nerve palsy that produces contralateral weakness of the lower face but spares the contralateral forehead. Lesion *B* produces a lower motor nerve palsy that produces total paralysis of the ipsilateral face.

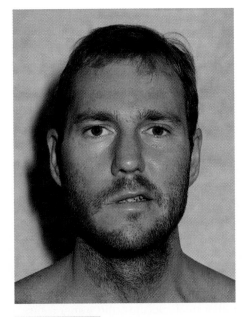

Figure 19–17

Right facial palsy.

Cranial Nerve IX: Glossopharyngeal

The glossopharyngeal nerve supplies sensation to the pharynx, posterior one third of the tongue, and tympanic membrane as well as secretory fibers to the parotid gland.

Test Sensory Function

Examination of the glossopharyngeal nerve involves the gag reflex. The examiner may use either a tongue blade or an applicator stick. By touching the posterior third of the tongue, the soft palate, or the posterior pharyngeal wall, the examiner should elicit a gag reflex. The sensory portion of the loop is through the glossopharyngeal nerve; the motor is mediated through the vagus nerve.

Another way of testing the nerve is to ask the patient to open the mouth widely and to say, "Ah . . . Ah. . . . " Symmetric elevation of the soft palate demonstrates normal function of cranial nerves IX and X. The uvula should remain in the midline.

Taste sensation of the posterior third of the tongue is not routinely tested.

Cranial Nerve X: Vagus

The vagus nerve supplies parasympathetic fibers to the viscera of the chest and abdomen; motor fibers to the pharynx and larynx; and sensory fibers to the external ear canal, meninges of the posterior cranial fossa, pharynx, larynx, and viscera of the body cavities above the pelvis.

Examination of the vagus nerve was performed with evaluation of the glossopharyngeal nerve.

Dysphonia or dysarthria may result from paralysis of the vagus nerve.

Cranial Nerve XI: Spinal Accessory

The spinal accessory nerve is a motor nerve that supplies the sternocleidomastoid and trapezius muscles.

Test Motor Function

The right spinal accessory nerve is examined by asking the patient to turn the head to the left against the resistance of the examiner's hand. This is shown in Figure 19–18. The left spinal accessory nerve is examined by reversing the directions.

An alternate test is to evaluate the trapezius muscles. The examiner places both hands on the trapezius muscles of the patient. Both muscles are palpated between the thumb and index fingers. The patient is then asked to shrug the shoulders against the resistance of the examiner's hands. Both sides should be equal. This technique is shown in Figure 19–19.

■ Cranial Nerve XII: Hypoglossal

The hypoglossal nerve supplies motor fibers to the muscles of the tongue. The examination of the hypoglossal nerve is performed by asking the patient to open the mouth, with the tongue resting quietly at the floor of the mouth. Inspection for *fasciculations** is performed. Fasciculations are indicative of a hypoglossal lower–motor-neuron lesion.

Test Motor Function

Ask the patient to open the mouth and stick out the tongue. Normally, the tongue is protruded and lies in the midline. This is shown in Figure 19–20. Deviation of the tongue to either side is abnormal. Because the tongue muscles push rather than pull, weakness of one side will result in the tongue's being pushed by the normal side to the side of the lesion.

Look at the tongue of the patient in Figure 19–21. Notice the marked scalloping of the tongue's surface. This is a patient with a chronic neurologic disease known as *amyotrophic lateral sclerosis,*† characterized by progressive degeneration of motor neurons. This patient had the typical features of a lower–motor-neuron bulbar palsy affecting the hypoglossal nucleus: wasting of the tongue with fasciculations.

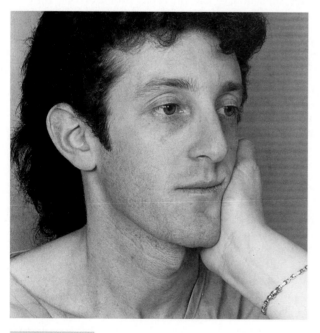

Figure 19–18

Technique for evaluating the spinal accessory nerve.

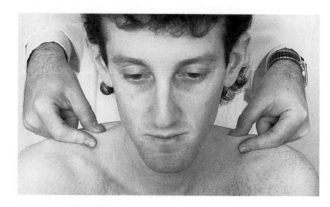

Figure 19–19

Alternate technique for evaluating the spinal accessory nerve.

---

* Spontaneous contractions of groups of muscles visible on inspection.

† This disease is also called *Lou Gehrig's disease,* after the famous baseball player who was one of its victims.

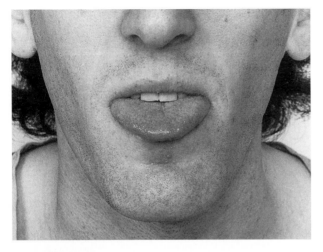

Figure 19–20

Technique for evaluating the hypoglossal nerve.

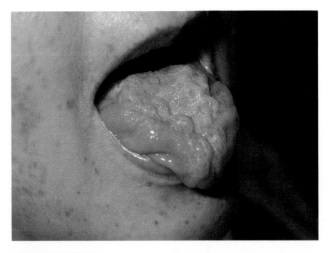

Figure 19–21

Amyotrophic lateral sclerosis. Note the scalloping of the tongue.

Motor Function

■ Principles of Testing Motor Function

The motor system is evaluated for the following:

- Muscle bulk
- Muscle strength
- Muscle tone

The motor examination begins with inspection of each area being examined. Compare the contours of symmetric *muscle masses*. Inspection is used to determine muscle atrophy and the presence of fasciculations.

Test *muscle strength* by having the patient move actively against your resistance. Compare one side with the other. The following is an arbitrary scale that is commonly used for the grading of muscle strength:

0: **Absent**   No contraction detected
1: **Trace**   Slight contraction detected
2: **Weak**   Movement with gravity eliminated
3: **Fair**   Movement against gravity
4: **Good**   Movement against gravity with some resistance
5: **Normal**   Movement against gravity with full resistance

If a muscle weakness is found, compare the proximal and distal strengths. In general, proximal weakness is related to muscle disease; distal weakness is related to neurologic disease.

Tone can be defined as the slight residual tension in a voluntarily relaxed muscle. Tone is assessed by resistance to passive movement. Ask the patient to relax. Perform passive motion of the muscle. Compare one side with the other. Upper motor neuron lesions produce spasticity,* hyperreflexia, clonus,† and Babinski's‡ sign. Lower motor neuron lesions produce atrophy, fasciculations, decreased tone, and hyporeflexia. Both types of lesions result in weakness. Fasciculations may become more apparent by gently tapping the muscle with a reflex hammer.

It is impractical to test all muscles during the neurologic examination. By testing key muscle groups, the examiner can determine whether a gross deficit exists. Further

---

* An increase in muscle tone that results in continuous resistance to stretching. Spasticity is generally worse at extremes of range.
† Spasm in which there is alternating rigidity and relaxation in rapid succession.
‡ Dorsiflexion of the big toe upon stimulating the sole of the foot.

testing of specific muscles and nerve roots may then be necessary. The student is referred to the many textbooks on neurology for these detailed examinations.

In the assessment of motor function, the upper extremities are examined first.

■ Inspect the Upper Extremities for Symmetry

Ask the patient to sit off the side of the bed facing you. Inspect both arms and hands for size differences, paying special attention to the size of the thumbs and the small muscles of the hands. Is muscle wasting present?

■ Test Flexion and Extension of the Arm

Test flexion and extension strength of the upper extremity by having the patient pull and push against your resistance. You might say, "Push down . . . relax." "Push up . . . relax." "Push back . . . relax." "Push forward . . . relax." Say "Relax" after each direction so that the patient will not continue to push or pull after you have removed your hands. After one side is tested, the other is tested, and the two sides are compared.

■ Test Arm Abduction

Ask the patient to extend the arms, with palms facing down. Place your hands at the lateral aspect of the patient's arms. Instruct the patient to abduct the arms against resistance. This tests abduction of the arm by the *axillary nerve* from roots C5–C6. This test is shown in Figure 19–22.

■ Test Forearm Flexion

Have the patient make a fist and flex the forearm. Hold the patient's fist or wrist. Ask the patient to pull the arm in against your resistance. This tests flexion of the forearm by the *musculocutaneous nerve* from roots C5–C6. This test is shown in Figure 19–23.

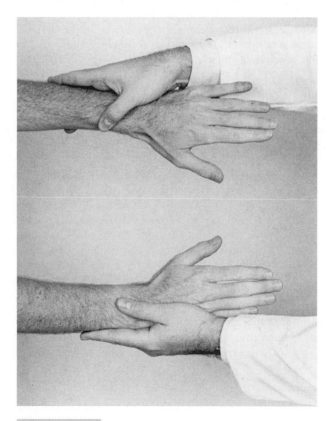

Figure 19–22

Technique for testing abduction of the arm.

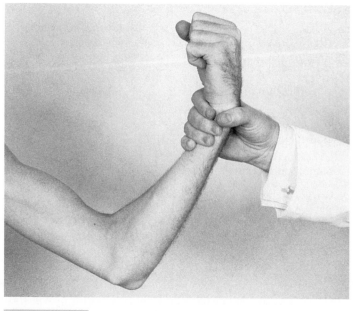

Figure 19–23

Technique for testing flexion of the forearm.

■ Test Forearm Extension

Ask the patient to abduct the arm and hold it midway between flexion and extension. Support the patient's arm by holding the wrist. Instruct the patient to extend the arm against your resistance. This tests extension of the forearm by the *radial nerve* from roots C6–C8. This test is shown in Figure 19–24.

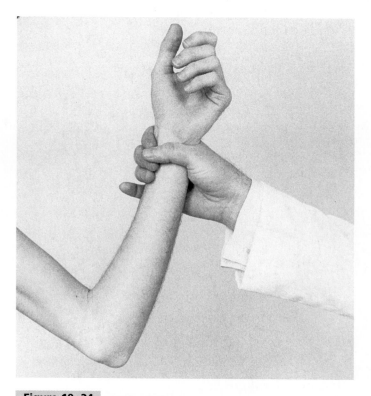

Figure 19–24

Technique for testing extension of the forearm.

■ Test Wrist Extension

Instruct the patient to make a fist and extend the wrist while you attempt to push it up. This tests extension of the wrist by the *radial nerve* from roots C6–C8. This test is shown in Figure 19–25.

■ Test Wrist Flexion

The patient is asked to make a fist and flex the wrist and you attempt to pull it down. This tests flexion of the wrist by the *median nerve* from roots C6–C7. This test is shown in Figure 19–26.

■ Test Finger Adduction

The patient is asked to grasp your extended index and middle fingers and to squeeze them as hard as possible. Compare the strengths of both hands. (It is important for the examiner to remove any finger rings, which may produce discomfort.) This tests adduction of the fingers by the *median nerve* from roots C7–T1. This procedure is shown in Figure 19–27.

■ Test Finger Abduction

Ask the patient to extend the hand with the palm down and to spread the fingers as widely as possible. Tell the patient to resist your attempt to bring the fingers together. This tests abduction of the fingers by the *ulnar nerve* from roots C8–T1. This is shown in Figure 19–28.

■ Test Thumb Adduction

The patient is instructed to touch the base of the little finger with the tip of the thumb against resistance while the thumbnail remains parallel to the palm. This tests adduction of the thumb by the *median nerve* from roots C8–T1. This test is shown in Figure 19–29.

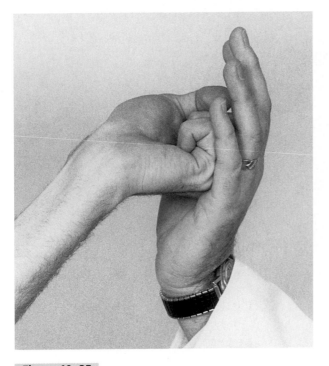

Figure 19–25

Technique for testing extension of the wrist.

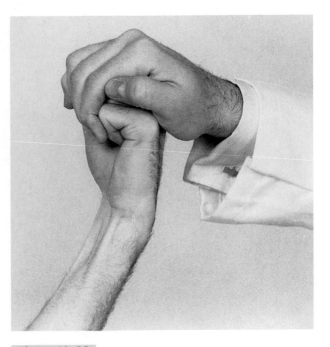

Figure 19–26

Technique for testing flexion of the wrist.

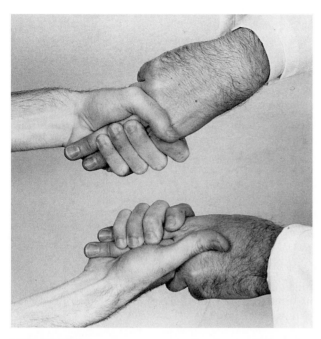

Figure 19-27

Technique for testing finger adduction.

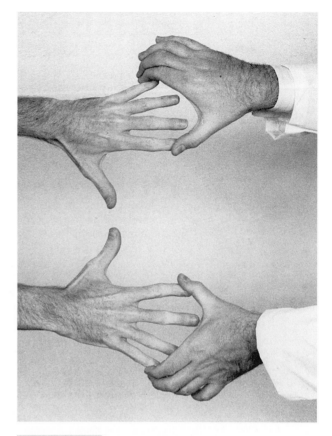

Figure 19-28

Technique for testing finger abduction.

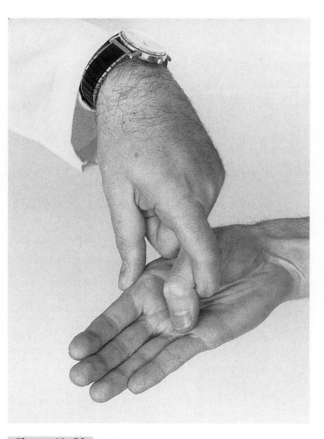

Figure 19-29

Technique for testing thumb adduction.

■ **Assess Upper Extremity Tone**

Tone is assessed in the patient's upper limbs by passive flexing and extending the limbs to determine the amount of resistance to the examiner's movements. Increased resistance, as in muscle rigidity or spasticity, means increased muscle tone. Decreased resistance, as in limpness or flaccidity, means decreased muscle tone. Normal tone has a smooth sensation. In extrapyramidal disease, palpation of a proximal muscle during passive movement will detect the presence of *cogwheeling,* which is a ratchety jerkiness to the motion.

■ **Inspect the Lower Extremities for Symmetry**

The lower extremities are now examined for muscle bulk and muscle wasting. This examination is performed with the patient lying on the back in bed. As with the upper extremities, proximal and distal muscle strengths are compared as well as the symmetry of one leg with the other.

■ **Test Hip Adduction**

Ask the patient to move the legs apart. Place your hands on the medial aspect of the patient's knees. Instruct the patient to close the legs against your resistance. This tests adduction of the hips by the *obturator nerve* from roots L2–L4. This procedure is shown in Figure 19–30.

■ **Test Hip Abduction**

Place your hands on the lateral margins of the patient's knees. Ask the patient to open the legs against your resistance. This tests abduction of the hips by the *superior gluteal nerve* from roots L4–S1. This test is shown in Figure 19–31.

■ **Test Knee Flexion**

Ask the patient to elevate a knee, with the foot resting on the bed. Instruct the patient to hold the foot down as you try to extend the leg. This tests flexion of the knee by the *sciatic nerve* from roots L4–S1. This test is shown in Figure 19–32.

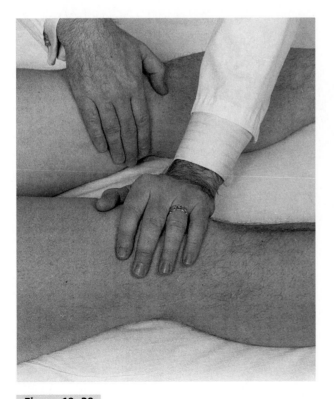

Figure 19–30

Technique for testing hip adduction.

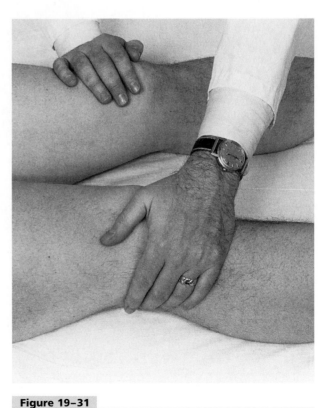

Figure 19–31

Technique for testing hip abduction.

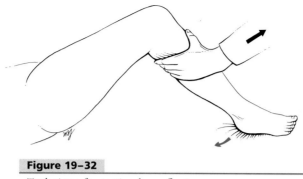

Figure 19–32

Technique for testing knee flexion.

■ **Test Knee Extension**

Instruct the patient to elevate the knee, with the foot resting on the bed. Place your left hand under the knee. Ask the patient to straighten the leg against the resistance of your right hand, which is placed on the patient's shin. This procedure tests extension of the knee by the *femoral nerve* from roots L2–L4. This test is shown in Figure 19–33.

■ **Test Ankle Dorsiflexion**

Place your hands on the dorsum of the foot, and ask the patient to dorsiflex the foot at the ankle against your resistance. This tests dorsiflexion of the ankle by the *deep peroneal nerve* from roots L4–L5. This maneuver is shown in Figure 19–34.

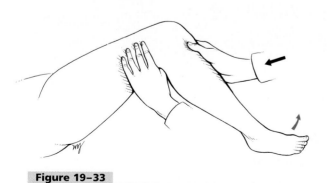

Figure 19–33

Technique for testing knee extension.

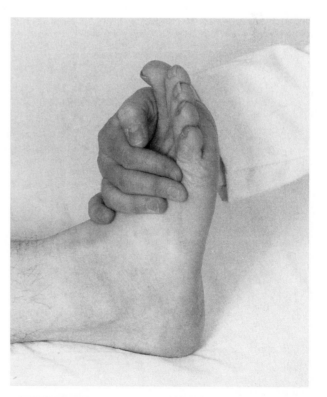

Figure 19–34

Technique for testing ankle dorsiflexion.

■ Test Ankle Plantar Flexion

Place your hand on the sole, and ask the patient to plantarflex the foot at the ankle against your resistance. This tests plantar flexion of the ankle by the *tibial nerve* from roots L5–S2. The test is shown in Figure 19–35.

■ Test Great Toe Dorsiflexion

Place your hand on the dorsal aspect of the patient's big toe. Ask the patient to dorsiflex the big toe against your resistance. This tests dorsiflexion of the big toe by the *deep peroneal nerve* from roots L4–S1. This test is shown in Figure 19–36.

■ Test Great Toe Plantar Flexion

Place your hand on the plantar surface of the patient's big toe. The patient is asked to plantarflex the great toe against your resistance. This tests plantar flexion of the great toe by the *posterior tibial nerve* from roots L5–S2. This test is shown in Figure 19–37.

■ Assess Lower Extremity Tone

Tone in the lower extremities is assessed as in the upper extremities.

Grasp the foot, and passively dorsiflex and plantarflex it several times, and end with dorsiflexion of the foot. If a sudden rhythmic involuntary dorsiflexion and plantar flexion occur, *ankle clonus* is present. This frequently occurs in conditions of increased tone.

If any abnormality is noted in the motor strength of the upper or lower extremity, a more detailed examination should be performed. Table 19–7 at the end of this chapter lists the muscle innervations and their actions.

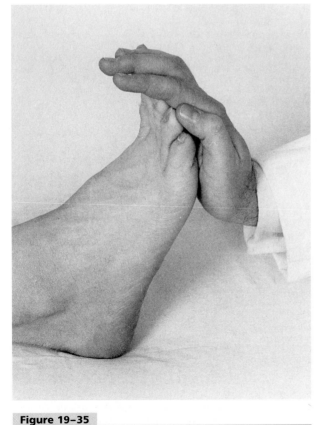

Figure 19–35

Technique for testing plantar flexion.

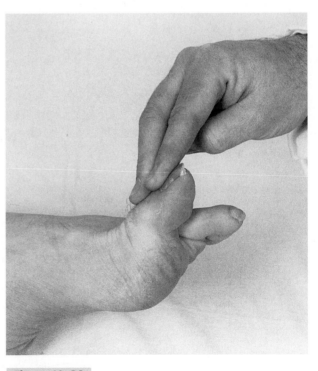

Figure 19–36

Technique for testing great toe dorsiflexion.

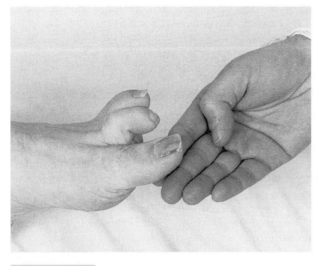

Figure 19-37

Technique for testing great toe plantar flexion.

Reflexes

▨ Basic Principles

Two main types of reflexes are tested. They are the *stretch,* or deep tendon, reflexes and the *superficial* reflexes.

To elicit a stretch reflex, support the joint being tested so that the muscle is relaxed. The reflex hammer is held between the thumb and the index finger and is swung by motion at the wrist, not the elbow. In general, the pointed end of a triangular reflex hammer is used. A gentle tap over the tendon being tested should produce muscle contraction. It is often necessary to palpate as well as observe the muscle to assess its contraction. Test each reflex, and compare it with the other side. Reflexes should be symmetrically equal.

There is a variation in the reflex response. Only with experience will the examiner be able to make an adequate assessment of normal reflexes. Reflexes are commonly graded on a scale from 0 to 4+ as follows:

0   No response
1+   Diminished
2+   Normal
3+   Increased
4+   Hyperactive

Hyperactive reflexes are characteristic of pyramidal tract disease. Electrolyte abnormalities, hyperthyroidism, and other metabolic abnormalities may be the cause of hyperactive reflexes. *Diminished* reflexes are characteristic of anterior horn cell disorders and myopathies. The examiner should always consider the strength of the reflex to the bulk of the muscle mass. A patient may have diminished reflexes as a result of a decrease in muscle bulk. Patients with hypothyroidism have decreased relaxation after a deep tendon reflex, which is termed a *hung* reflex.

In a patient with a diminished reflex, the technique of *reinforcement* may be useful. By asking the patient to perform isometric contraction of other muscles, the generalized reflex activity may be increased. In testing reflexes on the upper extremities, have the patient clench the teeth or push down on the bed with the thighs. In testing reflexes on the lower extremities, have the patient lock fingers and try to pull them apart at the time of testing. This procedure is sometimes called *Jendrassik's maneuver*. This is shown in Figure 19–38.

The deep tendon reflexes that are routinely tested are as follows:

- Biceps
- Brachioradialis
- Triceps
- Patellar
- Achilles

Test Biceps Tendon Reflex

The *biceps tendon* reflex is assessed by having the patient relax the arm and pronate the forearm midway between flexion and extension. The examiner should place a thumb firmly on the biceps tendon. The hammer is then struck on the examiner's thumb. This is shown in Figure 19–39. The examiner should observe for contraction of the biceps followed by flexion at the elbow. The examiner may also palpate the contraction of the muscle. This reflex tests the nerves at roots C5–C6.

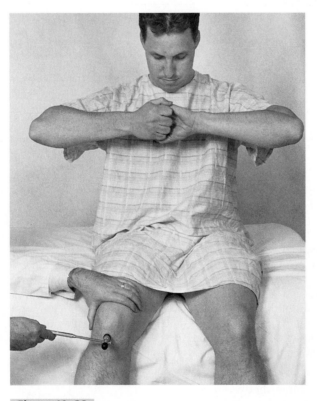

Figure 19–38

Jendrassik's maneuver.

Figure 19–39

Technique for testing for the biceps tendon reflex.

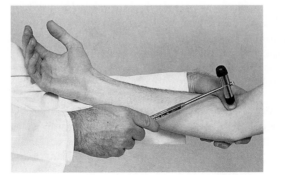

■ **Test Brachioradialis Tendon Reflex**

The *brachioradialis tendon* reflex is performed by having the patient's forearm in semiflexion and semipronation. The arm should be rested on the patient's knee. If a triangular reflex hammer is used, the wide end should strike the styloid process of the radius about 1–2 inches above the wrist. The examiner should observe for flexion at the elbow and simultaneous supination of the forearm. The position is shown in Figure 19–40. This reflex tests the nerves at roots C5–C6.

■ **Test Triceps Tendon Reflex**

The *triceps tendon* reflex is tested by flexing the patient's forearm at the elbow and pulling the arm toward the chest. The elbow should be midway between flexion and extension. Tap the triceps tendon above the insertion of the ulna's olecranon process about 1–2 inches above the elbow. There should be a prompt contraction of the triceps with extension at the elbow. This technique is shown in Figure 19–41. This reflex tests the nerves at roots C6–C8.

If the triceps reflex cannot be elicited by this maneuver, try to hang the patient's arm over your arm, as shown in Figure 19–42. Tapping the triceps tendon in this position will often elicit the reflex.

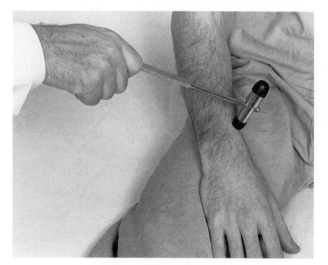

Figure 19–40

Technique for testing for the brachioradialis tendon reflex.

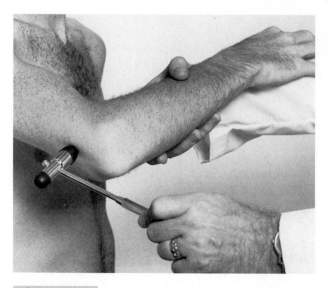

Figure 19–41

Technique for testing for the triceps tendon reflex.

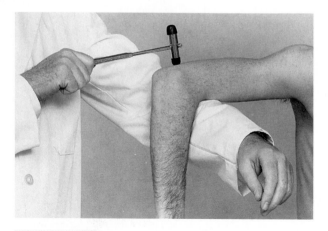

Figure 19–42

Another test for the triceps tendon reflex.

Test Patellar Tendon Reflex

Perform the *patellar reflex*, also known as the *knee jerk*, by having the patient sit with legs dangling off the side of the bed. Place your hand on the patient's quadriceps muscle. Strike the patellar tendon firmly with the base of the reflex hammer. A contraction of the quadriceps should be felt, and extension at the knee should be observed. This technique is shown in Figure 19–43. This reflex tests the nerves at roots L2–L4.

Test Achilles Tendon Reflex

The *Achilles reflex*, also known as the *ankle jerk*, is elicited by having the patient sit with feet dangling off the side of the bed. The leg should be flexed at the hip and the knee. The examiner should place a hand under the patient's foot to dorsiflex the ankle. The Achilles tendon is struck just above its insertion on the posterior aspect of the calcaneus with the wide end of the reflex hammer. This is shown in Figure 19–44. The result is plantar flexion at the ankle. This tests the nerves at roots S1–S2.

Another method of testing for the Achilles reflex is to have the patient lie in bed. Flex one of the patient's legs at the hip and knee, and rotate the leg externally so that it lies on the opposite shin. Again dorsiflex the ankle as the tendon is struck. This test is shown in Figure 19–45*A*.

A patient with a depressed Achilles reflex should be asked to kneel, if possible, on the bed with the feet hanging off the side, as shown in Figure 19–45*B*. Tap the Achilles tendon, and observe the reflex response in this position.

Test Superficial Reflexes

The most commonly tested superficial reflexes are the abdominal and the cremasteric. The *abdominal* superficial reflex is elicited by having the patient lie on the back. An applicator stick or tongue blade is quickly stroked horizontally laterally to medially toward the umbilicus. The result is a contraction of the abdominal muscles, with the umbilicus deviating toward the stimulus. The abdominal reflex is frequently not seen in obese individuals. The *cremasteric* superficial reflex in men is elicited by lightly stroking the inner aspect of the thigh with an applicator stick or tongue depressor. The result is a rapid elevation of the testicle on the same side. Although the superficial

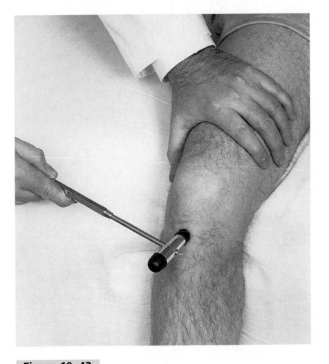

Figure 19–43

Technique for testing for the patellar tendon reflex.

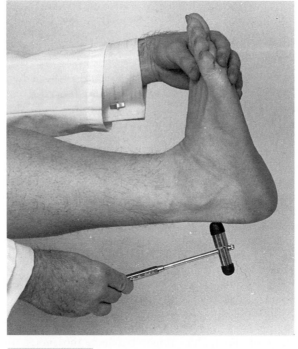

Figure 19–44

Technique for testing for the Achilles tendon reflex.

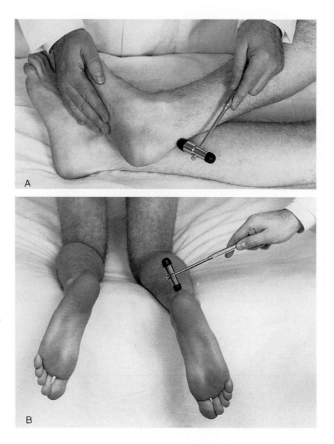

Figure 19–45

A, Alternative technique for evaluating the Achilles tendon reflex. *B,* Technique for assessing the Achilles tendon reflex when the reflex appears to be depressed.

reflexes are absent on the side of a corticospinal tract lesion, there is little clinical significance to their presence or absence. They are indicated here for completeness only.

■ Test for Abnormal Reflexes

Babinski's sign or *reflex* is a pathologic reflex. Normally, when the lateral aspect of the sole is stroked from the heel to the ball of the foot and curved medially across the heads of the metatarsal bones, there is plantar flexion of the big toe. This tests the nerve roots at L5–S2. The foot should be stroked with a noxious stimulus such as a key. A pin should *never* be used. In the presence of pyramidal tract disease, when the described movement is performed, there is a *dorsiflexion* of the big toe, with fanning of the other toes. This is Babinski's reflex. Because Babinski's sign is an abnormal reflex, one should comment only that Babinski's sign is present; it is never absent. It is correct to describe the plantar reflex as either plantar flexion (normal) or dorsiflexion (abnormal, Babinski's). The technique for evaluating the plantar reflex is shown in Figure 19–46.

Pyramidal tract disease is also suggested when the big toe dorsiflexes upon stroking the lateral aspect of the foot. This is *Chaddock's sign.* In the presence of pyramidal tract disease, downward pressure along the shin will also cause the big toe to dorsiflex. This is *Oppenheim's sign.* The elicitation of these signs is less sensitive than stroking the plantar surface.

Another abnormal reflex associated with pyramidal tract disease is *Hoffmann's sign.* To elicit this sign, the patient's hand is pronated, and the examiner grasps the terminal phalanx of the middle finger between the index finger and thumb. With a sharp jerk, the phalanx is passively flexed and suddenly released. A positive response consists of adduction and flexion of the thumb as well as flexion of the other fingers.

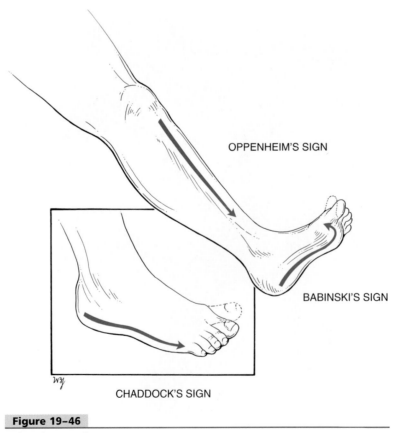

OPPENHEIM'S SIGN

BABINSKI'S SIGN

CHADDOCK'S SIGN

Figure 19–46

The plantar reflex.

Sensory Function

■ **Basic Principles**

The sensory examination consists of testing for the following:

- Light touch
- Pain sensation
- Vibration sense
- Proprioception
- Tactile localization
- Discriminative sensations (two-point discrimination, stereognosis, graphesthesia, and point localization)

In a patient without any symptoms or signs of neurologic disease, the examination for sensory function can be performed by quickly assessing the presence of normal sensation on the distal fingers and toes. The examiner can choose to test for light touch, pain, and vibration sense. If these are normal, the details of the rest of the sensory examination are not required. If symptoms or signs are referable to a neurologic disorder, complete testing is indicated.

As with the motor examination, the examiner compares side with side and proximal with distal. Neurologic disorders usually result in a sensory loss that is first seen more distally than proximally.

The hand is supplied by the median, ulnar, and radial nerves. The median nerve is the chief nerve of sensation because it supplies the palmar surfaces of the digits, the parts of the hand most commonly employed for feeling. The ulnar nerve supplies sensation only to the ulnar one-and-a-half fingers. The radial nerve has its sensory distribution to the dorsum of the hand. There is considerable overlap in innervation. The clinically most reliable cutaneous areas for testing these nerves are illustrated in Figure 19–47. These areas have the least likelihood of overlapping innervation.

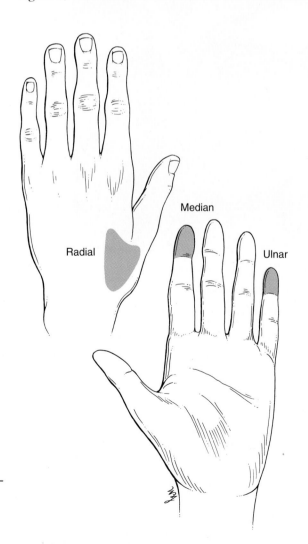

Radial

Median

Ulnar

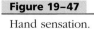
Figure 19–47

Hand sensation.

Test Light Touch

Light touch is evaluated by lightly touching the patient with a small piece of gauze. Ask the patient to close eyes and to tell you when the touch is felt. Try touching the patient on the toes and fingers. This is shown in Figure 19–48. If sensation is normal, continue with the next test. If sensation is abnormal, work proximally until a *sensory level* can be determined. A sensory level is a spinal cord level below which there is a marked decrease in sensation. Figure 19–49 shows the segmental distribution of the spinal nerves that transmit sensation to the spinal cord.

Test Pain Sensation

Pain sensation is tested by using a safety pin and asking the patient if it is felt. Ask the patient to close eyes. Open the safety pin and touch the patient with its tip. Tell the patient, "This is sharp." Now touch the patient with the blunt end of the pin and say,

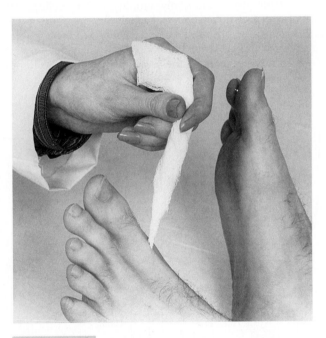

Figure 19–48

Technique for testing light touch.

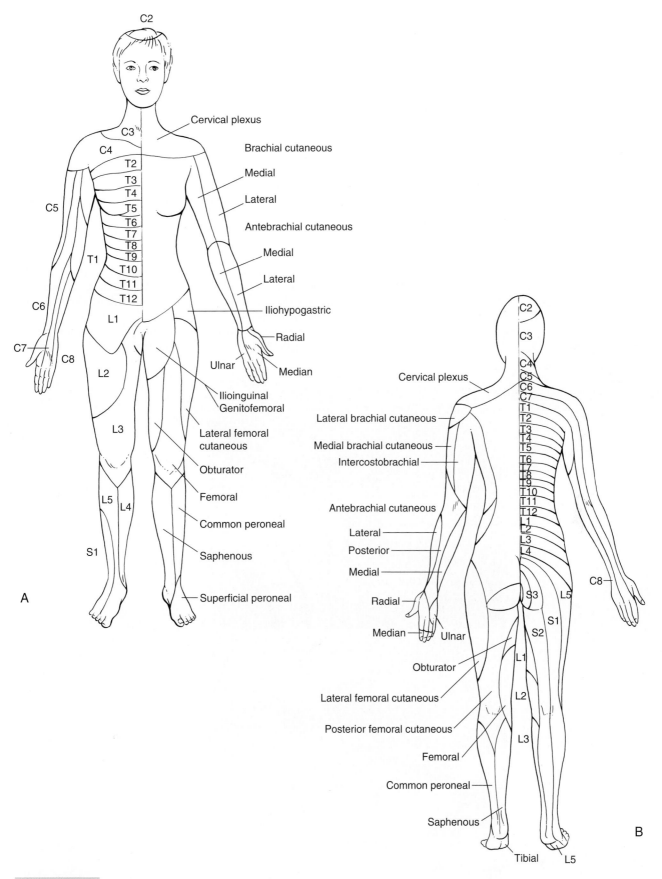

Figure 19–49

Segmental distribution of the spinal nerves. *A,* Distribution in the front. *B,* Distribution in the back.

"This is dull." This is shown in Figure 19–50. Start testing pain sensation on the toes and fingers and say, "What is this, sharp or dull?" If the patient has no loss of sensation, proceed with the next examination. If there is a sensory loss to pain, continue proximally to determine the sensory level. A new pin should be used for each patient.

Test Vibration Sense

Vibration sense is tested using a 128 Hz tuning fork. Tap the tuning fork on the heel of your hand, and place it on the patient on a bone prominence distally. Instruct the patient to inform you when the vibration is no longer felt. Ask the patient to close eyes. Place the vibrating tuning fork over the distal phalanx of the patient's finger and your own finger under the patient's finger, as shown in Figure 19–51A. In this manner, you will be able to feel the vibration through the patient's finger to determine the accuracy of the patient's response. After the fingers are tested, test the big toes as shown in Figure 19–51B. If there is no loss of vibration sense, proceed with the next examination. If a loss is present, determine the level.

Test Proprioception

Position sense, or proprioception, is tested by moving the distal phalanx. Hold the distal phalanx at its *lateral* aspects, and move the digit up while telling the patient, "This is up." Move the distal phalanx down, and tell the patient, "This is down." With the patient's eyes closed, move the distal phalanx up and down and finally stop and ask, "What is this, up or down?" This is shown in Figure 19–52A. Grasp only the *sides* of the digit so that the patient will not have a clue by the pressure exerted on the digit.

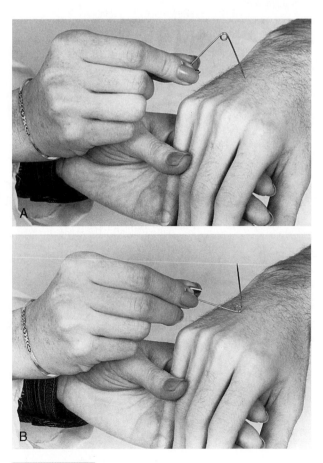

Figure 19–50

Technique for testing pain sensation. The examiner should hold the pin as shown in *A* and say, "This is sharp." "This is dull" is illustrated in *B*.

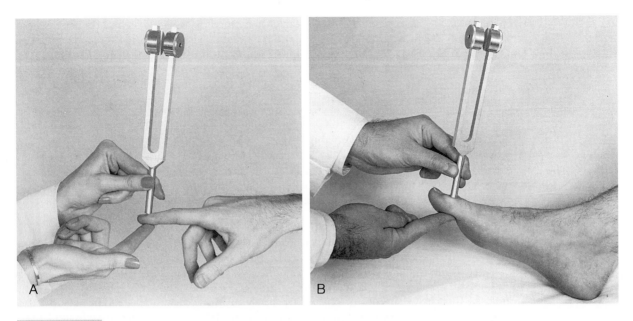

Figure 19–51

Technique for testing vibration sensation. *A,* Correct position for evaluating the vibration sensation in the finger. *B,* The technique for a toe.

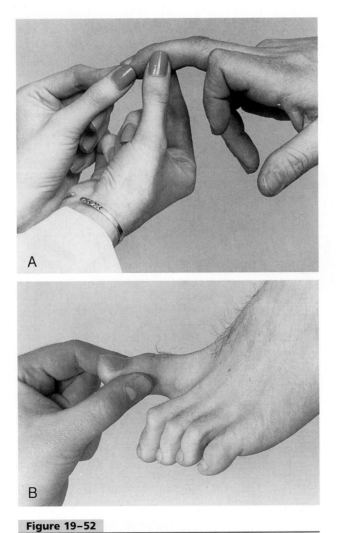

Figure 19–52

Technique for testing proprioception. *A,* Correct manner of holding the digit. *B,* Technique for the toe.

It is routine to test the terminal phalanx of a finger on each hand and the terminal phalanx of the toes (Fig. 19–52*B*). If no loss of position sense is detected, continue with the rest of the examination. A loss requires further evaluation to determine the level of loss of proprioception.

Test Tactile Localization

Tactile localization, also known as double simultaneous stimulation, is assessed by having the patient close eyes while identifying where your touch was felt. Touch the patient on the right cheek and the left arm. The patient is then asked, "Where did I touch you?" This is shown in Figure 19–53. Normally, patients will have no problem identifying both areas. A patient with a lesion in the parietal lobe may feel the individual touches but may "extinguish" the sensation on the side contralateral to the side of the lesion. This is the phenomenon termed *extinction*.

Test Two-Point Discrimination

Two-point discrimination tests the ability of a patient to differentiate one stimulus from two. Gently hold two pins 2–3 mm apart, and touch the patient's fingertip. Ask the patient to state the number of pins felt. This is shown in Figure 19–54. Compare this finding with the corresponding area on a fingertip on the other hand. Because different areas of the body have different sensitivities, you must know these differences. At the fingertips, two-point discrimination is 2 mm apart. The tongue can discriminate 1 mm; the toes 3–8 mm; the palms 8–12 mm; the back 40–60 mm. The fingertips of the two hands are compared. A lesion in the parietal lobe will impair two-point discrimination.

Test Stereognosis

Stereognosis is the integrative function of the parietal and occipital lobes in which the patient attempts to identify an object placed in the hands. Have the patient close eyes. Place a key, pencil, paper clip, or coin in the palm of the patient's hand, and ask what it is. Test the other hand and compare the findings.

Test Graphesthesia

Graphesthesia is the ability to identify a number "written" in the palm of one's hand. Ask the patient to close eyes and extend the hand. Use the blunt end of a pencil to

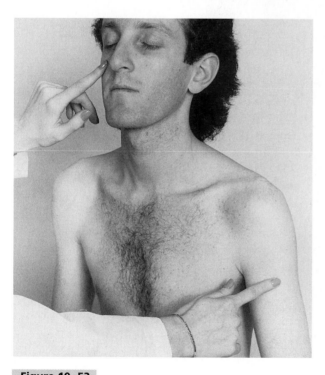

Figure 19–53

Technique for testing tactile localization.

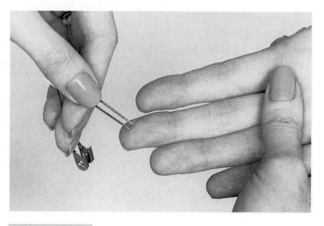

Figure 19–54

Technique for testing two-point discrimination.

"write" numbers from 0 to 9 in the palm. The numbers should be oriented facing the patient. This is shown in Figure 19–55. Normally, the patient will be able to identify the numbers. Compare one hand with the other. The inability to identify the numbers is a sensitive sign of parietal lobe disease.

■ Test Point Localization

Point localization is the ability of a person to point to an area where she or he was touched. Have the patient close eyes. Touch the patient. Ask the patient to open the eyes and point to the area touched. Abnormalities of the sensory cortex impair the ability to localize the area touched.

Cerebellar Function

Cerebellar function is tested by the following:

- The finger-to-nose test
- The heel-to-knee test
- Rapid alternating movement
- Romberg's test
- Gait

■ Perform the Finger-to-Nose Test

The finger-to-nose test is performed by asking the patient to touch the nose and the examiner's finger alternately as quickly, accurately, and smoothly as possible. The examiner holds a finger at arm's length from the patient. The patient is instructed to touch the finger and then the nose. This is repeated several times, after which the patient is asked to perform the test with eyes closed. This is demonstrated in Figure 19–56. Patients with cerebellar disease persistently overshoot the target, a condition known as *past pointing*. They may often have a tremor in addition as the finger approaches the target.

■ Perform the Heel-to-Knee Test

The heel-to-knee test is performed by having the patient lie on the back. The patient is instructed to slide the heel of one lower extremity down the shin of the other, starting at the knee. A smooth movement should be seen, with the heel staying on the shin.

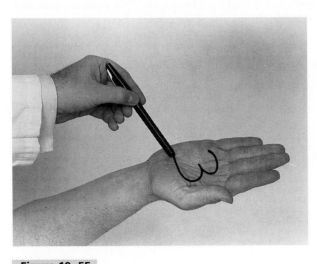

Figure 19–55

Technique for testing graphesthesia.

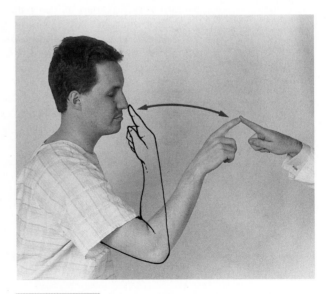

Figure 19–56

The finger-to-nose test.

This is shown in Figure 19–57. In patients with cerebellar disease, the heel wobbles from side to side.

Assess Rapid Alternating Movements

The ability to perform rapid alternating movements is called *diadochokinesia*. These motions may be tested in the upper extremity or in the lower extremity. The patient may be asked to pronate and supinate one hand on the other hand rapidly. Another technique involves having the patient touch the thumb to each finger as quickly as possible. The patient may also be asked to slap the thigh, raise the hand, turn it over, and slap the thigh again rapidly. This pattern is repeated over and over as quickly as possible. These techniques are illustrated in Figure 19–58. An abnormality in performing rapid alternating movements is called *adiadochokinesia*.

Perform Romberg's Test

Romberg's test is performed by having the patient stand in front of the examiner with feet together so that the heels and toes are touching. The examiner instructs the patient to extend the arms with palms facing upward and to close the eyes. If the patient can maintain this posture without moving, the test is negative. Romberg's test is positive if the patient begins to sway and has to move the feet for balance. Another common finding is for one of the arms to drift downward, with flexion of the fingers. This is called *pronator drift* and is seen in patients with a mild hemiparesis. Romberg's test examines the posterior columns rather than actual cerebellar function. The examiner should be at the patient's side during this test, because occasionally a patient will suddenly sway and fall if assistance is not provided.

Assess Gait

Foremost in the examination of cerebellar function is the observation of gait. The patient is asked to walk straight ahead while the examiner observes the gait. The patient is then instructed to return on tiptoes; walk away again on the heels; and finally return to the examiner by walking in tandem gait with one foot placed in front of the other; the heel of one foot touches the toes of each step. The examiner may wish to demonstrate this gait for the patient. The patient should have normal posture, and there should be normal associated movements of the arms. The examiner should pay special attention to the way in which the patient turns around. These maneuvers will often accentuate cerebellar ataxia as well as indicate weakness in the lower extremities.

Many neurologic disorders produce striking and characteristic gaits. The patient with *hemiplegia* tends to drag or to circumduct a weak and spastic leg. The arm is frequently flexed at the elbow across the abdomen as the patient walks. The patient with *Parkinson's disease* shuffles with short, hurried steps. The head is bowed, with the back bent over. The patient with *cerebellar ataxia* walks with a wide-based gait. Feet are very far apart as the patient staggers from side to side. The patient with *foot drop* has a characteristic slapping gait resulting from weakness of the dorsiflexors of the ankle. The patient with *sensory ataxia* has a high-stepping gait. This person slaps feet down firmly as if unsure of their location. Figure 19–59 illustrates these gaits.

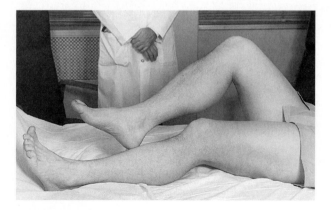

Figure 19–57

The heel-to-knee test.

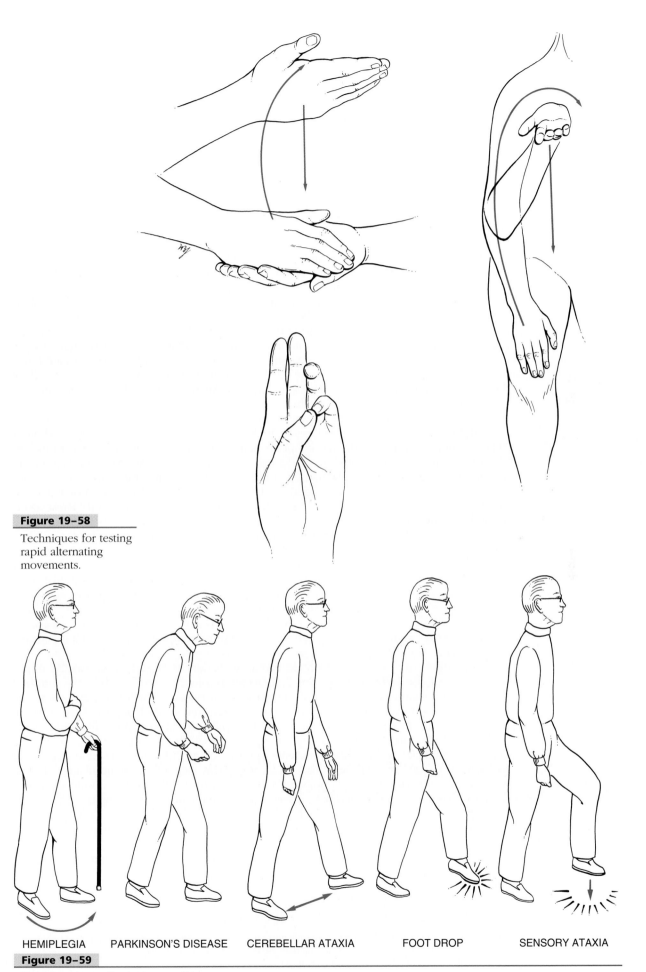

Figure 19–58

Techniques for testing rapid alternating movements.

HEMIPLEGIA PARKINSON'S DISEASE CEREBELLAR ATAXIA FOOT DROP SENSORY ATAXIA

Figure 19–59

Common types of gait abnormalities.

Clinicopathologic Correlations
The Comatose Patient

Coma is the state in which the patient is unable to respond to any stimuli. The causes of coma include the following:

- Meningeal infection
- Increased intracranial pressure of any cause
- Subarachnoid hemorrhage
- Focal cerebral lesion
- Brain stem lesion affecting the reticular system
- Metabolic encephalopathy*
- Status postseizure activity

If the patient's friends or family are available, speak with them. They can help in the evaluation of the patient by giving valuable information. Is there a history of hypertension, diabetes, epilepsy, substance abuse, or recent head trauma?

If there is any evidence of head trauma, x-ray views of the cervical spine must be taken before the examiner moves the patient's neck.

The physical examination of the comatose patient should start with inspection. The clothing, age, and evidence of chronic illness provide valuable clues as to the cause of the coma. Does the patient have gingival enlargement consistent with antiepileptic medical therapy?† Is there a characteristic odor to the breath? The sweet smell of ketones may be present in diabetic ketoacidosis. An odor of alcohol may be present. Are there stigmata of chronic liver disease?

What is the *posture* of the patient? Patients with cerebral hemispheric dysfunction or a destructive lesion of the pyramidal tracts maintain a *decorticate* posture, whereas those patients with a midbrain or pons lesion maintain a *decerebrate* posture. In decorticate rigidity, the arms are adducted, and the elbows, wrists, and fingers are flexed. The legs are internally rotated. In decerebrate rigidity, the arms are also adducted, but they are rigidly extended at the elbows and the forearms pronated. The wrists and fingers are flexed. In both postures, the feet are plantarflexed. These positions are shown in Figure 19–60.

The head should be evaluated for any areas of depression, as in a depressed skull fracture. Does the nose appear broken? Are there any broken teeth? Is there any clear, watery discharge from the nose or ear, suggestive of a leakage of cerebrospinal fluid?

The *respiratory pattern* should be evaluated. Central neurogenic hyperventilation is seen in lesions of the midbrain or pons. This type of respiration consists of rapid, deep, regular breathing. *Cheyne-Stokes* breathing is characterized by rhythmic changes in the breathing pattern. Periods of rapid breathing are separated by periods of apnea. Cheyne-Stokes breathing is associated with brain-stem compression or bilateral cerebral dysfunction.

The neurologic examination of the comatose patient is largely based on the pupillary size and the light reflexes. Small, reactive pupils are seen in bilateral cerebral dysfunction. Dilated pupils are seen following an overdose of hallucinogenic agents or central nervous system stimulants. A unilateral fixed and dilated pupil is suggestive of pressure on the ipsilateral oculomotor nerve. Pupillary dilatation precedes paralysis of the extraocular muscles. This is due to the fact that the pupillary nerve fibers are located superficial to the fibers innervating the extraocular muscles and are more vulnerable to extrinsic stresses. This is an important sign of uncal herniation. In the presence of normally reactive pupils with absent corneal reflexes and absent extraocular movement, consider a metabolic abnormality as the cause of the coma.

Descriptions of Tables

As was indicated earlier in the chapter, headache is an important symptom of neurologic disease. Table 19–2 provides a differential diagnosis of headaches.

---

*Common causes include electrolyte abnormalities, endocrine disorders, liver or kidney failure, vitamin deficiencies, poisoning, intoxications, and marked changes in body temperature.
† Commonly related to phenytoin (Dilantin) therapy.

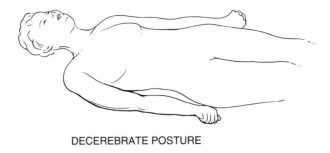

DECEREBRATE POSTURE

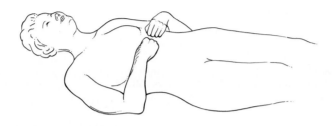

DECORTICATE POSTURE

Figure 19–60

Postures of comatose patients.

The correct assessment of a patient's motor activity can help localize the site of a lesion. The term *extrapyramidal* refers to those parts of the motor system that are not directly involved with the pyramidal tracts. The extrapyramidal system is composed of the basal ganglia, nuclei of the midbrain and reticular formation, and cerebellum. Table 19–3 lists the major areas and the specific motor problems associated with lesions of the lower motor neuron, the pyramidal tract, and the extrapyramidal tract. Table 19–4 summarizes the important signs and symptoms in five common chronic neurologic disorders.

Table 19–2   Differential Diagnosis of Headache

Type	Epidemiology	Location	Signs and Symptoms
Migraine	Family history Young adults Females	Bifrontal	Nausea Vomiting Possible neurologic deficits
Cluster	Adolescent males	Orbitofrontal Unilateral	Unilateral nasal congestion Lacrimation
Tension	Females	Bilateral Generalized or occipital	
Hypertensive	Family history	Variable	Hypertensive retinopathy Possible papilledema
Increased intracranial pressure		Variable	Nausea Vomiting Papilledema
Meningitis		Bilateral Often occipital	Nuchal rigidity Fever
Temporal arteritis*	Adults	Unilateral Over temporal artery	Tender temporal artery Loss of vision in ipsilateral eye

* See Chapter 23, The Geriatric Patient.

Table 19–3   Effects of Various Lesions

	Lower Motor Neuron	Pyramidal Tract	Extrapyramidal Tract
Major effect	Flaccid paralysis	Spastic paralysis Hyperactive reflexes	No paralysis
Muscle appearance	Atrophy Fasciculations	Mild atrophy from disuse	Rest tremor
Muscle tone	Decreased	Increased	Increased
Muscle strength	Decreased or absent	Decreased or absent	Normal
Coordination	Absent or poor	Absent or poor	Slowed

Table 19–4   Common Neurologic Conditions and Their Signs and Symptoms

Condition	Age of Onset (yr)	Sex	Signs and Symptoms
Multiple sclerosis	30–35	Women	Nystagmus Diplopia Slurring of speech Muscular weakness Paresthesias Poor coordination Bowel and bladder dysfunction
Amyotrophic lateral sclerosis	50–80	Men	Irregular twitching of involved muscles Muscular weakness Muscle atrophy* Absence of sensory or mental deficits
Parkinson's disease	60–80	Men	Rigidity Slowing of movements Involuntary tremor Difficulty in swallowing Tremor in upper extremities Jerky, "cogwheel" motions Slow, shuffling gait with loss of arm swing Mask-like facial expression Body in moderate flexion Excessive salivation
Myasthenia gravis	20–50	Women	Generalized muscular fatigue Bilateral ptosis† Diplopia Difficulty in swallowing Voice weakness
Huntington's chorea	35–50	Both sexes	Choreiform movements Brain failure Rapid movements Facial grimacing Dysarthria Personality change

* See Figure 19–21.
† See Figure 8–19.

A comparison of the effects of upper and lower motor neuron lesions is shown in Table 19–5.

Paraplegia and *quadriplegia* are upper motor neuron defects. They can also involve lower motor neurons. Injury of the spinal cord can produce partial or complete paralysis. In patients with cervical or thoracic lesions, spasticity will be present below the level of the lesion, and flaccidity will be present in all muscles supplied from reflex arcs at the level of the lesion. In the presence of sacral lesions, a flaccid paralysis results. Table 19–6 summarizes motor involvement in spinal cord lesions.

Table 19–5   **Comparison of Effects of Upper and Lower Motor Neuron Lesions**

Effect	Upper Motor Neuron Lesion	Lower Motor Neuron Lesion
Voluntary control	Lost	Lost
Muscle tone	Spastic, increased	Flaccid, decreased
Reflex arcs	Present	Absent
Pathologic reflexes	Present	Not present
Muscle atrophy	Little or none	Significant

Table 19–6   **Motor Involvement in Spinal Cord Lesions**

Affected Cord Segment	Motor Involvement
C1–4	Paralysis of neck, diaphragm, intercostals, and all four extremities
C5	Spastic paralysis of trunk, arms, and legs; partial shoulder control
C6–7	Spastic paralysis of trunk and legs; upper arm control; partial lower arm control
C8	Spastic paralysis of trunk and legs; hand weakness only
T1–10	Spastic paralysis of trunk and legs
T11–12	Spastic paralysis of legs
L1–S1	Flaccid paralysis of legs
S2–5	Flaccid paralysis of lower legs; bowel, bladder, and sexual function affected

Table 19–7   **Motor Function According to Cord Segments**

Area of Body	Action Tested	Cord Segment
Shoulder	Flexion, extension, or rotation of neck	C1–C4
Arm	Adduction of arm	C5–C8, T1
	Abduction of arm	C4–C6
	Flexion of forearm	C5–C6
	Extension of forearm	C6–C8
	Supination of forearm	C5–C7
	Pronation of forearm	C6–C7
Hand	Extension of hand	C6–C8
	Flexion of hand	C7–C8, T1
Finger	Abduction of thumb	C7–C8, T1
	Adduction of thumb	C8, T1
	Abduction of little finger	C8, T1
	Opposition of thumb	C8, T1
Hip	Flexion of hip	L1–L3
	Extension of leg	L2–L4
	Flexion of leg	L4–L5, S1–S2
	Adduction of thigh	L2–L4
	Abduction of thigh	L4–L5, S1–S2
	Medial rotation of thigh	L4–L5, S1
	Lateral rotation of thigh	L4–L5, S1–S2
	Flexion of thigh	L4–L5
Foot	Dorsiflexion of foot	L4–L5, S1
	Plantar flexion of foot	L5, S1–S2
Toe	Extension of great toe	L4–L5, S1
	Flexion of great toe	L5, S1–S2
	Spreading of toes	S1–S2

Often a patient may complain of a decreased ability to perform a task. Physical examination may reveal a decreased motor strength. Table 19–7 summarizes the major actions of the more common muscles and their corresponding cord segments.

Patients with *inflammation of the meninges* often complain of pain in the neck and a resistance to flexion of the neck. If meningitis is suspected, have the patient lie on the back. Place your hand behind the patient's neck and flex it until the chin touches the sternum. In patients with meningitis, there is neck pain and resistance to motion. There may also be flexion of the patient's hips and knees. This has been called *Brudzinski's nape of the neck sign*. Brudzinski described at least five different physical signs indicative of meningeal irritation. The one just described is the best known and most reliable of his signs. Another sign of meningeal irritation can be elicited while the patient lies on the back and you flex one of the patient's legs at the hip and knee. If pain or resistance is elicited as the knee is extended, a positive *Kernig's sign* is present.

The fundus of the eye may provide a clue as to the cause of the coma.

If there is no evidence of a fracture of the cervical spine, *oculocephalic reflexes* should be tested. If a comatose patient's head is rapidly turned to one side while the eyelids are held open, the eyes should move conjugately to the other side. This reflex is termed *doll's eyes*. In a patient with a lesion in the brain stem, the doll's eyes reflex is absent. The doll's eyes reflex can be elicited only in a comatose patient, because alert individuals will fixate on an object and override this reflex.

Caloric stimulation is used to enhance the doll's eyes reflex or to test movements in an individual with a broken cervical spine. The patient should be placed with the head flexed at 30°. This orients the semicircular canal in a horizontal position. A large bore syringe is filled with 20–30 mL of ice water, and the water is squeezed into one of the external auditory canals. The normal response is the development of nystagmus. Slowly the eyes will move conjugately to the ipsilateral side, followed by the rapid movement of the eyes back to the midline. Because nystagmus is named for the rapid component, the use of cold water causes nystagmus to the opposite side. If warm water is used, the eyes will show the rapid component toward the side being irrigated. This can easily be remembered by using the mnemonic *COWS*, which stands for *c*old *o*pposite, *w*arm *s*ame.

An absence of the caloric response is seen in patients with a disruption of the connections between the vestibular nuclei and the 6th nerve nucleus at the level of the brain stem.

Useful Vocabulary

Listed here are the specific roots that are important in order to understand the terminology related to neurologic diseases.

Root	Pertaining to	Example	Definition
esthe-	feeling	an*esthe*sia	Loss of feeling
-gnosia	recognition	a*gnosia*	Loss of the power to recognize sensory stimuli
myelo-	spinal cord	*myelo*gram	X-ray study of the spinal cord
-paresis	weakness	hemi*paresis*	Muscular weakness affecting half the body
-plegia	paralysis	ophthalmo*plegia*	Paralysis of the eye muscles
radicul(o)-	spinal nerve root	*radiculo*pathy	Disease of a spinal nerve root

Writing Up the Physical Examination

Listed here are examples of the write-up for the examination of the neurologic system.

- The patient is oriented to person, time, and place. Cranial nerves II–XII are intact. Motor examination reveals normal gait, normal heel-to-toe movement, and normal strength bilaterally. Reflexes are equal bilaterally and are within normal limits. The sensory examination is normal, with pain, light touch, and stereognosis intact. Cerebellar function is normal.
- The mental status examination is within normal limits. There is a marked weakness of the lower half of the right side of the face. The right nasolabial fold is flat, and the mouth droops downward on the right. There is no other cranial nerve abnormality. The motor and sensory examinations are within normal limits. Reflexes are normal. Romberg's test is negative.
- The patient has an expressive aphasia and a right hemiplegia with ipsilateral trigeminal hemiplegia. Reflexes in the right lower extremity are hyperactive compared with the left. Sensory examination is difficult to assess. Babinski's sign is present on the right side.
- Mental status is within normal limits. Motor examination and reflexes are equal bilaterally. There is a sensory level at L2 on the right and at L4 on the left. Vibration sense is impaired more on the right than on the left, as is position sense. Romberg's test is positive.

Bibliography

Adams RD, Victor M: Principles of Neurology. New York, McGraw-Hill, 1985.

Brazis PW, Masdeu JC, Biller J: Localization in Clinical Neurology. Boston, Little, Brown, 1985.

Chusid JG: Correlative Neuroanatomy and Functional Neurology. Los Altos, CA, Lange Medical Publishers, 1985.

Fowler TJ, May RW: Neurology. Littleton, MA, PSG Publishing, 1985.

Froehling DA, Silverman MD, Mohr DN, et al: Does this dizzy patient have a serious form of vertigo? JAMA 271:385, 1994.

Goldstein LB, Matchar DB: Clinical assessment of stroke. JAMA 271:1114, 1994.

Weiner WJ, Goetz CG (eds): Neurology for the Non-Neurologist. Philadelphia, Harper & Row, 1981.

CHAPTER 20

Putting the Examination Together

A physician is not only a scientist or a good technician. He must be more than that—he must have good human qualities. He has to have a personal understanding and sympathy for the suffering of human beings.

Albert Einstein
1879–1955

The Techniques

The previous chapters have dealt with the individual organ systems and the history and physical examinations related to each of them. The purpose of this chapter is to help the student assimilate each of the individual examinations into one that is complete and smoothly performed.

A complete examination is ideally performed in an orderly, thorough manner with as few movements as possible required of the patient. Most errors in performing a physical examination are due to a lack of organization and thoroughness, not to a lack of knowledge. Evaluate each part of the examination carefully before moving on to the next part. The most commonly observed errors in the physical examination are related to the following:

- Technique
- Omission
- Detection
- Interpretation
- Recording

Errors in *technique* are related to lack of order and organization of the examination, faulty equipment, and poor bedside etiquette. Errors of *omission* are common in the examination of the eye and nose; auscultation of the neck vessels, chest, and heart; palpation of the spleen; rectal and genitalia examinations; and the neurologic examination. Errors of *detection* are those in which the examiner fails to detect abnormalities that are present. Most commonly occurring errors of this type are those involving thyroid nodules, tracheal deviation, abnormal breath sounds, diastolic murmurs, hernias, and abnormalities of the extraocular muscles. Errors in *interpretation* of findings occur most commonly with tracheal deviation, venous pulses, systolic murmurs, fremitus changes, abdominal tenderness, liver size, eye findings, and reflexes. The most common types of *recording* errors are related to the description of heart size and murmurs, improper terminology, and obscure abbreviations.

The following examination sequence is the one the author uses. There is no right or wrong sequence. Develop your own approach. At the end of whichever technique you use, a complete examination should have been performed.

In most situations, the patient will be lying in bed when you arrive. After introducing yourself and taking a complete history, you should then inform the patient that you are ready to begin the physical examination. Start by washing your hands.

Patient Lying Supine in Bed

General Appearance

1. Inspect patient's facial expression (Chaps. 11, The Chest; 12, The Heart; and 15, The Abdomen)

◼ **Vital Signs (Chap. 12)**

1. Palpate blood pressure in right arm
2. Auscultate blood pressure in right arm
3. Auscultate blood pressure in left arm*

Have Patient Sit Up in Bed

◼ **Vital Signs**

1. Check for orthostatic changes in left arm (Chap. 12)

Have Patient Turn and Sit with Legs Dangling Off Side of Bed

◼ **Vital Signs**

1. Palpate radial pulse for rate and regularity (Chap. 13, The Peripheral Vascular System)
2. Determine respiratory rate and pattern (Chap. 11)

◼ **Head (Chap. 7, The Head and Neck)**

1. Inspect cranium
2. Inspect scalp
3. Palpate cranium

◼ **Face (Chaps. 6, The Skin and 7)**

1. Inspect face
2. Inspect skin on face

◼ **Eyes (Chap. 8, The Eye)**

1. Assess visual acuity, both eyes
2. Check visual fields, both eyes
3. Determine eye alignment, both eyes
4. Test extraocular muscle function, both eyes
5. Check pupillary responses to light, both eyes
6. Test for accommodation, both eyes
7. Inspect external eye structures, both eyes
8. Ophthalmoscopic examination, both eyes

◼ **Nose (Chap. 9, The Ear and Nose)**

1. Inspect nose
2. Palpate nasal skeleton
3. Palpate sinuses (frontal, maxillary), both sides
4. Inspect nasal septum, both sides
5. Inspect turbinates, both sides

◼ **Ears (Chap. 9)**

1. Inspect external ear structures, both sides
2. Palpate external ear structures, both sides
3. Evaluate auditory acuity, both sides
4. Perform Rinne's test, both sides
5. Perform Weber's test
6. Perform otoscopic examination, both sides
7. Inspect external canal, both sides
8. Inspect tympanic membrane, both sides

---

*If the blood pressure is elevated in the upper extremity, blood pressure in the lower extremity must be assessed to exclude coarctation of the aorta. The patient is asked to lie prone, and blood pressure by auscultation is determined (see Chapter 12).

■ **Mouth (Chap. 10, The Oral Cavity and Pharynx)**

1. Inspect outer and inner surfaces of lips
2. Inspect buccal mucosa
3. Inspect gingivae
4. Inspect teeth
5. Observe Stenson's and Wharton's ducts, both sides
6. Inspect hard palate
7. Inspect soft palate
8. Inspect tongue
9. Test hypoglossal nerve function (Chap. 19, The Nervous System)
10. Palpate tongue
11. Inspect floor of the mouth
12. Palpate floor of the mouth
13. Inspect tonsils, both sides
14. Inspect posterior pharyngeal wall
15. Observe uvula as patient says "Ah" (Chap. 19)
16. Test gag reflex (Chap. 19)

■ **Neck (Chap. 7)**

1. Inspect neck, both sides
2. Palpate neck, both sides
3. Palpate lymph nodes of head and neck, both sides
4. Palpate thyroid gland by anterior approach
5. Evaluate position of trachea (Chap. 11)
6. Evaluate mobility of trachea (Chap. 11)

■ **Neck Vessels (Chap. 12)**

1. Inspect height of the jugular venous pulsation, right side

■ **Neck* (Chap. 7)**

1. Palpate thyroid gland by posterior approach
2. Palpate for supraclavicular lymph nodes, both sides

■ **Posterior Chest (Chap. 11)**

1. Inspect back, both sides
2. Palpate back for tenderness, both sides
3. Evaluate chest excursion, both sides
4. Palpate for tactile fremitus, both sides
5. Percuss back, both sides
6. Evaluate diaphragmatic excursion, right side
7. Auscultate back, both sides
8. Palpate for costovertebral angle tenderness, both sides (Chap. 15, The Abdomen)

■ **Sacrum (Chap. 12)**

1. Test for edema

■ **Anterior Chest† (Chap. 11)**

1. Inspect patient's posture
2. Inspect configuration of chest
3. Inspect chest, both sides
4. Palpate chest for tactile fremitus, both sides

■ **Female Breast (Chap. 14, The Breast)**

1. Inspect breast, both sides
2. Inspect breast during maneuvers to tense pectoral muscles, both sides

---

* The examiner should now go to the back of the patient while the patient remains seated with legs dangling off the side of the bed.

† The examiner should now go to the front of the patient while the patient remains seated with legs dangling off the side of the bed.

■ **Heart (Chap. 12)**

   1. Inspect for abnormal chest movements
   2. Palpate for point of maximum impulse
   3. Ausculate for heart sounds, all four positions

■ **Axilla (Chap. 14)**

   1. Inspect axilla, both sides
   2. Palpate axilla, both sides
   3. Palpate for epitrochlear nodes, both sides (Chap. 13)

Have Patient Lean Forward

■ **Heart (Chap. 12)**

   1. Ausculate with diaphragm at cardiac base

Have Patient Lie Supine with Head of Bed Elevated About 30°

■ **Neck Vessels (Chap. 12)**

   1. Inspect the jugular venous wave form, right side
   2. Ausculate the carotid artery, both sides
   3. Palpate the carotid artery, each side separately

■ **Breasts, Male and Female (Chap. 14)**

   1. Inspect breast, both sides
   2. Palpate breast, both sides
   3. Palpate subareolar area, both sides
   4. Palpate nipple, both sides

■ **Chest (Chap. 11)**

   1. Inspect chest, both sides
   2. Evaluate chest excursion, both sides
   3. Palpate for tactile fremitus, both sides
   4. Percuss chest, both sides
   5. Ausculate breath sounds, both sides

■ **Heart (Chap. 12)**

   1. Inspect for movements
   2. Palpate for localized motion, all four positions
   3. Palpate for generalized motion, all four positions
   4. Palpate for thrills, all four positions
   5. Ausculate heart sounds, all four positions
   6. Time the heart sounds to the carotid pulse

Have Patient Turn on Left Side

■ **Heart (Chap. 12)**

   1. Ausculate with bell at cardiac apex

Have Patient Lie Supine with Bed Flat

■ **Abdomen (Chap. 15)**

   1. Inspect the contour of the abdomen
   2. Inspect the skin of the abdomen
   3. Inspect for hernias
   4. Ausculate the abdomen for bowel sounds, one quadrant
   5. Ausculate the abdomen for bruits, both sides
   6. Percuss the abdomen, all quadrants
   7. Percuss the liver
   8. Percuss the spleen
   9. Test superficial abdominal reflex (Chap. 19)

10. Palpate abdomen lightly, all quadrants
11. Palpate abdomen deeply, all quadrants
12. Exclude rebound tenderness
13. Check for hepatic tenderness
14. Evaluate the hepatojugular reflux (Chap. 12)
15. Palpate liver
16. Palpate spleen
17. Palpate kidney
18. Palpate aorta
19. Check for shifting dullness if ascites is suspected

■ **Pulses (Chap. 13)**

1. Palpate radial pulse, both sides
2. Palpate brachial pulse, both sides
3. Palpate femoral pulse, both sides
4. Palpate popliteal pulse, both sides
5. Palpate dorsalis pedis pulse, both sides
6. Palpate posterior tibial pulse, both sides
7. Time radial and femoral pulses, right side
8. Perform heel-to-knee test (part of neurologic examination: see Chap. 19)

■ **Male Genitalia (Chap. 16, Male Genitalia and Hernias)**

1. Inspect the skin and hair distribution
2. Observe the inguinal area while instructing the patient to bear down
3. Inspect the penis
4. Inspect the scrotum
5. Palpate for inguinal nodes, both sides
6. Elevate the scrotum and inspect the perineum

Have the Man Stand in Front of Seated Examiner

■ **Male Genitalia (Chap. 16)**

1. Inspect the penis
2. Inspect the external urethral meatus
3. Palpate the shaft of the penis
4. Palpate the urethra
5. Inspect the scrotum
6. Palpate the testicle, both sides
7. Palpate the epididymis and vas deferens, both sides
8. Observe the inguinal area while instructing the patient to bear down
9. Test superficial cremasteric reflex (Chap. 19)
10. Transilluminate any masses
11. Palpate for hernias, both sides

Have the Man Turn Around and Bend over Bed

■ **Rectum (Chap. 15)**

1. Inspect the anus
2. Inspect the anus while patient strains
3. Palpate the anal sphincter
4. Palpate the rectal walls
5. Palpate the prostate gland
6. Test stool for occult blood

The Woman Is Helped to Lithotomy Position

■ **Female Genitalia (Chap. 17, Female Genitalia)**

1. Inspect the skin and hair distribution
2. Inspect the labia majora
3. Palpate the labia majora
4. Inspect the labia minora, clitoris, urethral meatus, and introitus

5. Inspect the area of Bartholin's glands, both sides
6. Inspect the perineum
7. Test for pelvic relaxation
8. Perform speculum examination
9. Inspect cervix
10. Obtain Papanicolaou's (Pap) smear
11. Inspect vaginal walls
12. Perform bimanual examination
13. Palpate cervix and uterine body
14. Palpate adnexa, both sides
15. Palpate rectovaginal septum
16. Test stool for occult blood

Have Patient Sit on Bed with Legs Off Side

▓ Mental Status

1. Ask routine questions (Chaps. 1, The Interviewer's Questions; 19; and 23, The Geriatric Patient)

▓ Face (Chap. 19)

1. Test motor function of trigeminal nerve, both sides
2. Test sensory function of trigeminal nerve, both sides
3. Test corneal reflex, both eyes
4. Test facial nerve, both sides
5. Test spinal accessory nerve, both sides
6. Test double simultaneous stimulation, both sides
7. Perform finger-to-nose test

▓ Neck

1. Test range of motion (Chap. 18, The Musculoskeletal System)

▓ Hands and Wrists (Chaps. 18 and 19)

1. Inspect hand and wrist, both sides
2. Inspect nails, both sides (Chap. 6)
3. Palpate shoulder joint, both sides
4. Palpate interphalangeal joints, both sides
5. Palpate metacarpophalangeal joints, both sides
6. Test light touch, both sides
7. Test vibration sense, both sides
8. Test position sense, both sides
9. Test object identification, both sides
10. Test graphesthesia, both sides
11. Test two-point discrimination, both sides
12. Assess rapid alternating movements, both sides

▓ Elbows (Chap. 18)

1. Inspect elbow, both sides
2. Test range of motion, both sides
3. Palpate elbow, both sides
4. Test upper extremity strength, both sides
5. Test biceps reflex, both sides (Chap. 19)
6. Test triceps reflex, both sides (Chap. 19)

▓ Shoulders (Chap. 18)

1. Inspect shoulder, both sides
2. Test range of motion, both sides
3. Palpate shoulder joint, both sides

▓ Shins

1. Inspect skin, both sides
2. Test for edema, both sides (Chap. 12)

■ **Feet and Ankles (Chaps. 18 and 19)**

1. Inspect feet and ankles
2. Test range of motion, both sides
3. Palpate Achilles tendon, both sides
4. Palpate metatarsophalangeal joints, both sides
5. Palpate metatarsal heads, both sides
6. Palpate ankle and foot joints, both sides
7. Test light touch, both sides
8. Test vibration sense, both sides
9. Test position sense, both sides
10. Test lower extremity strength, both sides
11. Test ankle reflex, both sides
12. Test plantar response, both sides

■ **Knees (Chaps. 18 and 19)**

1. Inspect knee, both sides
2. Test range of motion, both sides
3. Palpate patella, both sides
4. Ballotte patella if effusion is suspected
5. Test patellar reflex, both sides

Have Patient Stand with Back to Examiner

■ **Hips (Chap. 18)**

1. Inspect hips
2. Test range of motion

■ **Spine (Chaps. 18 and 19)**

1. Inspect spine
2. Palpate spine
3. Test range of motion
4. Assess gait
5. Perform Romberg's test

The Written Physical Examination

After the examination has been completed, the examiner must be able to record objectively all the findings of inspection, palpation, percussion, and auscultation. Be precise in stating locations of abnormalities. Small drawings may be useful to describe a shape or location better. When describing the size of a finding, state the size in millimeters or centimeters rather than describing it as compared with a fruit or nut, as these can vary greatly in size. It is best not to use abbreviations; abbreviations may mean different things to different readers. However, the abbreviations used in the following examples are standard and may be used. Finally, do not make diagnostic statements in the write-up; save them for the summary at the end. For example, it is better to state that "a grade III/VI holosystolic murmur at the apex with radiation to the axilla" is present rather than "a murmur of mitral insufficiency."

Patient: John Henry*

General Appearance. The patient is a 65 year old white man who is lying in bed on two pillows and is in no acute distress. He is well developed and thin and appears slightly older than his stated age. The patient is well groomed, alert, and cooperative.

Vital Signs. Blood pressure (BP), 185/65/55 right arm (lying), 180/60/50 left arm (lying), 175/65/50 left arm (sitting); heart rate, 90 and regular; respirations, 16.

Skin. Pink, with small hyperkeratotic papules over the face; nail beds slightly dusky; hair thin on head; hair absent on lower portion of lower extremities; normal male escutcheon.

---

* This name is fictitious. Any similarity to a person living or dead with this name is purely coincidental.

Head. Normocephalic without evidence of trauma; no tenderness present.

Eyes. Visual acuity with glasses using near card: right eye (OD), 20/60, left eye (OS) 20/40; visual fields full bilaterally; extraocular movements (EOMs) intact; PERRLA (pupils are equal, round, and reactive to light and to accommodation); xanthelasma present bilaterally, L > R; eyebrows normal; bilateral arcus senilis present; conjunctivae pink without injection or discharge; opacities present in both lenses, R > L; left disc sharp with normal cup-to-disc ratio; normal arteriovenous (A-V) ratio OS; no A-V nicking present OS; there is a flame-shaped hemorrhage at the 6 o'clock position OS; several cotton-wool spots are also present at the 1 and 5 o'clock positions OS; right fundus not well visualized as a result of lenticular opacity.

Ears. Pinnae in normal position; no tenderness present; small amount of cerumen in left external canal; canals without injection or discharge; in Rinne's test, bone conduction (BC) > air conduction (AC) right ear, AC > BC left ear; in Weber's test, lateralization to the right ear; both tympanic membranes are gray without injection; normal landmarks seen bilaterally.

Nose. Nose straight without masses; patent bilaterally; mucosa pink with a clear discharge present; inferior turbinate on the right slightly edematous.

Sinuses. No tenderness detected over frontal and maxillary sinuses.

Throat. Lips slightly cyanotic without lesions; patient wears an upper denture; buccal mucosa pink without injection; all lower teeth are present and are in fair condition; no obvious caries; gingivae normal; tongue midline without fasciculations; no lesions seen or palpated on tongue; mild injection of posterior pharynx with yellowish-white discharge present on posterior pharynx and tonsils; tonsils minimally enlarged; uvula elevates in midline; gag reflex intact.

Neck. Supple with full range of motion; trachea midline and freely movable; small (1–2 cm) lymph nodes are present in superficial cervical and tonsillar node chains; thyroid borders palpable; no thyroid nodules or enlargement noted; no abnormal neck vein distention present; neck veins flat while patient is sitting upright.

Chest. Anteroposterior (AP) diameter increased; symmetric excursion bilaterally; tactile fremitus normal bilaterally; chest resonant bilaterally; vesicular breath sounds bilaterally; coarse breath sounds with occasional crackles present at the bases.

Breasts. Mild gynecomastia, L > R; no masses or discharge present.

Heart. Point of maximum impulse, 6th intercostal space (PMI 6ICS) 2 cm lateral to midclavicular line (MCL); normal physiologic splitting present; no heaves or thrills are present; S_1 and S_2 distant; a grade II/VI high-pitched holodiastolic murmur is heard at the 2ICS at the right upper sternal border; a grade I/VI medium-pitched systolic crescendo-decrescendo murmur is heard in the aortic area; the systolic murmur is midpeaking (Fig. 20–1).

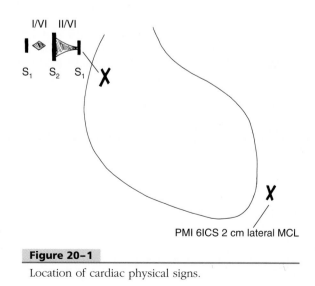

Figure 20–1

Location of cardiac physical signs.

Vascular. A carotid bruit is present on the right; no bruits are heard over the left carotid, renal, femoral, or abdominal arteries; lower extremities are slightly cool in comparison with the upper extremities; 1+ pretibial edema is present on the right lower extremity; 2+ pretibial edema is present on the left; mild venous varicosities are present from midthigh to calf bilaterally; no ulceration or stasis changes are present; no calf tenderness is present.

Abdomen. The abdomen is scaphoid; a right lower quadrant (RLQ) appendectomy scar and a left lower quadrant (LLQ) herniorrhaphy scar are present; both scars are well healed; a 3 × 3 cm mass is seen in the RLQ after coughing or straining; no guarding, rigidity, or tenderness is present; no visible pulsations are present; bowel sounds are present; percussion note is tympanitic throughout the abdomen except over the suprapubic region, where the percussion note is dull; liver span is 10 cm from top to bottom in the MCL; spleen percussed in left upper quadrant but not palpated; kidneys not felt; no costovertebral angle tenderness (CVAT) present; an easily reducible right indirect inguinal hernia is felt at the external ring.

Rectal. Anal sphincter normal; no hemorrhoids present; nontender prostate enlarged symmetrically; prostate firm without nodules felt; no luminal masses felt in rectum; stool negative for blood.

Genitalia. Circumcised male with normal genitalia; penis without induration; left hemiscrotum 4–5 cm below the right; palpation of left hemiscrotum reveals dilatation of the pampiniform plexus; soft testes 2 × 3 × 1 cm bilaterally.

Lymphatic. Nodes in anterior triangle chains already noted; two firm, 1 to 2 cm, rubbery, freely mobile nodes in left femoral area; no epitrochlear, axillary, or supraclavicular nodes felt.

Musculoskeletal. Distal interphalangeal joint enlargement on both hands, causing pain on making a fist, L > R; no tenderness or erythema present; proximal joints normal; neck, arms, hips, knees, and ankles with full range of active and passive motion; muscles appear symmetric; mild kyphosis present.

Neurologic. Oriented to person, place, and time; cranial nerves II–XII intact; gross sensory and motor strength intact; cerebellar function normal; plantar reflexes down; gait normal; deep tendon reflexes as shown in Table 20–1.

Summary. Mr. Henry is a 65 year old man in no acute distress. Physical examination reveals systolic hypertension, retinal changes suggestive of sustained hypertension, a mild cataract in his right eye, a conductive hearing loss in his right ear, tonsillopharyngitis, and gynecomastia. Cardiac examination reveals aortic insufficiency. Peripheral vascular examination reveals probable atherosclerotic disease of the right carotid artery and mild venous disease of the lower extremities. The patient has a right, easily reducible inguinal hernia. A left-sided varicocele is present. Mild osteoarthritis of the hands is also present.

Patient: Mary Jones*

General Appearance. The patient is a 51 year old black woman who is sitting up in bed in mild respiratory distress. She is obese and appears to be her stated age. She is well groomed and alert, but she constantly complains about her shortness of breath.

Table 20–1   Deep Tendon Reflexes of Patient John Henry

	Biceps	Triceps	Knee	Achilles
Right	1+	0	2+	1+
Left	2+	1+	3+	2+

* This name is fictitious. Any similarity to a person living or dead with this name is purely coincidental.

Vital Signs. BP, 130/80/75 right arm (lying), 125/75/70 left arm (lying), 120/75/70 (sitting); heart rate, 100 and regular; respirations, 20

Skin. Upper extremities slightly dusky as compared with lower extremities; good tissue turgor; patient is wearing a wig to cover her marked total baldness; normal female escutcheon.

Head. Normocephalic without evidence of trauma; face appears edematous; no tenderness noted.

Eyes. Visual acuity using near card: OD, 20/40, OS, 20/30; visual fields full bilaterally; EOMs intact; PERRLA; eyebrows thin bilaterally; conjunctivae red bilaterally with injection present; lenses clear; both discs appear sharp with some nasal blurring; the cup-to-disc ratio is 1:3 bilaterally, and the cups are symmetric; the retinal veins appear dilated bilaterally.

Ears. Pinnae in normal position; no mastoid or external canal tenderness; canals without injection or discharge; in Rinne's test, AC > BC bilaterally; in Weber's test, no lateralization; both tympanic membranes clearly visualized; normal landmarks seen bilaterally.

Nose. Straight without deviation; mucosa reddish pink; inferior turbinates within normal limits.

Sinuses. No tenderness detected.

Throat. Lips cyanotic; all teeth present except for all third molars, which have been extracted; occlusion normal; no caries seen; gingivae normal; tongue midline with markedly dilated tortuous veins on undersurface; no fasciculations of tongue noted; posterior pharynx appears within normal limits; uvula midline and elevates normally; gag reflex intact.

Neck. Full with normal range of motion; trachea midline but fixed; neck veins distended to angle of jaw while sitting upright; no adenopathy of neck noted.

Chest. AP diameter normal; symmetric excursion bilaterally; increased tactile fremitus at right base posteriorly corresponds to area of bronchial breath sounds; percussion note in this area is dull, all other chest areas are resonant; bronchophony and egophony present in area of bronchial breath sounds; crackles and wheezes present in area at right posterior base.

Breasts. Left mastectomy scar; right breast without masses, dimpling, or discharge.

Heart. PMI 5ICS MCL; normal physiologic splitting present; no heaves or thrills present; S_1 and S_2 within normal limits; no murmurs, gallops, or rubs present.

Vascular. There are no bruits present over the carotid, renal, femoral, or abdominal arteries; the extremities are without clubbing or edema.

Abdomen. The abdomen is obese without guarding, rigidity or tenderness; no visible pulsations are present; bowel sounds are normal; percussion note is tympanitic throughout the abdomen; liver span is 15 cm in the MCL; spleen not percussed or palpated; kidneys not palpated; no CVAT present.

Rectal. Refused.

Pelvic. Deferred until patient more stable.

Lymphatic. No adenopathy felt in the neck chains or in the epitrochlear, axillary, supraclavicular, or femoral regions.

Musculoskeletal. Marked edema of both upper extremities, L > R; neck, arms, knees, and ankles with full range of active and passive motion; muscles appear symmetric except for upper extremities.

Neurologic. Oriented to person, place, and time; cranial nerves II–XII intact; gross sensory and motor strength intact; cerebellar function normal; plantar reflex down bilaterally; deep tendon reflexes as shown in Table 20–2.

Summary. Ms. Jones is a 51 year old black woman, status post–left mastectomy, in respiratory distress. She is cyanotic and has evidence of vascular engorgement of the upper half of her body. Her trachea is fixed to the mediastinum. Chest examination reveals evidence of consolidation of the right lower lobe of her lung.

Table 20–2 Deep Tendon Reflexes of Patient Mary Jones

	Biceps	Triceps	Knee	Achilles
Right	2+	2+	2+	1+
Left	2+	1+	2+	2+

Bibliography

Wiener S, Nathanson M: Physical examination: Frequently observed errors. JAMA 236:852, 1976.

SECTION III

Evaluation of Specific Patients

CHAPTER 21

The Pregnant Patient

It was the best of times, it was the worst of times. . . .

Charles Dickens
1812–1870

General Considerations

In 1991, there were 4.1 million live births in the United States, which represented the largest number of births recorded since 1964. The fertility rate, which is the number of live births per 1000 females between the ages of 15 and 44 years, was 64.9 in 1986 and 70.9 in 1991. This increase was, in part, related to an increase in the number of women of childbearing age (postwar "baby boomers") as well as to a slight increase in their fertility.

A study by the World Health Organization estimated in 1991 that nearly 500,000 women die annually from pregnancy-related conditions. Most of these deaths occur in developing nations. It has been estimated that pregnancy-related deaths in Africa are 1 in 20. In the United States, the number of maternal deaths has decreased significantly since the 1930s. In 1935, there were 582.1 deaths per 100,000 live births; in 1991, the number was 9.1 deaths per 100,000 live births. The highest maternal mortality rate in the United States is seen in African-American women. Because of generally unfavorable economic and social conditions that are frequently present, African-American women tend to receive less antepartum care than do white women. Rates of mortality also vary with the age of the mother, regardless of race; among older women, the mortality rate is higher.

The major causes of maternal deaths in the United States from 1990 to 1995 were embolism (17%), hypertension (12%), ectopic pregnancy (10%), hemorrhage (9%), stroke (8%), complications from anesthesia (7%), abortion-related complications (5%), cardiomyopathy (4%), and infection (3.5%).

Any woman of reproductive age who presents with symptoms, even if not directly related to the abdomen, should be evaluated for pregnancy. *"Think pregnancy"* should be your motto in the evaluation of this patient. This is extremely important because the diagnosis or treatment of her medical or surgical problem may be deleterious to her developing fetus, if indeed she is pregnant. As discussed later in this chapter, many of the symptoms of pregnancy are nonspecific and could be interpreted erroneously if the pregnancy were not recognized. For example, the urinary frequency that is common in early pregnancy might easily be mistaken for cystitis. The patient might then receive an antibacterial agent such as a sulfonamide or a quinolone, which is potentially toxic to the developing fetus. When the urinary symptoms fail to respond to the medication, the patient might then be referred for an intravenous pyelogram, which adds the risk of radiation to the early pregnancy.

Structure and Physiology

The anatomy and the physiologic changes that occur in the nonpregnant woman have already been discussed. This chapter reviews the physiologic alterations resulting from pregnancy and functional pelvic anatomy.

Basic Physiology of Reproduction

When semen is deposited in the vagina, sperm travel through the cervix and uterus and into the fallopian tubes, where fertilization usually occurs if an egg is present. The majority of sperm deposited in the vagina die within 1–2 hours because of the normal acidic environment. The sperm are aided in their travel into the fallopian tubes by uterine and tubal contractions and favorable mucous conditions.

The fertilized ovum, or zygote, remains in the tube for about 3 days. While in the fallopian tube, the fertilized ovum divides repeatedly to form a round mass of cells called the *morula*. If there is an obstruction in the fallopian tube, the fertilized ovum may become trapped in the tube and attach itself to the lining of the tube, giving rise to an *ectopic,* or *tubal, pregnancy.* In a normal pregnancy, approximately 6–8 days after fertilization, the morula becomes a *blastocyst,* which migrates through the tube into the uterus, where it attaches itself to the endometrium, with the inner cell mass adjacent to the endometrial surface *(implantation).* Substances that destroy the surface epithelial cells are released, allowing the blastocyst to burrow into the endometrium. The endometrium then grows over the invading blastocyst.

The primitive *chorion,* the combination of *trophoblast* and primitive *mesoderm,* secretes a luteinizing hormone known as *human chorionic gonadotropin (hCG),* which controls the corpus luteum and inhibits pituitary gonadotropic activity. Quickly thereafter, as the invasion proceeds, maternal venous blood vessels are tapped to form lakes of blood, and *chorionic villi* develop. These can be identified as early as the 12th day after fertilization. These villi develop a leafy appearance and are called the *chorion frondosum.* By the 15th day after fertilization, the maternal arterial vessels are tapped, and by the 17th–18th day, a functioning placental circulation is established. At term, the uteroplacental blood flow is estimated to be about 550–705 mL/min. Figure 21–1*A* illustrates the path of sperm, fertilization, and implantation.

Decidua is the name given to the endometrium of pregnancy. There are three types, distinguished by location with regard to the growing embryo. The *decidua capsularis* is the overlying endothelium that covers the conceptus, and the *decidua basalis* is the decidual tissue lying between the blastocyst and the myometrium. The decidua of the remainder of the endometrial cavity is the *decidua vera.* Figures 21–1*B* and *C* show a cross section through the uterus of a pregnant woman and the different types of decidua in early pregnancy.

One of the first placental hormones produced by the developing trophoblastic tissue is hCG. This hormone is present as early as the 8th day after fertilization has taken place. The titers increase to a maximal level by about the 60th–70th day after fertilization and then decrease. The primary function of hCG is to maintain the corpus luteum during the first 2 months of pregnancy until the placenta can produce enough progesterone by itself. Other hormones, such as human placental lactogen, human chorionic thyrotropin, and adrenocorticotropic hormone, and estrogens are also produced by the placenta. It is beyond the scope of this book to discuss the actions of these hormones; the reader is referred to the references at the end of this chapter for further information.

Functional Anatomy of Birth

The pelvic cavity is bounded above by the plane of the *brim* (the inner sacral promontory to the upper and inner borders of the symphysis pubis), below by the plane of the *outlet* (the lower and inner borders of the symphysis pubis to the end of the sacrum or coccyx), posteriorly by the sacrum, laterally by the sacrosciatic ligaments and ischial bones, and anteriorly by the pubic rami.

The birth canal, through which the infant is delivered, may be thought of as a cylindrical passage with walls composed partially of hard parts (the bony pelvis) and partially of soft parts (the muscles of the pelvic floor and the pelvic ligaments). The cross section of the cylinder is oval, rather than circular, to accommodate the oval cross section of the entering fetal part (e.g., the head) as it descends through the pelvis as a result of the expulsive effect of uterine contractions.

This mechanism for delivery and its corresponding anatomy would be easily understood were it not for the fact that the long axis of the schematic oval, which lies transversely at the entrance to the pelvis, comes to lie in the anteroposterior axis in the

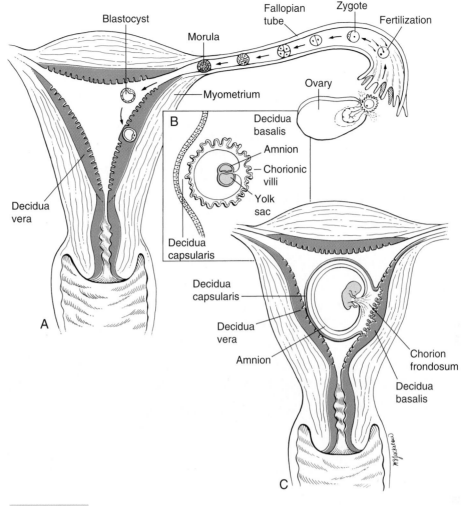

Figure 21–1

A, Fertilization and implantation. *B* and *C,* Cross-sectional view through uterus of a pregnant woman at approximately 8 days and 20 days, respectively.

midpelvis. The entering fetal part must therefore descend in a spiral path as it progresses through the birth canal.

The process of birth varies greatly, depending on the relationships—*lie, presentation, attitude,* and *position*—of the fetus to the maternal anatomy. It is important to define these relationships accurately in order to follow the birth process.

The term *lie* refers to the relation of the long axis of the fetus to that of the mother. In over 99% of full-term pregnancies, the lie is in the same plane as or parallel to the long axis of the mother, a longitudinal lie. In rare instances, the long axis of the fetus is perpendicular to the maternal pelvis, a transverse lie.

The term *presentation* refers to the part of the fetus in the lower pole of the uterus overlying the pelvic brim (e.g., cephalic, vertex, breech) and can be felt through the cervix. Usually the fetus's head is flexed so that the chin is in contact with the chest. In this case, the occipital fontanelle is the *presenting part,* and the presentation is referred to as a vertex presentation.

The *attitude,* or *habitus,* of the fetus is the posture of the fetus: flexion, deflexion, or extension. In most cases, the fetus becomes bent over so that the back is convex, the head is sharply flexed on the chest, the thighs are flexed over the abdomen, and the legs are bent at the knees. This is the description of the fetal attitude of flexion. Figure 21–2 illustrates these postures.

The *position* is the relationship of an arbitrarily chosen portion of the presenting part of the fetus to the maternal pelvis. For example, in a vertex presentation, the chosen portion is the fetal *occiput;* in a breech presentation, it is the *sacrum;* and in a face presentation, it is the chin, termed the *mentum.* The maternal pelvis is divided into eight parts for the purpose of further defining position. These divisions are shown in Figure 21–3.

Because the arbitrarily chosen portion of the presenting part may be either left or right, the portion can be described as left occiput (LO), right occiput (RO), left sacral (LS), right sacral (RS), left mental (LM), and right mental (RM). This part is also directed anteriorly (A), posteriorly (P), or transversely (T). For each of the three presentations (vertex, breech, and face), there are, therefore, six varieties of position. For example, in a vertex presentation, if the occiput is in the left anterior segment of the maternal pelvis, the position is described as *left occiput anterior (LOA).* The common clinical vertex positions are illustrated in Figure 21–4. "Left" and "right"

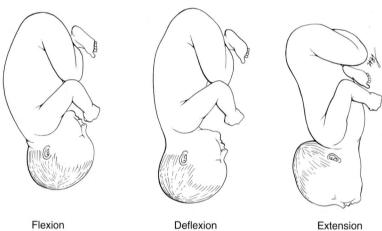

Figure 21–2

Types of fetal positions.

Flexion   Deflexion   Extension

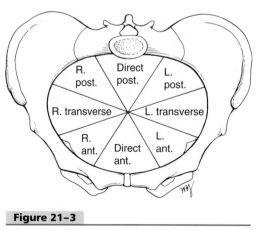

Figure 21–3

Division of maternal pelvis as seen from above.

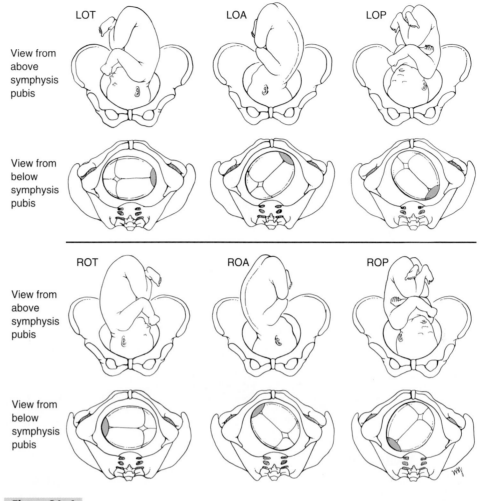

Figure 21–4

Common clinical vertex positions. For each position shown, the top diagram is the view from above the symphysis pubis; the bottom is the view from below the symphysis pubis. "Right" and "left" refer to the mother's side. "Anterior," "posterior," and "transverse" refer to the maternal pelvis. Highlighted area is fetal occiput.

always denote the side of the mother. Likewise, "anterior," "posterior," and "transverse" refer to the mother's pelvis.

The term *station* characterizes the level of descent of the presenting part of the fetus; "0 station" signifies that the fetal occiput has reached the level of the maternal ischial spines and that the widest transverse part of the baby's head *(biparietal diameter)* is at the level of the pelvic brim. This is also known as *engagement.* If the vertex is at "− 1 station," it means that the fetal occiput is at a plane 1 cm above the level of the maternal ischial spines (and that the biparietal diameter is therefore 1 cm above the pelvic brim), and the baby's head is thus not engaged.

There are four basic pelvic configurations: *gynecoid, anthropoid, android,* and *platypelloid.* These are based on the shape of the brim, midpelvis, and outlet. Any pelvis is likely to combine features of more than one configuration. Figure 21–5 illustrates these basic types and summarizes the differences in pelvic anatomy.

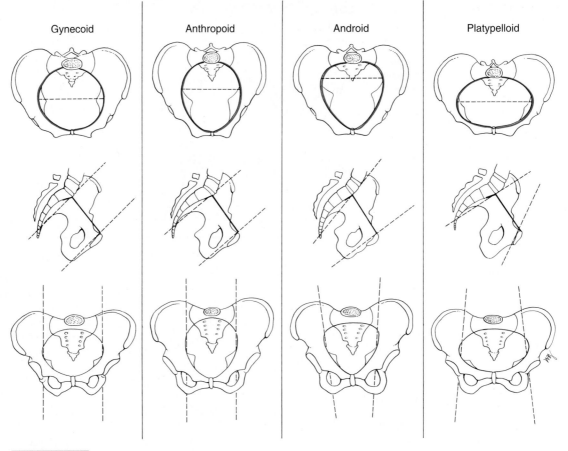

| Gynecoid | Anthropoid | Android | Platypelloid |

Figure 21–5

Basic types of pelvic anatomy. Top view is from above, looking down at inlet; middle view is from the side; bottom view is from the front.

Review of Specific Symptoms

The most common symptoms of pregnancy are the following:

- Amenorrhea
- Nausea
- Breast changes
- Heartburn
- Backache
- Abdominal enlargement
- Quickening
- Skin changes
- Disturbances in urination
- Vaginal discharge
- Fatigue

Amenorrhea

Amenorrhea results from the high levels of estrogen, progesterone, and hCG, which increase the uterine endometrium and do not allow the endometrium to slough as menstrual bleeding.

Nausea

Nausea, with or without vomiting, is the so-called *morning sickness of pregnancy.* As the name implies, the symptom is usually worse during the early part of the day and usually passes in a few hours, although it may last longer. More than 50% of all pregnant women in their first trimester have gastrointestinal symptoms. Although the cause is unknown, high levels of estrogen and of hCG have been implicated in its development. The pregnant woman is also hypersensitive to odors, and she may experience alterations in taste. Morning sickness usually improves after 12–16 weeks, when the hCG levels fall. Severe vomiting may occur, resulting in dehydration and ketosis, but is much less common, occurring in fewer than 2% of pregnancies.

Breast Changes

Several changes in the breast occur with pregnancy. One of the earliest symptoms is an increase in the vascularity of the breast, associated with a sensation of heaviness, almost pain. This occurs at about the 6th week. By the 8th week, the nipple and areola have become more pigmented, and the nipple becomes more erectile. The Montgomery tubercles become prominent as raised pinkish-red nodules on the areola. By the 16th week, a clear fluid called *colostrum* is secreted and may be expressed from the nipple. By the 20th week, further pigmentation and mottling of the areola have developed. Figure 21–6 illustrates the changes in the breast.

Heartburn

Heartburn in pregnancy occurs because progesterone causes relaxation of the gastro-esophageal sphincter. Another cause of heartburn in the 3rd trimester is the pushing upward of the enlarged uterus. This upward displacement exerts pressure on the stomach. There is a decrease in gastric motility as well as a decrease in gastric acid secretion, which delays digestion.

Backache

As a result of secretion of estrogen and progesterone, the pelvic joints relax, and the increased uterine weight accentuates lordosis. The abdominal muscles stretch and lose tone.

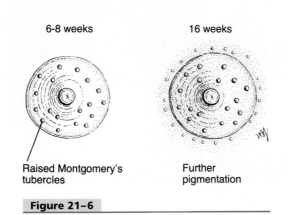

6-8 weeks   16 weeks

Raised Montgomery's tubercles   Further pigmentation

Figure 21–6

Breast changes during pregnancy.

Abdominal Enlargement

The uterus rises out of the pelvis and into the abdomen by the 12th week of gestation, and an increase in abdominal girth is usually apparent by the 15th week. This enlargement is usually more apparent earlier in multiparous women, in whom some of the tone of the abdominal muscles was lost in previous pregnancies.

Quickening

Quickening is the sensation of fetal movement. It is a faint sensation initially. Quickening usually begins at 20 weeks in the primigravida but is felt 2–3 weeks earlier in the multipara. Although an important symptom, quickening is not a reliable sign of pregnancy because a woman can convince herself of its presence.

Skin Changes

In addition to the skin changes of the breast already discussed, hyperpigmentation is common, especially in women with dark hair and a dark complexion. The linea alba darkens to become the *linea nigra,* as shown in Figure 21–7A. Areas prone to friction (e.g., medial thighs, axillae) also tend to darken. New pigmentation on the face, called *chloasma,* also commonly develops on the cheeks, forehead, nose, and chin. These skin changes are caused by the presence of high levels of ovarian, placental, and pituitary hormones. A patient with chloasma is shown in Figure 21–7B.

"Stretch marks," or *striae gravidarum,* are irregular, linear, pinkish-purple lesions that develop on the abdomen, breasts, upper arms, buttocks, and thighs. They are due to tears in the connective tissue below the stratum corneum. Figures 21–8 and 21–9 show striae gravidarum of the abdomen and breast, respectively. The linea nigra is also present on the patient in Figure 21–8. Figure 21–10 illustrates the common skin changes seen in pregnancy.

Transverse grooving, as well as increased brittleness or softening of the nails, may occur. Eccrine sweating progressively increases throughout pregnancy, whereas apocrine gland activity decreases. Hirsutism, caused by increased androgen secretion, may also occur on the face, arms, legs, and back.

Disturbances in Urination

Beginning at the 6th week, urinary bladder symptoms are common. Increased frequency of urination is thought to be caused by increased vascularity of the bladder as well as by pressure of the enlarging uterus on the bladder. As the uterus rises above

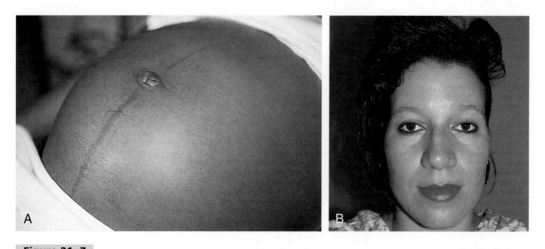

A   B

Figure 21–7

Skin changes due to high levels of ovarian, placental, and pituitary hormones. *A,* Linea nigra. *B,* Chloasma.

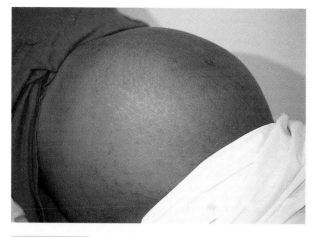

Figure 21-8

Striae gravidarum of the abdomen. Note also the linea nigra.

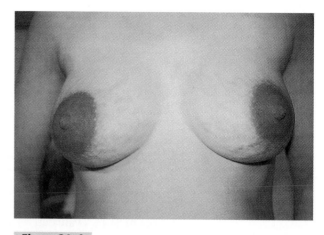

Figure 21-9

Striae gravidarum of the breasts. Note also the marked pigmentation of the areolae.

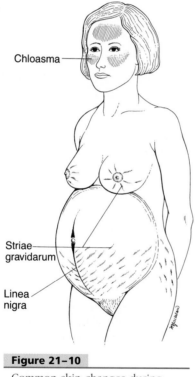

Figure 21-10

Common skin changes during pregnancy.

the pelvis, the symptoms tend to remit. Near term, however, urinary symptoms recur as the fetal head settles into the maternal pelvis and impinges on the volume capacity of the urinary bladder.

Vaginal Discharge

An asymptomatic, white, milky vaginal discharge is common as the elevated estrogen levels increase the production of cervical mucus and secretions from the vaginal walls.

Fatigue

Easy fatigability is common during early pregnancy. Some physicians believe that estrogen has a soporific effect and is the cause of the fatigue.

Several other symptoms are frequently seen in pregnant women. These include varicose veins, headache, leg cramps, swelling of the legs and hands, constipation, bleeding gums, insomnia, and "dizziness."

Obstetric Risk Assessment

The medical history of the pregnant woman is similar to that of the nonpregnant woman. In addition, the interviewer must assess obstetric risk. The following major risk factors must be evaluated:

- Age
- Parity
- Height
- Pregnancy weight
- Diabetes
- Hypertension and renal disease
- Hemoglobinopathy
- Isoimmunization
- History of previous pregnancies
- Sexually transmitted infections
- Other infections
- Tobacco use
- Alcohol use
- Drug use

Age

Older women have an increased risk of conceiving fetuses with chromosomal abnormalities. The chance of having a chromosomally abnormal child is about 1 in 200 at age 35 and reaches about 1 in 20 at age 44. Women younger than the age of 20 years generally give birth to more premature infants and to infants of low birth weight than do women aged 25–35 years.

Parity

Women who have had more than five children are at increased risk of *placenta previa* and *placenta accreta,* possibly because of scarring of the endometrium. Postpartum hemorrhage and uterine rupture are also more common in this group of women.

Height

Women who are less than 5 feet tall generally have small pelves and therefore may be prone to *cephalopelvic disproportion** and may require a cesarean section.

Pregnancy Weight

Perinatal mortality is increased among women whose initial prepregnancy weight is less than 120 pounds, especially if their weight gain during pregnancy is less than 11 pounds.

---

* Disparity between the size of the maternal pelvis and the fetal head that precludes vaginal delivery.

History of Diabetes, Hypertension, and Renal Disease

Women with diabetes, hypertension, or renal disease are at an increased risk of fetal intrauterine growth retardation (IUGR), premature labor, toxemia, and abruptio placentae. Diabetes mellitus occurs in 2–3% of all pregnancies and is thus the most common medical complication of pregnancy.

Hemoglobinopathy and Isoimmunization

Determine the presence of any hemoglobinopathy, because pregnancy can precipitate an exacerbation of the anemia. Women who are Rh-negative must be monitored closely throughout pregnancy if they have Rh antibodies from isoimmunization, because severe hemolytic anemia may develop in the fetus before delivery.

History of Previous Pregnancies

A history of traumatic or 2nd trimester abortions increases the possibilities of cervical injury and subsequent incompetence of the cervix, an often preventable cause of 2nd trimester miscarriage. A history of premature delivery (newborn's weight less than 2500 g) or immature delivery (less than 1000 g) increases the probability of recurrent early delivery. These patients require particularly close surveillance. A history of unexplained pregnancy loss in the 3rd trimester should be an alert to undiagnosed medical problems in the mother, such as gestational diabetes or systemic lupus erythematosus. Previous cesarian section requires exact information as to the reason for the procedure and the type of uterine incision in order to make a proper assessment about whether or not a patient is a candidate for a vaginal birth after a previous cesarian.

Sexually Transmitted Infections

Because medical therapy for a human immunodeficiency virus (HIV)–positive mother can reduce transmission of the infection to the fetus by more than two thirds, it is obvious that identification of the HIV-positive mother is essential. Although HIV testing cannot be required of the mother, it is mandatory that she be counseled about the value of testing. A history of genital herpes simplex will require screening for recurrences near the time of delivery because they may necessitate cesarian delivery to prevent transmission to the neonate.

Other Infections

Questioning regarding exposure to rubella, chickenpox, or parvovirus (fifth disease) is critical. Antibody titers may be necessary to determine.

Tobacco, Alcohol, and Drug Use

Tobacco, alcohol, and drug use and exposure to toxic substances in the work place or at home and exposure to other teratogenic agents must be determined. Women who smoke cigarettes place their fetuses at a higher risk of complications and should be encouraged to stop. The fetus is more likely to exhibit IUGR and to become hypoxic during labor as a result of reduction in placental exchange. Special note must be made of *any* drugs taken during pregnancy. Ideally, this information should be obtained before the woman conceives so that she can be properly counseled.

Any of these hazards is liable to increase the risk of maternal and/or fetal morbidity and mortality and should be evaluated.

A question that most women have after being told that they are pregnant is "When am I due?" To calculate the expected date of confinement (EDC), first determine the date of the onset of the last menstrual period (LMP) and then calculate the EDC as follows:

LMP	12/29/97
Go back 3 months	9/29/97
Add 1 year	9/29/98
Add 7 days	10/06/98 = EDC

Alternatively, the EDC can be calculated by adding 9 months and 7 days to the first day of the LMP. This calculation is based on a gestation of 280 days and is known as *Nägele's rule*. By knowing the EDC, the examiner can predict the size of the uterus on physical examination, provided that the LMP is correct and conception actually occurred. If the size of the uterus differs significantly from that expected according to the EDC, the causes must be determined. Ultrasonography and other diagnostic tests can be helpful in dating a pregnancy.

Impact of Pregnancy on a Female

Pregnancy may be one of the most exciting time in a woman's life or one of the worst. Even the woman who experiences joy from becoming pregnant may suffer from anxiety during her pregnancy. "Will the baby be normal?" "How will I tolerate labor?" "How will the baby change my life?" "I've put on so much weight. Will I ever be able to take it off?" These are just a few of the many questions asked commonly by pregnant women, and the issues are the cause of much of their anxiety. Another common cause for anxiety is a woman's body image as her pregnancy progresses. Pregnancy may worsen an existing psychiatric illness or may actually produce it.

Pregnancy and the postpartum period are often stressful enough to induce psychiatric illness. It has been estimated that in one of every five pregnant women, some sort of mental health problem develops during pregnancy. In addition, a severe psychotic episode occurs in 1–2 women per 1000 live births.

Depression is common during pregnancy; almost 15% of all pregnant women suffer from some degree of depression during pregnancy, and 8% suffer from it in the postpartum period. The *postpartum blues* may be related to the let-down after delivery, the loss of sleep during labor, anxiety about abilities to take care of the child, perineal pain, feeding difficulties, and appearance. Fortunately, postpartum depression is usually self-limited and remits within a week. Women at greatest risk for the development of postpartum depression are those with an unwanted pregnancy and those with marital difficulties. Sympathetic reassurance and support can help a woman return to her baseline state.

In previously psychotic patients, depression or schizophrenia is likely to occur during the postpartum period. Confusion, paranoid delusions, and disorientation may result. An important symptom is an aversion to the baby. Because child abuse is common in this group of patients, patients with the symptom must be identified quickly.

Physical Examination

The equipment necessary for the examination of the pregnant woman is the same as for the nonpregnant woman. In addition, specialized instruments such as an ultrasonic scan, ultrasonic Doppler scan, or fetoscope may be used for listening to the fetal heart. The ultrasonic scan can detect the fetal heart beat as early as weeks 6–7; an ultrasonic Doppler scan is used at about week 10; and a fetoscope or stethoscope can be used after the 20th week to auscultate the fetal heart beat.

Always try to make the patient as comfortable as possible. She should be examined in comfortable surroundings, with attention to privacy. Discuss with her all of the procedures that you will perform. The patient's gown should open in the front for ease of examination. Draping the patient is the same as discussed in the previous chapters. If the patient is in advanced pregnancy, avoid having her lie for a long period on her back, because the gravid uterus will diminish venous return and produce supine hypotension. It is useful for the woman to urinate before the pelvic examination. As always, wash your hands before beginning the examination. Make sure that your hands are warm and dry.

Because the examination of the pregnant woman is identical to other examinations described in the other chapters of this book, only the special techniques and the modifications of the examination are discussed here.

The Initial Comprehensive Evaluation

There are three main goals to the initial evaluation:

1. Determine the health of the mother and fetus
2. Determine the gestational age of the fetus
3. Initiate a plan for continuing care

The physical examination must include the following:

- Determination of height and weight
- Assessment of blood pressure
- Inspection of the teeth and gums
- Palpation of the thyroid gland
- Auscultation of the heart and lungs
- Examination of the breasts and nipples
- Examination of the abdomen
- Examination of the legs for varicosities and edema
- Examination of the pelvis
- Inspection of the vagina and cervix
- Cytologic study (Papanicolaou's [Pap] smear)
- Swab for *Chlamydia* and gonorrhea

Whenever possible, an ultrasonogram should be performed at about 16–20 weeks to confirm that the pregnancy is progressing normally, to check for multiple fetuses, to estimate the maturity of the fetus, and to recognize any major abnormality.

Head, Eyes, Ears, Nose, Throat, and Neck

Inspect the face. Is chloasma present? What is the texture of the hair and skin? Inspect the mouth. What is the condition of the teeth and gums? Palpate the thyroid. Is it enlarged symmetrically?

Chest

Inspect, palpate, and auscultate the chest. Is there any evidence of labored breathing?

Heart

Palpate for the point of maximum impulse (PMI). Is it displaced laterally? During the latter stages of pregnancy, the gravid uterus pushes up on the diaphragm, and the PMI is displaced laterally. Auscultate the heart. Systolic ejection murmurs are common during pregnancy as a result of the hyperdynamic state. Diastolic murmurs are always pathologic.

Breasts

Inspect the breasts. Are they symmetric? Notice the presence of vascular engorgement and pigmentary changes. Are the nipples everted? An inverted nipple may interfere with a woman's plans to breast-feed. Palpate the breasts. The normal nodularity of breast tissue is accentuated during pregnancy, but *any discrete mass should be considered pathologic until proved otherwise.*

Abdomen

Inspect for the linea nigra and striae gravidarum. Notice the contour of the abdomen. Palpate the abdomen. Fetal movement may be felt by the examiner after 24 weeks. Are there uterine contractions? Hold your hand on the abdomen as the uterus relaxes.

Use a tape measure to assess the fundal height. The measurement should be taken from the top of the symphysis pubis in a straight line to the top of the fundus, with the bladder empty. Figure 21–11 shows the technique. Between 18 and 32 weeks, the superior-inferior measurement in centimeters should equal the number of weeks of gestation. The uterus rises up and enters the abdomen at 12 weeks. It reaches the umbilicus at 24 weeks and is just under the costal margin by 36 weeks. The reduction in fundal height that usually occurs between the 38th and 40th weeks is called *lightening* and results from the descent of the fetus into the pelvis, or "dropping." Figure 21–12 shows the approximate size of the uterus by weeks.

Auscultate the fetal heart and determine the *fetal heart rate (FHR)* and note its location. Throughout pregnancy, the FHR is approximately 120–160 per minute. From weeks 12 to 18, the FHR is usually detected in the midline of the lower abdomen. After 30 weeks, the FHR is best heard over the fetal chest or back. Knowing the location of the fetal back is helpful in determining where to listen for the FHR.

Female Genitalia

Inspect the external genitalia. Are any lesions present? Inspect the anus. Are varicosities present?

With gloves on, perform a speculum examination as described in Chapter 17, Female Genitalia. Inspect the cervix. A dusky blue color is characteristic of pregnancy and occurs by weeks 6–8 of gestation. Is the cervix dilated? If so, fetal membranes may be seen within. Note the character of the vaginal secretions. Obtain cytologic studies for a Pap test and a swab for *Chlamydia* and gonorrhea. As the speculum is removed, inspect the vaginal walls. The vaginal walls are commonly blue-violaceous in pregnancy. Withdraw the speculum carefully.

Perform a digital bimanual examination, paying special attention to the consistency, length, and dilatation of the cervix; the fetal presenting part (in advanced pregnancy); the structure of the pelvis; and to any abnormalities of the vagina and perineum. Is the cervix closed? A nulliparous cervix should be closed, whereas a multiparous cervix may allow the tip of a finger through the external os. Estimate the length of the cervix by palpating the lateral side of the cervix from the cervical tip to the lateral fornix. Only at term should the cervix shorten, or efface. The normal length of the cervix is 1.5–2.0 cm.

Palpate the uterus for size, consistency, and position. An early sign of pregnancy, at about 6–12 weeks, is the softening of the entire isthmus of the cervix and is known

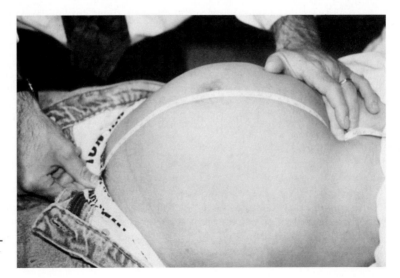

Figure 21–11

Technique for measuring fundal height.

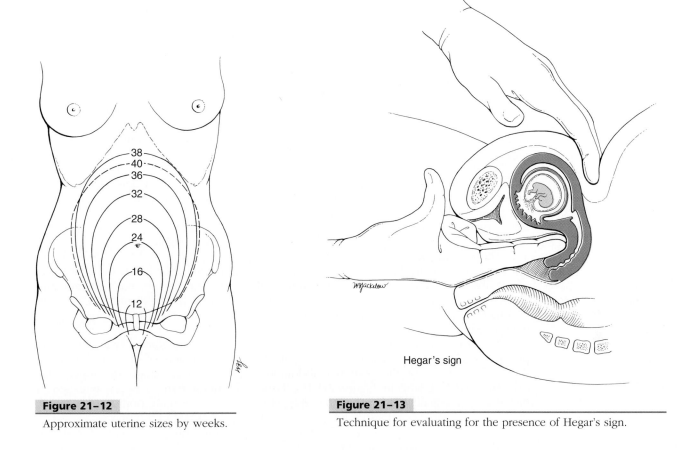

Figure 21–12

Approximate uterine sizes by weeks.

Figure 21–13

Technique for evaluating for the presence of Hegar's sign.

as *Hegar's sign*. During the bimanual examination of the uterus, the examiner will notice an extreme softening of the lower uterine segment. This produces a sensation of the close proximity of the fingers of the vaginal (internal) and abdominal (external) hands. The technique for evaluating for the presence of Hegar's sign is illustrated in Figure 21–13. Bimanual palpation of the uterus is useful up to about 12–14 weeks' gestation. After that, the uterus can be palpated abdominally. Fetal parts are usually palpated from about 26–28 weeks' gestation by abdominal examination (described later).

Palpate the adnexa. Early in pregnancy, the corpus luteum may be palpable as a cystic mass on one ovary. As you withdraw your hand from the vagina, evaluate the pelvic muscles.

A rectovaginal examination is not indicated unless the woman has a retroverted, retroflexed uterus.

Extremities

Inspect for varicosities. Is edema present?

This completes the routine initial examination.

Subsequent Antenatal Examinations

Subsequent antenatal examinations are important for screening for impaired fetal growth, malpresentation, anemia, preeclampsia, and other problems. All parts of the examination just outlined are routinely performed during each visit. This section concerns the abdominal examination.

The physical examination should confirm that fetal growth is consistent with gestational age. Attention should then be given to assessing the lie and presentation of the fetus. From the 28th week of gestation and on to term, the following four maneuvers, known as *Leopold's maneuvers,* provide vital information for the examiner about these important questions. The patient lies supine for these maneuvers.

The *first maneuver* is used to evaluate the upper pole and defines the fetal part in the fundus of the uterus. Stand facing the patient at her side, and gently palpate the upper uterine fundus with your fingers to ascertain which fetal pole is present. This technique is demonstrated in Figure 21–14. Usually, the fetal buttocks are felt at the upper pole. They feel firm but irregular. In a breech presentation, the head is at the upper pole. The head feels hard and round and is usually movable.

The *second maneuver* is used to locate the position of the fetal back. Standing in the same place as in the first maneuver, place the palms of your hands on either side of the abdomen, and apply gentle pressure to the uterus to identify the fetal back and limbs, as shown in Figure 21–15. On one side, the fetal back is felt: rounded, smooth, and hard. On the other side are the limbs, which are nodular or bumpy, and kicking may be felt.

The *third maneuver* is to palpate the lower pole of the fetus. From the same position as the first two maneuvers, use your thumb and fingers of one hand to grasp the lower portion of the maternal abdomen just above the symphysis pubis. This maneuver is illustrated in Figure 21–16. If the presenting portion is not engaged, a movable part, usually the head of the fetus, is felt. If the presenting portion is engaged, this maneuver indicates that the lower pole of the fetus is fixed in the pelvis.

The *fourth maneuver* is performed to confirm the presenting portion and to locate the side of the cephalic prominence. You should now stand beside the patient, facing her feet. Place your hands on either side of the lower abdomen. With the tips of your

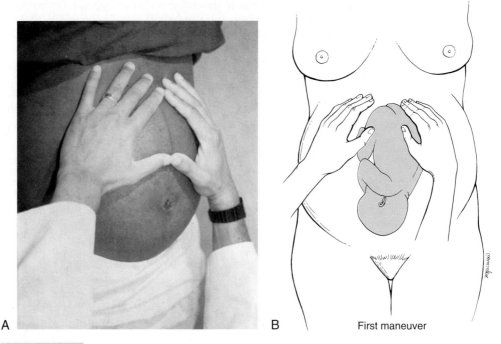

A   B   First maneuver

Figure 21–14

Leopold's first maneuver. *A,* Position of hands on abdomen. *B,* Illustration of relationship of hands and fetus.

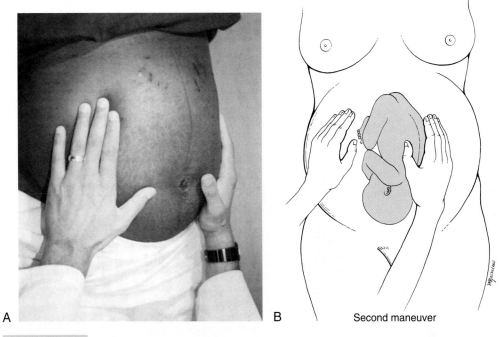

Figure 21–15

Leopold's second maneuver. *A,* Position of hands on abdomen. *B,* Illustration of relationship of hands and fetus.

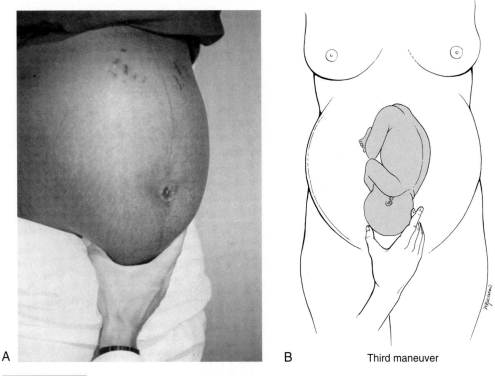

Figure 21–16

Leopold's third maneuver. Relationship of hand and fetal presenting part. *A,* Position of hand on abdomen. *B,* Illustration of relationship of hand and fetus.

fingers, exert a deep pressure in the direction of the pelvic inlet as indicated in Figure 21–17. If the presenting portion is the head and the head is flexed normally, one hand will be stopped sooner by the cephalic prominence, and the other hand descends further into the pelvis. In a vertex presentation, the cephalic prominence is on the same side as the fetal small parts. In a vertex presentation with the head extended, the prominence is on the side of the back.

Labor is the process of birth. The diagnosis and the mechanism of labor are complex topics and are beyond the scope of this book. The reader is referred to the references at the end of this chapter for discussion of these topics.

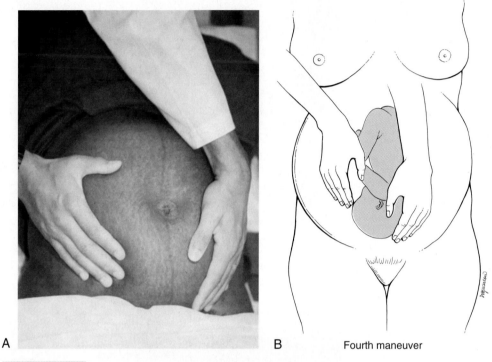

A   B   Fourth maneuver

Figure 21–17

Leopold's fourth maneuver. Relationship of hands and fetal presenting part. *A,* Position of hands on abdomen. *B,* Illustration of relationship of hands and fetus. Note that the examiner's right hand is stopped higher by the cephalic prominence.

Clinicopathologic Correlations

Bleeding during pregnancy is common. The causes may be benign or serious and are different according to the stage of pregnancy.

First trimester bleeding may indicate implantation of the ovum, or it may indicate cervicitis, vaginal varicosities, or, more serious, a threatened, inevitable, incomplete, or complete abortion.

A *threatened abortion* should always be considered when vaginal bleeding occurs in the first 20 weeks of pregnancy.

An *inevitable abortion* can be diagnosed if a patient presents during the first half of pregnancy with bleeding and crampy abdominal pain in association with a dilated cervix and/or a gush of fluid (rupture of membranes) without passing of the products of conception.

An *incomplete* or *complete abortion* occurs when part or all of the products of conception are extruded through the cervix and into the vagina and are passed out of the body.

Second or *3rd trimester bleeding* is seen in about 3% of all pregnancies. About 60% of these bleeding episodes result from placenta previa or abruptio placentae. Both of these conditions may gravely endanger the mother and fetus.

The incidence of *placenta previa* is about 1 in 100 deliveries and is more common among multiparas than in primagravidas. Placenta previa is characterized by painless vaginal bleeding in association with a soft, nontender uterus. The hemorrhage usually does not occur until the end of the 2nd trimester or later. Although there are several types of placenta previa, the symptoms arise from the abnormal location of the placenta over or near the internal os of the cervix. Of all patients with placenta previa, 90% have at least one antepartum hemorrhage. There is also a 20% incidence of premature labor.

Abruptio placentae is the premature separation of a normally situated placenta. It also has an incidence of 1 in 100 deliveries. The symptoms include mild to severe pain with or without external bleeding in association with increasing uterine tone and tenderness. Fetal distress may or may not occur. The incidence of abruptio placentae is higher among women with high parity. It is also more common among African-American women than among white or Latino women. Hypertension is, by far, the most commonly associated condition. Cigarette smoking and cocaine abuse have also been linked to an increased risk of abruptio placentae. Women with a history of abruptio placentae are at significant risk of recurrent abruption in a subsequent pregnancy.

Vasa previa is another serious, but fortunately rare, condition, in which some of the fetal vessels in the membranes cross the region of the internal os. These vessels occupy a position in front of the presenting portion of the fetus. Rupture of the membranes may be accompanied by rupture of the fetal vessel, causing fetal blood loss and possible exsanguination.

Postpartum hemorrhage is the most common cause of serious bleeding in obstetric patients and one of the leading causes of maternal death. It is defined as blood loss in excess of 500 mL during the first 24 hours after delivery. The most common causes are uterine atony and laceration of the vagina and/or cervix. There are many causes for uterine atony: complications of general anesthesia, overdistention of the uterus by a large fetus or twins, prolonged labor, rapid labor, augmented labor, high parity, retained products of conception, coagulation defects, sepsis, ruptured uterus, chorioamnionitis, and drugs such as aspirin and nonsteroidal anti-inflammatory agents. It has been estimated that postpartum hemorrhage occurs in 8% of all pregnancies.

Pseudocyesis, or false pregnancy, is said to occur in 1 in 5000 pregnancies. These nonpregnant women present with many of the classic symptoms of pregnancy and often report fetal movement. They may exhibit weight gain and amenorrhea. Many of these patients are psychotic and may be schizophrenic. They are fixated on their alleged pregnancy. Aggressive psychiatric help is usually required.

Useful Vocabulary

Listed below are the specific roots that are important in order to understand the terminology related to the pregnant patient.

Root	Pertaining to	Example	Definition
-par(ere)	parity	multi*para*	A woman who has two or more pregnancies that resulted in viable offspring
-gravid	pregnancy	primi*gravida*	A woman pregnant for the first time
part-	partus	*part*urient	Giving birth; a woman in labor
puer-	puerperium	*puer*pera	A woman who has just given birth
-cyesis	pregnancy	pseudo*cyesis*	False pregnancy
-tocia	labor	dys*tocia*	Abnormal labor
-natal	birth	pre*natal*	Before birth
lochi-	postpartum vaginal discharge	*lochi*orrhea	Abnormally profuse discharge of lochia

Writing Up the Physical Examination

Listed here are examples of the write-up for the assessment of the pregnant patient.

■ Patient is a 32 year old white female, para 2-0-0-2 (see Chapter 17, Female Genitalia). Her larger infant weighed 7 pounds 4 ounces. Both deliveries were normal, spontaneous, and vaginal. LMP = 8/1/97. EDC = 5/8/98. Blood pressure is 125/80. Examination of the head, eye, ear, nose, throat, and neck is unremarkable except for presence of chloasma. Breasts are symmetrically enlarged with venous pattern visible. Colostrum expressed. Chest is clear to percussion and auscultation. Heart rate is 100 and regular. Heart sounds are normal. A grade II/VI midsystolic murmur is heard at the aortic area. No gallops are present. Examination of the abdomen reveals a 32 week gestation and is appropriate for dates. There are reddish, slightly depressed streaks on the lower abdomen. Movement of the fetus is felt. The fetus is in a longitudinal lie in a vertex presentation, with its back to the left. Fetal heart rate is 150 and is heard through the back of the fetus, 2 cm to the left of midline in the lower left quadrant. 1^+ pretibial edema is present bilaterally.

■ Patient is a 29 year old African-American female, para 2-1-1-3. Her first pregnancy was full-term, delivered by cesarean section because of a double footling breech presentation; weight, 7 pounds 2 ounces. Her next two pregnancies were vaginal deliveries following cesarean section. The first infant weighed 7 pounds 7 ounces, and the second one weighed 5 pounds 6 ounces. Patient had one elective termination of pregnancy at 8 weeks between her first and second children. LMP = 9/3/97. EDC = 6/10/98. Blood pressure is 135/75. Thyroid is mildly enlarged symmetrically without nodularity. Multiple spider angiomas are present over the face, neck, upper chest, and arms. Breasts are symmetrically enlarged, with increased pigmentation of the areolae present. Striae gravidarum are present on the breasts. Chest is clear to percussion and auscultation. Heart rate is 90 and regular. S_1 and S_2 are normal. No murmurs, gallops, or rubs are heard. Uterus is felt in the abdomen at about a 16-week gestation, which is consistent with dates. Fetal heart rate is 160 with ultrasonic Doppler scan and is located in the midline of the lower abdomen. Bimanual examination reveals a soft lower uterine segment. External os admits a fingertip. Cervix is approximately 2 cm in length. Uterus is globular and smooth. Adnexa are unremarkable. Rectovaginal examination not performed. No edema present. Mild varicosities of both lower extremities are present.

Bibliography

Andolsek KM: Obstetric Care: Standards of Prenatal, Intrapartum and Postpartum Management. Philadelphia, Lea & Febiger, 1990.

Chamberlain G, Dewhurst J, Harvey D: Obstetrics, 2nd ed. London, Gower Medical Publishing, 1991.

Cunningham FG, MacDonald PC, Gant NF, et al: Williams Obstetrics, 19th ed. Norwalk, CT, Appleton & Lange, 1993.

Dawes MC, Ashurst H: Routine weighing in pregnancy. Br Med J 304:487, 1992.

Dunnihoo DR: Fundamentals of Gynecology & Obstetrics, 2nd ed. Philadelphia, J.B. Lippincott, 1992.

Herbert WNP, Bruninghaus HM, Barefoot, AB, et al: Clinical aspects of fetal heart auscultation. Obstet Gynecol 69:574, 1987.

Miller AWF, Callander R: Obstetrics Illustrated, 4th ed. Edinburgh, Churchill Livingstone, 1989.

Public Health Service, U.S. Department of Health and Human Services: Caring for Our Future: The Content of Prenatal Care. Washington, DC, U.S. Government Printing Office, 1989.

CHAPTER 22

The Pediatric Patient

Children are not like men nor women; they are almost as different creatures, in many respects, as if they never were to be the one or the other; they are as unlike as buds are unlike flowers, and almost as blossoms are unlike fruits.

Walter Savage Landor
1775–1864

General Considerations

Since the late 1920s, awareness of the importance of child health care has increased. In addition to better control of infectious disease and the great strides in technology, the importance of the behavioral and social aspects of a child's health is now recognized. Despite the many advances and the marked reduction in infant mortality rates, of all the infant deaths less than 1 year of age, more than 70% occur within the 1st month of life.* Of these deaths, 85% occur within the 1st week and 40% within the 1st day of life.

The previous chapters discuss the history and physical examination as they relate to adult patients. This chapter discusses the differences of physical diagnosis in the pediatric age group. The field of pediatrics is broad and encompasses birth through adolescence. During this period, there are enormous changes in children's emotional, social, and physical development, all of which require thorough discussions.

This chapter is organized somewhat differently than the previous chapters. The first section is devoted to the pediatric history, which is similar in most pediatric age groups. The sections that follow are devoted to the physical examinations of the following age groups:

- Newborn period (birth–1 week)
- Infancy (1 week–1 year)
- Early childhood (1–5 years)
- Late childhood (6–12 years)
- Adolescence (12–18 years)

Most of this chapter is devoted to the first three groups because the examination of children from ages 6 through adolescence is similar in order and techniques to examination of adults.

The Pediatric History

The pediatric history, like the adult history, is obtained before the examination is performed. During this period, the child can get accustomed to the interviewer. Unlike the adult history, however, much of the pediatric history is taken from the parent or the guardian. If the child is old enough, interview the child as well.

Good communication with the child is the key to a successful work-up just as with an adult. An infant communicates by crying and, in so doing, indicates that something is wrong. Although older children can communicate through language, they often use crying as a response to pain or to express emotional unrest. This mode of communication deserves attention. Newborns often communicate by cooing and babbling. This form of communication generally represents contentment.

In the early stages, children use sounds to mimic words as well as use gestures to communicate language. At about 10–12 months of age, children usually speak their

---

* Data from National Center for Health Statistics, 3700 East-West Highway, Hyattsville, MD 20782.

first word, usually "dada" or "mama." By 2 years of age, their vocabulary may contain more than 200 words. By 3 years of age, children are able to put together sentences of 5 or 6 words from a 1500 word vocabulary. By the time they are 6 years of age, they are able to communicate in longer sentences, with a vocabulary of several thousand words.

The examiner must pay attention to everything a child says. The interactions of the child with the interviewer can be mutually beneficial. Children are sensitive to the tone of the examiner's voice, which must be modulated with care.

A good relationship with a child begins by making friends with him or her. Not wearing a white coat may alleviate some of the child's fears. One of the best ways to make a child feel comfortable is through praise. When one is talking to a child, it is useful to say, "Thank you for holding still. That makes the examination easier." The use of "You're a good boy" or "You are such a sweet girl" should be kept to a minimum because this may only produce embarrassment. Therefore, praise should be given for a child's behavior and not for his or her personality.

While the history is being taken from the parent or child, it is often helpful to establish physical contact with the child. Touching an arm or rubbing his or her back goes a long way in establishing good rapport.

Although most of the history is obtained from the parent or the guardian, some questions are asked of the child. There are two simple rules in asking questions of children:

1. Don't ask too many questions too quickly.
2. Use simple language.

Interviewers are often amazed by how well a child can respond to questions phrased according to these rules. It is useful to spend time observing the child at play while interviewing a parent. It is also rewarding to allow a toddler to play with a stethoscope, tongue blade, or penlight to "make friends" with the equipment that will be used later in the physical examination.

The pediatric history consists of the following:

■ Chief complaint
■ History of the present illness
■ Past medical history
■ Immunizations
■ Birth history
■ Growth and development
■ Nutrition
■ Social history
■ Family history
■ Review of symptoms

Basically, the *chief complaint* and the *history of the present illness* are obtained in the same manner as with the adult patient.

The *past medical history* section contains more detailed information about *immunizations* and the severity and complications of any of the *childhood illnesses* than the adult counterpart. The current recommended immunization schedule is shown in Table 22–1. Ask the following questions:

"Has the child had DPT* shots? How many? What were the dates?"
"Was the child given the polio vaccination by mouth? How many times? What were the dates?"
"Has the child had shots against measles? mumps? German measles (rubella)? HIB?"† If so, record the dates for each.
"Has the child had any reactions to previous shots?"
"Has the child had a test for tuberculosis? When? What was the result?"

---

* Diphtheria, pertussis, and tetanus.

†*Haemophilus influenzae* type B vaccine; this is recommended for children from the ages of 2 to 6 years. HIB is the most frequent cause of meningitis and is a leading cause of epiglottis, septic arthritis, cellulitis, pericarditis, sepsis, and pneumonia in children younger than the age of 6 years. Children younger than 18 months of age demonstrate poor immunologic response to this polysaccharide vaccine; therefore, it is generally not given until 2 years of age.

Table 22-1   Recommended Childhood Immunization Schedule

Birth	HBV (hepatitis B virus vaccine)
2 months	DPT (diphtheria, pertussis vaccine, tetanus toxoids)
	OPV (oral poliovirus vaccine)
	HIB (*Haemophilis influenza* type B conjugate vaccine)
	HBV
4 months	DPT
	OPV
	HIB
6 months	DPT
	OPV[1]
	HIB[2]
	HBV[1]
12-15 months	HIB
	MMR (measles, mumps, rubella vaccine)
12-18 months	DPT
4-6 years	DPT
	OPV
	MMR[3]
14-16 years	DT (diphtheria and tetanus toxoids)

[1] The third dose of OPV and HBV may be given at any time from 6–18 months of age.
[2] There are several HIB vaccines available. If the child was given PRP-OMP vaccine at 2 and 4 months, the third dose is not required.
[3] The second dose of MMR may be given at either 4–6 or 11–12 years of age.

> *"Has the child had any other shots? BCG?* pneumococcal? hepatitis B?"*
> *"Has the child had any other vaccinations or tests?"*
> *"Has the child had any of the following illnesses: measles? chickenpox? whooping cough? mumps? diphtheria? German measles? strep diseases? rheumatic fever? pneumonia? tuberculosis?"* If so, ask about severity and complications.
> *"Has the child had any serious accidents? surgery? any other medical problem?"*
> *"Has the child had any convulsions?"*
> *"Has the child exhibited any appetite for unusual things such as clay, chalk, or peeling paint?"*
> *"Does the child have asthma?"*

Another question to ask is, "Does the child have difficulty in keeping up with other children?" The answer to this question may provide valuable information about the child's development from the parent's perspective.

Allergies are pertinent to the past medical history. Determine the existence of allergies to penicillin, foods, or other substances. The most common problem associated with allergies to medications is the development of a rash. Rashes, however, are common in children and may have occurred coincidentally at the time the medication was prescribed. Therefore, determine whether the medication was the *cause* of the rash. It is also well known that certain viral states "sensitize" a patient to a medication. The medication may be given at other times without any problems. Whenever a parent describes a "medication allergy," ask the following questions:

> *"How do you know the child is allergic to _____?"*
> *"What was the rash like?"*
> *"Did the child have any problems other than the rash?"*
> *"How long after starting the medications did the rash appear?"†*
> *"After the medication was stopped, how long did the rash last?"*
> *"Has the child ever had the medication again with recurrence of the rash?"*

An important part of the pediatric history is the *birth history*. An opening such as "How was your pregnancy?" may be all that is needed to start this part of the medical

---

* Bacille Calmette-Guérin; this is used for protection from the complications of primary tuberculosis. This vaccine is not given in the United States but is commonly used in Europe and in Central and South America.
† The typical *ampicillin rash* occurs around 7–8 days after the drug is started and is not considered a penicillin allergy.

history. Determine any maternal problems, medications taken, illnesses, bleeding, or whether x-ray films were taken during the pregnancy. Ask the following questions:

"Did you have any illnesses during your pregnancy?" If so, ask the patient to describe them.

"How much weight did you gain during your pregnancy?"

"During your pregnancy, did you take any drugs, recreational or otherwise? drink alcohol? have any x-rays? have any abnormal bleeding?"

"Were you told during your pregnancy that you had high blood pressure? diabetes? protein in your urine?"

"How long was your labor? Were there any unusual problems with it?"

"What type of delivery did you have, vaginal or cesarean?" If cesarean, ask whether the procedure was performed because of a previous cesarean birth.

"What was the child's birth weight?"

"Did the baby come out head first or feet first?"

"Were forceps used during the delivery?"

"Were you told of any abnormalities at birth?"

"Were you told the Apgar* scores?"

"Did the child experience any problems in the newborn nursery, such as breathing difficulties? color? feeding?"

"Did the child receive oxygen in the nursery?"

"Did the child go home with the mother?" If not, ask why not.

The *child's characteristics during infancy* indicate early developmental progress. The *developmental milestones* are useful for helping determine normal patterns. These developmental milestones reflect the child's ability in four areas: gross motor, language, fine motor, and personal development. The following questions should be asked:

"Was the child breast-fed? bottle-fed? For how long?"

"Would you describe your child as active, average, or quiet?"

"Has the child ever had a problem with vomiting? diarrhea? constipation? colic?"

"Has the child ever failed to make progress or ever lost any ability he or she once had?"

"When did the child first sleep through the night?"

"At what age did the child sit without support? wave 'bye-bye'? recognize objects by names? walk without support? learn to talk? walk up and down stairs without support? learn to dress himself? learn to tie shoes? make sentences of 3 to 5 words?"

"At what age was the child toilet-trained?"

"How old a child do you think he or she is acting like now?"

The *Denver Developmental Screening Test* was developed to detect developmental delays in the first 6 years of a child's life, with special emphasis on the first 2 years. It is standardized on the basis of findings from a large group of children in the Denver area. The four main areas of development indicated previously are tested. Figure 22–1 shows this test, on pages 588–589. A line is drawn from top to bottom according to the age of the child. Test each of the milestones crossed by this line. Each milestone has a bar that indicates the percentage of the "standard" population that should be able to perform this task. Failure to perform an item passed by 90% of children is significant. Two failures in any of the four main areas indicate a developmental delay. This test is a screening device for developmental delays; it is not an intelligence test.

The *current functioning of the child* provides insight into present characteristics. The child's social, motor, and language developments as well as maturation are reflected in current behavior. A nice way to broach this topic is to ask, "How would you describe your child as a person?" On the basis of the parent's response, it is useful to ask these questions:

"What do you enjoy the most about your child? the least?"

"Does your child usually complete what he or she starts?"

"How does your child get along with other children his or her age?"

---

* A rapid determination of the child's cardiopulmonary status at birth. This is discussed later in the chapter.

"How many hours of sleep does your child get each night?"
"Does the child have any recurrent nightmares?"
"Does the child have temper tantrums?"
"What type of responsibility can he or she be given?"
"How old was your child when he or she started school?"
"In what grade is he or she now?"
"How is he or she doing in school?"
"Has he or she ever been left back?"
"What is your child's grade level for reading? math?"
"What does your child enjoy during his or her free time?"
"What kinds of things scare him or her?"
"How does the child get along with his or her brothers and sisters?"

It is useful to ask whether the child has any disturbing habits. This question allows the parent or guardian to vent any previously unexpressed concerns. This may be asked as follows:

"Is there anything about the child's behavior that worries you or that is different from that of other children?"

Age-appropriate questions relating to *nutrition* are important. Long-term consequences of malnutrition include defective neurologic development, stunting of growth, and decreased immunocompetence. Overeating with an unbalanced diet is equally important. Therefore, an awareness of nutrition during infancy and childhood is vital. For the newborn, determine the following:

"Is the child being breast-fed?" If so, *"How often?"* *"Is supplemental fluoride being given?"*
*"How many ounces of formula is the baby given a day?"**

Until a baby is 1 year of age, breast milk or infant formula should be his or her main food. Cow's milk may be fine for older children, but it is too hard on an infant's digestive system. In addition, it does not meet the child's nutritional needs during the 1st year of life. There are some major differences between cow's milk and breast milk: cow's milk has too much protein, too little iron, and too much sodium; the amount of vitamin C, copper, and zinc in cow's milk is too low for developing infants; and the type of fat in cow's milk is poorly absorbed by babies.

Determine how many ounces of milk and juice a toddler drinks. Inquire about the daily consumption of vegetables, fruit, and protein. In evaluating older children and adolescents, ask the same questions in addition to asking about the consumption of junk foods and vitamin supplementation.

Differentiate diarrhea from liquid stools. If the baby is breast-fed, the stools are usually yellow or mustard-colored liquid. If the baby is bottle-fed, the stools are more likely to be yellowish tan. Babies frequently have green, brown, or grayish stools. Normal stools may be loose or liquid in consistency, especially in nursing babies; this is not the same as diarrhea. With diarrhea, the stools are more frequent and all liquid, and watery rings are commonly left in the baby's diaper. Minor changes in the stool are common. Normal babies have several bowel movements a day but may go 1 or 2 days without a bowel movement. Small, pebble-like stools indicate constipation.

The *social history* should include the parents' occupations as well as the current living conditions. Ask these questions:

"In how many rooms do you live?"
"What is the condition of the paint and plaster in your home?"
"Are there any pets?"
"Who lives in the house?"
"Does the child sleep in his or her own room?"
"Is the child cared for in any other house?"
"Who supervises the child during the day?"
"How does the family have fun together?"
"Do both the child's parents share in family life?"
"Has the child had any known exposure to lead?"

Text continued on page 590

----

* The normal newborn can take 15–20 ounces a day.

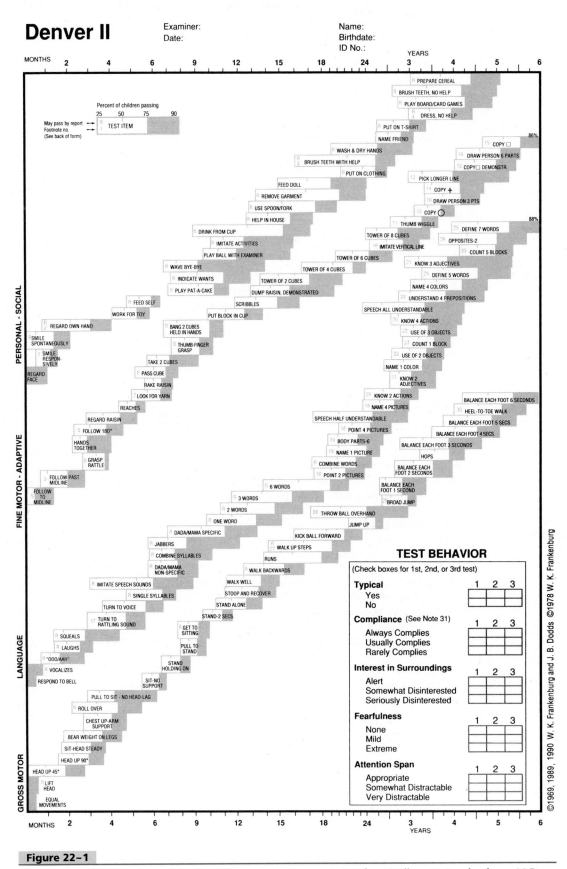

Figure 22-1

Denver Developmental Screening Test. (Reprinted with permission from William K. Frankenburg, M.D., Denver Developmental Materials, Inc., Denver, CO.)

DIRECTIONS FOR ADMINISTRATION

1. Try to get child to smile by smiling, talking, or waving. Do not touch him/her.
2. Child must stare at hand several seconds.
3. Parent may help guide toothbrush and put toothpaste on brush.
4. Child does not have to be able to tie shoes or button/zip in the back.
5. Move yarn slowly in an arc from one side to the other, about 8" above child's face.
6. Pass if child grasps rattle when it is touched to the backs or tips of fingers.
7. Pass if child tries to see where yarn went. Yarn should be dropped quickly from sight from tester's hand without arm movement.
8. Child must transfer cube from hand to hand without help of body, mouth, or table.
9. Pass if child picks up raisin with any part of thumb and finger.
10. Line can vary only 30 degrees or less from tester's line. /
11. Make a fist with thumb pointing upward and wiggle only the thumb. Pass if child imitates and does not move any fingers other than the thumb.

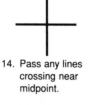

12. Pass any enclosed form. Fail continuous round motions.
13. Which line is longer? (Not bigger.) Turn paper upside down and repeat. (pass 3 of 3 or 5 of 6)
14. Pass any lines crossing near midpoint.
15. Have child copy first. If failed, demonstrate.

When giving items 12, 14, and 15, do not name the forms. Do not demonstrate 12 and 14.

16. When scoring, each pair (2 arms, 2 legs, etc.) counts as one part.
17. Place one cube in cup and shake gently near child's ear, but out of sight. Repeat for other ear.
18. Point to picture and have child name it. (No credit is given for sounds only.)
    If less than 4 pictures are named correctly, have child point to picture as each is named by tester.

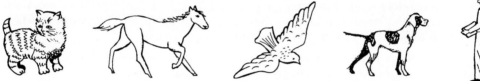

19. Using doll, tell child: Show me the nose, eyes, ears, mouth, hands, feet, tummy, hair. Pass 6 of 8.
20. Using pictures, ask child: Which one flies?... says meow?... talks?... barks?... gallops? Pass 2 of 5, 4 of 5.
21. Ask child: What do you do when you are cold?... tired?... hungry? Pass 2 of 3, 3 of 3.
22. Ask child: What do you do with a cup? What is a chair used for? What is a pencil used for?
    Action words must be included in answers.
23. Pass if child correctly places and says how many blocks are on paper. (1, 5).
24. Tell child: Put block **on** table; **under** table; **in front of** me, **behind** me. Pass 4 of 4.
    (Do not help child by pointing, moving head or eyes.)
25. Ask child: What is a ball?... lake?... desk?... house?... banana?... curtain?... fence?... ceiling? Pass if defined in terms of use, shape, what it is made of, or general category (such as banana is fruit, not just yellow). Pass 5 of 8, 7 of 8.
26. Ask child: If a horse is big, a mouse is __? If fire is hot, ice is __? If the sun shines during the day, the moon shines during the __? Pass 2 of 3.
27. Child may use wall or rail only, not person. May not crawl.
28. Child must throw ball overhand 3 feet to within arm's reach of tester.
29. Child must perform standing broad jump over width of test sheet (8 1/2 inches).
30. Tell child to walk forward, 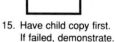 heel within 1 inch of toe. Tester may demonstrate. Child must walk 4 consecutive steps.
31. In the second year, half of normal children are non-compliant.

OBSERVATIONS:

Figure 22–1

Continued

The effects of lead poisoning are more pervasive and longer lasting in children than previously believed and may contribute to the increased high school–dropout rate. Even moderate levels of lead may contribute to reading disabilities. Low levels have been linked to lower intelligence and to speech and hearing deficits. Prenatal exposure and exposure in children age 2–3 years are of particular concern. The Centers for Disease Control and Prevention estimate that nearly 750,000 children in the United States have excessive lead in the bloodstream.

Children with sensory deprivation frequently go to their rooms and rock back and forth. A nonthreatening approach to finding out whether a child does this would be to say,

> *"Some children have a habit of rocking back and forth when they are alone. Have you ever noticed your child doing this?"*

The pediatric *family history* is basically the same as in the adult history. Obtain the names of both parents. Do not assume that a man and a woman who are with a child are the parents or that they are married. Always ask who the child's parents are. Determine consanguinity. Diseases with familial tendencies, such as diabetes, coronary artery disease, hypertension, and cancer, should be determined in the history. Always ask whether there is a genetic or familial pattern of any diseases in any relative. These diseases include hemophilia, Tay-Sachs disease, muscular dystrophy, and Huntington's chorea. If there is an abnormal genetic history, a complete family tree should be drawn. An example of a family tree is shown in Figure 22–2.

The health of all siblings should be ascertained. Note who the parents of all siblings are.

The *review of systems* is essentially the same as in the adult history. In the child's history, however, there should be increased emphasis on the symptoms related to the *respiratory, gastrointestinal,* and *genitourinary* systems. The high incidence of symptoms and diseases related to these systems obligates the interviewer to be methodical in these areas. Ask the following questions:

> *"Does your child have frequent sore throats? headaches? ear infections? nosebleeds? draining ears? cough? pneumonias? runny nose?"*
> *"Does your child snore? wheeze?"*

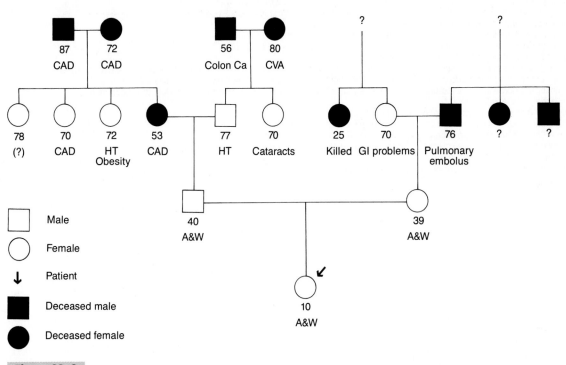

Figure 22–2

A family tree. *Abbreviations:* A&W = alive and well; CAD = coronary artery disease; HT = hypertension; Ca = cancer; CVA = cerebral vascular accident.

"Have you noticed your child stop breathing for more than 5 seconds?"*
"Has your child ever awakened from sleep gasping for breath?"
"Have you noticed your child sleeping restlessly?"
"Have you been told that your child sleeps while in school?"†
"Does the child breathe through the mouth?"
"How is the child's appetite?"
"Does your child have frequent stomach aches? diarrhea? constipation? vomiting?"
"Has the child ever complained of burning while urinating?"
"Has your child ever produced red urine?"
"Does the child urinate frequently?"

The final question in the review of systems allows the parent to discuss anything that is of concern to the parent that has not already been discussed. An example of such a question is the following:

"Is there anything else about your child that you would like to tell me?"

Adolescent patients are too old to be considered children but too young to be considered adults. It is during adolescence that the second major growth spurt, both emotional and physical, occurs. Adolescents have many problems. They may be developing physically faster or slower than their friends; in either case, they are different and uncomfortable. They have many concerns about the changes occurring in their bodies. There are many psychosocial adjustments during adolescence; these include establishments of self-image and adult sexual role, achievement of independence from parents, and choosing a career. Adolescents have many questions but frequently have difficulty obtaining answers because they may be too embarrassed to ask their parents. Usually the interview and physical examination of adolescents are performed without the parent or guardian. The interviewer should assure the patient that the interview will be strictly confidential insofar as the patient's health is not in jeopardy. With this as an introduction, most adolescents feel comfortable discussing their problems because confidentiality is ensured.

Depression is common among the adolescent population, especially in girls. Worry about their bodies is one reason adolescence is more emotionally stressful for girls than for boys. Although depression rates before puberty are the same in boys and girls, the rates are higher among girls at around ages 12–13 years. Several studies have shown that girls' preoccupation with how they look accounts for most of the incease. They frequently are convinced that they are too short or too tall, that their hair is too curly or too straight, that they are too fat, or that they have a bad complexion. There are some common signs of depression in adolescents. Although both boys and girls may show these symptoms, they tend to be more common in one sex or the other.

More Common Among Girls
Body-image distortion
Loss of appetite and weight
Lack of satisfaction

More Common Among Boys
Irritability
Social withdrawal
Drop in school performance

The interviewer should broach the major general areas of concern and allow the adolescent to respond. An approach to interviewing the adolescent might be to ask some or all of the following questions:

"Most adolescents have some concerns about the size and development of their
   bodies. What thoughts do you have?"
"Do you think there is something wrong with your body development?"
"Do you think there is something seriously wrong with your health?"
"Do you think there is anything wrong with your feelings about sex?"

---

* This is a feature of sleep apnea.
† Often a sign that the child may have sleep apnea and restless sleeping at night.

"How would you describe yourself? your moods?"
"Stress affects everyone. What makes you feel most stressed?"

Adolescents often have many questions regarding recreational drugs, birth control, and venereal disease but are afraid to ask their parents. The interviewer can play a key role in helping the adolescent through this trying period. Many times it is more useful to ask about birth control or sexual activity *during* the physical examination when the examination of the appropriate body area is being performed. Adolescents usually believe that this discussion is relevant to this part of the examination. Ask specific questions of teenagers. The interviewer should ask these questions:

"Do you have any questions you would like to ask me about 'street drugs'? birth control? venereal disease?"
"What do your friends think about drugs? sex? drinking?"
"Do you have a girlfriend or boyfriend?"
"Is it an exclusive (close) relationship?"
"Have you ever had sex?" If so, *"What type of birth control do you use?"*

The patient's description of a "friend's" feelings often reveals some of the patient's concerns. Establishing rapport and then using an open, straightforward approach goes a long way in developing a good doctor-patient relationship, one that may last several decades.

Incest and sexual abuse are not uncommon. In more than 80% of all cases of sexual abuse, the molester is not a stranger. All children should be told that their bodies are personal and that no one has the right to touch them or make them feel uncomfortable. Children need to know that there are different types of touch: *good* touches are hugs, kisses, and pats; *confusing* touch is tickling or rubbing; *bad* touch is hitting, hurting, spanking, or touching or fondling the "private parts" of their bodies. Listen carefully to a child who describes any type of sexual abuse. Children do not confabulate sexually explicit stories. If the child is older than 3 years of age, ask the following:

"Has anyone touched your body in any way that made you feel uncomfortable or confused?"

It is useful to ask a child to show you on a doll where the person touched him or her. Male and female dolls that are anatomically correct are often used by pediatricians for this purpose when they ask about sexual abuse.

The child who has been sexually or physically abused may exhibit behavior such as aggression, moodiness, irritability, hysteria, withdrawal, regression, memory loss, insecurity, and clinging. In addition, the child may exhibit some of the following physical changes: torn and/or bloody clothing, bruises or other suspicious injuries, difficulty in walking or sitting, loss of appetite, stomach problems, genital soreness or burning, difficulty in urination, vaginal or penile discharge, excessive bathing, or a desire not to bathe at all. For the older child in school, additional problems may result, such as a drop in academic performance, prevarication, stealing, or even running away from home.

Examination of the Newborn

The newborn is assessed immediately after birth to determine the integrity of the cardiopulmonary systems. The infant is placed on a warmer, where the initial examination is conducted. Start the examination by carefully washing your hands.

The initial examination consists of evaluation of five signs:

- Color
- Heart rate
- Reflex irritability
- Muscle tone
- Respiratory effort

Dr. Virginia Apgar developed a scale for rating the newborn 1 and 5 minutes after birth. The *Apgar scale* is shown in Table 22–2. Each of the tests is scored from 0 to 2.

Table 22–2   The Apgar Test

Sign	Score		
	0	1	2
Color	Blue, pale	Pink body with blue extremities	Completely pink
Heart rate	Absent	Below 100	Over 100
Reflex irritability*	No response	Grimace	Sneeze or cough
Muscle tone	Flaccid	Some flexion of the extremities	Good flexion of the extremities
Respiratory effort	Absent	Weak, irregular	Good, crying

The acronym APGAR is useful for remembering the examinations of the APGAR test:

*A*ppearance: color
*P*ulse: heart rate
*G*rimace: reflex irritability
*A*ctivity: muscle tone
*R*espiratory: respiratory effort

* This is determined by placing a soft catheter into the external nares.

At 1 minute, a total score of 3 to 4 indicates severe cardiopulmonary depression, and the infant requires immediate resuscitative measures; a score from 5 to 6 indicates mild central nervous system depression. The tests are repeated at 5 minutes; a score equal to or greater than 8 indicates a grossly normal cardiopulmonary examination.

General Assessment

After the Apgar score has been assessed, the *gestational age* should be determined. Because menstrual dates are frequently inaccurate, make an objective determination of the gestational age, which is an indicator of the maturity of the newborn. The standardized scoring system for assessing gestational age is the *Dubowitz Clinical Assessment*. This is based on 10 neurologic signs and 11 external signs, such as skin texture, breast size, and genitalia development. The neurologic scoring system is shown in Figure 22–3, and the external criteria are shown in Table 22–3.

The total scores of the neurologic and external signs are summed. The total is then correlated with the gestational age, according to the graph shown in Figure 22–4. A total score of 46–60 is associated with a gestational age of 37–41 weeks. A child with a gestational age from 37 to 41 weeks is denoted a *term infant*. Gestational ages of less than 37 weeks are *pre-term;* those greater than 41 weeks are *post-term*.

The newborn infant is also weighed, but weight alone does not totally relate to maturational age. The birth weight is correlated with gestational age according to the standard classification of Battaglia and Lubchenco, which is shown in Figure 22–5. By this method, the infant is classified as being small, appropriate, or large for gestational age. If the birth weight is from the 10th to the 90th percentile, the infant is *appropriate for gestational age (AGA)*. If the birth weight is less than the 10th percentile on the intrauterine growth curve, the newborn is classified *small for gestational age (SGA)*. If the birth weight is greater than the 90th percentile, the newborn is called *large for gestational age (LGA)*. According to the standard shown in Figure 22–5, *term* is defined as a gestational age from 38 to 42 weeks.

The value of weight–gestational age determination lies in its ability to predict certain risk groups. Children born in the LGA group are at risk for hypoglycemia and polycythemia. The SGA classification may be an indication of congenital anomalies, hypoglycemia, or congenital infections. All pre-term newborns are at risk for hyaline membrane disease, hypoglycemia, and hypocalcemia.

The remainder of the examination is usually performed in the warmed environment of the nursery, often within 24 hours after birth.

The *respiratory rate* and degree of *respiratory effort* are carefully assessed while the baby is undressed. The respiratory rate of a newborn varies from 30 to 50 per minute. Observe the respiratory rate for 1–2 minutes, because periods of apnea and periodic

Text continued on page 598

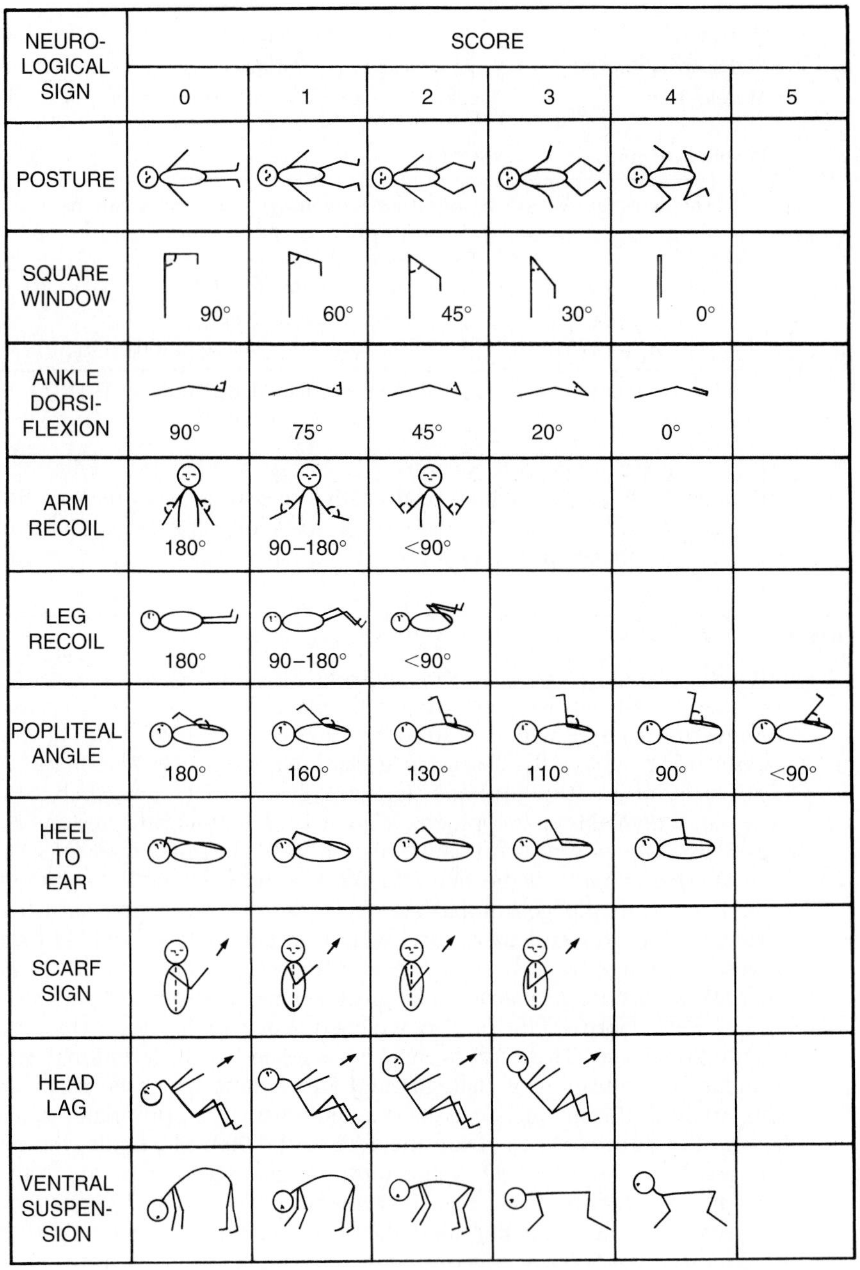

NEURO-LOGICAL SIGN	SCORE					
	0	1	2	3	4	5
POSTURE						
SQUARE WINDOW	90°	60°	45°	30°	0°	
ANKLE DORSI-FLEXION	90°	75°	45°	20°	0°	
ARM RECOIL	180°	90–180°	<90°			
LEG RECOIL	180°	90–180°	<90°			
POPLITEAL ANGLE	180°	160°	130°	110°	90°	<90°
HEEL TO EAR						
SCARF SIGN						
HEAD LAG						
VENTRAL SUSPEN-SION						

Figure 22–3

Figure 22-3

The Dubowitz Clinical Assessment. Some notes on techniques of assessment of the neurologic criteria:

Posture: Observed with infant quiet and in supine position. Score 0: Arms and legs extended; 1: beginning of flexion of hips and knees, arms extended; 2: stronger flexion of legs, arms extended; 3: arms slightly flexed, legs flexed and abducted; 4: full flexion of arms and legs.

Square Window: The hand is flexed on the forearm between the thumb and index finger of the examiner. Enough pressure is applied to get as full a flexion as possible, and the angle between the hypothenar eminence and the ventral aspect of the forearm is measured and graded according to diagram. (Care is taken not to rotate the infant's wrist while performing this maneuver.)

Ankle Dorsiflexion: The foot is dorsiflexed onto the anterior aspect of the leg, with the examiner's thumb on the sole of the foot and other fingers behind the leg. Enough pressure is applied to get as full flexion as possible, and the angle between the dorsum of the foot and the anterior aspect of the leg is measured.

Arm Recoil: With the infant in the supine position, the forearms are first flexed for 5 seconds, then fully extended by pulling on the hands, and then released. The sign is fully positive if the arms return briskly to full flexion (score 2). If the arms return to incomplete flexion or the response is sluggish, it is graded as score 1. If they remain extended or are only followed by random movements, the score is 0.

Leg Recoil: With the infant supine, the hips and knees are fully flexed for 5 seconds, then extended by traction on the feet, and released. A maximal response is one of full flexion of the hips and knees (score 2). A partial flexion is scored 1, and minimal or no movement is scored 0.

Popliteal Angle: With the infant supine and the pelvis flat on the examining couch, the thigh is held in the knee-chest position by the examiner's left index finger and thumb supporting the knee. The leg is then extended by gentle pressure from the examiner's right index finger behind the ankle, and the popliteal angle is measured.

Heel to Ear Maneuver: With the baby supine, draw the baby's foot as near to the head as it will go without forcing it. Observe the distance between the foot and the head as well as the degree of extension at the knee. Grade according to diagram. Note that the knee is left free and may draw down alongside the abdomen.

Scarf Sign: With the baby supine, take the infant's hand and try to put it around the neck and as far posteriorly as possible around the opposite shoulder. Assist this maneuver by lifting the elbow across the body. See how far the elbow will go across and grade according to illustrations. Score 0: elbow reaches opposite axillary line; 1: elbow between midline and opposite axillary line; 2: elbow reaches midline; 3: elbow will not reach midline.

Head Lag: With the baby lying supine, grasp the hands (or the arms if a very small infant) and pull him or her slowly towards the sitting position. Observe the position of the head in relation to the trunk and grade accordingly. In a small infant, the head may initially be supported by one hand. Score 0: complete lag; 1: partial head control; 2: able to maintain head in line with body; 3: brings head anterior to body.

Ventral Suspension: The infant is suspended in the prone position, with the examiner's hand under the infant's chest (one hand in a small infant, two in a large infant). Observe the degree of extension of the back and the amount of flexion of the arms and legs. Also note the relation of the head to the trunk. Grade according to diagrams.

If score differs on the two sides, take the mean.

(Reprinted with permission from Dubowitz LMS, Dubowitz V, Goldberg C: Clinical assessment of gestational age in the newborn infant. J Pediatr 77:1–10, 1970.)

Table 22–3   Scoring System for External Criteria of Gestational Age

External Sign	Score* 0	1	2	3	4
Edema	Obvious edema of hands and feet; pitting over tibia	No obvious edema of hands and feet; pitting over tibia	No edema		
Skin texture	Very thin, gelatinous	Thin and smooth	Smooth; medium thickness. Rash or superficial peeling	Slight thickening. Superficial cracking and peeling, especially of hands and feet	Thick and parchment-like; superficial or deep cracking
Skin color	Dark red	Uniformly pink	Pale pink; variable over body	Pale; pink only over ears, lips, palms, or soles	
Skin opacity (trunk)	Numerous veins and venules clearly seen, especially over abdomen	Veins and tributaries seen	A few large vessels clearly seen over abdomen	A few large vessels seen indistinctly over abdomen	No blood vessels seen
Lanugo (over back)	No lanugo	Abundant; long and thick over whole back	Hair thinning, especially over lower back	Small amount of lanugo and bald areas	At least half of back devoid of lanugo
Plantar creases	No skin creases	Faint red marks over anterior half of sole	Definite red marks over >anterior half; indentations over <anterior third	Indentations over >anterior third	Definite deep indentations over >anterior third
Nipple formation	Nipple barely visible; no areola	Nipple well defined; areola smooth and flat, diameter <0.75 cm	Areola stippled, edge not raised, diameter <0.75 cm	Areola stippled, edge raised, diameter >0.75 cm	
Breast size	No breast tissue palpable	Breast tissue on one or both sides <0.5 cm diameter	Breast tissue both sides; one or both 0.5–1.0 cm	Breast tissue both sides; one or both >1 cm	
Ear form	Pinna flat and shapeless, little or no incurving of edge	Incurving of part of edge of pinna	Partial incurving whole of upper pinna	Well-defined incurving whole of upper pinna	
Ear firmness	Pinna soft, easily folded, no recoil	Pinna soft, easily folded, slow recoil	Cartilage to edge of pinna, but soft in places; ready recoil	Pinna firm, cartilage to edge; instant recoil	
Genitals Male Female (with hips half abducted)	Neither testicle in scrotum Labia majora widely separated, labia minora protruding	At least one testicle high in scrotum Labia majora almost cover labia minora	At least one testicle fully descended Labia majora completely cover labia minora		

* If score differs on two sides, take the mean.
From Dubowitz LM, Dubowitz V, Goldberg C: Clinical assessment of gestational age in the newborn infant. J Pediatr 77:1–10, 1970. Developed from Farr V, Mitchell RG, Neligan GA, et al: The definition of some external characteristics used in the assessment of gestational age in the newborn infant. Develop Med Child Neurol 8:507–511, 1966.

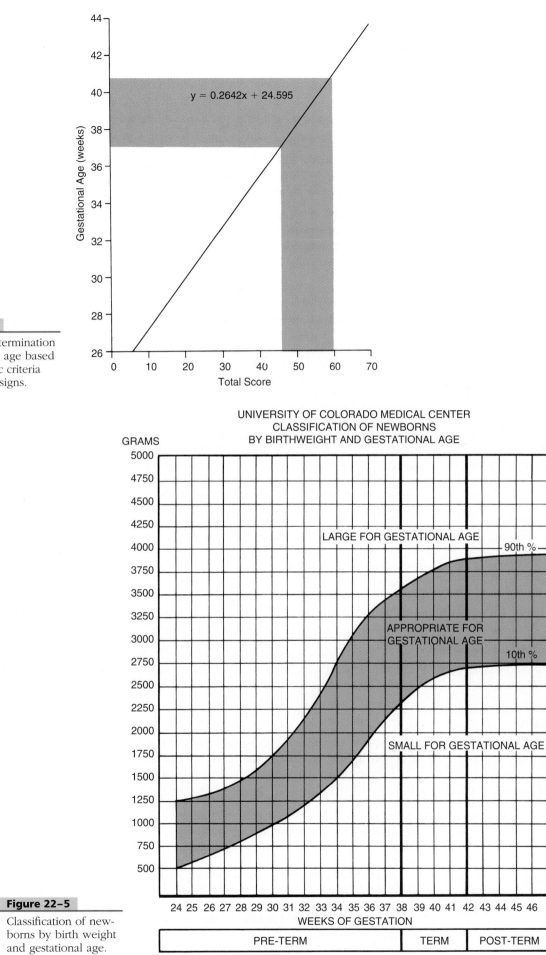

Figure 22–4

Graph for determination of gestational age based on neurologic criteria and external signs.

$y = 0.2642x + 24.595$

Gestational Age (weeks)

Total Score

UNIVERSITY OF COLORADO MEDICAL CENTER
CLASSIFICATION OF NEWBORNS
BY BIRTHWEIGHT AND GESTATIONAL AGE

GRAMS

LARGE FOR GESTATIONAL AGE

90th %

APPROPRIATE FOR
GESTATIONAL AGE

10th %

SMALL FOR GESTATIONAL AGE

WEEKS OF GESTATION

PRE-TERM | TERM | POST-TERM

Figure 22–5

Classification of newborns by birth weight and gestational age.

597

breathing are common, especially among pre-term infants. Look for grunting respirations and for retractions, each of which is evidence of respiratory distress.

Measure the *temperature* by using a rectal thermometer. The infant is placed in a prone position on an examining table or in the examiner's lap. The infant's buttocks are spread, and a well-lubricated thermometer is inserted slowly through the anal sphincter to approximately 1 inch. After 1 minute, it may be read. Newborn infants often have relative thermal instability, and for this reason, the ambient temperature should also be determined.

Determine the *pulse* by auscultation of the heart. The average heart rate of a newborn ranges from 120 to 140 per minute. There are wide fluctuations; the rate increases to as fast as 190 during crying and decreases to as low as 90 during sleep. A heart rate below 90 is of concern.

Basic *measurements of the head and chest* are taken next. The head is measured at its greatest circumference around the occipitofrontal area. In general, three measurements are taken, the largest of which is recorded. The head circumference is usually 13.0–14.5 inches (34–37 cm). The chest circumference is normally smaller than the head circumference by 2–3 cm. The chest measurement is taken at the level of the nipples midway between inspiration and expiration. By the time the newborn is 1 year of age, the chest circumference will exceed the head circumference. A second measurement is the *ratio of the upper to the lower* half of the body. The distance from the crown to the pubic symphysis and from the pubic symphysis to the heel should be compared. In the newborn, this ratio is 1.7 : 1; in the adult, the ratio is 1 : 1. A third measurement is the *arm span*. Normally the arm span equals the crown-to-heel length. Although all measurements are important, the determination of the head and chest size are the only routine measurements performed at this time.

Note the *posture*. The normal newborn lies on one side with the arms and legs flexed. A term infant who lies on his or her back with arms and legs abducted in a frog position has an abnormal posture. However, this posture can be consistent with prematurity.

Note the *movements*. Normally, all four limbs should be moving in a random and asymmetric manner. Fine movements of the face and fingers are usually present. Abnormal movements include jerky, symmetric, coarse movements. All extremities should be moving, with full range of motion seen at some time. Injury to the *brachial plexus* may cause paralysis of the upper arm. This injury may result from lateral traction on the head and neck during delivery of the shoulder. *Erb's palsy* produces an inability to abduct the arm at the shoulder, to rotate the arm externally, and to supinate the forearm. This injury to the 5th and 6th cervical nerves results in a characteristic position of arm adduction, forearm pronation, and arm internal rotation. *Klumpke's paralysis* results from injury to the 7th and 8th cervical nerves, producing paralysis of the hand and forearm. The arm is limp at the side. Involvement of the 1st thoracic nerve with Klumpke's paralysis may also result in ipsilateral ptosis and miosis. The prognosis of any brachial plexus palsy depends on whether the nerve or nerves were lacerated or only bruised. If the palsy is related only to edema of the nerve fibers and not to actual injury, function usually returns within a few months.

Skin

Skin color in newborns is partially related to the amount of fat present. Pre-term infants generally appear redder because they have less subcutaneous fat than do term infants.

The newborn has vasomotor instability, and the color of the skin may vary greatly from time to time and from one area of the body to another. It is often noted that when the infant is lying on one side for a time, a sharp color demarcation appears: the lower half of the body becomes red, and the upper half is pale. This has been termed the *harlequin color change* and is benign. This color change is seen in 10–15% of infants, especially in premature infants. The attacks may persist from 30 seconds to 30 minutes.

Inspect for *cyanosis* or *acrocyanosis*. Acrocyanosis is a benign condition in which the extremities are cyanotic and cool, but the trunk is pink and warm. This condition is common among newborns.

Is *plethora* present? Plethora in the newborn usually indicates high levels of hemoglobin.

Is *pallor* present? Pallor may be associated with anemia or, more commonly, with cold stress and peripheral vasoconstriction. Pallor may also represent asphyxia, shock, or edema. It should be recognized that the presence of pallor may mask cyanosis in the newborn with circulatory failure.

Is there any evidence of *birth trauma,* manifested by petechiae, ecchymoses, or lacerations?

Physiologic jaundice is found in almost 50% of all term newborns by the 3rd or 4th day of life. This finding is even more prevalent among pre-term infants. Icterus appearing before the 3rd day may indicate a blood-group incompatibility and hemolytic disease.

Observe the *pigmentation.* Large, slate-blue, well-demarcated areas of pigmentation near the buttocks are called *mongolian spots* and have little meaning. Within the first few years of life, these spots usually fade and may disappear. Mongolian spots are present in more than 80% of African-American and Asian-American babies but in fewer than 10% of white newborns. *Telangiectases* on the eyelids, glabella, or nape of the neck are common and frequently disappear during the first few years of life. They are often referred to as "stork bites" or "angel kisses" by the public.

Vascular nevi may be isolated defects or part of a syndrome. They may be flat and are commonly caused by dilated capillaries, or they may be mass lesions and consist of large, blood-filled cavities. The *port wine stain* or *nevus,* also known as the *nevus flammeus,* consists of dilated capillaries and appears as a pink-to-purple macular lesion of variable size. It can often be as large as one half of the body. The face is a common site. If the eye is involved, *glaucoma* should be ruled out. Figure 22–6 shows a child with a port wine stain involving the ophthalmic division of the trigeminal nerve. Often, children with a port wine stain in this area have associated capillary hemangiomas of the ipsilateral meninges and cerebral cortex, a condition known as *Sturge-Weber syndrome.* Mental retardation, seizures, hemiparesis, contralateral hemianopsia, and glaucoma are often seen in the first few years of life. The *strawberry hemangioma* is a bright red, protuberant lesion seen commonly on the face, scalp, or back. It may be present at birth, but it more commonly develops within the first few months of life. It may expand rapidly, reach a stationary period, and then regress. Most strawberry hemangiomas become involuted by the time the child is 5 years of age. The *cavernous hemangioma* is a bluish cystic lesion that is more diffuse and ill-defined than the strawberry hemangioma. Like the strawberry hemangioma, the cavernous hemangioma has a growth phase followed by a period of involution. If located near the trachea, life-

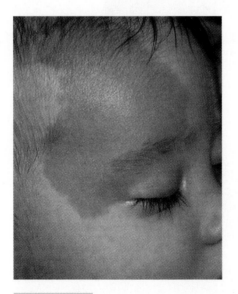

Figure 22–6

Port wine stain.

threatening compression may result when the hemangioma enlarges. Look at Figure 22–7. This child has a combination of a strawberry and a cavernous hemangioma. The strawberry lesion overlies the cavernous hemangioma. Figure 22–8 shows a child with a mixed hemangioma. Palpable hemangiomas occur in 10–12% of infants by the end of the 1st month of life, despite the fact that they are rarely present at birth. The hemangioma shown in this figure has both superficial capillary and deep cavernous components. This lesion involuted by the 3rd year of life of the child. Although these lesions usually resolve by the 7th year of life, they may leave scarring, loose skin, and telangiectasias.

Is a *rash* present? *Erythema toxicum* is a common rash among newborns. It is a self-limited benign eruption of unknown cause, consisting of erythematous macules, papules, and pustules. The lesions may appear anywhere on the body except on the palms and soles. It is most commonly seen during the first 3–4 days of life but may be present at birth. Erythema toxicum is shown in Figure 22–9.

Milia on the face are commonly seen in almost 50% of all newborns. Milia appear as tiny whitish papules on the cheeks, nose, chin, and forehead and usually disappear by 3 weeks of life.

At 3–4 days of life, *staphylococcal pustulosis* may occur. This manifests as pustular skin lesions found mainly around the groin and umbilicus.

Congenital infections of the fetus may manifest with cutaneous symptoms. *Congenital rubella* may manifest with purpura. Another cutaneous sign of congenital rubella is the *blueberry muffin* lesion. These lesions are bluish-red macules ranging in size from 2 to 8 mm. They are noted at birth or within the first 24 hours and appear on the face, neck, trunk, or extremities. Figure 22–10 shows a child with classic "blueberry muffin" rash of congenital rubella.

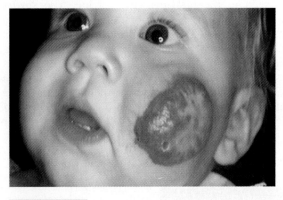

Figure 22–7

Strawberry hemangioma overlying cavernous hemangioma.

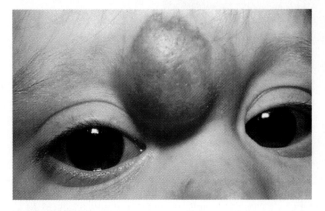

Figure 22–8

Mixed hemangioma.

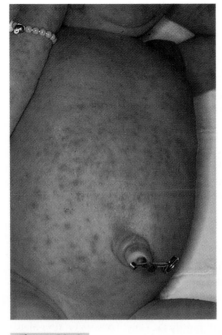

Figure 22–9

Erythema toxicum.

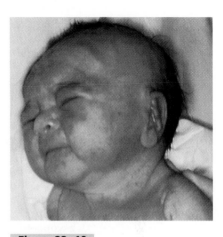

Figure 22–10

Congenital rubella.

Congenital syphilis may present as an erythematous maculopapular rash that later becomes brown or becomes a hemorrhagic vesicular rash.

Scattered superficial bullae on the upper extremities and lips are termed *sucking blisters* and are presumed to be caused by vigorous sucking in utero. These are most commonly seen on the radial aspect of the forearms, the thumbs, and the center of the upper lip. Resolution without sequelae is the rule.

Is *hair* present? A newborn's skin may be covered with fine, soft, immature hair, known as *lanugo hair.* Lanugo hair frequently covers the scalp and brow in premature infants but is usually absent in term infants. Lanugo hair may be present on the ears and shoulders. Inspect the lumbosacral area for tufts of hair. Hair in this area suggests the presence of an occult spina bifida or a sinus tract. Examine the *fingernails.* In the post-term infant, the fingernails are long and may be stained yellow by meconium, if meconium was present in the amniotic fluid.

Examine the *dermatoglyphics* of the fingers, palms, and soles. In addition to identification, these patterns are of importance as indicators of genetic abnormalities. Normal finger dermatoglyphic patterns are the loop, whorl, and arch. The loop is normally the most prevalent pattern. The arch is the least prevalent pattern, and the presence of more than four arches is generally abnormal. A single palmar crease, known as a *simian crease,* is frequently found in individuals with chromosomal abnormalities such as trisomy 21.

Head

Examination of the head involves a thorough assessment of its shape, symmetry, and fontanelles. The skull may be *molded,* especially if the labor was prolonged and the head was engaged for a long period. The skull of a child born by cesarean section has a characteristic roundness.

In the newborn, the *fontanelles* are frequently felt as ridges as a result of the overriding of the cranial bones by molding of the skull as it passes through the vaginal canal. Palpate the fontanelles. The *anterior fontanelle* is located at the junction of the sagittal and coronal sutures, is usually 4–6 cm in diameter, and appears diamond-shaped. The *posterior fontanelle* is located at the junction of the sagittal and lambdoid sutures, is smaller than the anterior fontanelle, and measures 1–2 cm in diameter. Normally, the fontanelles are flat. A bulging fontanelle may indicate increased intracranial pressure; a depressed fontanelle may be seen in dehydration. Normally during crying, the fontanelles bulge. Pulsations of the fontanelles reflect the pulse. The anterior fontanelle normally closes by 18 months, but there is a wide range of normality; the posterior fontanelle should be closed by 2 months of age. The locations of the fontanelles are shown in Figure 22–11.

A *caput succedaneum* is edema of the soft tissues over the vertex of the skull that is related to the birth process. This swelling crosses the sutures and disappears after a few days. The capute succedaneum should be differentiated from a *cephalohematoma,* which is a subperiosteal hemorrhage limited to one cranial bone, usually the parietal. There is no discoloration of the overlying scalp, and the swelling does not cross the suture line. The swelling is usually not visible until several hours after birth.

Inspect the skull for *symmetry.*

Transillumination of the skull is utilized to detect subdural effusions and congenital defects such as porencephalic cysts, which are cysts in the brain parenchyma that communicate with the arachnoid space. Transillumination is performed by using a strong light source and shining it against the skull in several areas. A soft foam collar should be placed at the lighted end. A 2–3 cm halo around the circumference of the light when placed in the frontoparietal area is normal; a 1–2 cm halo in the occipital area is also normal. Localized bright spots may indicate a disorder. Hydrocephaly is indicated by a glow over the entire skull.

Inspect the *face* for symmetry. The eye creases should be equal. Observe the infant as he or she sucks or cries. The mouth should remain on a level plane. If it is asymmetric, suspect a facial paralysis. The face may reveal abnormal features such as *epicanthal folds, widely spaced eyes,* or *low-set ears,* each of which may be associated with congenital defects.

Eyes

Several attempts to evaluate the eyes of the newborn may be necessary. Eyelid edema related to the birth process, medications, or infection makes this part of the examination difficult.

Inspect the eyes for *symmetry.* The eyes should be the same size and should be at the same depth in the orbits. Bulging eyes may be a sign of congenital glaucoma. Microcornea may result from congenital rubella.

Inspect the *eyelids* for evidence of trauma. Use a soft cloth to gently remove the vernix caseosa and any conjunctival exudate. Newborns rarely have eyebrows, but long eyelashes are frequently present. Medial epicanthal folds are seen frequently in individuals with trisomy 21.

The best method of evaluating the eyes of a newborn is to hold the infant at arm's length while slowly rotating him or her in one direction. The infant's eyes usually open spontaneously.

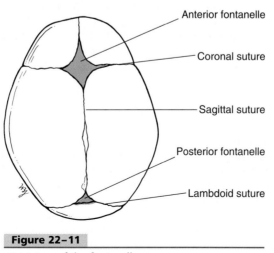

Anterior fontanelle

Coronal suture

Sagittal suture

Posterior fontanelle

Lambdoid suture

Figure 22–11

Location of the fontanelles.

Inspect the *cornea.* The cornea should be clear. Cloudiness of the cornea or a corneal diameter that is greater than 1 cm may indicate congenital glaucoma.

Inspect the *iris.* The iris of a newborn is pale because full pigmentation does not occur before 10–12 months of life. Is an abnormal ventral cleft present in the iris? This cleft, known as a *coloboma,* is associated with defects in the lens and retina. A coloboma is commonly associated with chromosomal abnormalities such as trisomy 13 or 18. Is there a ring of whitish dots at the periphery of the iris? These dots are best seen in slit-lamp examination by an ophthalmologist, but the ring is sometimes visible to the naked eye. These dots, called *Brushfield's spots,* may be associated with trisomy 21 or may be normal.

Inspect the *conjunctivae.* Small conjunctival hemorrhages are common. As a result of the erythromycin drops* instilled at birth, there may be some inflammation of the conjunctivae as well as edema of the eyelids in the neonate.

The *pupils* of neonates are usually constricted until about the 3rd week of life. Pupillary responses are not to be interpreted in this age group.

Rotate the infant slowly to one side. The eyes should turn in the direction to which he or she is being turned. At the end of the motion, the eyes should quickly look back in the opposite direction after a few quick, nonsustained nystagmoid movements. This is termed the *rotational response.*

Place the infant back on his or her back.

In order to test for *visual acuity* in the newborn, the examiner must rely on indirect methods such as the response to a bright light, known as the *optical blink reflex.* This reflex is normally observed when a bright light is shined on each eye: the newborn blinks and dorsiflexes the head. Although never actually tested, the visual acuity of the newborn has been estimated to be approximately 20/600.

A *funduscopic examination* of all infants is important. However, very often the examination can be postponed until the infant is 3–4 months of age, when he or she may be more cooperative. The examination may be postponed only after the presence of intraocular disorder has been excluded. In all newborns, the presence of the *red reflex* bilaterally suggests grossly normal eyes and the absence of glaucoma or intraocular disorders. Determine the presence of the red reflex by holding the ophthalmoscope 10–12 inches away from the eyes. The presence of the red reflex indicates that there is no serious obstruction to light between the cornea and the retina. If a red reflex is absent, funduscopic examination is required at this time.

To inspect the retina, instill a mydriatic into the eyes. Place one drop each of phenylephrine 2.5% and tropicamide (Mydriacyl) 1% into each eye and wait 15–20 minutes. At the end of this period, place the infant flat on his or her back and ask the parent or a nurse for assistance. Use a pacifier to help quiet the child. Hold the ophthalmoscope in the same manner as when examining an adult. The cornea can usually be visualized when the ophthalmoscope is set at +20 diopters, the lens visualized at +15 diopters, and the retina visualized at 0 diopters.

Inspect the *optic disc* and the *vessels.* In the newborn, the disc appears paler than in the adult. The pinpoint light reflex at the fovea is absent because the fovea is not fully developed until 4–5 months of age. Are any *hemorrhages* present? Papilledema is rarely seen in children younger than the age of 2–3 years. Because the fontanelles are open until this age, any increased intracranial pressure will be dissipated by these open sutures and the optic discs will be spared. Is there any *abnormal pigmentation* present? Congenital rubella and toxoplasmosis are often associated with abnormal pigmentation of the retina. Ophthalmoscopic examination of newborns is difficult. Multiple attempts may be required.

Ears

Inspect the *external ear.* An imaginary line drawn from the inner and outer canthus of the eye toward the vertex should be at the level of or below the level of the superior attachment of the ear. Low-set ears are often associated with congenital kidney defects or other chromosomal disorders. Frequently, the ears may be misshapened as a result of intrauterine positioning. Such misshapening usually rapidly resolves within 1–2 days.

---

* As prophylaxis against gonorrheal conjuctivitis, also known as *ophthalmia neonatorum.*

Are any *skin tags* present? A skin tag or cleft that is present in front of the tragus often represents a remnant of the first branchial cleft.

Hearing in newborns may be tested by utilizing the primitive acoustic blink reflex. Blinking of the eyes in response to snapping of fingers or a loud noise indicates that the newborn can hear. This is a crude test with low sensitivity. A negative response should be further tested with a specific pure-tone screening device.

The *external canal* should be inspected. Hold the otoscope (as indicated in Chapter 9, The Ear and Nose) by bracing it against the child's forehead. Because the external canal of the newborn is directed downward, insert the otoscope by pulling the pinna gently downward. The external canal is usually filled with vernix caseosa, and so the tympanic membrane may not be seen. If the tympanic membrane is seen, only the most superior portion is usually visualized. The tympanic membrane may appear to be bulging with amniotic fluid behind it. This is a normal condition. Rotation of the tympanic membrane to a normal anatomic position occurs within 6–12 weeks.

Nose

Inspect for a *congenitally deviated septum*.

Patency of the nasopharynx is determined by passing a soft, sterile, number 14 French catheter through each external naris and advancing it into the posterior nasopharynx. This test rules out the presence of unilateral or bilateral *choanal atresia,* which is a cause of severe respiratory distress in newborns. Newborns are nasal breathers, and obstruction to nasal flow can cause considerable distress.

Mouth and Pharynx

Test the *sucking reflex*. Put on a glove, and insert your index finger into the newborn's mouth. A strong sucking reflex should be present. The sucking reflex is strong at 34 weeks' gestation and disappears at 9–12 months.

Inspect the *gingivae*. The gums should be raised, smooth, and pink.

Inspect the *tongue*. The frenulum may be short or may extend almost to the tip of the tongue. Because the production of saliva is limited in the first few months of life, the presence of excessive saliva in the mouth is suggestive of *esophageal atresia*.

Inspect the *palate*. Is there a *cleft palate?* A *bifid uvula* may be associated with a submucous cleft palate. Is the palate *high-arched? Petechiae* are commonly found on the hard and soft palates. Pinhead, whitish-yellow, rounded lesions on either side of the raphe on the hard palate are *Epstein's pearls*. These are mucous retention cysts and disappear within the first few weeks of life. Similar cysts may be present on the gingivae. A patulous white membrane on the tongue or palate may represent *thrush,* or oral candidiasis. Inspect for *neonatal teeth*. These teeth have a poor root system and may have to be removed to prevent accidental aspiration.

Inspect the *oropharynx*. This can be performed while the infant is crying. Tonsillar tissue is not visible in the newborn. Small ulcers or clusters of small, whitish-yellow follicles on an erythematous base are commonly seen on the anterior tonsillar pillars. The cause is unknown, and they disappear within the first week of life.

Listen to the child's *cry*. Evaluate the cry for its nature, pitch, intensity, and effort. A healthy child has a strong cry, indicative of normal functioning airways. The cry varies in intensity with breathing. A high-pitched, shrill cry is seen in diseases associated with increased intracranial pressure. Children born to drug-addicted mothers often have a high-pitched cry. A low-pitched, hoarse cry that is infrequent and low in intensity is often associated with hypothyroidism or hypocalcemic tetany. A "cri du chat" cry sounds like a cat mewing and may be associated with chromosomal abnormalities. Absence of crying is suggestive of severe illness or mental retardation.

Neck

The neck of a newborn appears relatively short. Is the neck *symmetric* with regard to the midline? Rotate the infant's head. The normal infant's head should be easily rotated to either side so that the chin can touch either shoulder. *Torticollis* is a condition in which the head is tilted to one side while the chin is rotated to the other shoulder. In the newborn, a hematoma of the sternocleidomastoid muscle as a result of a birth injury may produce this condition. Palpate for a mass in the area of the sternocleidomastoid muscle if torticollis is present.

Palpate the *clavicles* to rule out a fracture. You should feel for the crepitus of a fractured clavicle. Clavicular fractures as a result of a birth injury usually occur at the junction of the middle and outer third of the bone. Decreased motion in the upper extremity may be associated with a clavicular fracture.

Palpate for *masses*. A midline mass may be a thyroglossal cyst.

Is *webbing* of the neck present? Webbing is a feature of *Turner's syndrome* and other congenital abnormalities.

Chest

Observe the *respiratory rate* while the infant is undisturbed. At several hours of age, the rate may vary from 20 to 80 per minute with an average of 30 to 40. Because of the wide variations, respirations should be counted for 1–2 minutes.

Inspect the *respiratory pattern*. The breathing pattern of newborns is almost entirely diaphragmatic. Irregular, shallow respirations are common in newborns. *Periodic breathing* is characterized by brief periods of apnea lasting 5–15 seconds and is not associated with bradycardia. *True apnea* has a duration of more than 20 seconds and is associated with bradycardia. The latter is more commonly found in premature infants with pulmonary disease. Infants with true apnea are at high risk for the sudden infant death syndrome. The presence of a *respiratory grunt, retractions* of the chest, or *flaring* of the nostrils indicates respiratory distress.

Inspect for *deformities*. The most important chest deformity in newborns is asymmetry that is due to unequal chest expansion on the other side. Other deformities seen in adults, such as pectus excavatum and pectus carinatum, cannot be detected in newborns.

Percussion of the chest is performed by using either one finger to tap the chest or the method discussed for the adult (see Chapter 11, The Chest). Normally, the thorax of a newborn is hyperresonant throughout. Dullness may indicate an effusion or consolidation.

Auscultate the chest with either the bell or the small diaphragm of the stethoscope. Bronchovesicular breath sounds should be easily heard throughout the lung fields and are higher in pitch than in adults. In general, auscultation of the chest in newborns is of low sensitivity.

Breast

Inspect the breasts. The breasts of both male and female newborns are enlarged. Commonly, a milky discharge from the nipple, known as *witch's milk,* may be present. This is the effect of maternal estrogen and is present for 1–2 weeks after birth.

Supernumerary nipples may be present along the milk line. They may or may not have areolae. They may often be mistaken for congenital nevi and have no clinical significance.

Heart

Inspect for *cyanosis*. If cyanosis is present within the first hours or days of birth, suspect atresia of one of the heart valves, transposition of the great vessels, or persistent fetal circulation.

Inspect for evidence of *congestive heart failure*. In newborns, the most important signs of heart failure are persistent tachycardia of 200 beats per minute, tachypnea, and an enlarged liver. Crackles are not sensitive indicators of heart failure in newborns. Heart failure during the first few days of life is frequently caused by hypoplastic left heart syndrome.

Palpate for the *point of maximum impulse*. In newborns less than 48 hours old, the point of maximum impulse is often in the xiphoid region. After this period and for several years, the point of maximum impulse should be in the fourth left intercostal space just lateral to the midclavicular line. A right-sided point of maximum impulse suggests *dextrocardia*.

Auscultate the heart in the same locations as in adults by using the small diaphragm and bell of the stethoscope. Because the respiratory rate is so rapid in newborns, it is often difficult to distinguish respiratory from cardiac events. Sometimes occluding the nares for a few seconds may help to elucidate the sounds. Auscultation in newborns has a low degree of sensitivity in detecting congenital heart disease. Many "normal" murmurs heard in the early neonatal period are related to the marked changes in circulation after birth. It has been suggested that there is less than a 1 in 10 chance that the presence of a murmur heard in the neonatal period is the consequence of actual congenital heart disease. The continuous machinery murmur of a *patent ductus arteriosus* is commonly heard at birth but disappears by the 2nd or 3rd day of life as the ductus spontaneously closes. This condition is frequently associated with a hyperdynamic precordium. If any murmurs are present, however, they should be noted and described as indicated in Chapter 12, The Heart.

Pulses

Palpate the femoral pulses. A delay in the femoral pulse in comparison with the radial pulse should raise the suspicion of coarctation of the aorta. Bounding pulses may indicate a patent ductus arteriosus.

Abdomen

Inspect the abdomen. The abdomen of a newborn is protuberant as a result of the poor development of the abdominal musculature. If the abdomen is scaphoid, there should be a high index of suspicion that a diaphragmatic hernia is present and that the abdominal organs may be located in the chest.

Is an *umbilical hernia* present? The abdominal wall is relatively weak in newborns, especially in premature infants. Umbilical hernias are common in African-American infants. An umbilical hernia in a non–African-American child may be an indication of hypothyroidism.

Inspect the *umbilical cord stump*. Is there evidence of yellow staining by meconium as a result of fetal distress? The normal umbilical cord contains two ventrally placed thick-walled arteries and one dorsally placed thin-walled vein. Newborns with a single artery often have congenital renal abnormalities. Drainage of a clear discharge from the umbilicus is suggestive of the presence of a patent urachus* or a possible omphalomesenteric duct.

Auscultate the abdomen. The abdomen of newborn infants is tympanitic, with metallic tinkling sounds being heard every 15–20 seconds.

Palpate the abdomen. To relax the abdomen, use your left hand to hold the hips and knees in a flexed position while the child is sucking, and palpate with your right hand. In general, the liver edge may be felt as much as 2 cm below the right costal margin in the newborn. A liver edge more than 3 cm below the right costal margin suggests hepatomegaly. The liver span can be measured by percussion, and this measurement is more accurate than abdominal measurements because respiratory conditions could inflate the lungs and push a normal liver down into the abdominal cavity. Palpation of the spleen tip is less common.

Palpate the *kidneys*. Place your left hand under the right side of the child's back, and lift upward. At the same time, place your right hand in the right upper quadrant, and palpate for the right kidney. Reverse hands to palpate the left kidney.

Unless clinically indicated, the *rectum* is not examined. Patency of the gastrointestinal tract is confirmed by the passage of meconium, which usually occurs within the first 12 hours after birth. If there is an absence of a meconium stool in the first 24 hours, suspect either cystic fibrosis or Hirschsprung's disease. In either case, examine the rectum. Glove and well-lubricate your right fifth finger and insert it into the infant's rectum while your left hand holds the infant's feet together and flexes the hips. Your left hand may now be used for bimanual palpation of the infant's abdomen in conjunction with your right hand. Palpate for any masses. When your finger is removed from the infant's rectum, some rectal bleeding may occur.

---

* A canal in the fetus that connects the urinary bladder to the allantois.

Genitalia

Inspect the external genitalia for *ambiguity*.

In the full-term male, the scrotum is relatively large and rugated. The foreskin of the penis is tight and adherent to the glans penis. Inspect the glans for the location of the external urethral meatus. *Hypospadias* is a condition in which the meatus is located in an abnormal ventral position. The meatus may be found anywhere from the tip of the penis to the scrotum. It is important to detect hypospadias in the neonatal period because it represents a contraindication to circumcision. Erection is common and has no clinical significance. The testicles should be descended into the scrotum or the inguinal canals. Palpate the testicles by a downward movement, which counteracts the active cremasteric reflex. Are any masses present? *Hydroceles* or *hernias* are common in newborns. A hydrocele should be evaluated until the child is 6 months of age. If by this time it is still present, the hydrocele usually must be repaired. A hernia should be repaired as soon as possible.

In the full-term female, the labia majora should cover the labia minora and clitoris. There should be a fingertip space between the vagina and the anus. If not, the possibility of sexual ambiguity exists. A whitish serosanguineous vaginal discharge is common during the first few days of life and is due to the estrogen effect. The examiner should inspect the *urethral meatus* and *vaginal orifice* by placing a gloved thumb and index finger on the child's perineum while pressing downward and laterally on the buttocks.

In the male or female infant born after a breech presentation, the external genitalia are often erythematous and edematous as a result of the trauma related to the birth process.

Musculoskeletal Examination

The purpose of the musculoskeletal examination of the newborn is to detect gross abnormalities. The appearance of the extremities at birth usually reflects the positioning of the child within the uterus, a condition known as *intrauterine packing*.

Inspect the *extremities* and *digits*. Are all four extremities and 20 digits present?

Palpate the *clavicle* if this has not already been performed. An area of crepitance over the distal third is suggestive of a fractured clavicle. Decreased motion in the upper extremity may also be associated with a clavicular fracture.

Check for a *brachial palsy*, which has been discussed earlier.

The most important part of the musculoskeletal examination of the newborn is the evaluation of the lower extremities. The *hips* are examined for the possibility of dislocation. Inspect the contours of the legs while the child is lying supine. The presence of asymmetric skin folds on the medial aspect of the thigh is suggestive of a proximally dislocated femur. The perineum should not be visible when the child is in this position, because the normal position of the thighs should cover most of it. If it is visible, suspect *bilateral* hip dislocations.

Place the infant's feet side by side with the soles on the examination table, allowing the hips and knees to flex. Observe the relative height of the knees. If one knee is at a lower level, you should suspect that the shorter knee is secondary to a dislocation of the hip on that side, a congenitally short femur, or both. If both knees are at the same height, either both hips are normal or both hips are dislocated.

After inspection of the knee heights, each hip is examined to determine joint stability. Flex the newborn's legs at the hips. Hold the legs by placing your thumbs over the lesser trochanters and your index fingers over the greater trochanters, and press downward* toward the examination table. Then simultaneously abduct the hips to almost 90°. The presence of a palpable or audible click suggests a dislocated hip as the femoral head suddenly snaps back into the acetabulum. This test is called *Ortolani's test*. The test should be performed *gently* on a quiet infant. After the neonatal

---

*This downward maneuver is *Barlow's variation*. The normal hip will not dislocate as a result of this pressure.

period, Ortolani's test result may be a false negative. The Ortolani test is illustrated in Figure 22–12.

Inspect the *feet*. Observe the foot at the sole. An imaginary line drawn from the center of the heel through the center of the metatarsal-tarsal line should bisect either the second toe or the space between the second and third toes. If the line crosses more laterally, the forefoot is adducted (turned inward) in relation to the hindfoot. This is the common condition known as *metatarsus adductus* and is often the result of intrauterine packing. This condition may resolve spontaneously within the first few years of life but may require early casting or exercises for passive correction.

The most serious foot deformity at birth is the *clubfoot,* also known as *talipes equinovarus.* The entire foot is deviated toward the midline. There is forefoot adduction, fixed inversion of the hindfoot, and internal tibial torsion. These deformities cannot be corrected passively. The Achilles tendon is foreshortened, and the foot assumes the position of a horse's hoof, hence the prefix "equino-." The calf muscles on the affected side are also smaller than on the unaffected side. Immediate therapy is required. If not corrected by casting or splinting, surgery may be necessary at a later date. See Figure 22–13. The 3 week old infant was born with bilateral club feet and bilateral hip dislocations.

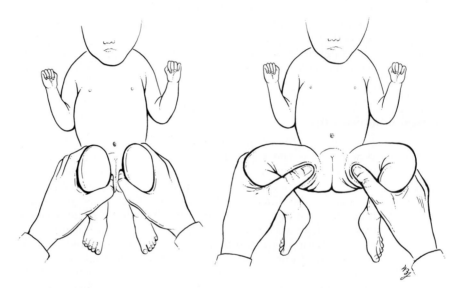

Figure 22–12

The Ortolani test.

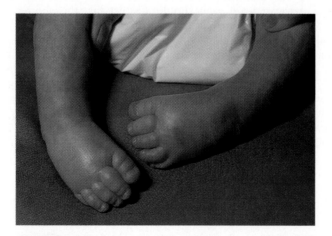

Figure 22–13

Talipes equinovarus.

Neurologic Examination

Careful inspection is the most important aspect of the neonatal neurologic examination. The inspection should include the following:

- Posture
- Symmetry of extremities
- Spontaneous movements
- Facial expressions and symmetry
- Eye movements and symmetry

Notice the *position* of the newborn. Is hyperextension of the neck present? This sign is frequently present in severe meningeal or brain-stem irritations. What is the position of the thumb? The *cerebral thumb sign* is the finding of the thumb curled under the flexed fingers. It is associated with many cerebral abnormalities.

The *motor* examination consists of testing the *range of motion* of all joints. Assess muscle tone and compare one side with the other. Compare the muscle sizes and strengths. Compare the resistance to passive stretch.

The *sensory* examination is generally omitted because it has low sensitivity among newborns.

Testing the *cranial nerves* is also difficult in newborns. A simple test for the 12th cranial nerve consists of pinching the nostrils of the newborn. A reflex opening of the mouth with extension and elevation of the tongue in the midline is the normal response. Deviation of the tongue to one side indicates a lesion on that side.

Because the corticospinal tracts are not fully developed in newborns, the response to testing of the deep tendon reflexes is variable and neither sensitive nor specific. *Babinski's reflex* is usually present in newborns and is tested as in adults. Babinski's reflex may normally be present until children are about 4 years of age.

Test for *infantile automatisms*. These are primitive reflex phenomena that may be present at birth, depending on gestational age, but disappear soon thereafter. There are many, and not all have to be tested. The most important automatisms include the following:

- Rooting response
- Plantar grasp
- Palmar grasp
- Moro's reflex
- Galant's reflex
- Perez's reflex
- Placing response
- Stepping response

The rotational response, optical blinking reflex, acoustic blink response, and sucking response are also automatisms and were discussed earlier in this chapter.

The following reflexes are elicited while the newborn infant is lying supine on the examination table.

The *rooting response* is elicited by having the infant lie with hands held against the chest. The examiner should touch the corner of the infant's mouth or cheek. The normal response is turning of the head to the same side and opening of the mouth to grasp the finger. This reflex is absent in infants with severe central nervous system disease. If only the upper lip is touched, the head will retroflex; if only the lower lip is touched, the jaw will drop. The rooting response is good at 32 weeks' gestation and usually disappears after 3–4 months. This primitive response is to ensure nursing.

The *plantar grasp* is elicited by flexing the leg at the hip and knee. Dorsiflex the infant's foot with your hand. The normal response is plantar flexion of the toes over the hand. This response disappears after 9–12 months.

The *palmar grasp* is elicited by stabilizing the infant's head in the midline. Place your index finger into the palm of the newborn from the ulnar side. The normal response is flexion of all the fingers to grasp the index finger. If the reflex is sluggish, allow the child to suck, which normally facilitates the grasp response. The palmar grasp is usually established by 32 weeks of gestation and usually disappears after 3–5 months. The absence of this response in the newborn or its persistence after 5 months is suggestive of cerebral disease. The newborn commonly holds the hand in a fist. After 2 months, however, the presence of this sign suggests neurologic disease.

The infant is now picked up and held supine in the examiner's hands.

Moro's reflex, or the *startle reflex,* is elicited by supporting the infant's body in the right hand and supporting the head by the left hand. The head is suddenly allowed to drop a few centimeters. Moro's reflex consists of symmetric abduction of the upper extremities at the shoulders and extension of the fingers. Adduction of the arm at the shoulder completes the reflex. The infant usually then emits a loud cry. Moro's reflex is one of the most important motor automatisms. The normal response indicates an intact central nervous system, which is usually complete by 28 weeks of gestation. The reflex normally disappears by 3–5 months of age. Persistence past 6 months may indicate neurologic disease.

The infant is now turned over and held in the prone position in one of the examiner's hands.

Galant's reflex is elicited by stroking one side of the back along a paravertebral line 2–3 cm from the midline from the shoulder to the buttocks. The normal response is lateral curvature of the trunk toward the stimulated side, with the shoulder and hip moving toward the side stroked. Galant's reflex normally disappears after 2–3 months. This reflex is absent in infants with transverse spinal cord lesions.

Perez's reflex is elicited by placing your thumb at the infant's sacrum and rubbing your thumb firmly along the spine toward the infant's head. The normal response is extension of the head and spine with flexion of the knees. Frequently, the newborn also urinates. This reflex is normally present until 2–3 months of age. Its absence suggests severe neurologic disease of the cerebrum or cervical spinal cord or a myopathy.

The child is now laid down on the examination table and then picked up by the examiner, holding the infant upright. The examiner's hands should be around the infant's chest, with the heart supported.

The *placing response* and the *stepping response* are elicited by allowing the dorsum of one of the infant's feet to touch the undersurface of a table top lightly. The normal placing response is for the infant to flex the knee and hip and place the stimulated foot on top of the table simultaneously. This response is then tested with the other foot. Placement of the soles of the feet on top of a table will elicit the stepping response, which is the alternating movements of both legs. Both these responses are best observed after 4–5 days of life and disappear after 2–5 months. If paresis of the lower extremities is present, these responses will be absent.

Examination of the Infant

Infants aged 1 week to 6 months can be examined on the examination table with a parent standing nearby. It may be easier to perform part of the examination while the infant is in the parent's arms or lap. Infants from the ages of 6 months to 1 year are best examined on the parent's lap.

Observe the infant's activity and alertness.

The more difficult portions of the examination, such as the evaluation of the pharynx and the otoscopic examination, should be performed last. Take advantage of any time when the infant is quiet to listen to the lungs and heart.

Before starting the examination, wash your hands in warm water.

General Assessment

Is any distinctive *body odor* present? Inborn errors of metabolism are associated with characteristic odors, such as the odor of *maple syrup* in maple syrup urine disease, *sweaty feet* in isovaleric acidemia, *fish* in methionine metabolism aberrations, and *acetone* in diabetic ketoacidosis. These odors, however, are rarely observed.

The average pulse of a child during the first 6 months of life is 130, with a range of 80–160 at rest. The average resting heart rate during the second 6 months of life is 110, with a range of 70–150. The normal respiratory rate varies from 20 to 40. Blood pressure is difficult to assess in this age group but may be determined by the *flush method*. In this technique, the arm is elevated while the uninflated *infant cuff* is applied to the arm. The arm is then "milked" from the fingers to the elbow so that blanching is noted. The cuff is inflated to just beyond an estimated blood pressure. The pale arm is then placed at the infant's side. The cuff pressure is then allowed to fall

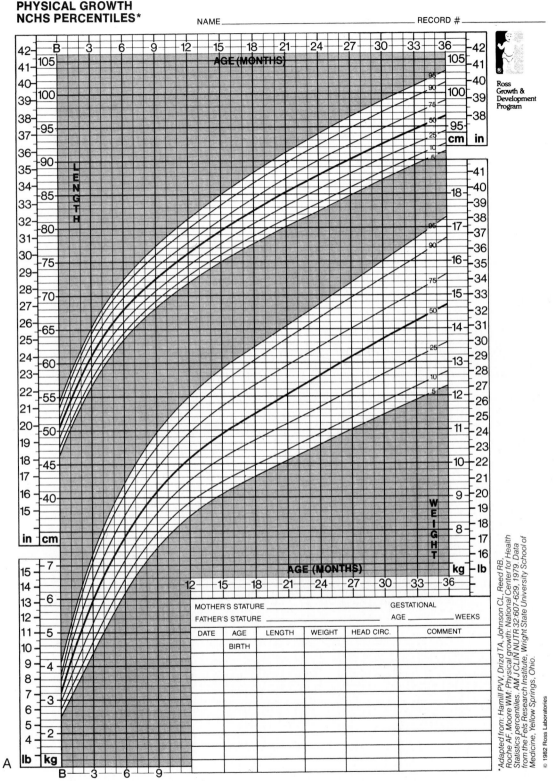

**BOYS: BIRTH TO 36 MONTHS
PHYSICAL GROWTH
NCHS PERCENTILES***

Figure 22–14

National Center for Health Statistics (NCHS) growth charts, birth to age 36 months. *A,* The NCHS percentiles for boys. *B,* The statistics for girls.

slowly. A sudden flush of color occurs at a level slightly lower than the true systolic pressure. The systolic blood pressure determined by the flush method of a 1 day old infant is 50 mm Hg. By the 2nd week of life, the systolic blood pressure has risen to 80 mm Hg. By the end of the 1st year, the systolic blood pressure is 95 mm Hg. A more accurate Doppler blood pressure assessment is available for critical determinations.

Determine the infant's *length* and *weight*. Plot these measurements on the standard growth charts. Growth charts are used to determine whether a child is growing and developing according to a group of standards. More important than a single value is the use of these charts to follow the rate of change at subsequent examinations. The National Center for Health Statistics publishes a variety of growth charts for boys and girls of two age groups: birth to 36 months and 2–18 years. Examples of these charts are shown in Figures 22–14 and 22–15.

Text continued on page 617

BOYS: BIRTH TO 36 MONTHS
PHYSICAL GROWTH
NCHS PERCENTILES*

NAME_____ RECORD #_____

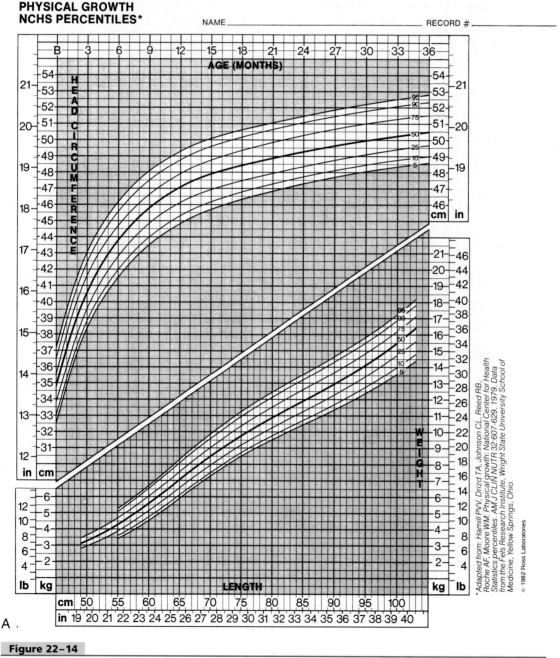

A.

Figure 22–14

Continued

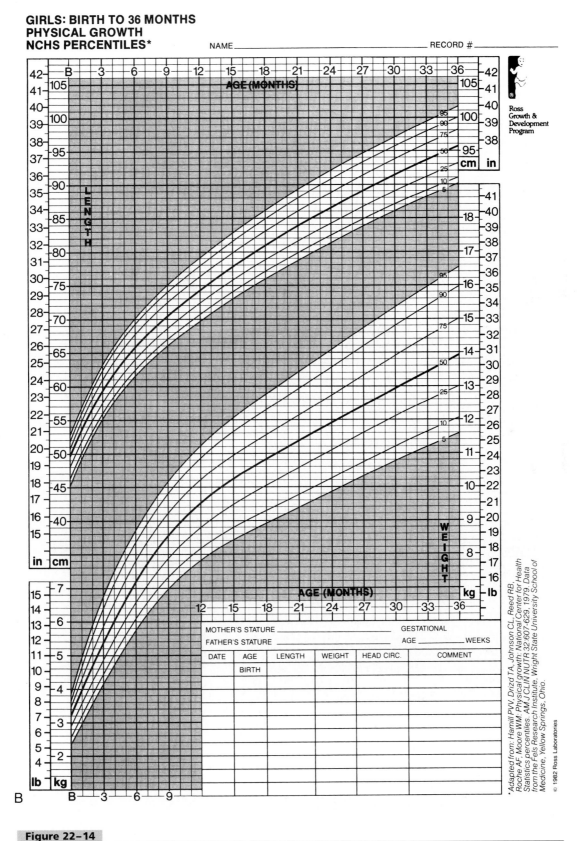

GIRLS: BIRTH TO 36 MONTHS PHYSICAL GROWTH NCHS PERCENTILES*

Figure 22–14

Continued

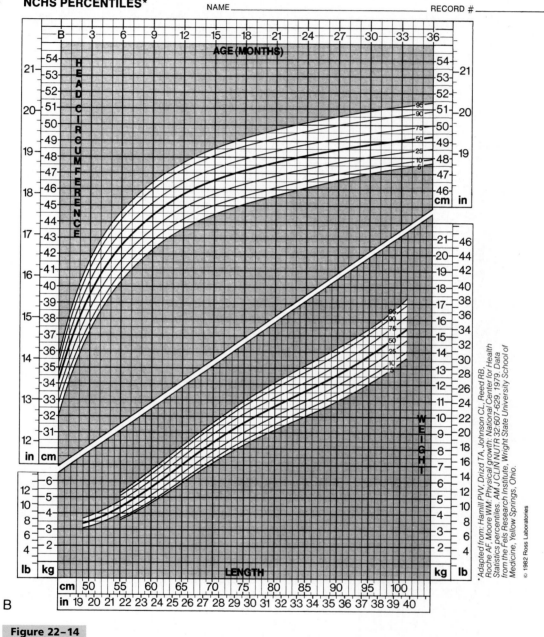

GIRLS: BIRTH TO 36 MONTHS
PHYSICAL GROWTH
NCHS PERCENTILES*

Figure 22–14

Continued

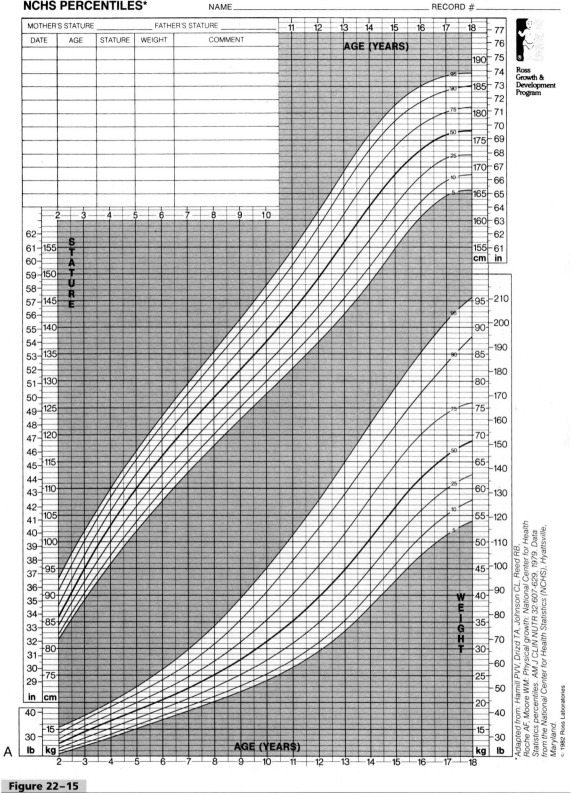

Figure 22–15

National Center for Health Statistics (NCHS) growth charts, ages 2–18 years. *A,* The NCHS percentiles for boys. *B,* The statistics for girls.

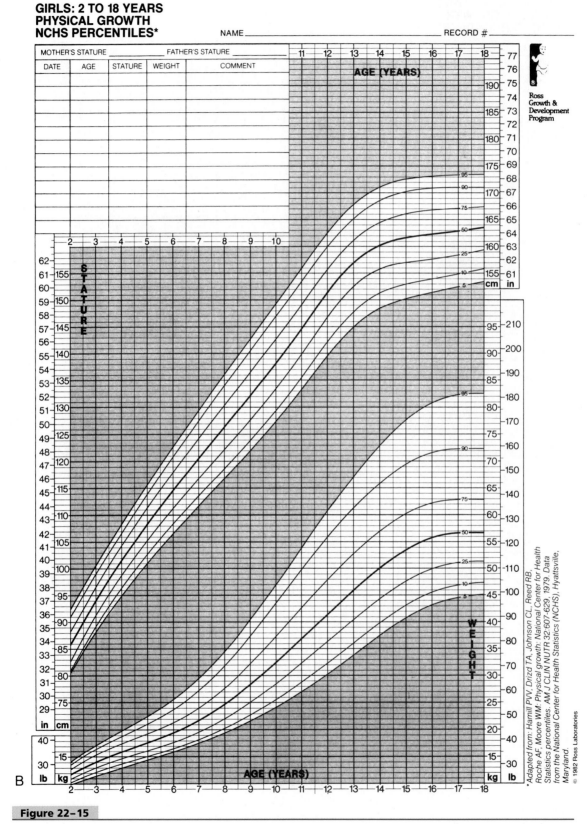

**GIRLS: 2 TO 18 YEARS
PHYSICAL GROWTH
NCHS PERCENTILES***

Figure 22–15

Continued

Somatic growth is one of the most important parts of the pediatric examination. These parameters must be determined at every visit. Deviations from the standard curves are often early sensitive indicators of a pathologic process. Children with a discrepancy between length and weight by more than two percentage lines also require further evaluation.

Skin

Inspect for dermatologic conditions. *Infantile eczema* is a type of seborrheic dermatitis that begins within the 1st month of life and is most troublesome during the 1st year of life. An initial manifestation is often a crusting of the scalp known as *cradle cap*. The greasy, salmon-colored, pruritic, sharply delimited oval scales involve the face, neck, axillae, and groin. Often the entire body is involved with the dry, scaly, nonpruritic dermatitis. Figure 22–16 shows a child with infantile eczema. Notice the weeping dermatitis on the cheeks and forehead. Seborrheic dermatitis may be differentiated from atopic dermatitis by its early onset, a lack of pruritus, and the absence of vesicles.

Atopic dermatitis is the most common cause of eczema in children. It is characterized by pruritus, erythematous papules and vesicles, serous discharge, and crusting. The atopic skin is dry and itchy. The usual site in children of 6 months of age is the face, whereas the extensor surfaces of the arms and legs are the most common sites in 8–10 month old infants. Patients with atopic dermatitis tend to have an extra groove of the lower eyelid, called the *atopic pleat*. This suggestive feature is shown in the 6 month old child with atopic dermatitis in Figure 22–17.

Are any *vascular lesions* present?

Palpate the skin and assess *skin turgor*. Pull up 1–2 inches of skin over the abdomen and release it. It should quickly return to its normal position. A decreased response is termed *tenting* and suggests dehydration.

Is there any evidence of physical *child abuse?* Are any bruises, welts, lacerations, or unusual scars present? Inspect the buttocks and lower back for evidence of bruises. Paired, crescent-shaped bruises facing each other on any part of the body may represent human bite marks. Is there evidence of traumatic alopecia from pulling out of the hair? The damaged hair is broken at various lengths. Are circular, punched-out lesions of uniform size present? These may represent cigarette burns. A circular-type burn on the buttocks and thighs may result from the infants being immersed in scalding hot

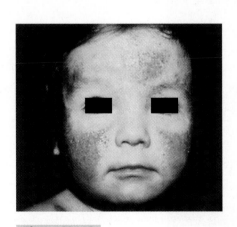

Figure 22–16

Infantile eczema.

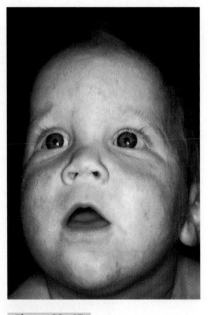

Figure 22–17

Atopic pleat.

water. Look at the child in Figure 22–18. This child has first- and second-degree burns on the penis, thighs, and inguinal and suprapubic areas. The buttocks and sacrum were spared. These burns were caused by holding the child under scalding hot water from the faucet. The diagnosis of physical child abuse is especially important in the first 6 months of life, because the risk of a fatal outcome is very high if the diagnosis is missed. In a case of suspected child abuse, conduct several laboratory tests, such as a platelet determination, to rule out any organic cause of increased bruising. If child abuse is verified, health authorities should be notified.

Head

Measure the *occipitofrontal* head circumference, as indicated previously, and chart it on the standard growth charts (see Fig. 22–14). A head that is growing too rapidly should be evaluated for *hydrocephaly. Microcephaly* is a defect in which the head size is three standard deviations below the normal mean and is related to a defect in brain growth. Check for asymmetry.

Is the *face* symmetric? An easy way to determine facial paralysis as a result of a birth injury is to observe the child when he or she cries. The weakened or paralyzed side appears expressionless in comparison with the normal side.

Eyes

In an infant older than 3 weeks of age, check the *pupillary responses*. A sluggishly reacting pupil is suggestive of congenital glaucoma.

The production of tears begins at about 2–3 months of age, but the nasolacrimal duct is not fully patent until 5–7 months of age. If chronic tearing is present, the nasolacrimal duct may not be patent. In this case, massaging over the nasolacrimal sac may yield a purulent or mucoid discharge, which suggestst the diagnosis of nasolacrimal obstruction.

Visual acuity is assessed by qualitative observations. By the age of 4 weeks, the infant should be capable of fixation on a target. By 6 weeks, coordinated eye movements in following an object should be present. At the age of 3 months, the normal infant can visually follow an object moving across the midline. Convergence is also present by this time. The presence of *optokinetic nystagmus* indicates a complete pathway from the retina to the occipital visual cortex. This response can best be elicited in children 3 months of age and more by using a long, striped cloth and

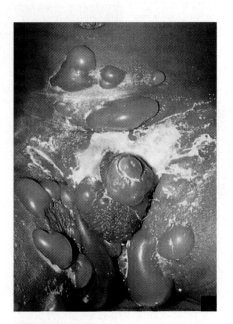

Figure 22–18

Hot-water immersion burns.

passing it rapidly from one side to the other in the child's view. The development of nystagmus as the child attempts to maintain fixation on a stripe is the normal response, indicating normal visual pathways. At 5–6 months of age, the child should be able to focus on objects but is farsighted. The child should be able to reach out for an object and grasp it. Recognition of objects and faces by 4–6 months of age suggests normal visual acuity.

Observe *ocular motility* in a child 3 months of age or older. Have the child follow an object into the various positions of gaze. Alignment of the eyes is best determined by the symmetry of the *corneal light reflex* and the *alternate cover test,* which were described in Chapter 8, The Eye. The child is most susceptible to *amblyopia* within the first 2 years of life, although the risk is present until ages 6–7 years.

Nose

Elevate the tip of the nose to view the nasal septum, floor of the nose, and the turbinates. Are any masses or *foreign bodies* present? A foreign body should be suspected in any child with a chronic nasal discharge.

Neck

Palpate for lymphadenopathy in the same areas as in the adult.

Any child with an acute illness should be examined for *nuchal rigidity,* resulting from meningeal irritation. The Brudzinski and Kernig tests are described in Chapter 19, The Nervous System.

Chest

The examination of the chest is best performed while the infant is either sleeping or held by a parent.

Often the tracheal breath sounds are transmitted down to the chest. Do not misinterpret these sounds as crackles.

Is the child in *respiratory distress?* The most important signs of distress are the use of accessory muscles, head bobbing, and flaring of the nasal alae. Intercostal retractions are also commonly present.

Percuss and auscultate the lung fields.

Heart

Inspect for *cyanosis.* If cyanosis develops within the first few weeks of life, there is probably a serious anatomic anomaly such as transposition of the great vessels or severe tetralogy of Fallot.*

Inspect for evidence of *congestive heart failure.* The most important signs are persistent tachycardia, tachypnea, and an enlarged liver. A persistent tachycardia of more than 200 in newborns or more than 150 in children up to 1 year of age should alert the examiner. Persistent *diaphoresis,* or a failure to thrive, is also an important sign associated with congestive heart failure. If heart failure develops within the first week or two, a complex defect such as a ventricular septal defect, a patent ductus arteriosus, or a coarctation of the aorta should be suspected. A truncus arteriosus will also produce heart failure during this period.

Palpate for the *point of maximum impulse.*

Auscultate as in newborns. An S$_3$ and an S$_4$ are common in this age group. As previously noted, the clinical significance of a murmur heard, especially in the first few weeks of life, must be carefully assessed. (A summary of pathologic murmurs heard in the pediatric age group is summarized in Table 22–4 in the Clinicopathologic Correlations section of this chapter.)

---

*Tetralogy of Fallot consists of pulmonic stenosis, an overriding aorta, a ventricular septal defect, and right ventricular hypertrophy; these conditions arise from an abnormal septation of the truncus arteriosus.

Abdomen

Inspect the *umbilicus.* Observe the abdomen for any masses. An umbilical hernia is common in this age group, especially in darker-skinned children. Large peristaltic waves moving from the left to the right in the upper abdomen are occasionally seen in the infant with *pyloric stenosis.*

In a newborn after the umbilical cord stump has fallen off, the examiner must check for an *umbilical granuloma,* which should be cauterized with silver nitrate.

Auscultate the abdomen, percuss the abdomen, and palpate the abdomen, using light and deep palpation. Are any masses present?

Palpate for the *liver, spleen,* and *kidneys.* The estimated liver span of a 6 month old infant varies from 2.5 to 3.0 cm. At 1 year of age, the span is approximately 3 cm. The spleen is commonly palpable 1–2 cm below the left costal margin during the 1st month of life.

Genitalia

Inspect the external genitalia. Check for *ambiguous genitalia.* Is diaper rash present?

The foreskin is not fully retractable until 1 year of age. Diaper rash can cause *balanitis,* which is an acute inflammation of the glans penis. Males who are uncircumcised may develop *phimosis* after balanitis.

Observe the position of the *urethral meatus.*

Inspect the *scrotum.* Is unilateral swelling present? Enlargement may represent a hernia or a hydrocele. Transilluminate any mass. Remember that hydroceles transilluminate, but hernias do not. Auscultate the mass. Listening to a hernia-containing bowel may reveal bowel sounds.

Palpate the testes. Are they both in the scrotum? Can an undescended testicle be palpated in the inguinal canal? If not, while the infant is lying on the examination table, press on the abdomen while trying to palpate the undescended testicle in the inguinal canal with the other hand.

In the female infant, is a vaginal *discharge* present? Commonly, there is a whitish, often blood-tinged, discharge lasting for 1 month after birth. This is related to the placental transfer of maternal hormones.

Inspect the *perineum* for rashes or lesions.

Musculoskeletal Examination

Palpate the *clavicle.* At 1 month of age, the presence of a callus formation suggests a healed clavicular fracture.

The *hips* must be reexamined for dislocation at every routine visit for the 1st year of life. The technique was described in the section on Examination of the Newborn.

Neurologic Examination

By the 4th month, when the supine infant is pulled into a sitting position, no head lag should be present. By the 8th month, the infant should be able to sit without support.

Coordination of the hands begins at about 5 months, when infants can reach and grasp objects. By 7 months, they can transfer these objects from hand to hand. At 8–9 months, they should be able to use a pincer grip to pick up small objects.

Ears

The child can either be placed on the examination table or held by a parent. To examine the right ear, use your left hand to pull the pinna out, back, and down as the right hand holds the otoscope firmly against the child's forehead. Always use the largest speculum possible. The speculum is introduced slowly into the external canal. Cerumen, if present, should be removed only by someone with experience in such removal. The *tympanic membrane* should be easily visualized.

Is the tympanic membrane erythematous? Bulging? Check for a light reflex. Its presence, however, does not rule out otitis media. Are air-fluid levels visible behind the drum? These signs suggest otitis media.

Mouth and Pharynx

The examination of the mouth and pharynx is the last part of the examination in this age group.

The child should be seated on the parent's lap, with the parent holding the child's head. The crying infant can usually be examined without the tongue depressor. The frightened child with the mouth firmly closed can be examined if you hold the child's nose; this will make the child open the mouth. The tongue depressor can then be slipped between the teeth and over the tongue. Be quick if you must be forceful.

Inspect the *gingivae*. Gingival ulceration is frequently the result of *primary* herpetic infection. Small, discrete, whitish vesicles are also present before ulceration. They are found on the buccal mucosa, palate, and tongue. Severe cases can produce lesions around the mouth.

Are any *teeth* present? The first teeth to erupt are the lower central incisors at about 6 months. These are followed by the lower lateral incisors at 7 months and the upper central teeth at 7–8 months. The upper lateral teeth begin to erupt at about 9 months. Increased salivation occurs temporarily with the eruption of new teeth. (A summary of the chronology of dentition is in Table 22–5 at the end of the chapter.)

Examination of the Young Child

The child 1–5 years of age needs to be relaxed in order for an adequate examination to be performed. It is important to children in this age group that you speak softly and demonstrate the parts of the examination on dolls or toy animals, on yourself, or on the parent. Allowing the child to hold the stethoscope or penlight will often distract him or her enough so that other parts of the examination can be performed. The child will soon learn that the light and stethoscope need not be feared. Play with the child. Have the child "blow out" the light. Let the child use the stethoscope as a telephone. Above all, *talk* to the child. It is amazing how easily an examination can often be performed by telling the young child a simple fantasy about imaginary animals. Ask the child questions about these characters. A reassuring voice goes a long way in making the child comfortable. As you proceed with the examination, describe to the child what is being done, such as, "I'm now going to listen to your heart beating." Children also seem to feel that a conversation with their parent during the examination is reassuring. Youngsters respond best to the examiner who is not wearing a white coat. Children younger than the age of 3 years are best examined on the parent's lap.

The child should be completely undressed for the examination. If the child is modest, remove only the clothing that is necessary for the examination. Modesty varies greatly among children in this age group. Respect the child's modesty.

Start the examination by washing your hands in warm water. In addition to being clean, the warm hands are more comfortable for the child. If the child is on an examination table, have the parent stand at the child's feet. Any child in respiratory distress is easiest to examine in the position of most comfort, usually sitting or lying prone.

The child should always be told what to do instead of being asked to do something. For example, it is better to say, "Please turn on your back," instead of, "Would you please turn on your back?"

In a child who appears to be *uncooperative,* auscultation of the heart and lungs should be performed *first,* because this requires the child's cooperation and should be performed early when the child may be more cooperative. Because the sight of medical instruments is likely to frighten a child, use them last. Proceed with the examination in the following order for the cooperative child:

- Take measurements
- Inspect the skin
- Examine the head
- Inspect the feet and hands
- Examine the neck
- Examine the chest
- Examine the heart
- Examine the abdomen

- Examine the genitalia
- Examine the eyes
- Examine the nose
- Examine the ears
- Examine the mouth and pharynx
- Measure blood pressure, if indicated
- Assess deep tendon reflexes, if indicated
- Take the temperature, if indicated

General Assessment

The heart rate of a child 1–5 years of age ranges from 80 to 140; the average rate is 100. The respiratory rate varies from 30 to 40. Blood pressure assessment by auscultation is usually possible with children older than the ages of 3–4 years and should be performed on all children. Inform the child that the cuff will get tight for a few moments. The size of the cuff is important. The cuff must cover two thirds of the distance between the antecubital fossa and the shoulder. A cuff that is too small will result in falsely high readings; conversely, a cuff that is too large will result in readings that are falsely low. The techniques of palpatory and auscultatory blood pressure determination are used as in adults. The National Heart, Lung, and Blood Institute has published standards of blood pressure measurements in boys and girls from the ages of 2 to 18 years. Figure 22–19 shows these percentile charts for boys and girls, respectively, taken in the right arm with the child seated.

Determine the *height, weight,* and *head circumference,* and plot these values on the standard growth charts (see Figs. 22–14 and 22–15).

Skin

The examination of the skin is the same for children as for adults.

Careful descriptions of the numerous rashes seen in this age group are paramount for the diagnosis. There are many exanthematous diseases of childhood. These rashes

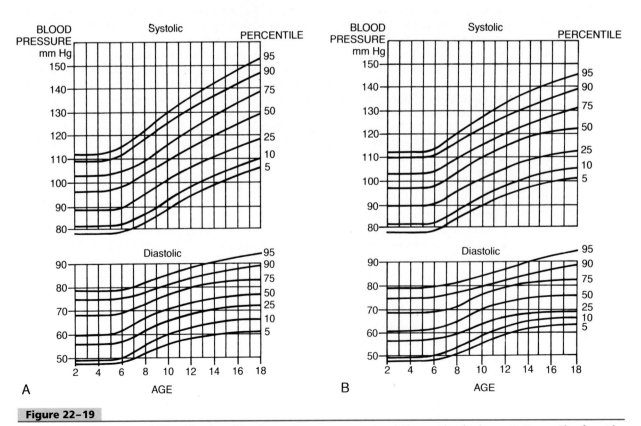

Figure 22–19

National Heart, Lung, and Blood Institute blood pressure measurements. *A,* Percentiles for boys. *B,* Percentiles for girls.

may consist of macules, papules, vesicles, pustules, or petechiae. (A summary of the most important viral and bacterial diseases is given in Table 22–6 at the end of the chapter.)

Impetigo is one of the most common skin conditions of children in this age group. It is a highly contagious, superficial skin infection caused by either a beta-hemolytic streptococcus, *Staphylococcus aureus,* or both. The primary lesion is a pustule; once it has ruptured, it produces a honey-colored crust. The lesions may be seen on any part of the body, but the face is a common location. The child shown in Figure 22–20 has the classic weeping, encrusted lesions of impetigo.

Examine the spine. Tufts of hair along the spine, especially over the sacrum, may mark the location of a *spina bifida occulta.*

Is there evidence of *trauma* or *child abuse?* The signs of physical child abuse were discussed in the previous section.

Head

Examine the *lymph nodes.* All of the chains (as indicated in Chapter 7, The Head and Neck) must be examined. Small (2–4 mm), movable, nontender, discrete nodes are commonly found. Warm, tender nodes usually indicate infection.

Inspect the *shape of the head.*

Palpate the *sutures* in the 1–3 year old child. Are they depressed? Elevated?

Palpate over the *frontal* and *maxillary sinuses* in children older than the age of 2 years. Tenderness may indicate sinusitis.

Inspect the area of the *parotid glands.* Localized swelling can best be detected by telling the child to look up to the ceiling while he or she is seated. Note any swelling below the angle of the jaw. Palpate the area. An enlarged parotid gland often pushes the pinna of the ear away from the side of the head when the child is observed from behind.

Musculoskeletal Examination

Observe the *gait* by telling the child to walk back and forth with shoes or socks on. Having the child walk on a cold floor without socks or shoes may actually distort the gait. "In-toeing" and "out-toeing" are common in children. Most such gaits are physiologic variants that arise from in utero positioning and resolve spontaneously during the active growing period.

Tell the child to stand in front of you, and inspect the legs. Is bowing present? Commonly, a child may appear bowlegged *(genu varum)* for 1–2 years after starting to walk. Knock-knees *(genu valgum)* are also frequently seen in children 2–4 years of age. The normal gait of a child 2–4 years of age is wide-based, with a prominent lumbar lordosis.

The child with a *limp* should be examined for evidence of trauma or localized bone tenderness. The presence of a limp and knee pain in a child, especially a boy,

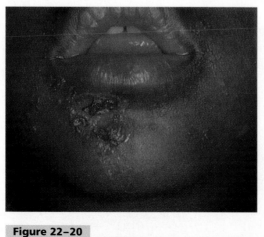

Figure 22–20

Impetigo.

3–8 years of age is indicative of *Legg-Calvé-Perthes disease,* which is aseptic necrosis of the femoral head. The *irritable hip* syndrome, or toxic synovitis, is another cause of a limp in this age group. This condition affects both sexes equally.

The Trendelenburg test (as described in Chapter 18, The Musculoskeletal System) should be performed if weakness of the gluteus medius is suspected.

Inspect the child's shoes. Is there evidence of abnormal wear?

Neurologic Examination

The development of speech, reading abilities, and the ability to manipulate small objects, throw a ball, and understand simple directions are the best indicators of a normally developing neurologic system.

Deep tendon reflexes are generally not tested unless there is reason to suspect that there may be a developmental abnormality. If they are tested, use the same techniques as described in Chapter 19, The Nervous System.

Neck

Inspect the size and shape of the neck. Check for a *thyroglossal duct cyst.* The young child in Figure 22–21 has a midline thyroglossal duct cyst.

Palpate the anterior and posterior triangles for lymphadenopathy as in adults. Cervical adenopathy is associated with inflammation of the sinuses, ears, teeth, or pharynx. Group A beta-hemolytic streptococci are the most frequent causes of pharyngitis in children. Streptococcal pharyngitis is also the cause of rheumatic fever. In the prediction of a positive bacterial culture, the most important diagnostic sign is reported to be tender anterior cervical lymphadenopathy (Rowe and Stone, 1977).

Palpate the *sternocleidomastoid muscle.*

Inspect the location of the *trachea.* Is it midline?

Palpate the *thyroid gland.* This is usually best felt with the child in a supine position by using your thumb and index fingers to feel for the gland.

Chest

Inspect the shape of the chest.

Determine the *respiratory rate.* The respiratory rate of a 6 year old child is 16–20 per minute.

Palpate the chest for dullness, as described earlier. Tactile fremitus is a technique of low sensitivity in childhood.

Percuss the chest, using the same technique as in adults. Because the chest wall is thinner in children than in adults, the percussion notes are more resonant in children than in adults. Percuss gently, because overly vigorous percussion may produce vibrations over a large area and obscure an area of dullness.

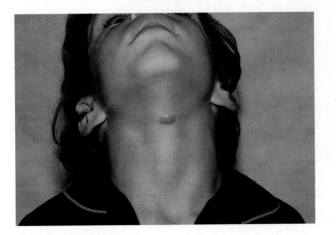

Figure 22–21

Thyroglossal cyst.

Auscultation is best performed by listening to the child when he or she is unaware of this portion of the examination. Telling a child to "take a deep breath" frequently results in the child's holding the breath. With a cooperative child, you can hold the youngster's nose while telling him or her to breathe in and out. Are the breath sounds normal? Are there any adventitious sounds? Breath sounds in the child sound louder than in the adult as a result of the chest's configuration.

Heart

In the cardiac examination of the young child, follow these procedures:

1. Inspect the precordium.
2. Palpate for any lifts, heaves, or thrills.
3. Auscultate in the same areas as described in Chapter 12. Describe any murmurs or abnormal sounds.

Abdomen

The examination of the abdomen is often one of the earlier parts of the examination of the young child, because this requires no instruments other than the stethoscope and is usually painless.

Inspect the abdomen. As children grow older, the protuberant abdomen becomes more scaphoid, except in children who are obese.

Inspect the *umbilicus*. Tell the child to cough. Are there any bulging masses at the umbilicus?

Auscultate for peristaltic sounds. Are any *bruits* present? The presence of an abdominal bruit may suggest coarctation, especially in the presence of upper extremity hypertension and reduced or delayed femoral pulses. Use the stethoscope to listen over the kidneys posteriorly. The presence of a bruit in this location is suggestive of renal artery stenosis.

Percuss the abdomen for abnormal dullness.

Light palpation is performed as described in the adult examination. Is tenderness noted? Observe the patient's face while palpating. Facial expressions are more useful than asking the child, "Does this hurt?"

Deep palpation is also performed as in adults.

Palpate the *liver* and *spleen* as described in Chapter 15, The Abdomen. The liver span of a 3 year old is approximately 4 cm. By 5 years of age, the span has increased to 5 cm.

The *kidneys* are frequently palpable by ballottement in the child up to 5–6 years of age. Place your left hand under the right costal margin at the costovertebral angle. Your right hand is placed over the midposition of the right abdomen. Tap firmly on the abdomen to try to feel the size of the kidney. The hands should be reversed to feel the left kidney.

Palpate the *femoral pulses*. Place the tips of your fingers along the inguinal ligament, midway between the symphysis pubis and the iliac crest. Time the pulse with the radial pulse; they should peak at the same time.

Palpate the femoral *lymph nodes*. It is common to find several 0.5–1.0 cm nodes.

Inspect the *anus*. Is diaper rash present? Is there evidence of excoriations? Pinworm infestation commonly causes pruritus and excoriations.

Rectal examination is usually not part of the standard examination in this age group. Only children with abdominal pain or symptoms referable to the lower gastrointestinal tract require a rectal examination. Instruct the child to lie on his or her back and flex the knees. Tell the child that the examination will be like "taking your temperature." You should use your fifth finger, gloved and well-lubricated, for the examination. Tenderness and sphincter tone are determined as well as the presence of a mass.

Genitalia

If the child is a male, inspect the *penis*. Check for *phimosis*. By the end of the 1st year, the foreskin can be retracted in most uncircumcised males. By the age of 4 years, the foreskin should be easily retractable in 80% of all uncircumcised males.

Inspect the *urethral meatus*.

Inspect the *scrotum*. Is there any unilateral enlargement present? Suspect a hydrocele or hernia if the scrotum appears large. Transilluminate and auscultate any scrotal mass.

Palpate the *testicles*. Are both present in the scrotum? In this age group, the testicles are often retracted into the inguinal canal. If one or both testicles are not felt in the scrotum, tell the child to sit on a chair with his feet on the seat. Instruct him to grab his knees. Repeat the palpation. This additional abdominal pressure may force a retracted or undescended testicle into the scrotum. Warm hands and a warm room often aid in this procedure.

Another useful maneuver to counteract an active cremasteric reflex is to have the child lie down and flex his leg at the knee, placing his foot on the opposite leg. This "tailor position" will bring the tendon of the sartorius muscle over the inguinal canal and prevent an active reflex from retracting the testicle.

Palpation for an *inguinal hernia* can usually be performed in children age 4 years and older. The procedure is the same as in adults and should be performed with the child standing.

In the female, inspect the *vaginal area*. Is a *rash* present? Rashes may be related to bubble baths. Is a *discharge* present? A discharge in girls age 2–6 years is commonly related to a vaginal foreign body. A nasal speculum is often used to inspect the vagina for the cause of the discharge. Look for an intact hymen and a smooth vaginal opening. Be on the lookout for sexual abuse. The most important signs of abuse include difficulty in walking, vaginal or anal infections, genital irritation or swelling, torn or stained underclothes, vaginal or anal bleeding, and bruises.

Eyes

Visual acuity in children 1–3 years of age is assessed by their ability to identify brightly colored objects and to circumnavigate the examining room. Further visual acuity testing may be performed by using Snellen's eye chart and asking the child which way the letter faces: up, down, to the right, to the left. Visual acuity for a 3 year old child is 20/40; at age 4–5 years, 20/30.

Confrontation visual field testing is performed only in children older than the age of 4 years in whom there is a suspicion of decreased acuity. The test is conducted as in adults, except that a small toy is used instead of finger counting. The toy is brought in from the periphery of the child's vision, and the child is instructed to tell the examiner when he or she sees it.

Check *ocular motility*. Are the eyes straight? Be aware that the child with large epicanthal folds that partially cover the globe may be thought to have strabismus. The eyes should be parallel in all fields of gaze. Shine a light from 2 feet away, and have the child look at it. The light should fall in the center of both pupils. Hold the patient's head, and turn it to the right and then to the left while the position of the light is maintained. Is the corneal reflection symmetric in both eyes as the head is turned? If there is asymmetry, perform the *cover test* as described in Chapter 8, The Eye.

Is the eye red? One of the most common problems of the eyes in this age group is the *red eye*. The causes are numerous and include conjunctivitis, obstruction of the nasolacrimal duct, chalazion, local trauma, allergy, and toxin exposure.

Nose

Inspect the nostrils. Is *flaring* of the nostrils present? Flaring occurs in any type of respiratory distress.

Inspect the tip of the nose. Is there a permanent transverse crease near the lower part of the nose directing the tip upward? This is commonly seen in allergy sufferers. This unmistakable sign of an allergy sufferer is caused by the *allergic salute;* using a palm or an extended forefinger to rub the nose upward and outward.

Elevate the tip of the nose and inspect the nasal mucosa. Are secretions present? Purulent secretions from above and below the middle turbinate suggest sinusitis. Watery discharge may indicate allergy or viral upper respiratory infections. Epistaxis is generally due to local trauma. In children with head trauma, the presence of a clear discharge from the nose suggests cerebrospinal fluid leakage.

Check for *nasal polyps*. These may be associated with allergies or cystic fibrosis.

Ears

Is any *discharge* present? Purulent discharges may be related to bacterial infection. Eczema may cause a flaking of and cracking behind the ears. A bloody discharge may be caused by irritation, injury, a foreign body, or a basilar skull fracture.

Use the otoscope to inspect the *external canal* and *tympanic membrane*. A cooperative 2–3 year old child may be either sitting or lying prone on the examination table with the head turned to one side. An uncooperative child can be held in a parent's arms or prone. The otoscope should be held as indicated previously. Use the largest-sized speculum. Insert the speculum tip to only a half inch.

Inspect the tympanic membrane. Redness is the most common abnormality of the membrane. Infection, trauma, or even crying may be responsible. In suppurative otitis media, the drum bulges outward and becomes diffusely erythematous, hearing is decreased, and the light reflex may be lost. Is the tympanic membrane perforated? Does the tympanic membrane move with insufflation? An immobile drum is seen in suppurative or serous otitis media.

Palpate the *mastoid tip*. Is it tender? Tenderness suggests mastoiditis.

Are *posterior auricular lymph nodes* present? These nodes are classically found in children with rubella. They are also found in children with measles, roseola, chickenpox, or inflammations of the scalp.

Check *hearing*. Hearing is necessary for normal development of language beyond the one-word stage. As a screening test, occlude one ear, and whisper a number into the child's ear. Ask the child what number he or she heard. Repeat the test with the other ear. If a hearing loss is suspected, perform the Weber and Rinne tests as described in Chapter 9, The Ear and Nose. If there is a hearing loss, the child should be scheduled for audiometric testing as soon as possible.

Mouth and Pharynx

The evaluation of the mouth and pharynx is usually the last part of the examination of the small child.

Inspect the *lips* for any lesions and color.

Tell the child, "Open your mouth. I am going to count your teeth."

Inspect the *teeth* for number and caries. The first lower molars erupt at the age of about 1 year. These are followed by the first upper molars at 14 months, lower cuspids at 16 months, upper cuspids at 18 months, second lower molars at 20 months, and finally the second upper molars at 2 years. This completes the primary dentition of 20 teeth. Flattened edges are seen in children who grind their teeth. (Table 22–5 at the end of this chapter summarizes the ages of tooth eruption.)

Multiple caries are often an indication of *milk caries*. They are caused by the child's going to sleep with a bottle of milk or juice in the mouth. The child shown in Figure 22–22 has severe milk caries that necessitate removal of all her primary dentition.

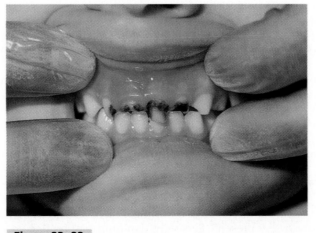

Figure 22–22

Milk caries.

Inspect the *bite*. Maxillary protrusion is termed *overbite* and is the normal position; mandibular protrusion is termed *underbite*.

Have the child bite down while you inspect the occlusion. Normally, the upper teeth override the lower teeth.

Inspect the *gingivae* for any lesions.

Inspect the *buccal mucosa*. In measles, on the 2nd or 3rd day of the disease, pinpoint white spots are often seen on the buccal mucosa at the level of the lower teeth. These spots are called *Koplik's spots* and are pathognomonic for measles. Vesicles on an erythematous base suggest *herpes simplex* infection. Similar vesicles on the soft palate suggest *herpangina* caused by coxsackievirus infections. Red spots about 1–3 mm on the buccal mucosa and palate are an early sign of rubella.

Inspect the *tongue*. Geographic tongue is a normal variation (see Fig. 10–24*A*). Dryness is seen in dehydration and in chronic mouth breathers. Strawberry tongue is indicative of scarlet fever.

The child should be seated during this part of the examination for best visualization of the posterior pharynx. Tell the youngster that you are going to look in his or her throat and that he or she should open the mouth as widely as possible. If the child is uncooperative, lay him or her down on the back on the examination table. The parent should stand at the head of the table. The child's hands are raised over the head, and the parent squeezes the child's elbows against the head so that the head does not move. The examiner can then lean over the child, holding a tongue blade in one hand and a light in the other.

Inspect the *posterior pharynx*. Inspect the size of the *tonsils*. Tonsillar size is estimated on a scale from 1+ to 4+, 4+ indicating that the tonsils meet in the midline. "Kissing" tonsils may be indicative of obstructive apnea. Is a purulent exudate present? Is a membrane present? Membranes are seen in diphtheria and *Candida* infections.

Are *petechiae* present? Streptococcal pharyngitis is often associated with petechiae.

Inspect the *posterior pharyngeal wall*. A cobblestone appearance suggests chronic postnasal drip.

Examination of the Older Child

Children age 6–12 years are usually easy to examine. They understand the purpose of the examination and rarely present any problems. It is often very helpful to engage a child in conversation regarding school, friends, and hobbies. Conversation will help to relax the child even if the child does not appear apprehensive.

Allow the child to wear a gown or drape.

The order of the examination is essentially the same as in adults. If the child is complaining of pain in a certain area, that area should be examined last.

As with younger children, brief explanations about each part of the examination should be given to older children.

Wash your hands with soap and warm water before beginning the examination.

General Assessment

In children 6–12 years of age, the *temperature* may be taken orally. The pulse of an average child in this age group varies from 75 to 125, and the respirations vary from 15 to 20.

Blood pressure should be obtained in all children in this age group by the methods described in Chapter 12, The Heart. Use the correct cuff size.

Measure the height and weight, and chart these on the child's record.

Skin

Inspect the skin for any evidence of fungal disease, especially between the toes.

Are any *rashes* present? Persistent dandruff may be tinea and not seborrhea. Seborrhea is most commonly seen in infancy and adolescence.

Eyes

The examination of the eyes is essentially the same as in adults, with emphasis on *visual acuity*. A test with a standard Snellen's eye chart is necessary.

Ears

The examination of the ears is as in adults, with emphasis on *auditory acuity*. Audiometric testing should be performed on all school-aged children.

Nose

The examination of the nose is essentially the same as in the adult.

Mouth and Pharynx

The *teeth* should be examined with respect to their condition and spacing. Have the child bite down, and observe the *bite*. (See Table 22–5, which summarizes the ages at which shedding of the primary teeth occurs as well as the ages of secondary teeth eruption.)

Inspect the *tongue* for dryness, size, and lesions. Deep furrows are common and have no clinical significance.

Inspect the *palate* for petechiae.

Inspect the *tonsils* for enlargement, injection, and exudation.

Neck

Palpate the *thyroid* for nodules. The thyroid is rarely palpable in normal children in this age group.

Palpate for *lymphadenopathy*. Anterior cervical nodes are seen in association with upper respiratory infections and dental infections. Posterior adenopathy is seen with infections of the middle ear and scalp. Generalized adenopathy is seen in viral diseases such as infectious mononucleosis, measles, and rubella.

Is the *trachea* midline?

Chest

The examination of the chest is the same as in adults.

Heart

The examination of the heart is the same as in adults.

Abdomen

The order of the abdominal examination is the same as in adults. The span of the liver at age 8 years is 5.0–5.5 cm; at age 12 years, the span is approximately 5.5–6.5 cm.

Genitalia

The age of development of the secondary sexual characteristics varies greatly. As indicated in Chapter 14, The Breast, development of the breast in girls may begin as early as age 8 years and continues for the next 5 years. The development of pubic hair in girls occurs at the same time. Testicular development in boys begins somewhat later, at about 9–10 years. Pubic hair starts to develop in boys at about age 12 years and continues to develop until age 15 years. The growth of the penis begins about a year after the beginning of testicular enlargement, at age 10–11 years. Whereas the growth spurt of girls occurs at about age 12 years, this spurt is not seen until around age 14 years in boys.

Sex maturity ratings for males and females were established by Tanner (1962). In the male, the growth of pubic hair and the development of the penis, testes, and scrotum are used to assign sex maturity rating in values from 1 to 5. The examiner should record two ratings, one rating for the pubic hair and the other rating for the genitalia. If the development of the penis differs from that of the testes and scrotum, the two ratings should be averaged. The sex maturity ratings for genital development in boys are illustrated and summarized in Figure 22–23.

Genital Development Stages: Boys

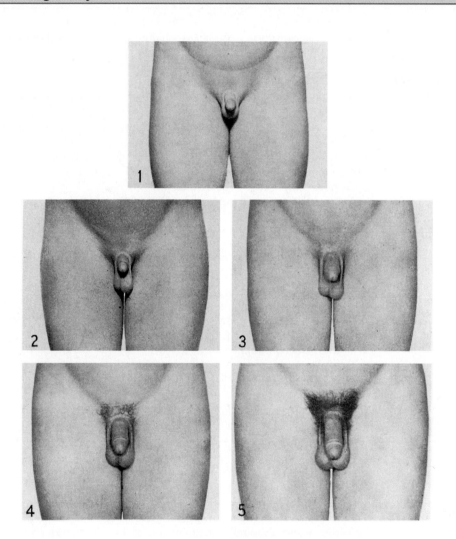

Stage	Characteristics
1	Prepubertal. Testes, scrotum, and penis are about the same size and proportion as in early childhood.
2	Enlargement of the testes and scrotum. Scrotal skin reddens and coarsens. Little changes in size of penis.
3	Enlargement of penis, which occurs mainly in length. Further growth of testes and scrotum.
4	Further enlargement of penis with growth in width and length. Enlargement of glans penis. Scrotal skin darkens.
5	Adult genitalia.

Figure 22–23

Genital development in boys. Numbers indicate sex maturity ratings.

The sex maturity ratings for the pubic hair stages for boys and girls are illustrated and summarized in Figure 22–24.

The sex maturity ratings for girls are based on the growth of pubic hair and the development of the breasts. Five stages are also observed for each. The examiner

Pubic Hair Stages: Boys and Girls

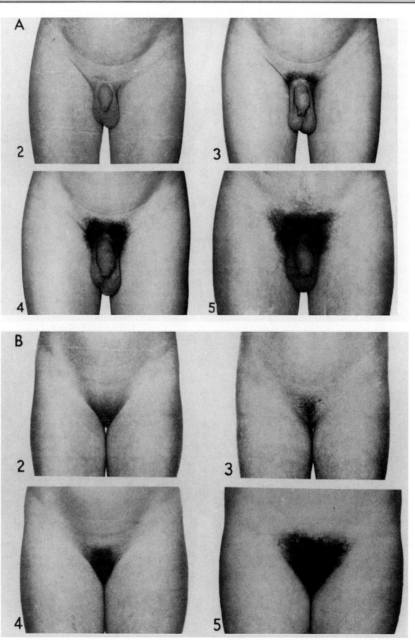

Stage	Characteristics
1	Prepubertal. No true pubic hair.
2	Sparse growth of slightly pigmentated, downy hair. Only slightly curled. Hair mainly at base of penis or along labia.
3	Increase in hair, which is becoming coarser, curled, and darker.
4	Adult-type hair, but limited in area. No spread to medial surface of thighs.
5	Adult-type hair with spread to thighs.

Figure 22–24

Pubic hair development. *A,* Development in boys. *B,* Development in girls. Numbers indicate sex maturity ratings.

should record two ratings, one for the breasts and the other for the pubic hair. The sex maturity ratings for breast development in girls are illustrated and summarized in Figure 22–25.

Breast Development Stages: Girls

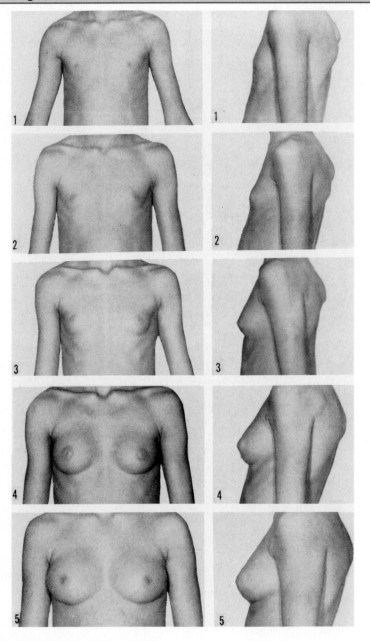

Stage	Characteristics
1	Prepubertal. Elevation of papilla only.
2	Breast bud stage. Elevation of breast and papilla as a small mound. Enlargement of diameter of areola.
3	Further enlargement of breast and areola with no separation of contours.
4*	Areola projected above level of breast as a secondary mound.
5	Mature stage. Recession of areola mound to the general contour of the breast. Projection of only papilla.

* This stage does not occur in all girls. In approximately 25% of girls, it is absent. In addition, many adult women have a persistence of this stage throughout life.

Figure 22–25

Breast development in girls. Numbers indicate sex maturity ratings.

A summary of the developmental sequence for boys is diagrammed in Figure 22–26; a summary for girls is given in Figure 22–27.

The youngster should be given a gown to avoid embarrassment in front of a parent.

Inspect the *external genitalia.* Is *pubic hair* present? What are the *sex maturity ratings?* Are any lesions present? Is there evidence of sexual abuse?

Palpate the testes. Is an *inguinal hernia* present?

Pelvic examinations are not routine in this age group, unless clinically indicated. Vaginal bleeding in girls younger than the age of 9 years is due to infection from foreign objects in over 66% of cases. Trauma accounts for an additional 16%.

Musculoskeletal Examination

The most important goal of the musculoskeletal examination of children age 6–12 years is to detect *scoliosis.* Scoliosis is the most common spinal deformity, especially in

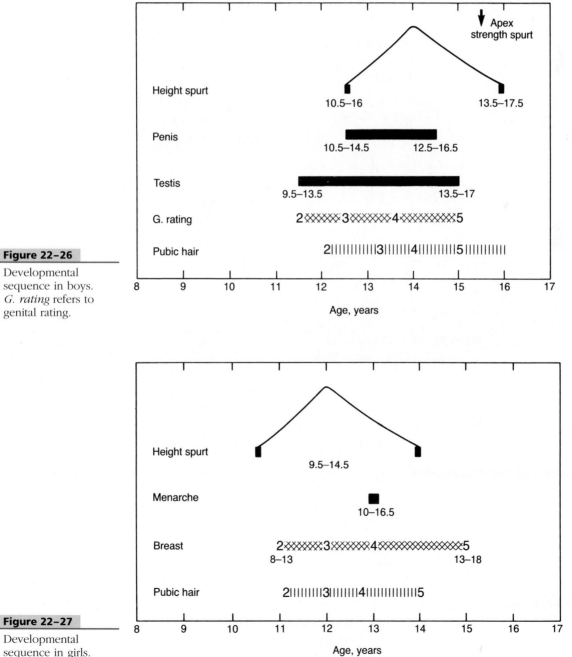

Figure 22–26

Developmental sequence in boys. *G. rating* refers to genital rating.

Figure 22–27

Developmental sequence in girls.

pubertal girls. Have the patient stand stripped to the waist. Inspect the back. Are the shoulders or scapulae at the same height? Is the occiput aligned over the intergluteal cleft? Ask the child to bend down and try to touch the toes, allowing the arms to hang freely. A unilateral elevation of the lower ribs is seen in patients with scoliosis. This is shown in Figure 22–28. Another similar method for detecting scoliosis is for you to mark the spinous processes with a pen while the child is standing in front of you. Then ask the child to bend forward from the waist. A deviation of the marks to either side suggests scoliosis. Unfortunately, none of the methods for detecting scoliosis has been shown to have adequate sensitivity or specificity.

A limp and knee pain in a child 9–16 years of age must be considered a result of a slipped epiphysis of the hip until proved otherwise. The pathognomonic sign of a slipped epiphysis is the hip going into external rotation as it is flexed.

Neurologic Examination

The neurologic examination is essentially the same as outlined in Chapter 19, The Nervous System. However, in children of this age group, the complete neurologic examination is indicated only when there is evidence of developmental abnormalities.

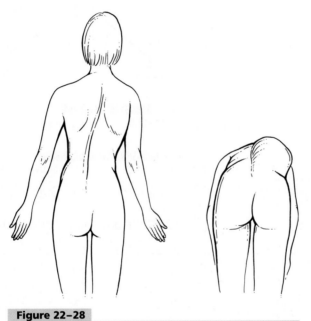

Figure 22–28

Technique for testing for scoliosis.

Examination of the Adolescent

The examination of adolescents is exactly the same as that of adults. It is appropriate for the examiner to ask the parent to leave during the examination and perhaps even for the history.

Because the examination is so similar to that of adults, only the dissimilarities are described in this section.

General Assessment

The average *heart rate* of the adolescent is 60 to 100 beats per minute. The respiratory rate varies from 12 to 18 respirations per minute by 16 years.

Blood pressure is important to determine by the methods discussed in Chapter 12, The Heart.

Skin

Examination of the skin of adolescents usually reveals evidence of *pubertal changes*. These include acne, areolar pigmentation, functioning of the apocrine sweat glands, pigmentation of the external genitalia, and the development of axillary and pubic hair.

Breast

Determine the *Tanner sex maturity rating* of the breasts in girls.

Breast development occurs in both boys and girls. The boy with unilateral gynecomastia should be reassured that this change is part of normal puberty and will be transient.

Asymmetric breast development in girls is common. Reassure the patient that puberty is progressing normally.

Abdomen

The abdominal examination is the same as in the adult. The liver span of a 16 year old varies from 6 to 7 cm.

Genitalia

Determine the *sex maturity ratings* of the pubic hair and genitalia for male patients. Determine the sex maturity rating of the pubic hair for female patients.

The examiner should evaluate the patient and try to reassure him or her that the body changes are related to normal puberty.

If an internal pelvic examination is necessary for the female adolescent, an extremely gentle approach is required. The use of a Pedersen speculum often renders the examination less uncomfortable. A female nurse is always required to be present if the examiner is a male.

Musculoskeletal Examination

Knee pain in the adolescent is usually the result of trauma. Partial avulsion of the tibial tubercle associated with a painful swelling in that area is called *Osgood-Schlatter disease*. This common condition is seen more commonly in pubertal boys and is usually self-limited.

Clinicopathologic Correlations

Viral exanthematous diseases of childhood are extremely common. There are immunizations for many of them. In the early years of this century, pediatricians frequently referred to many childhood diseases by number. Scarlet fever and measles were numbers one and two, respectively; rubella became known as the third disease; fourth disease was probably a combination of scarlet fever and rubella and did not represent a distinct entity; fifth disease is known as *erythema infectiosum;* finally, sixth disease is known as roseola.

Fifth disease was linked in 1983 to human parvovirus B19. Erythema infectiosum is a moderately contagious disease affecting school-aged children, with an asymptomatic "slapped cheek" erythema on the face and an erythematous maculopapular, lacy, serpiginous blanching rash on the trunk and extremities. The rash, sometimes pruritic, lasts 2–40 days, with an average time of 11 days. There is no gender predilection.

Fever is generally absent or low-grade. Figure 22–29 shows the classic "slapped cheek" rash on a child with fifth disease.

Herpes simplex virus is a common cause of painful oral lesions in children, especially toddlers and those of school age. Figure 22–30 shows a 6 year old boy with herpetic gingivostomatitis. Extensive perioral vesicles, pustules, and erosions are common. The gingivae become markedly edematous, erythematous, and bleed easily. Fever, irritability, and cervical and submaxillary lymphadenopathy are common. The acute phase lasts 4–9 days and is self-limited. The vesicles rupture and become encrusted. Desquamation and healing are usually complete in 10–14 days

Kawasaki's disease, or mucocutaneous lymph node syndrome, is an acute febrile illness of young children. Almost all children are younger than the age of 5 years and most are younger than 3 years of age. The cause is unknown, although a viral or rickettsial agent has been suspected. The male-to-female ratio is 2.5:1, and the overall frequency is highest among Asians. Kawasaki's disease is the most frequent cause of acquired heart disease in children from 1 to 5 years of age. The histopathologic condition is a vasculitis with a predilection to aneurysmal disease of the coronary arteries. This coronary thromboarteritis carries a morbidity rate as high as 30%. The annual incidence in the United States is estimated to be 4.5–8.5 per 100,000 children. The illness occurs most commonly during winter and spring.

High fever, around 40°C, is usually the first sign and should be present for at least 5 days. Within a few days, an irregular, erythematous, macular eruption develops over the trunk and legs. Figure 22–31 shows the typical rash in a patient with Kawasaki's disease. Erythema multiforme can also be seen. Palmoplantar desquamation is common; this is one of the most characteristic features of the disease. Figure 22–32 shows this desquamation on the hands of a child with Kawasaki's disease. The conjunctiva becomes injected, and the tongue becomes strawberry-colored. Peripheral edema and cervical adenopathy are frequently seen early in the disease. Arthritis is present in 40% of cases. Although most individuals affected recover without sequelae, death occurs in approximately 2% of patients due to coronary arteritis. The diagnostic criteria for Kawasaki's disease are

Fever for at least 5 days
Presence of four of the following:
     Bilateral conjunctival injection
     Changes in the mucosa of the oropharynx
     Changes of the extremities (e.g., edema, erythema, or desquamation)
     Rash (not vesicular), primarily truncal
     Cervical adenopathy

Early involvement of the cardiovascular system is manifested by tachycardia and often an S₃ gallop. An apical holosystolic murmur is common. Early intervention with intrave-

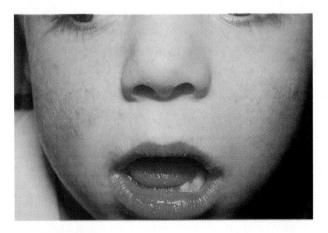

Figure 22–29

"Slapped cheek" rash of fifth disease.

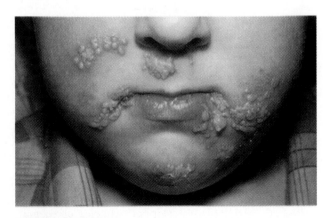

Figure 22–30

Herpetic gingivostomatitis.

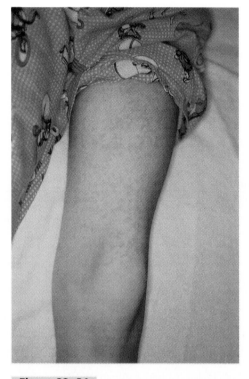

Figure 22–31

Rash in a patient with Kawasaki's disease.

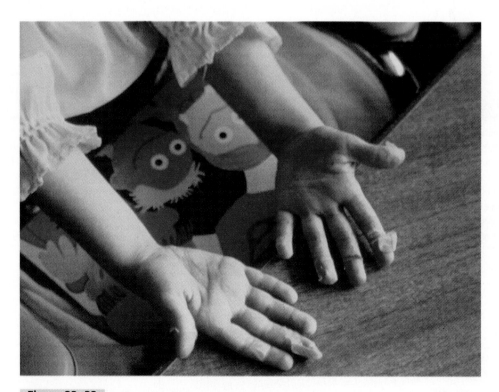

Figure 22–32

Desquamation on the hands of child with Kawasaki's disease.

nous gamma globulin and antiplatelet therapy has been shown to significantly reduce coronary abnormalities.

Heart murmurs are common in the pediatric age group. Some are more serious than others. Table 22–4 summarizes the more common murmurs and associated findings. Table 22–5 lists the chronology of dentition. Table 22–6 lists the more common exanthematous diseases of childhood.

Table 22–4   Cardiovascular Murmurs of Childhood

Condition	Cycle	Location	Radiation	Pitch	Other Signs
Ventricular septal defect	Pansystolic	Left sternal border at the 4th or 5th intercostal space	Over the precordium, rarely to the axilla	High	Thrill at left lower sternal border
Mitral insufficiency	Pansystolic	Apex	Axilla	High	S_1 decreased S_3
Pulmonic stenosis	Systolic ejection	Left 2nd or 3rd intercostal space	Left shoulder	Medium	Widely split S_2 Right-sided S_4 Ejection click
Patent ductus arteriosus	Continuous	Left 2nd intercostal space	Left clavicle	Medium	Machinery-like, harsh Thrill
Venous hum	Continuous	Medial third of clavicles, often on the right	1st and 2nd intercostal spaces	Low	Can be obliterated by pressure on the jugular veins

Table 22–5   Chronology of Dentition

	Deciduous Teeth				Permanent Teeth Eruption	
	Eruption Maxillary (mo)	Eruption Mandibular (mo)	Shedding Maxillary (yr)	Shedding Mandibular (yr)	Maxillary (yr)	Mandibular (yr)
Central incisors	6–8	5–7	7–8	6–7	7–8	6–7
Lateral incisors	8–11	7–10	8–9	7–8	8–9	7–8
Canines	16–20	16–20	11–12	9–11	11–12	9–11
First premolars	—	—	—	—	10–11	10–12
Second premolars	—	—	—	—	10–12	11–13
First molars	10–16	10–16	10–11	10–12	6–7	6–7
Second molars	20–30	20–30	10–12	11–13	12–13	12–13
Third molars	—	—	—	—	17–22	17–22

Table 22–6   Exanthematous Diseases of Childhood

Disease	Cutaneous Lesion	Location	Mucous Membranes	Systemic Components
Chickenpox (varicella)	Maculopapular; "tear-drop" vesicles on an erythematous base	Trunk, face, and scalp; centrifugal* spread	Yes	Mild febrile disorder; malaise; rash preceded by a 24 hr prodrome of headache and malaise; all stages and sizes of lesions found at the same time and in the same area; pruritus
Measles (rubeola)	Erythematous, maculopapular, purplish red	Scalp, hairline, forehead, behind ears, upper neck; rash starts on head and spreads rapidly to upper extremities and then to lower extremities; rash often slightly hemorrhagic; as rash fades, brown discoloration occurs and then disappears within 7–10 days	Yes†	Prodrome of 3–4 days of high fever, chills, headache, malaise, cough, photophobia, conjunctivitis; 2 days before the rash develops, Koplik's† spots may be seen
Rubella (German measles)	Rose-pink, small irregular macules and papules;§ rash is the first evidence of the disease	Hairline, face, neck, trunk, extremities; centripetal‡ spread; rapidly involves body in 24 hr and tends to fade as it spreads	Yes§	Mild fever present, if any; headache, sore throat, mild upper respiratory infection; presence of suboccipital and posterior auricular lymph nodes
Erythema infectiosum (see Fig. 22–29)	Erythematous malar blush	Face, upper arm, thighs; sudden rash in an asymptomatic child giving a "slapped cheek" appearance; maculopapular rash on upper extremities the next day; several days later, a lacy rash on proximal extremities	No	Mild fever, mild pruritus
Roseola infantum (exanthema subitum)	Macules, rose pink, 2–3 mm; rash appears at end of febrile period; duration of rash only 24 hr	Trunk	Rarely	Sudden onset; high fever
Scarlet fever	Fine punctate, erythematous lesion that blanches on pressure	Face, along skin folds, buttocks, sternum, between scapulae	Yes‖	Disease results from toxin produced by group A streptococci as a result of pharyngeal infection;‖ abrupt onset of fever, headache, sore throat, vomiting; 12–48 hr later, rash appears

* Moving outward from the center.
† Koplik's spots are highly diagnostic; these appear on the buccal mucosa opposite the first molar teeth; they often appear as bluish-white pinpoint papules on an erythematous base.
‡ Moving toward the center.
§ Forschheimer's sign consists of petechiae or reddish spots on the soft palate during the 1st day of the illness.
‖ Bright red lesions, often on tonsils and soft palate.

Bibliography

Behrman RE, Kliegman RM, Arvin AM (eds): Nelson Textbook of Pediatrics, 15th ed. Philadelphia, W.B. Saunders Co., 1996.
Green M, Haggerty RJ: Ambulatory Pediatrics IV. Philadelphia, W.B. Saunders Co., 1990.
Gundy JH: Assessment of the Child in Primary Health Care. New York, McGraw-Hill, 1981.
Hurwitz S: Clinical Pediatric Dermatology, 2nd ed. Philadelphia, W.B. Saunders Co., 1993.
Marshall WA, Tanner JM: Variations in the pattern of pubertal changes in boys. Arch Dis Child 45: 22, 1970.
Rowe RT, Stone RT: Steptococcal pharyngitis in children. Clin Pediatr 16:933, 1977.
Tanner JM: Growth at Adolescence, 2nd ed. Oxford, Blackwell Scientific Publications, 1962.

CHAPTER 23

The Geriatric Patient

Old age isn't so bad when you consider the alternative.

Maurice Chevalier
1888–1972

General Considerations

The "geriatric patient" is a member of a group of individuals 65 years of age and older. The individuals experience considerable variation in general health, mental status, functional ability, personal and social resources, marital status, living arrangements, creativity, and social integration. The age range of this rapidly growing population spans more than 40 years. The world's geriatric population is currently increasing at a rate of 2.5% per year, significantly faster than the overall total population. It is estimated that, in the developed nations of the world, there are 146 million people aged 65 years and older. This group will increase to 232 million by the year 2020.

In 1989 in the United States, 12.5% of the population was 65 years of age and older; this proportion had increased from 4.1% in 1900. A decreasing rate of mortality, especially from heart disease and stroke, and a reduction in risk factors such as smoking, high blood pressure, and high serum cholesterol levels have contributed to this increased survival. Elderly women outnumber elderly men 1.5 : 1 overall and 3 : 1 among individuals 95 years of age and older.

In 1995, more than 35 million Americans were older than 65 years of age. The population older than 85 years of age represents the fastest growing segment of the U.S. population. This "graying of America" is expected to continue. By the year 2020, one fifth of the population will be older than the age of 65 years. These statistics are extremely important in view of the cost of medical care for this population. Currently, 32% of all health-care dollars is spent on the geriatric population, which comprises only 12% of the total population.

Some other statistics are important. Eighty-nine percent of the elderly is white. African-Americans constitute 12% of the U.S. population but only 8% of the older age groups. In 1986, most older men (77%) were married, whereas most older women (52%) were widows. Fifteen percent of older men live alone, in comparison with 40% of women. Nursing home residents account for 5% of the population older than 65 years of age. Approximately 12% of the population older than 65 years of age continue to work; 25% is self-employed, in comparison with 10% of the total population. Five percent of the geriatric population—nearly 1 million individuals—is victimized by abuse or neglect. The U.S. Bureau of the Census estimates that 1 million Americans will be 100 years of age or older by the year 2050 and that nearly 2 million will be that age by the year 2080.

Structure and Physiology

This section covers some of the many anatomic and physiologic changes that are attributed to aging, as well as some of the physical findings that result.

Skin

There is atrophy of the epidermis, hair follicles, and sweat glands, which results in thinning skin. The skin becomes fragile and discolored. Wrinkling and dryness result from reduced skin turgor. In addition, the nails become thin and brittle with marked ridging. There is decreased vascularity of the dermis, which contributes to prolonged healing time. There are common pigmentary changes, such as the development of *senile lentigenes,* or liver spots. These brown macules are commonly found on the backs of the hands, on the forearms, and on the face. They are caused by localized mild epidermal hyperplasia, in association with increased numbers of melanocytes and increased melanin production. Figure 23–1 shows senile lentigenes on the forearms of an 87 year old woman.

Another common skin change is *senile (solar) keratosis,* which is a well-defined, raised papule or plaque of epidermal hyperkeratosis. The surface scale varies in color from yellow to brown. These lesions are common on the face, neck, trunk, and hands. Figure 23–2 shows several senile keratoses on an 82 year old man.

There is commonly a degeneration of the elastic fibers and collagen of the skin, resulting in a loss of elasticity and the development of *senile purpura.* These purple

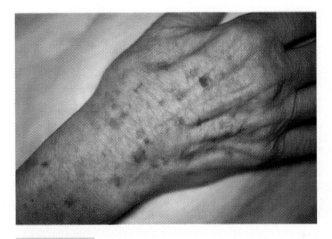

Figure 23–1

Senile lentigenes in an 87 year old woman. Notice the brownish-black well-demarcated macules.

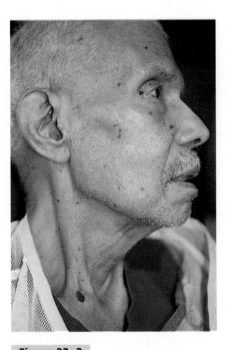

Figure 23–2

Raised senile keratoses on the face and neck of an 82 year old man.

macules, commonly seen on the backs of the hands or on the forearms, result from blood that has extravasated through capillaries that have lost their elastic support. Figure 23–3 shows senile purpura on the forearm of a 90 year old woman.

Sebaceous gland hyperplasia, especially on the forehead and nose, is common. These yellowish glands range in size from 1 to 3 mm and have a central pore. It is important to differentiate these benign lesions from basal cell carcinomas.

Hair loses its pigment, which commonly results in *"graying" of the hair.* With the reduction in the number of hair follicles, there is *hair loss* all over the body: head, axillae, pubic area, and extremities. With the reduction in estrogens, an increase in hair may actually develop in many older women, especially on the chin and upper lip. A 79 year old woman with chin hairs is shown in Figure 23–4.

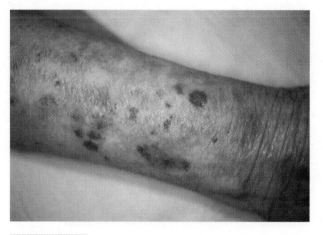

Figure 23–3

Senile purpura on the forearm of a 90 year old woman. Note the red macules and the loss of turgidity of the skin.

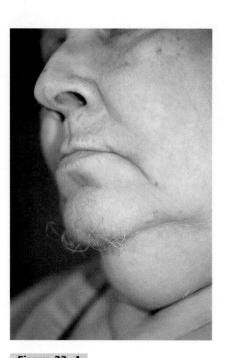

Figure 23–4

Chin whiskers on a 79 year old woman.

As a result of reduction in subcutaneous tissue, there is less insulation and less padding over bony surfaces. This predisposes to hypothermia and the development of *pressure sores,* or *decubitus ulcers.* Figure 23–5 shows a pressure sore that developed on an 85 year old man within 1 week. The man was seen 1 week earlier when a small, intact erythematous area was noticed over his sacral area. He was brought back to the emergency room 7 days later with the decubitus ulcer seen in this figure. The ulceration has eroded through the skin and muscle, into the sacrum, and into the bowel, with the development of a rectovesicular fistula.

Eyes

As a result of a reduction of orbital fat, the eyes appear sunken. Laxity of the eyelids, or *senile ptosis,* often develops. *Ectropion* or *entropion* may develop, from the lower eyelid's falling away or falling inward, respectively. There may also be a clogging of the lacrimal duct, resulting in *epiphora,* or tearing. Fatty deposits in the cornea may produce an *arcus senilis,* seen in Figure 8–24. Inadequate production of mucous tears by the conjunctiva may predispose to *corneal ulcers, exposure keratitis,* or *dry eye syndrome.*

An accumulation of yellow pigment in the lens alters color perception. A loss of elasticity in the lens results in *presbyopia.* Nuclear sclerosis of the lens develops into *cataract* formation. Patients experience a decrease in visual acuity and commonly complain of a sensitivity to glare from interior lights, from sunlight, or from reflection from floors.

Degenerative changes in the iris, vitreous humor, and retina may impair visual acuity, reduce the fields of vision, and lead to the development of floaters *(muscae volentes). Senile macular degeneration* and *retinal hemorrhages* are other medically significant causes of decreases in visual acuity.

Ears

Degeneration of the organ of Corti may result in *presbycusis,* an impaired sensitivity to high-frequency tones. Patients experience a slowly progressive type of hearing loss with a consistent pattern of pure tone loss. *Otosclerosis* may produce *conductive deafness,* as does the excessive cerumen accumulation so commonly seen in older individuals. A degeneration of the hair cells in the semicircular canals may produce *dizziness.*

Nose and Throat

Atrophic changes occur in the mucosa of the nose and throat. Taste and, especially, smell may be altered, particularly in institutionalized individuals. A decrease in mucus

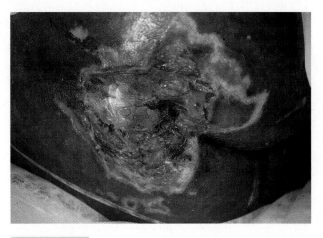

Figure 23–5

A stage IV pressure sore in the sacral area of an 85 year old man. Note the sacrum *(white area)* and necrotic surrounding muscles.

production predisposes older patients to upper respiratory infections. A loss of elasticity in the laryngeal muscles may produce tremulousness and high pitch of the voice.

Mouth

Loss of teeth from dental caries or periodontal disease is common. *Gingival recession* may produce problems with dentures and a malalignment of bite. Atrophic changes in the salivary glands cause dryness of the mouth, known as *xerostomia,* a common complaint among the elderly.

Lungs

A loss of elasticity in the pulmonary septa and atrophy of the alveoli cause a coalescence of the alveoli, with a reduction in vital capacity and oxygen diffusion. There are decreases in forced vital capacity and expiratory flow rate. A degeneration of bronchial epithelium and mucous glands increases the susceptibility to infections. Skeletal changes also contribute to a decrease in vital capacity.

Cardiovascular

A loss in the elasticity of the aorta may cause aortic dilatation. The semilunar and atrioventricular valves may degenerate and become regurgitant. Alternatively, these valves may become sclerotic, which causes stenosis of the valves. Degeneration or calcification of the conducting system may cause *heart block* or *arrhythmias.*

Noncompliance of the peripheral arteries may cause *hypertension* with a *widened pulse pressure.* Systolic blood pressure rises progressively with age, whereas diastolic pressure levels off in the 6th decade of life; these developments lead to an increased prevalence of isolated systolic hypertension. Coronary atherosclerosis may produce angina, *myocardial infarction,* or nonspecific symptoms such as confusion or tiredness.

There are also decreases in plasma volume, ventricular filling time, and baroreflex sensitivity.

Breasts

The amount of glandular tissue decreases, and the tissue is replaced by fatty deposits. As a result of a loss of elastic tissue, the breasts become pendulous, and the ducts may be more palpable.

In men, *gynecomastia* may result from a change in the metabolism of sex hormones by the liver.

Gastrointestinal System

Atrophy of the gastrointestinal mucosa occurs with a reduction in the number of stomach and intestinal glands, causing alterations in secretion, motility, and absorption. Changes in elastic tissue and colonic pressures may result in diverticulosis, which can lead to diverticulitis. Pancreatic acinar atrophy is common, as are decreases in hepatic mass, hepatic blood flow, and microsomal enzyme activity. These decreases result in an increased half-life of lipid-soluble drugs.

Genitourinary System

There is a decrease in the number of glomeruli and a thickening of the basement membrane in Bowman's capsule, resulting in a reduction in renal function. Degenerative changes occur in the renal tubules, as does a reduction in the actual number of tubules. Renal blood flow is reduced to half by the age of 75 years. Vascular changes may also contribute to a reduced glomerular filtration rate.

In men, *prostatic atrophy* or *prostatic hypertrophy* develops. Benign prostatic hypertrophy is present in 80% of all men older than the age of 80 years. The penis decreases in size, and the testicles hang lower in the scrotum.

In postmenopausal women, the reduction in estrogen is associated with an increase in *osteoporosis.* The labia and clitoris are reduced in size, and the vaginal mucosa becomes thin and dry. The uterus and ovaries also decrease in size.

As discussed previously, pubic hair decreases in amount and becomes gray.

Endocrine System

There is decreased metabolism of thyroxine and decreased conversion of thyroxine to triiodothyronine. Because of a reduction in pancreatic beta cell secretion, *hyperglycemia* may result. The hypothalamus and the pituitary gland secrete reduced amounts of hormones. An increase in secretion of antidiuretic hormone and atrial natriuretic hormone may alter fluid balance. There are also increased levels of norepinephrine.

Musculoskeletal System

There is general atrophy of muscles, causing a decline in strength. *Muscle wasting* is seen most commonly in the distal extremities, especially in the dorsal interosseous muscles.

Osteoclastic activity is greater than osteoblastic activity. An enlargement of the cancellous bone spaces and a thinning of the trabeculae result in osteoporosis. *Kyphosis* and a loss of height are common. Degenerative changes and a loss of elastic tissue occur in joints, ligaments, and tendons. This frequently results in *joint stiffness*. Degenerative changes in bone may result in bone cysts and erosions, making these bones prone to *fracture*. *Osteoarthritis* is common. Thinning of cartilage and synovial thickening produce joint stiffness and pain. Range of motion is also reduced, perhaps because of pain.

Figure 18–57 shows Heberden's and Bouchard's nodes, which have already been described, in an 86 year old woman with osteoarthritis.

Nervous System

Changes in brain function may adversely affect memory and intelligence, although other skills such as language and sustained attention may remain. Significant variability exists among individuals, and many elderly individuals continue to perform at levels that are comparable to or that exceed those of much younger people.

Brain weight is frequently reduced 5–7% as a result of atrophy of selected areas. There is a decrease in blood flow to the brain by 10–15%. Vascular change of atherosclerosis can result in *multiple infarcts* or *transient ischemic attacks*.

Reflexes are commonly reduced; the gag reflex is frequently absent. The Achilles tendon reflex is often symmetrically reduced or absent. Primitive reflexes, such as snout or palmomental, may be present in *normal* elderly persons.

Hematopoietic System

There is an increase in the amount of marrow fat and a decrease in the amount of active bone marrow.

Immune System

There is a decreased number of newly formed T lymphocytes and a reduced capability of T lymphocytes to proliferate in response to mitogens or antigens. Humoral immunity is impaired, and suppressor T lymphocytes are decreased in number.

Basic Principles of Geriatric Medicine

First, there is an *altered presentation of disease*. The actual symptom may not be a symptom of the organ system involved with the disease. For example, if a person in his or her 50s were to have a heart attack, the individual, unless diabetic, would usually suffer from chest pain. This is not the case in the geriatric age group. It is well documented that 70% of nondiabetic individuals older than the age of 70 years do not have chest pain with a myocardial infarction. Such patients may present instead with breathlessness, falling, confusion, or palpitations.

Another illustration of alterations in symptoms is the geriatric patient with diabetes mellitus. Ordinarily, because of lack of insulin, younger patients become acidotic and ketotic, with a smell of ketones on their breath. They may also exhibit shallow, rapid respirations. Older patients with uncontrolled diabetes mellitus may not become ketotic and acidotic. Instead, the syndrome of hyperosmolar, nonketotic coma may ensue. These patients, who do not have the smell of ketones on their breath and are not acidotic, are hyperosmolar and may have serum glucose levels in excess of 600 or 700 mg/dL. They may even present in coma.

A third example is a patient with hyperthyroidism. The geriatric patient with hyperthyroidism might not present with the tachycardia, sweats, or anxiety states that are seen in younger individuals with increased thyroid activity. The geriatric patient may instead appear depressed and apathetic.

An older patient with acute appendicitis might not suffer from abdominal pain, and an older patient with pneumonia might not have shortness of breath; confusion may be the only symptom.

A second principle is the *nonspecific presentation of disease.* When an elderly person becomes ill, a family member commonly reports that the patient "just hasn't gotten out of bed." The patient may go to bed and stay there. The patient may not want to eat and may have only nonspecific complaints.

A third principle is the *underreporting of illness.* When an interviewer asks a geriatric patient about various symptoms, the patient may fail to report blindness caused by a cataract, deafness caused by otosclerosis, pain in the legs at night, urinary incontinence, constipation, confusion, and so forth. The geriatric patient may believe that these symptoms are normal for a 75 or 80 year old person. Abdominal pain and other gastrointestinal complaints such as increased gas are commonly mistaken by geriatric patients as a normal part of aging. Sometimes a patient may say, "Nothing can be done about it, so I don't want to bother anyone by mentioning it."

A fourth principle is the recognition that *multiple pathologic conditions may be present* in a geriatric patient. Such a patient may therefore have been given multiple medications or therapies. One medicine may have deleterious effects on a patient if some other condition exists. Of course, this can occur with any aged patient, but it is more likely to occur in older patients who probably have several pathologic conditions.

A fifth principle is *polypharmacy,* which is defined as three or more medicines. It is critically important that the interviewer see and know of all the medications being taken by the patient. Instruct the patient or family to bring in all medications, both prescription and nonprescription, and ask the patient how he or she is taking them. There is commonly a significant discrepancy between the written prescription and the dosage that the patient actually takes.

Americans older than the age of 65 years use about 25% of all prescription medications consumed in the United States, and at any one time, the average geriatric patient uses 4.5 prescription medications. The average nursing home resident consumes the most medications, averaging eight medications at any one time. The use of mood-altering drugs is common in the geriatric population. Approximately 7% of nursing home residents are taking three or more psychoactive drugs.

Finally, what is the patient's *chief complaint?* This is sometimes referred to as "the myth of the chief complaint." Many geriatric patients do not have a single complaint. There may be several problems related to their many conditions. In fact, as already discussed, if a chief complaint is indeed given, it may bear no relationship to the organ system involved. *Be careful in the evaluation of the chief complaint when dealing with the older patient.*

Expectations of geriatric patients are different from those of patients in other age groups. Whereas in younger patients the emphasis is on diagnosis and cure, the goal in the care of older patients is to improve function. You should strive to prolong the period of optimal physical, mental, and social activity. In the event of terminal illness, you should ensure as little mental and physical distress as possible and provide appropriate emotional support to the patient and family.

The Geriatric History

The main components of the medical history are basically the same for geriatric patients as for younger patients, except for the chief complaint and the family history.

With the exception of a family history of Alzheimer's disease, the family history is less important for geriatric patients than for younger patients. For example, the fact that a family member died of a myocardial infarction at age 60 years is relatively unimportant for a patient who is already in his or her 80s. It is also often difficult for an older patient to remember the causes of and ages at death of relatives.

Before beginning the history, determine whether there is an impairment of hearing, vision, or cognition. A quick check of these three functions is mandatory. Ask the patient whether he or she uses any assistive devices (e.g., hearing aid, glasses, cane, walker, wheelchair). If so, evaluate the condition of the device. Is the patient using the device properly? Ask the patient how the device was obtained; often these devices have been given to the patient by friends or family members or have been left by deceased spouses.

If there is a hearing impairment, sit facing the patient, as close as possible and at ear level with the patient. Make sure that the patient is wearing, if required, the hearing aid or other assistive device. Try to minimize both audible and visual distractions. Speak in a slow, low-pitched, and moderately loud voice. Allow the patient to observe your lips as you talk. Finally, confirm with the patient that he or she is being understood by repeating portions of the history.

Because many older patients have a memory deficit or dementia, it is frequently necessary to obtain a confirming history from another family member or caregiver.

All support systems must be evaluated. These include family, friends, and professional services.

Ascertain diet, because many older patients have poorly balanced diets.

A *comprehensive geriatric assessment* is an essential component of the history. It ensures that the many complex health-care needs are evaluated and met. Every geriatric history must include a comprehensive assessment of activities. Measures of the patient's ability to perform basic activities, called *activities of daily living (ADL)*, must be gathered. These include measures of bathing, dressing, toileting, continence, feeding, and transferring in and out of bed or on and off a chair. The ability to perform more complex tasks, called *instrumental activities of daily living (IADL)*, is also assessed. These tasks include food preparation, shopping, housekeeping, laundry, financial management, medicine management, use of transportation, and use of the telephone.

Other areas that must be evaluated for all geriatric patients are the following:

1. Abuse and neglect
2. Affective disorder
3. Caregiver stress
4. Cognitive impairment
5. Decubitus ulcers
6. Dental impairment
7. Discussion of advance directives*
8. Falls
9. Feeding impairment
10. Gait abnormalities
11. Health maintenance
12. Hearing impairment
13. Incontinence (fecal and urinary)
14. Infections (recurrent)
15. Nutritional assessment
16. Osteoporosis
17. Podiatric disorders
18. Polypharmacy
19. Preoperative evaluation, if appropriate
20. Rehabilitation needs
21. Sleep disorders
22. Visual impairment

Certain questionnaires and scales have been validated in the elderly and may be used to *screen patients for affective disorders* such as depression or dementia. An

---

* These include living wills, resuscitation, and proxy appointments.

example is the Yesavage Geriatric Depression Scale, which consists of 30 items (Table 23–1) and in which each of the patient's answers that matches the scoresheet is scored 1 point. A total score from 0 to 9 indicates no depression; from 10 to 19, mild depression; and from 20 to 30, severe depression.

The presentation of depression is not always classic, especially in older individuals. Symptoms that suggest psychomotor retardation, such as listlessness, decreased appetite, cognitive impairment, and decreased energy, may be important clues.

Finally, an *assessment of mental status* is required for all older patients. Memory deficits and decreased intellectual functioning influence the reliability of the medical history; therefore, evaluate mental status early in your assessment. Casual conversation is rarely sufficient for detecting cognitive impairment in the elderly. All older patients should be screened with the use of a validated instrument such as the Folstein Mini-Mental State (Table 23–2). A score of 30 points is possible. A score greater than 24

Table 23–1   Yesavage Geriatric Depression Scale

1. Are you basically satisfied with your life?	yes/no
2. Have you dropped many of your activities and interests?	yes/no
3. Do you feel that your life is empty?	yes/no
4. Do you often get bored?	yes/no
5. Are you hopeful about the future?	yes/no
6. Are you bothered by thoughts you can't get out of your head?	yes/no
7. Are you in good spirits most of the time?	yes/no
8. Are you afraid that something bad is going to happen to you?	yes/no
9. Do you feel happy most of the time?	yes/no
10. Do you often feel helpless?	yes/no
11. Do you often get restless and fidgety?	yes/no
12. Do you prefer to stay at home, rather than going out and doing new things?	yes/no
13. Do you frequently worry about the future?	yes/no
14. Do you feel you have more problems with memory than most?	yes/no
15. Do you think it is wonderful to be alive now?	yes/no
16. Do you often feel downhearted and blue?	yes/no
17. Do you feel pretty worthless the way you are now?	yes/no
18. Do you worry a lot about the past?	yes/no
19. Do you find life gets very exciting?	yes/no
20. Is it hard for you to get started on new projects?	yes/no
21. Do you feel full of energy?	yes/no
22. Do you feel that your situation is hopeless?	yes/no
23. Do you think that most people are better off than you are?	yes/no
24. Do you frequently get upset over little things?	yes/no
25. Do you frequently feel like crying?	yes/no
26. Do you have trouble concentrating?	yes/no
27. Do you enjoy getting up in the morning?	yes/no
28. Do you prefer to avoid social gatherings?	yes/no
29. Is it easy for you to make decisions?	yes/no
30. Is your mind as clear as it used to be?	

Scoresheet*

1. No	2. Yes	3. Yes	4. Yes	5. No
6. Yes	7. No	8. Yes	9. No	10. Yes
11. Yes	12. Yes	13. Yes	14. Yes	15. No
16. Yes	17. Yes	18. Yes	19. No	20. Yes
21. No	22. Yes	23. Yes	24. Yes	25. Yes
26. Yes	27. No	28. Yes	29. No	30. No

Reprinted from Yesavage JA, Brink TL, Rose, TL, et al: Development and validation of a geriatric depression rating scale: A preliminary report. J Psychiatr Res 17:37–49, 1983. Copyright 1983, with kind permission from Pergamon Press Ltd., Headington Hill Hall, Oxford 0X3 0BW, UK.

* See text for interpretation.

Table 23–2   **Folstein's "Mini-Mental State"**

Maximum Score	Score	
		Orientation
5	( )	What is the (year) (season) (date) (day) (month)?
5	( )	Where are we (state) (county) (town) (hospital) (floor)?
		Registration
3	( )	Name 3 objects: 1 second to say each. Then ask the patient all 3 after you have said them. Give 1 point for each correct answer. Then repeat them until he learns all 3. Count trials and record. **Trials**
		Attention and Calculation
5	( )	Serial 7's. 1 point for each correct. Stop after 5 answers. Alternatively, spell "world" backwards.
		Recall
3	( )	Ask for the 3 objects repeated above. Give 1 point for each correct.
		Language
9	( )	Name a pencil, and watch (2 points)
		Repeat the following "No ifs, ands or buts." (1 point)
		Follow a 3-stage command:
		"Take a paper in your right hand, fold it in half, and put it on the floor" (3 points)
		Read and obey the following: **CLOSE YOUR EYES** (1 point)
		Write a sentence (1 point)
		Copy design (1 point)
_____		**Total score**
		ASSESS level of consciousness along a continuum _____
		Alert Drowsy Stupor Coma

Instructions for Administration of Mini-Mental State Examination

Orientation

(1) Ask for the date. Then ask specifically for parts omitted, e.g., "Can you also tell me what season it is?" 1 point for each correct.

(2) Ask in turn "Can you tell me the name of this hospital?" (town, county, etc.). 1 point for each correct.

Registration

Ask the patient if you may test his memory. Then say the names of 3 unrelated objects, clearly and slowly, about one second for each. After you have said all 3, ask him to repeat them. This first repetition determines his score (0–3) but keep saying them until he can repeat all 3, up to 6 trials. If he does not eventually learn all 3, recall cannot be meaningfully tested.

Attention and Calculation

Ask the patient to begin with 100 and count backwards by 7. Stop after 5 subtractions (93, 86, 79, 72, 65). Score the number of correct answers.

If the patient cannot or will not perform this task, ask him to spell the word "world" backwards. The score is the number of letters in correct order. E.g., dlrow = 5, dlorw = 3.

Recall

Ask the patient if he can recall the 3 words you previously asked him to remember. Score 0–3.

Language

Naming: Show the patient a wrist watch and ask him what it is. Repeat for pencil. Score 0–2.

Repetition: Ask the patient to repeat the sentence after you. Allow only one trial. Score 0 or 1.

3-Stage command: Give the patient a piece of plain blank paper and repeat the command. Score 1 point for each part correctly executed.

Table continued

Table 23–2 *Continued*
Instructions for Administration of Mini-Mental State Examination
Language

Reading: On a blank piece of paper, print the sentence "Close your eyes" in letters large enough for the patient to see clearly. Ask him to read it and do what it says. Score 1 point only if he actually closes his eyes.

Writing: Give the patient a blank piece of paper and ask him to write a sentence for you. Do not dictate a sentence; it is to be written spontaneously. It must contain a subject and verb and be sensible. Correct grammar and punctuation are not necessary.

Copying: On a clean piece of paper, draw intersecting pentagons, each side about 1 in., and ask him to copy it exactly as it is. All 10 angles must be present and 2 must intersect to score 1 point. Tremor and rotation are ignored.

Estimate the patient's level of sensorium along a continuum, from alert on the left to coma on the right.

Reprinted from Folstein MF, Folstein SE, McHugh PR: "Mini-mental state": A practical method for grading the cognitive state of patients for the clinician. J Psychiatr Res 12:189–198, 1975. Copyright 1975, with kind permission from Pergamon Press Ltd., Headington Hill Hall, Oxford 0X3 0BW, UK.

probably indicates no cognitive impairment. Patients with scores from 20 to 24 need further cognitive testing, unless educational, language, or cultural reasons are thought to play a role in the lowness of the score. Scores of less than 20 indicate cognitive impairment.

Impact on the Patient of Growing Old

Growing old can bring great joy and satisfaction: free time to start new hobbies or new occupations; time to travel; time to meet new friends; time to write about lifelong experiences; time to become creative; time to impart wisdom to younger generations; time to enjoy grandparenthood, great-grandparenthood, or even great-great-grandparenthood. Of the 80% of individuals older than the age of 65 years, 94% are grandparents and 46% are great-grandparents. Becoming a grandparent can give the older person a new lease on life and allow him or her to relive the memories of earlier years. Old age can allow the individual to use the knowledge attained throughout life for goals that, perhaps because of time or financial constraints, were unable to be achieved earlier. All this is true if the patient's health permits it. The physical and mental health of the person may, however, limit enjoyment of this period of life.

As already discussed, many physical changes occur with aging. Specific disabilities, such as locomotor afflictions, may be particularly handicapping in the presence of normal cognitive functioning. Loss of vision or hearing can lead to social isolation. These physical changes can have a profound effect on the emotional health of the individual. The loss of friends and loved ones may take its toll on the patient as well.

Of the 30 million Americans older than the age of 65 years, it is estimated that 12–15% suffer from some functional psychiatric disorder, ranging from anxiety and depression to severe delirium and other psychotic states. Depression may result from loss, which is common among the more frequent problems of the geriatric patient: loss of health, a friend, a spouse, a relative, or loss of status or participation in society. These losses and others can be devastating to the older patient.

The patient may feel trapped within an aged body. Grief, a sense of helplessness, or a sense of emptiness can develop. Guilt feelings may also develop: "Why did I outlive . . . ?" In older individuals, as in children, being left alone provokes terror and anger because of a sense of vulnerability. Depression and loss of self-esteem may contribute to suicide, rates of which are highest among older white men in their 80s.

Finally, concerns and fears related to their own death are important. Interesting is the fact that most older individuals fear death less than do younger persons. What older persons fear is not when they will die but *how* they will die. Will they be in pain? Will they be alone? The health-care provider must address these issues directly so that the anxiety and depression so commonly related to these issues can be allayed.

Physical Examination

The physical examination of the geriatric patient is no different from that already described in the chapters in Part II of this book. Special attention, however, should be given to the following areas.

Disrobing may be embarrassing for the older patient, especially because examiners are usually much younger than the patients. Modesty must be respected. Make sure that only the area being examined is exposed. Try to make sure that the room is warm; older individuals tend to chill easily. Finally, remember that putting on a robe or gown for a younger patient may not present any difficulty, but for an older patient who may have difficulty in moving, perhaps because of arthritis, it may be a real problem.

Assessment of Vital Signs

Perform routine evaluation, including that of orthostatic changes in pulse and blood pressure. Be careful if the patient complains of dizziness or chest discomfort. If the patient becomes orthostatic, have the patient lie down immediately. Obtain body temperature. If the patient is hypometabolic, as happens in hypothyroidism or in exposure hypothermia, the temperature may be less than 36°C. In the geriatric population, a normal temperature is commonly found in patients with severe infections. Accurate weights should be taken and observed over time.

Skin

Observe the skin for any malignant changes, pressure sores, evidence of pruritus, and ecchymoses suggestive of falls or abuse.

Head, Eye, Ear, Nose, Throat, and Neck

Evaluate the patient for any evidence of skull trauma. Palpate the superficial temporal arteries, which are located anterosuperior to the tragus. In patients who complain of visual symptoms, headaches, and/or polymyalgic symptoms, polymyalgia rheumatica and/or temporal (giant cell) arteritis should be suspected (see the Clinicopathologic Correlations section at the end of this chapter).

Is entropion or ectropion present? Determine visual acuity, if this was not already tested. Eye movement should be checked for gaze palsies. The ability to gaze upward declines with increasing age. Are cataracts present? Examine the retina, if a cataract does not exist. Is macular degeneration present?

Is cerumen impacted in the external canal? Evaluate auditory acuity, if this was not already done.

Ask the patient to remove any dentures, if present. Examine the mouth for dryness, lesions, condition of teeth, oral ulcers, and malignancies. Poor-fitting dentures may cause weight loss as a result of difficulty in eating and chewing. Examine the tongue for malignancy.

Auscultate the neck. Are carotid bruits present? Palpate the thyroid. Are nodules present? Is the thyroid diffusely enlarged?

Breasts

Examine the breasts for dimpling, discharge, and masses. The incidence of breast cancer increases with advancing age. The highest incidence occurs among women aged 85 years and older.

Chest

Inspect the shape of the chest. Is kyphoscoliosis present? Auscultate the chest. Are any adventitious sounds present?

Cardiovascular System

Evaluate the point of maximum impulse. Is it displaced laterally? Auscultate the heart in the four main positions. Are any murmurs, rubs, or gallops heard? Systolic murmurs are heard in 55% of all older adults.

Are the peripheral pulses present? Loss of peripheral pulses is common and may have little clinical significance, especially if the patient does not complain of intermittent claudication. Is there evidence of peripheral vascular disease?

Abdomen

Perform routine palpation and percussion of the abdomen. Is the bladder enlarged? Is a pulsatile abdominal mass present? Palpate for inguinal and femoral hernias. Is there evidence of urine leakage on the undergarments? Perform a rectal examination. Examine the stool for blood. In a man, is the prostate enlarged?

Musculoskeletal Examination

Examine the joints. Ask the patient to stand up from a seated position, and observe for any difficulties. Can the patient lift the hands over the head to brush his or her hair?

The extremities should be examined for arthritis, impaired range of motion, and deformities. The feet should be inspected for nail care, calluses, deformities, and peripheral pulses.

Neurologic Examination

Evaluate mental status, if this was not already done. Check vibration sensation. Lack of this is the most commonly found deficit in otherwise healthy elderly individuals. Test reflexes. Asymmetry is suggestive of stroke, myelopathy, or root compression. Evaluate for rigidity. Cogwheel rigidity is suggestive of Parkinson's disease. Perform Romberg's test. Evaluate gait.

Any patient presenting with a change in function must be evaluated for dementia, depression, and Parkinson's disease.

Evaluate motor strength, tone, and rapid alternating movements.

Clinicopathologic Correlations

Many organ system problems are seen in the geriatric age group. This section covers several disorders and functional states that are especially common in the older age group and are not discussed in other chapters of this book.

Senile macular degeneration affects nearly 10% of the geriatric population and a higher proportion of women than of men. It represents the most common cause of legal blindness in the United States. There is painless and progressive loss of central vision. The patient frequently complains of difficulty in reading. Because only the macula is involved, peripheral vision is spared, and complete blindness does not result.

Temporal arteritis and *polymyalgia rheumatica* are diseases unique to the geriatric age group and most likely are manifestations of a condition known as *giant cell arteritis*. Polymyalgia rheumatica is estimated to occur in 40–50% of patients with temporal arteritis. Both of these conditions are three- to fourfold more frequent among women than among men.

The symptoms of temporal arteritis include headache, which is frequently associated with scalp tenderness; the temporal artery may also be tender; and there are several generalized symptoms, which include fever, weight loss, anorexia, and fatigue. Visual disturbances include loss of vision, blurred vision, diplopia, and amaurosis fugax. Sometimes patients may also complain of pain on chewing food. The diagnosis is made from temporal artery biopsy, which has a sensitivity of 90% and a specificity of 100%.

Many patients with polymyalgia rheumatica complain of symmetric pain, especially in the morning, and stiffness of the neck, shoulders, lower back, and pelvic girdle.

They often find it difficult to brush their hair. The proximal muscle groups of the upper extremities and pelvic girdle are commonly affected.

Pressure sores, or *decubitus ulcers,* affect up to 3 million individuals yearly. The annual health-care expenditures for these lesions is in excess of 5 billion dollars. It has been estimated that the cost to heal one decubitus ulcer ranges from $5,000 to $50,000. In long-term health-care facilities, the prevalence of decubitus ulcers is 15–25%, whereas the prevalence in the community is 5–15%. There are literally thousands of legal court cases yearly as a result of the development of pressure sores and the related morbidity and mortality rates. Bacteremia is common, and osteomyelitis occurs in more than 25% of all patients with nonhealing decubitus ulcers.

Decubitus ulcers result from prolonged pressure over a small area of the body. It is thought that this pressure causes a decrease in perfusion to the area, leading to the accumulation of toxic products, with subsequent necrosis of skin, muscle, subcutaneous tissue, and bone. Moisture, caused by fecal or urinary incontinence or by perspiration, is also implicated because it causes maceration of the epidermis and allows tissue necrosis to occur. Shearing force is also a factor. Shear is generated when the head of a bed is elevated, causing the torso to slide down and transmit pressure to the sacrum. Poor nutritional status and delayed wound healing are other widespread contributing factors.

The four clinical stages of decubitus ulcers are as follows:

Stage I	Nonblanchable erythema
Stage II	Ulcer extending up to subcutaneous fat
Stage III	Ulceration extending through subcutaneous fat without involving muscle or bone
Stage IV	Ulceration extending into muscle or bone

Ulcers covered by superficial necrosis must undergo débridement before they can be staged. The patient in Figure 23–5 presented with a stage I pressure sore, and 1 week later, when this photograph was taken, the sore had rapidly advanced to a stage IV lesion. The patient died of sepsis 4 days after the photograph was taken.

Prevention of decubitus ulcers is extremely important in the care of a bedridden patient. Repositioning or rotating the patient at least every 2 hours, minimizing moisture, practicing basic skin care, and improving the nutritional state are important.

Urinary incontinence is an important problem in the geriatric age group. It occurs in 15–30% of community-dwelling individuals 65 years of age and older. Among institutionalized patients, the prevalence is 40–60%. In 1995, the total cost of health care for urinary incontinence was more than 15 billion dollars.

There are many causes of urinary incontinence. Some causes are decreased bladder capacity, increased residual volume, and pelvic relaxation. Resnick and Yalla (1987) summarized the major transient causes of urinary incontinence by the mnemonic "DIAPPERS":

D Delirium and/or dementia
I Infections (urinary)
A Atrophic vaginitis or urethritis; atonic bladder
P Psychologic causes such as depression; prostatitis
P Pharmacologic agents such as anticholinergics, psychotropics, alcohol, diuretics, opiates, and alpha adrenergic agents
E Endocrine abnormalities such as diabetes and hypercalcemia
R Restricted mobility
S Stool impaction

Dementia, according to the American Psychiatric Association's *Diagnostic and Statistical Manual of Mental Disorders, 3rd Edition—Revised (DSM-III-R)* criteria, is characterized by an acquired and persistent impairment in short- and long-term memory and other disturbances, such as impairment in language (e.g., reading, writing, fluency, naming, repetition), concentration ability, visuospatial function (e.g., drawing, copying), emotions, and personality, despite a state of clear consciousness. The prevalence of dementia in the general population older than 65 years of age is estimated to be 15–50%. In chronic care facilities, the prevalence is higher than 50% of all hospitalized patients.

The most common causes of dementia are strokes and Alzheimer's disease. The course and onset of the symptoms often provide clues to the cause of dementia. Sudden onset is practically always related to a cerebrovascular accident. A subacute, insidious course may be related to tumor, Jakob-Creutzfeldt disease, or Alzheimer's disease. Dementia with rigidity and bradykinesis strongly suggests Parkinson's disease. Dementia in association with urinary incontinence and a spastic-like, magnetic gait is seen in hydrocephalus. The development of dementia after a fall should raise suspicion of a subdural hematoma.

Falls are a common problem in the geriatric age group. Most falls are not associated with fractures, but most hip fractures (more than 90%) are associated with falls. Falls are the result of a decline in vision, gait, balance, sensory perception, strength, and coordination and are often precipitated by medications. Most falls are sustained by patients who have taken long-acting sedatives/hypnotic agents, antidepressants, or major tranquilizers. *Whenever possible, therefore, try to reduce the number of medications.*

Falls are the leading cause of death from injury in individuals 65 years of age and older. Two thirds of reported injury-related deaths in patients age 85 years and older are caused by falls. A fear of falling is also common; 50–60% of all patients older than the age of 65 years have this fear.

Bibliography

Allman RM: Pressure ulcers among the elderly. N Engl J Med 320:850, 1989.

Breslow L, Somers AR: The lifetime health-monitoring program. N Engl J Med 296:601, 1977.

Brocklehurst JC: Textbook of Geriatric Medicine and Gerontology, 3rd ed. Edinburgh, Churchill Livingstone, 1985.

Butler RN, Lewis M, Sunderland T: Aging and Mental Health: Positive Psychosocial and Biomedical Approaches. New York, Macmillan, 1991.

Calkins E, Ford AB, Katz PR: Practice of Geriatrics. Philadelphia, W.B. Saunders Co., 1992.

Evans JG, Williams TF (eds): Oxford Textbook of Geriatric Medicine. Oxford, England, Oxford University Press, 1992.

Ferri FF, Fretwell MD: Practical Guide to the Care of the Geriatric Patient. St. Louis, Mosby-Year Book, 1992.

Folstein MF, Folstein SE, McHugh PR: "Mini-mental state": A practical method for grading the cognitive state of patients for the clinician. J Psychiatr Res 12:189, 1975.

Hazzard WR, Andres R, Bierman EL, et al (eds): Principles of Geriatric Medicine and Gerontology, 2nd ed. New York, McGraw-Hill, 1990.

Katz S, Stroud MW III: Functional assessment in geriatrics. A review of progress and directions. J Am Geriatr Soc 37:267, 1989.

Pfeiffer E: A short psychiatric evaluation schedule. In Brain Function in Old Age (Bayer Symposium VII). New York, Springer Verlag, 1979.

Resnick NM, Yalla SV: Aging and its effect on the bladder. Semin Urol 5:82, 1987.

Rowe JW, Besdine RW: Geriatric Medicine, 2nd ed. Boston, Little, Brown, 1988.

Schrier RW: Geriatric Medicine. Philadelphia, W.B. Saunders, Co., 1990.

Tideksaar R: Falling in Old Age: Its Prevention and Treatment. New York, Springer, 1989.

Wilcock GK, Gray JAM, Longmore JM: Geriatric Problems in General Practice. Oxford, England, Oxford University Press, 1991.

Williams ME: Urinary incontinence in the elderly. Ann Intern Med 97:895, 1982.

Wolf RS: Elder abuse: Ten years later. J Am Geriatr Soc 36:758, 1988.

Yesavage JA, Brink TL, Rose TL, et al: Development and validation of a geriatric depression rating scale: A Preliminary report. J Psychiatr Res 17:37, 1983.

CHAPTER 24

The Acutely Ill Patient

Ther is no thing more precious here than tyme.   [There is nothing more precious here than time.]

Saint Bernard
1090–1153.

The objective of this chapter is to provide a practical approach to the acutely ill patient. The emphasis is on diagnosis, *not* on therapy. In the assessment of the acutely ill patient, time is a critical factor. Unlike assessment of the stable patient, the evaluation of the acutely ill patient does not involve achieving a specific diagnosis but rather identifying a pathophysiologic abnormality that may appear to be identical for several diagnoses. In the evaluation of the acutely ill patient, always ask yourself, "What is the most serious threat to life, and have I ruled it out?" Remember, also, that *your* health is important. Exposure to body substances places you at risk. The minimum isolation precaution for an emergency response is the wearing of latex gloves.

When delivering health care in the field, and perhaps even in the hospital, as you approach the apparent victim, always perform a brief evaluation to determine whether you are in a safe environment; if not, protect yourself and your patient to limit exposure to possible injury. This may be a rare situation, but in circumstances in which it is likely that the rescuer may be injured or killed while rendering care, the rescuer should wait until the situation can be made safe. It does not help the patient or the rescuer to be injured. For example, in an automobile accident, the patient trapped in a car that is in a busy traffic lane should *not* be given first aid until safety flares or cones can be placed to prevent secondary accidents.

During this evaluation, search for other victims who may be hidden from view as you approach the scene of the accident. You will also be able to appreciate the mechanism(s) of injury and attempt to memorize the scene for later reconsideration in the emergency department and perhaps as a witness for the injured plaintiff.

The task for the clinician in approaching most, if not all, patients in acute situations is, first, to ascertain that these patients are not in cardiopulmonary arrest or do not have major perturbations of their vital signs to the point that their continued viability is threatened. The general approach to these acute undefined encounters is to consider the patient unstable until you can confirm, through a series of diagnostic steps, that the patient is well enough for you to take the time to perform a more rigorous and complete history and physical examination.

This strategy leads you to rapidly access and move through a series of simple algorithms, which are grouped into two categories termed the *primary* and *secondary surveys*. The primary survey is a check for conditions that are an immediate threat to the patient's life. This initial assessment should take no longer than 30 seconds. The primary survey is subdivided into a *Cardiopulmonary Resuscitation (CPR) Survey* and a *Key Vital Functions Assessment.* The algorithms for the primary survey are shown in Figures 24–1 and 24–2. The secondary survey is a check for conditions that could become life-threatening problems if not recognized and attended to. An acutely ill patient is anxious and frightened; a calm and reassuring voice can go a long way toward comforting the patient. It is always easier to care for a more relaxed patient than an anxious one.

The primary and secondary surveys are used for both adult and pediatric patients, as well as for medical and injury-related problems. The treatment process is integrated into the diagnostic process. For example, if the patient is not breathing, then ventilations are begun immediately, before moving on to the next diagnostic step in the algorithm.

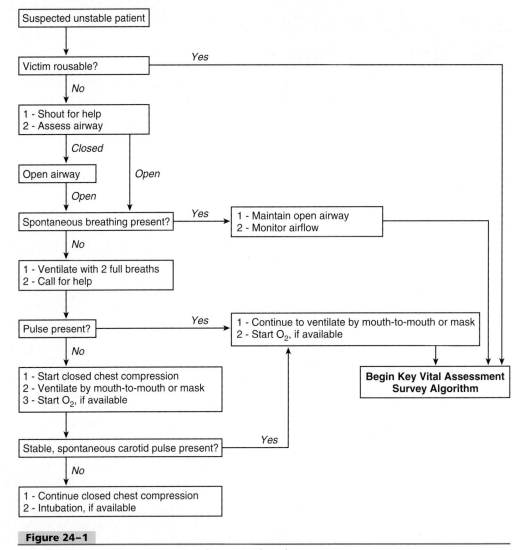

Figure 24–1

Cardiopulmonary Resuscitation (CPR) Survey Algorithm.

The first task is to recognize an acutely ill patient. An unusual appearance or behavior may be the only signs. These include breathing difficulties, clutching the chest or throat, slurring of speech, confusion, unusual odor to the breath, sweating for no apparent reason, or an uncharacteristic skin color (e.g., pale, flushed, or bluish).

Primary Survey

CPR Survey

It should not be assumed that any patient who is not obviously interacting with his or her environment is simply sleeping. For the purpose of this approach, the patient is in cardiopulmonary arrest, until it is proved otherwise. As you approach the patient, observe the patient closely, looking for spontaneous breathing or movements. If these are not discernible, stimulate the patient by talking loudly to him or her. If necessary, shout "ARE YOU OKAY?"

If there is no response, obtain an open airway by the chin-lift/head-tilt maneuver and look, listen, and feel (feel air movement against your cheek) for breathing. To open an unconscious victim's airway, hyperextend the head and lift the chin; place one hand on the forehead and the other behind the occiput and tilt the head backward. This maneuver moves the tongue away from the back of the throat, allowing air to pass around the tongue and into the trachea. Caution should be exercised with any patient in whom there is a suspected neck injury. With such a patient, try to open the

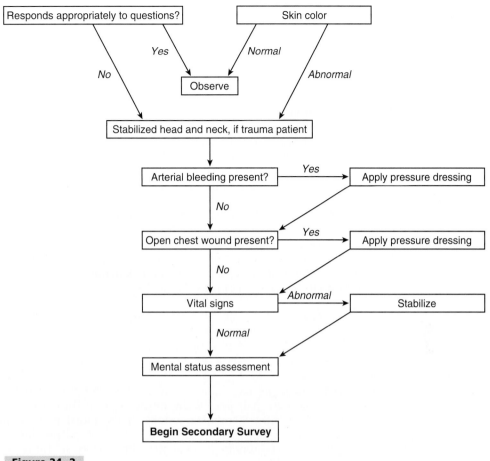

Figure 24–2

Key Vital Functions Assessment Algorithm.

airway by lifting the chin without tilting the head backward; grasp the lower teeth and pull the mandible forward. If necessary, tilt the head back very slightly. If a patient is wearing dentures, remove them only if they occlude the airway.

If there is no evidence of spontaneous breathing, deliver two full breaths using mouth-to-mouth ventilation. Next, call for help in any way you can without leaving the patient, as your patient is *in extremis;* it is unlikely that you can manage the entire resuscitation by yourself.

Determine whether there is spontaneous cardiac function by feeling for a carotid pulse, or in an infant, palpate the precordium for a cardiac impulse. If there is no pulse, begin external chest compression, and intersperse it with your ventilations—in other words, begin CPR.

Key Vital Functions Assessment Survey

Once it has been determined that the patient does not need CPR or the patient has recovered spontaneous cardiopulmonary activity, ascertain whether key life-sustaining functions are adequate and stable or require augmentation or other supportive measures. In the initial overview of the patient, two observations can save a great deal of time and will help avoid unnecessary or untimely interventions. Thus, if the patient's central nervous system is functioning as manifested by the patient's ability to respond appropriately to questions, it is unlikely that the key vital functions are so deranged as to require immediate intervention. Similarly, if the patient's skin is warm, dry, and of normal color, it is likely that there is adequate oxygenation and flow of blood to the periphery. In shock, peripheral blood flow is shunted centrally; thus, skin changes are early indicators of hypovolemic or cardiogenic (low cardiac output) shock. The key diagnostic signs in the skin that are associated with these major acute cardiopulmonary derangements include gray, mottled, or cyanotic color; cold skin temperature; and markedly sweaty skin. The latter sign, termed *diaphoresis,* is caused by the activation of the sympathetic nervous systems by any major threat to homeostasis.

At this point in the algorithm, in a patient who has sustained a possible head injury, immobilize the patient's head and neck by using boards, tape, bulky dressing, or towels or by assigning someone to hold the head immobile. Once the evaluation is completed and the imaging studies are performed, where necessary, the patient can be freed of restriction to movement. Once immobilized, the patient's demobilization requires careful decision-making.

The next two orders of priority are the search for, and the management of, arterial bleeding and open chest injuries. The latter are termed *sucking chest wounds* because they allow air to enter the pleural space, leading to collapse of the underlying lung (pneumothorax). Arterial bleeding and a sucking chest wound can cause death in a very short period, and both are treated by application of a pressure dressing to occlude the area.

At this point in the algorithm, the patient has been stabilized to the point where formal vital signs can be obtained. In the field, these include the patient's mental status, the respiratory rate and pattern, pulse, blood pressure, and in some circumstances, the body temperature. Mental status can be assessed according to the AVPU system, or more traditionally categorized as alert, lethargic, stuporous, or comatose. The AVPU mnemonic for level of consciousness is:

> **A**—Patient is *a*lert
> **V**—Patient responds to a *v*erbal stimulus
> **P**—Patient responds to a *p*ainful stimulus
> **U**—Patient is *u*nresponsive

The blood pressure can be estimated by the pulse wave fullness and by assessing which pulses are palpable. If the radial pulse at the wrist is palpable, then the blood pressure is at least 80 mm Hg systolic. If the radial pulse is impalpable and only the femoral pulse is perceptible, then the systolic blood pressure is from 60 to 70 mm Hg. If a vital sign is abnormal, treat the abnormality to bring it back to normal. If the patient is breathing spontaneously at a rate of 5 breaths per minute, augment and assist the patient's breathing so that the depth and rate of breathing are normalized. This can be accomplished by applying interspersed mouth-to-mouth ventilations, utilizing a self-inflating bag-valve-mask device, or by performing endotracheal intubation and placing the patient on a ventilator. In a similar fashion, the blood pressure can be supported by raising the legs, thus emptying the blood stored in the venous system back into the central circulation. The trauma victim should have a cardiopulmonary examination as well. You are seeking to rule in, or rule out, a tension pneumothorax (shift of the heart away from the tension, increased breath sounds over the side with the tension pneumothorax, distended neck veins, subcutaneous emphysema), cardiac tamponade (distended neck veins, distant heart sounds, hypotension, pulsus paradoxus, normal breath sounds), and chest wall disruption (paradoxical movement of a flail segment).

Secondary Survey

In the secondary survey, take a history from the patient, the patient's relatives, emergency room personnel, or bystanders. The secondary survey is a systematic method for determining whether other conditions or injuries are present and if they need attention. This survey consists of a rapid interview, a check of the vital signs, and a focused physical examination. Here the mnemonic AMPLE can be helpful in gathering pertinent information.

> **A** — *a*llergies
> **M** — *m*edications currently being taken
> **P** — *p*ast medical history
> **L** — *l*ast meal
> **E** — *e*vents preceding the event

A critical piece of information in a trauma patient is the mechanism of injury. Did the patient sustain blunt trauma, or was a weapon used to cause a penetrating injury? In a vehicular accident, ascertain whether the patient was ejected from the car, was wearing a seat belt, and whether there were other injuries or fatalities in the accident. In addition, trauma victims must have all their bones and joints, including the rib cage and pelvis, facial bones, and skull palpated and gently compressed to determine if there is a fracture step-off or crepitation; also check for stability of structure and for function. A screening neurologic examination is necessary to determine whether there are focal cranial nerve, motor, or sensory findings. Most multisystem trauma patients require a rectal examination to determine the presence of blood, tenderness, or upward displacement of the prostate. The latter is a sign of urethral injury.

In performing the physical examination on an injured patient, the patient, if alert, can direct you to the appropriate body areas to be evaluated. The assessment of the patient involves examination of three main regions: the head and neck, the torso, and the extremities. Can the patient move the neck? Ask the patient to move the neck *slowly*. Can the shoulders be moved? Ask the patient to take a deep breath and then blow it out. Does this elicit any pain? Is the patient able to move the fingers? Can the arms be bent? Can the patient move the toes? ankles? Can the patient bend the legs? If the patient can move all extremities without experiencing pain, help the patient up to a sitting position slowly. If the patient cannot move a body part or can do so only with pain, reassess the airway, breathing, and circulation, and get immediate assistance. Continue to observe the patient's level of consciousness, breathing, and skin color.

Head and Neck

Look at the victim's face. Evaluate skin color and temperature. Is there evidence of *raccoon eyes* or *Battles' sign*? A patient with raccoon eyes is shown in Figure 8–16. Periorbital ecchymoses, or raccoon eyes, are seen 6–12 hours after a fracture of the base of the skull. Battles' sign is ecchymosis behind the ear(s) caused by basilar skull or temporal bone fractures; this sign may take 24–36 hours to develop. Palpate the head.

Examine the eyes for pupillary size and responsiveness to light. Are the pupils equal? Are the pupils pinpoint? Is there a unilateral dilated pupil? Are the pupils fixed? Table 24–1 reviews the eye signs in a comatose patient.

Is there a discharge from the ears, nose, or mouth?

Table 24–1   Eye Signs in a Comatose Patient*

Eye Sign	Possible Causes
Pupils reactive, eyes directed straight ahead, normal oculocephalic reflex (OCR)†	Toxic/metabolic
Pinpoint pupils	Narcotic poisoning (OCR intact)
	Pontine or cerebellar hemorrhage (OCR absent)
	Thalamic hemorrhage
	Miotic eye drops
Disconjugate deviation of eyes	Structural brain-stem lesion
Conjugate lateral deviation of eyes	Ipsilateral pontine infarction
	Contralateral frontal hemispheric infarction
Unilateral dilated pupil, fixed pupil with no consensual responses	Supratentorial mass lesion
	Impending brain herniation
	Posterior communicating aneurysm
Bilateral midposition pupils, fixed pupils	Midbrain lesion
	Impending brain herniation
Raccoon eyes (periorbital ecchymoses)	Fracture of the base of the skull

* Eye signs are difficult to evaluate in patients with artifical lenses, prosthetic eyes, contact lenses, or cataracts, or after cataract surgery.

† "Doll's eyes": Rotate the head quickly but gently from side to side. In an unconscious patient with an intact brain stem, the eyes move conjugately in a direction opposite the head turning.

Inspect the neck. Is the trachea deviated? Suspect a chest injury, such as a tension pneumothorax, if the trachea is not midline. Palpate the neck for crepitus, which is indicative of air under the skin from a rupture of the lung.

Abdomen

Inspect the abdomen. Is abdominal distention present? Is there evidence of blunt abdominal trauma, such as an ecchymosis, an abrasion, or an abdominal wound? *Cullen's sign* is a bluish discoloration around the umbilicus indicative of intra-abdominal bleeding or trauma. A *Grey Turner sign* is ecchymotic discoloration around the flanks which is suggestive of retroperitoneal bleeding. The presence of swelling or ecchymosis often occurs late; therefore, its presence is extremely important.

Gently palpate the abdomen, noting the presence of tenderness. If the patient is a woman of childbearing age, always consider the possibility that she may be pregnant.

Inspect the anus and the perineum. Inspect the urethral meatus for blood.

Perform a rectal examination to assess anal sphincter tone, to determine whether blood is present, and to verify that the prostate is in its normal position.

Pelvis

Use the heels of your hands to apply gentle downward pressure on the anterosuperior iliac spine and on the symphysis pubis. Is tenderness present? If so, a fracture to the pelvic ring may be present.

Extremities

Inspect and palpate all extremities for evidence of injury. Try to determine whether the patient can move all extremities. Palpate all peripheral pulses.

Back

Inspect the back, looking for obvious signs of injury. This can be done by gently insinuating your hands beneath the back and neck without moving the patient. If this cannot be done, then the patient should be gently "log-rolled" onto the side. To do this, you will need at least four assistants: one to control the head and neck, two to roll the patient onto the side, and one to cautiously move the lower extremities. Figure 24–3 shows this "log-roll" procedure.

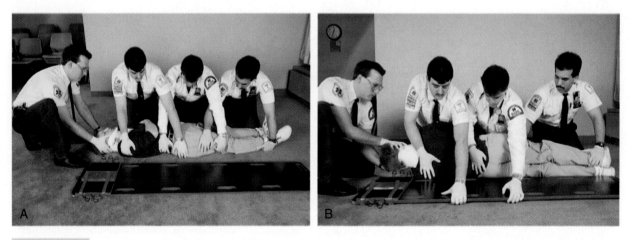

Figure 24–3

Log-roll procedure. *A*: (1) Apply a cervical spine immobilization device and place the patient's arms at the side. Note that one emergency management technician (EMT) maintains cervical immobilization manually throughout this procedure. (2) Three EMTs can be positioned at the side of the patient at the level of the chest, hips, and lower extremities while the long spine board is positioned on one side of the patient. (3) Check the patient's arm on the side of the EMTs for injury before log-rolling the patient, and then align the lower extremities. Note: The EMT at the lower extremities holds the patient's lower leg and thigh region; the EMT at the hips holds the patient's lower legs and places the other hand on the top of the patient's buttocks, and the EMT at the chest holds the patient's arms against the body and at the level of the lower buttocks. *B*: (4) On command from the EMT at the head, all EMTs should rotate the patient toward themselves, keeping the body in alignment. (5) The EMTs then reach across with one hand and pull the board beneath the patient's arm. (6) On command from the EMT at the head, they gently roll the patient onto the board, then roll the board to the ground. (7) Strap the patient's torso and extremities securely to the board, and immobilize the head.

Vital Signs

Reassess vital signs.

The history obtained from the acutely ill patient conforms closely to the standard history, but it is abbreviated to allow rapid diagnostic and management decisions to be made. The physical examination of the acutely ill nontrauma patient includes a cardiopulmonary examination and examinations of the abdomen and the peripheral pulses.

The Pediatric Emergency

When assessing the acutely ill child, always consider the similarities and differences of the pediatric age group as compared with the adult patient; approach the pediatric emergency as an emergency in an adult but recognize the smaller size of the patient and the difference in the physiologic responses to acute illness and injury. The primary assessment of the child is the same as that of the adult.

The most important life-threatening pediatric emergency is *respiratory distress*. Respiratory distress in the pediatric patient may arise from a variety of conditions that result from upper or lower airway disease. Common pediatric respiratory problems of the upper airway include croup (laryngotracheobronchitis), epiglottitis, foreign bodies, and bacterial tracheitis. Lower airway obstruction may result from asthma, pneumonia, bronchiolitis, and foreign bodies.

The hallmarks of respiratory distress are tachypnea, nasal flaring, retractions, stridor, cyanosis, head bobbing, prolonged expiration, and grunting. Children with upper airway disease almost always exhibit stridor. In a child with stridor, distinguish between croup and epiglottitis; a child with epiglottitis may have a rapid progression to respiratory failure. Fortunately, the incidence of epiglottitis has decreased, presumably due to the *Haemophilus influenzae* type B (HIB) vaccine. *If epiglottitis is suspected, do not examine the airway without being prepared to intervene in airway stabilization on an emergency basis.* Manipulation of the child's airway can lead to complete airway obstruction. Table 24–2 compares some of the important differences between epiglottitis and croup.

The peak time for foreign-body aspiration is from 1 to 2 years of age. In a child, consider relief of airway obstruction if

- choking is present
- the cough becomes ineffective
- breathing becomes stridorous
- there is loss of consciousness
- the child becomes cyanotic

Immediately place the child face down, with the head lower than the torso, over your arm, which is placed on your thigh. Support the head of the child by holding the

Table 24–2   Differentiation Between Epiglottitis and Croup

Characteristics	Epiglottitis	Croup
Cause	*H. influenza* type B	Viral, usually parainfluenza virus
Age of child	Any age (peak 3–7 years)	3 months–3 years
Clinical appearance	Toxic	Not toxic
Season	No seasonal preference	Autumn and winter
Clinical onset	Rapid	Insidious
Upper respiratory tract infection	Rare	Common
Fever	>104°F (40°C)	<103°F (39.5°C)
Sore throat	Severe	Variable
Cough	Not "barking," throughout the day	"Barking," during the night
Drooling	Prominent	None
Stridor	Inspiration	Inspiration and expiration
Position	Sitting forward with neck extended and mouth open	Variable
Epiglottis	Bright red	Normal

child's jaw. Deliver five forceful back blows with the heel of your hand between the child's scapulae. Turn the child onto the back while holding the child's head. Place two fingertips on the middle portion of the sternum, one fingerbreadth below the nipples. Depress the sternum 1 inch. Repeat this maneuver up to five times. Attempt to remove any visible material from the pharynx. Repeat the back blows and chest thrusts until the object is dislodged.

If the child becomes unconscious, check the mouth for a foreign body, and then perform mouth-to-mouth breathing. Gently tilt the child's head back while placing the other fingers under the jaw at the chin, and lift the chin upwards. Seal the child's mouth and nose with your mouth. Deliver two breaths, watching the chest rise. Repeat the back blows and chest thrusts. Have someone call for help.

Dehydration is another important pediatric emergency. The most common causes are vomiting and diarrhea. In a child with mild dehydration (<5%), there may be only a slight decrease in mucous membrane moisture. In severe dehydration (15%), the following will commonly be found:

- Parched mucous membranes; no tears
- Markedly decreased skin turgor
- Sunken fontanelles
- Sunken eyeballs
- Tachypnea
- Capillary refill* >2 seconds
- Cool and clammy skin
- Orthostatic hypotension; systolic <80 mm Hg
- Tachycardia; >130 beats per minute

Immediate intravenous infusion of isotonic fluids should be started in children with severe dehydration.

The secondary assessment as outlined earlier and the AVPU mnemonic are just as important for the child as for the adult. Table 24–3 provides a useful reference for CPR.

Table 24–3   Cardiopulmonary Resuscitation Reference Chart

	Infant (less than 1 year of age)	Child (older than 1 year of age)	Adult
If victim has a pulse, give one breath every:	3 seconds	3 seconds	5–6 seconds
If victim has **no** pulse, locate compression landmark:	1 fingerbreadth below the nipple line	Same as adult	One finger on sternum
Compressions are perfomed with:	Two or three fingers on sternum	Heel of hand on sternum	Two hands stacked, with heel of one hand on sternum
Rate of compressions per minute:	>100	100	80–100
Compression depth:	½–1″	1–1½″	1½–2″
Ratio of compressions to breaths with:			
one rescuer	5:1	5:1	15:2
two rescuers	5:1	5:1	5:1

---

* Capillary refill is an assessment of perfusion. It is the time required for a patient's skin color to return to normal after the nailbed has been pressed. The normal refill time is less than 2 seconds.

Bibliography

American Heart Association: Standards and guidelines for cardiopulmonary resuscitation (CPR) and emergency cardiac care (ECC). JAMA 268:2171, 1992.

American Red Cross: First Aid: Responding to Emergencies. St. Louis, Mosby-Year Book, 1991.

Barkin RM, Rosen P (eds): Emergency Pediatrics: A Guide to Ambulatory Care, 3rd ed. St. Louis, Mosby, 1990.

Fleisher GR, Ludwig S (eds): Textbook of Pediatric Emergency Medicine, 3rd ed. Baltimore, Williams & Wilkins, 1993.

Henry MC, Stapleton ER (eds): EMT Prehospital Care, 2nd ed. Philadelphia, W.B. Saunders Co., 1997.

Ho MT, Saunders CE (eds): Current Emergency Diagnosis and Treatment, 3rd ed. Norwalk, CT, Appleton & Lange, 1990.

McSwain NE, White RD, Paturas JL, et al: The Basic EMT: Comprehensive Prehospital Patient Care. St. Louis, Mosby Lifeline, 1997.

Revere C, Hasty R: Diagnostic and characteristic signs of illness and injury. J Emerg Nurs 19:2, 1993.

Rund DA, Barkin RM, Rosen P, et al (eds): Essentials of Emergency Medicine, 2nd ed. St. Louis, Mosby, 1996.

Stine RJ, Chudnofsky CR, Aaron CK (eds): A Practical Approach to Emergency Medicine, 2nd ed. Boston, Little, Brown & Co., 1994.

Tintinalli JE, Krome RL, Ruiz (eds): Emergency Medicine: A Comprehensive Study Guide, 3rd ed. New York, McGraw-Hill, Inc., 1992.

Putting the Data to Work

CHAPTER 25

Diagnostic Reasoning in Physical Diagnosis*

Medicine is a science of uncertainty and an art of probability. One of the chief reasons for this uncertainty is the increasing variability in the manifestations of any one disease.

Sir William Osler
1849–1919

Art, Science, and Observation

This is one of the most important chapters of the book, because it considers the methods and concepts of evaluating the signs and symptoms involved in diagnostic reasoning. The previous chapters discuss the "science" of medicine by explaining the techniques for interviewing and performing the physical examination. The ability to make the "best" decision in the face of uncertainty is the "art" of medicine. But there are rules and standards for the practice of this art, and these are the focus of this chapter.

The primary steps in this process involve the following:

- Data collection
- Data processing
- Problem list development

Data collection is the product of the history and the physical examination. These can be augmented with laboratory test results, such as blood chemistry profiles, complete blood count, bacterial cultures, electrocardiogram, and chest x-ray films. The history, which is the most important element of the database, accounts for more than 70% of the problem list. The physical examination contributes an additional 20–25% of the database; less than 10% of the database is related to laboratory testing.

Data processing is the clustering of data obtained from the history, physical examination, and laboratory studies. It is rare that patients have a solitary symptom or sign of a disease. They more commonly complain of multiple symptoms, and the examiner may find several related signs during the physical examination. It is the job of the astute observer to fit as many of these clues together into a meaningful pathophysiologic relationship. This is data processing.

The interviewer obtains a history of, for example, dyspnea, cough, earache, and hemoptysis. The symptoms of dyspnea, cough, and hemoptysis can be grouped together as symptoms suggestive of possible cardiopulmonary disease. The symptom of earache does not fit with the other three symptoms and may indicate another problem. For another patient who complains of epigastric burning relieved by eating and whose stool is found to have blood, this symptom and sign should be studied together. These data likely represent an abnormality of the gastrointestinal tract, possibly a duodenal ulcer. Although patients usually have multiple symptoms or signs from a pathologic condition, they may not always manifest all the symptoms or signs of the disease being considered. The presence of polyuria and polydipsia in a patient with a family history of diabetes is adequate to raise the suspicion that a lateral rectus palsy may be related to diabetes, even if diabetes has not previously been diagnosed in this patient. In yet another patient, a 30-pound weight loss, anorexia, jaundice, and a left supraclavicular

---

* In collaboration with Jerry A. Colliver, Ph.D., and Ethan D. Fried, M.D. Dr. Colliver is Director of Statistics and Research Consulting and Professor of Medical Education at Southern Illinois University School of Medicine. Dr. Fried is Assistant Professor of Medicine at the State University of New York, Health Science Center at Brooklyn, and Associate Chairman of Medicine at The Brookdale University Hospital and Medical Center.

lymph node is suggestive of gastric carcinoma with liver metastasis to the porta hepatis. This illustrates the process of data-processing multiple symptoms into a single diagnosis; the process has sometimes been referred to as *Occam's razor*. This rule tries to explain all the symptoms by one diagnosis. Although it is a useful rule to keep in mind, it is not always a correct one.

Problem list development results in the summary of the physical, mental, social, and personal conditions affecting the patient's health. The problem list may contain actual diagnosis or only a symptom or sign that cannot be clustered with other bits of data. The date on which each problem developed is noted. The list reflects the level of understanding of the patient's problems, and the problems should be listed in order of importance. Table 25–1 is an example of a problem list.

The presence of a symptom or sign related to a specific problem is a *pertinent positive;* the absence of a symptom or sign that, if present, would be suggestive of a diagnosis is a *pertinent negative.* A pertinent negative may be just as important as the presence of a symptom or sign. The fact that a key finding is not present helps to rule out a certain diagnosis. For example, a history of gout and increased uric acid level are pertinent positives in a man suffering from excruciating back pain radiating to his testicle. This patient may be suffering from renal colic secondary to a uric acid kidney stone. The absence of tachycardia in a woman with weight loss and a tremor makes a diagnosis of hyperthyroidism less than likely; the presence of tachycardia would strengthen the diagnosis of hyperthyroidism.

An important consideration in any database is the patient's demographic information: *sex, age, ethnicity,* and *area of residence.* A *man* with a bleeding disorder from birth is likely to have hemophilia. A *65 year old* person with exertional chest pain is probably suffering, statistically, from coronary artery disease. An *African-American* with episodes of severe bone pain may be suffering from sickle cell anemia. A person living in the *San Joaquin Valley* who suffers from pulmonary symptoms may have coccidioidomycosis. The use of this information often suggests a unifying diagnosis, but the absence of a "usual" finding should never totally exclude a diagnosis.

It has been said, "Common diseases are common." This apparently simplistic statement has great merit because it underlines the fact that the observer should not assume an exotic diagnosis if a common one accurately explains the clinical state. (In contrast, if a common diagnosis cannot account for all the symptoms, look for another, less common diagnosis.) It is true that "Uncommon signs of common diseases are more common than common signs of uncommon diseases."

Finally, "A rare disease is *not* rare for the patient who has the disease." If the symptoms and signs in a patient suggest an uncommon condition, that specific patient may be the 1 in 10,000 with the disease. Nevertheless, statistics based on population groups provide a useful guide in approaching clinical decision-making for the individual patient.

Table 25–1　Example of a Problem List

Problem	Date	Resolved
1. Chest pain	6/28/96	
2. Acute inferior myocardial infarction	1/30/95	2/15/95
3. Colonic cancer	4/30/93	6/3/93
4. Diabetes mellitus	1987	
5. Hypertension	1983	
6. "Red urine"	6/10/95	
7. Problems with son's drug abuse	1/95	

Diagnostic Reasoning from Signs and Symptoms

Unfortunately, decisions in medicine can rarely be made with 100% certainty. Probability weights the decision. Only if the cluster of symptoms, signs, and laboratory tests is unequivocal can the physician be certain of a diagnosis. This does not occur often. How, then, can the physician make the "best" decision—best in light of current knowledge and research?

Laboratory tests immediately come to mind. But signs and symptoms obtained from the patient's history and physical examination perform the same function as laboratory tests, and the information and results obtained from signs, symptoms, and tests are evaluated in the same way and are subject to the same rules and standards of evidence for diagnostic reasoning. And signs and symptoms actually account for more of the developing problem list (90% or more) when compared with laboratory test resuults (less than 10%).

Sensitivity and Specificity

Throughout this text, signs and symptoms have been described according to their *operating characteristics: sensitivity* and *specificity*. These operating characteristics, which also apply to laboratory tests, indicate the usefulness of the sign, symptom, or test to the physician in making a diagnosis. *Sensitivity* is equal to the true positive rate, or the proportion of positive test results in individuals with a disease. Sensitivity, therefore, is based solely on patients with the disease. *Specificity* is equal to the true negative rate, or the proportion of negative test results in individuals without a disease. Specificity, therefore, is based only on individuals without the disease. A *false positive* refers to a positive test result in an individual without the disease or condition. Thus, a sign, symptom, or test with 90% specificity can correctly identify 90 out of 100 normal individuals; the other 10 individuals are false positives, and the false-positive rate is 10%. If a test or observation is negative in a person with the disease, the result is termed a *false negative*.

The *2 × 2* table is useful for representing the relationship of a test, symptom, or sign to a disease. D+ indicates the presence of the disease; D− indicates the absence of the disease; T+ is a positive test result or the presence of a symptom or sign; T− is the absence of a positive test result or the absence of a symptom or sign. Each of the cells of the table represents a set of patients. Consider the following 2 × 2 table:

	With Disease D+	Without Disease D−
Test Positive T+	True Positive (TP)	False Positive (FP)
Test Negative T−	False Negative (FN)	True Negative (TN)

Sensitivity is defined as the number of true positives divided by the number with disease (i.e., the total of the true positives and the false negatives):

$$\text{Sensitivity} = \text{TP/(number with disease)} = \text{TP/(TP + FN)}$$

Specificity is defined as the number of true negatives divided by the number without disease (i.e., the total of false positives and true negatives):

$$\text{Specificity} = \text{TN/(number without disease)} = \text{TN/(FP + TN)}$$

Substituting numbers:

	D+	D−
T+	65 (65%) (TP)	100 (10%) (FP)
T−	35 (35%) (FN)	900 (90%) (TN)
	100	1000

The upper left cell indicates that 65 of 100 patients with a certain disease (65%) had a certain positive test result or symptom or sign. Thus, the test has a true positive rate of .65, or a sensitivity of 65%.

The true negative rate is .90, as indicated in the lower right cell; this shows that 900 of 1000 individuals without the disease (90%) did not have a positive test result or symptom or sign. Therefore, the specificity of the test is 90%.

The false-positive rate is .10, showing that 100 of 1000 in the normal population (10%) had the finding for some reason, without having the disease in question. This is shown in the upper right cell.

Finally, the lower left cell indicates that the test result, symptom, or sign is absent in 35 of 100 patients with the disease. Thus, the false-negative rate is 35%.

Notice that the true positive rate plus the false negative rate equals 1.0; the false-positive rate plus the true negative rate also equals 1.0. If the disease is aortic stenosis and the symptom is syncope in the cited table, 65% of patients with aortic stenosis have syncope, and 35% do not; 90% of individuals without aortic stenosis do not have syncope and 10% do.

Likelihood Ratio

Because sensitivity and specificity are used to measure different properties, a symptom, sign, or test will have both sensitivity and specificity values: high sensitivity and high specificity, low sensitivity and low specificity, high sensitivity and low specificity, and low sensitivity and high specificity. Sensitivity and specificity are often combined to form the likelihood ratio (LR), which provides a unitary measure of the operating characteristics of a sign, symptom, or test. The LR is defined as the ratio of sensitivity to one minus specificity. In other words, the LR is simply the ratio of the true positive rate to the false-positive rate.

$$LR = sensitivity/(1 - specificity)$$
$$= TP\ rate/FP\ rate$$

Thus, the likelihood ratio indicates the proportion of accurate to inaccurate positive test results. In the preceding example of syncope and aortic stenosis, where sensitivity = TP rate = .65 and 1 minus specificity = FP rate = .10, the likelihood ratio would be equal to .65/.10 or 6.5. In other words, a positive result on a sign, symptom, or test is 6.5 times more likely in patients with disease than in individuals without disease. In the example, the proportion with syncope would be 6.5 times greater in patients with aortic stenosis than in individuals without. Tests or signs with likelihood ratios greater than ten are generally highly useful because they provide considerable confidence in diagnostic reasoning.

Ruling in and Ruling out Disease

Sensitivity and specificity (and the likelihood ratio) refer to properties of the symptom, sign, or test, that are invariant across different populations. This particularly applies to populations that differ with respect to prevalence of the disease or condition in question. Sensitivity is based solely on patients with disease, and specificity is based solely on individuals without disease. Thus, the relative sizes of the disease and no disease groups in the population of concern—which is the basis for the computation of prevalence—play no role in the computation of sensitivity and specificity. Sensitivity and specificity are simply the operating characteristics of the test and as such provide general information about the usefulness of the test for diagnostic reasoning *with any population of patients*. But in actual clinical practice, the physician is concerned with the patient and whether the patient's test results are predictive of disease. How certain can the physician be that a patient has a disease if the test result is positive or if a symptom or sign is present? How certain can a physician be that a person is healthy if a test result is negative or if a symptom or sign is absent? Typically, these questions are answered by computing the positive and negative predictive values, which are based on sensitivity and specificity, but also take into account the prevalence of disease in the population of which the patient is a member.

But first, consider two special cases of diagnostic reasoning in which clinical decisions can be made based on only a knowledge of sensitivity and specificity. If the sensitivity of a given symptom, sign, or test is quite high, 90% or greater, and the patient has a negative result, the physician can somewhat confidently rule out disease because so few patients with disease get a negative test (<10%). Sackett* devised the following acronym for this special case: **S**ensitive signs when **N**egative help to rule **out** the disease (**SnNout**), because in the absence of a highly sensitive sign, a person is most likely not to have the disease. The second special case occurs if the specificity of a given test, symptom, or sign is quite high, 90% or greater, and the patient has a positive result. The physician can then somewhat confidently rule in disease because so few individuals without disease get a positive test (<10%). Sackett's acronym: **S**pecific signs when **P**ositive help to rule **in** the disease (**SpPin**), because in the presence of a highly specific sign, a person is most likely to have the disease.

Positive and Negative Predictive Values

SnNout and SpPin are quite useful in these two special cases, but more generally the clinician wants to predict the actual probability of disease for a patient with a positive result, or the probability of no disease for an individual with a negative result. The former is estimated by the *positive predictive value* (PV+), which is equal to the number of true positives divided by the total number of positive results in the population of which the patient is a member (the true positives plus the false positives):

$$PV+ = TP/\text{all positives} = TP/(TP + FP)$$

The positive predictive value is the *frequency of disease* among patients with positive test results. Stated another way, it is the probability that a patient with a positive test result actually has the disease. The *negative predictive value* (PV−) is equal to the number of true negatives divided by the total number of negative results in the patient's population (the true negatives plus the false negatives):

$$PV- = TN/\text{all negatives} = TN/(TN + FN)$$

The negative predictive value is the *frequency of nondisease* in individuals with negative test results. Stated another way, it is the probability of not having the disease if the test is negative or if the symptom or sign is absent.

For example, assume that the above 2 × 2 table represents the entire population of interest to the clinician. The PV+ is calculated as follows:

$$PV+ = 65/(65 + 100)$$
$$= .39$$

*Sackett DL: A primer on the precision and accuracy of the clinical examination. JAMA 267:2638, 1992.

and the PV— is as follows:

$$PV- = 900/(35 + 900)$$
$$= .96$$

Thus, the predicted probability that a person with a positive result in fact has the disease is 39%. The predicted probability that a person with a negative result does not have the disease is 96%. In the hypothetical example, the probability that a patient with syncope actually has aortic stenosis is only 39%, whereas the probability that a person without syncope does not have aortic stenosis is 96%. The high PV— of 96% is consistent with the large test specificity of 90%.

Prevalence

Clearly, the sensitivity and specificity of a test, sign, or symptom are important factors in predicting the probability of disease, given the test results. So too is the prevalence of the disease in the population of which the patient is a member. The prevalence of disease refers to the proportion with disease in the population of interest. In a 2 × 2 table that represents the entire population (or a representative sample), prevalence is equal to the number with disease (TP + FN) divided by the total number in the population (TP + FP + FN + TN). Again, assuming that the preceding 2 × 2 table represents the entire population of concern, prevalence is calculated as follows:

$$\text{Prevalence} = (65 + 35)/(65 + 100 + 35 + 900)$$
$$= 100/1100$$
$$= .09$$

Of the population, 9% has the disease in question.

Two intuitive examples illustrate the role of prevalence in predicting the probability of disease. Consider the value of the symptom of chest pain for predicting the probability of coronary artery disease. The first patient is a 65 year old man with chest pain. The prevalence of coronary artery disease in a population of 65 year old men is high. Therefore, the presence of chest pain has a high positive predictive value for this patient, and it is very probable that coronary artery disease exists in this patient. However, the absence of chest pain has a low negative predictive value, indicating that, because the prevalence is high, coronary artery disease may nevertheless exist even in the absence of symptoms.

In contrast, consider the positive predictive value of chest pain in a 20 year old woman. In this age group, the prevalence of coronary artery disease is low, so the probability that this patient's chest pain represents coronary artery disease is low. The presence of chest pain in a 20 year old person has a low positive predictive value. However, the absence of chest pain has a high negative predictive value, indicating that coronary artery disease is unlikely to be present.

Figure 25–1 illustrates the effect upon the predictive values of changing the prevalence. The most significant increase in the positive predictive value of a test, symptom, or sign occurs when the disease is less common. Small changes in prevalence, at this end of the curve, make great changes in the positive predictive value. Conversely, the most significant increase in the negative predictive value occurs when the disease is most prevalent. Slight decreases in the prevalence of common diseases produce significant increases in the negative predictive value. The higher the prevalence, the higher the positive predictive value will be and the lower the negative predictive value will be.

Differences in prevalence rates may be related either to the clinical setting in which the patient is seen or to the specific demographic characteristics of the patient. For example, a physician performing routine examinations in an outpatient clinic will find a prevalence of disease different from that found by a physician working only with inpatients in a hospital specializing in that disease. The demographic characteristics of the patient refers to age, sex, and race, and these characteristics play a major role in the prevalence of many diseases. Both the clinical setting and the characteristics of the patient help to determine the usefulness of the sign, symptom, or laboratory test, because they affect both the positive and the negative predictive values of the finding.

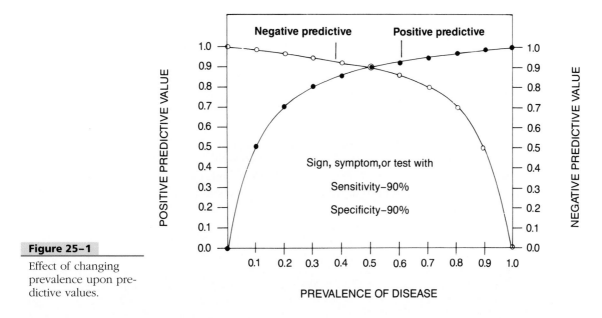

Figure 25–1

Effect of changing prevalence upon predictive values.

Bayes' Theorem

The formulas for PV+ and PV− are appropriate only if data in the 2 × 2 table are for the entire population or a representative sample of that population, in which case the prevalence of disease in the population is accurately reflected in the table. More typically, the sensitivity and specificity of the test, sign, or symptom are determined independently of the prevalence of disease, which must be ascertained by the physician for the specific patient in question (e.g., prevalence of disease for the patient's gender group, age group, or ethnicity group, or for inpatients versus outpatients). Thus, the positive and negative predictive values are typically computed with Bayes' theorem, which expresses PV+ and PV− as a function of sensitivity, specificity and prevalence. To understand Bayes' theorem, consider the following tree diagram, Figure 25–2:

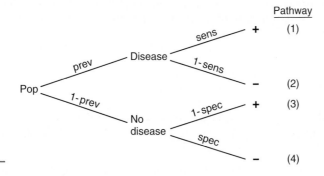

Figure 25–2

- Starting on the left, the diagram shows that the population consists of those with disease and those without the disease.
- *Prev* is the proportion with disease;
  1 − prev is the proportion without disease.
- Moving to the right, the diagram shows that patients with disease can have positive or negative results, and those without disease can also have positive or negative results.
- *Sens* is the proportion of diseased patients with positive results;
  1 − sens is the proportion of diseased patients with negative results.
- *Spec* is the proportion of nondiseased patients with negative results;
  1 − spec is the proportion of nondiseased patients with positive results.

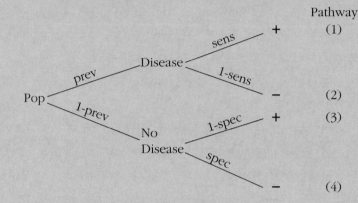

- PV+ refers in general to patients with positive results, which is represented in the diagram by pathways (1) and (3).
- PV+ in particular refers to patients with positive tests who also have disease, which is represented in the diagram by pathway (1).
- PV+ specifically is the proportion of patients with positive tests who also have disease. This can be obtained by dividing the term represented by pathway (1) by the sum of the terms represented by pathways (1) and (3):

$$PV+ = \frac{(1)}{(1) + (3)} = \frac{prev \times sens}{(prev \times sens) + (1 - prev)(1 - spec)}$$

- PV− can be obtained by dividing the term represented by pathway (4) by the sum of the terms represented by pathways (2) and (4):

$$PV- = \frac{(4)}{(2) + (4)} = \frac{(1 - prev)(spec)}{(prev)(1 - sens) + (1 - prev)(spec)}$$

Consider again the example of syncope in patients with aortic stenosis, using the data in the 2 × 2 table. But now, do *not* assume that the data represent the entire population; assume that the data for the diseased and nondiseased groups were obtained separately, meaning that the prevalence of disease cannot be determined from the table, although sensitivity and specificity can. Now assume that the prevalence of aortic stenosis is 80% in a given patient population. The sensitivity of syncope related to aortic stenosis remains 65% and the specificity 90%, as indicated in the table. Using Bayes' theorem, the PV+ and the PV− are calculated as follows:

$$PV+ = \frac{(.80)(.65)}{(.80)(.65) + (1 - .80)(1 - .90)}$$

$$= 96\%$$

$$PV- = \frac{(1 - .80)(.90)}{(.80)(1 - .65) + (1 - .80)(.90)}$$

$$= 39\%$$

Thus, a positive finding of syncope would increase the probability that the patient has aortic stenosis from 80% (the prevalence or unconditional probability of aortic stenosis in the general population) to 96% (the conditional probability of aortic stenosis given the presence of syncope). A negative finding for syncope would increase the probability of absence of stenosis from 20% (1 − prevalence in the general population) to 39% (the conditional probability of no stenosis given the absence of syncope). The absence of syncope in this patient has reduced the probability of aortic stenosis from 80% to 61% (100% − 39%).

Pursuing this example, now assume that the prevalence of aortic stenosis is only 20% in another patient population, but that sensitivity and specificity remain at 65% and 90%, respectively. Bayes' theorem now shows the PV+ and the PV− are:

$$PV+ = \frac{(.20)(.65)}{(.20)(.65) + (1 - .20)(1 - .90)}$$
$$= 62\%$$

$$PV- = \frac{(1 - .20)(.90)}{(.20)(1 - .65) + (1 - .20)(.90)}$$
$$= 91\%$$

Notice that the PV+ has fallen from 96% (when prevalence was 80%) to 62% (with prevalence reduced to 20%). When the prevalence of a disease is quite low, the positive predictive value of a test, sign, or symptom is extremely low even if the sensitivity and specificity are high. Also, notice that PV− has increased from 39% (when prevalence was 80%) to 91% (with prevalence reduced to 20%). Low prevalence of disease implies high values for negative predictive value. In general, with more disease (Prev ↑), more people with positive results will have the disease (PV+ ↑), and more people with negative results will have the disease (and fewer will not have the disease [PV− ↓]). In brief, as Prev ↑, PV+ ↑ but PV− ↓.

■ Nomogram

To simplify matters, a Bayes nomogram is given in Figure 25–3, which can be copied and used in the clinic or office. The nomogram provides the predictive values without

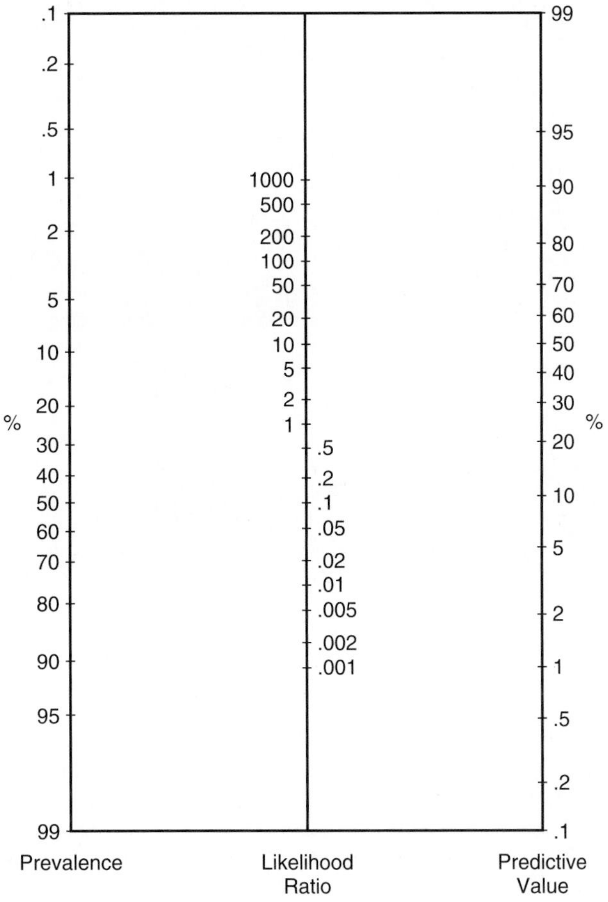

Figure 25–3

A nomogram for applying likelihood ratios.

requiring the calculations of Bayes' theorem. To use the nomogram, first locate on the relevant axes the points that correspond to (1) the prevalence of disease for the patient's population and (2) the likelihood ratio for the sign, symptom, or test. Recall that the likelihood ratio is the ratio of the TP rate (sensitivity) to the FP rate (1− specificity). Next, place a straight edge on the nomogram to connect the points. The PV+ is given by the point at which the straight edge intersects the predictive value axis. For example, with Prev = .80 and LR = .65/.10 = 6.50, the PV+ = .96 as computed above with Bayes' theorem. To determine the PV−, use 1− prevalence and TN rate/FN rate instead of prevalence and the likelihood ratio.

Multiple Signs and Symptoms

Typically, diagnostic reasoning is based on multiple signs and symptoms and possibly laboratory test results, and the multiple findings must be combined to evaluate a diagnostic possibility. For example, consider the following clinical situation. A 21 year old asymptomatic woman finds a thyroid nodule on self-examination, and she is referred to an endocrinologist for evaluation. The physician describes the thyroid nodule as hard to palpation and fixed to the surrounding tissue. In this physician's practice, the prevalence of thyroid cancer is 3%. What is the chance that this nodule is cancerous?

To start, you can consider each finding separately. First, evaluate the predictive value of the presence of a palpable hard nodule. The sensitivity and specificity of this finding are 42% and 89%, respectively. With a prevalence of malignancy of 3%, Bayes' theorem (or the nomogram) shows that the PV+ = 11% and the PV− = 98%. For the second finding, fixation of the nodule to the surrounding tissue, sensitivity is 31% and specificity is 94%. Again with prevalence equal to 3%, Bayes' theorem (or the nomogram) shows PV+ = 14% and PV− = 98%.

But what about the presence of both: a hard nodule that is also fixed to the surrounding tissue? And the presence of either a hard or a fixed nodule? Or the presence of neither? What are the predictive values of these combined findings? If it is assumed that the multiple signs, symptoms, and tests are independent (i.e., their findings are unrelated), the predictive values of these combined findings can be determined by extending the Bayesian tree diagram by adding a second finding, as shown in Figure 25−4.

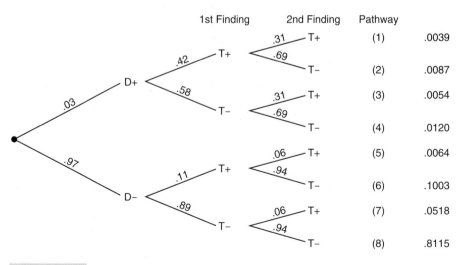

Figure 25–4

D+, with disease; D−, without disease; T+, positive test; T−, negative test.

Thus, Bayes' theorem can be used to compute the positive predictive values of the combined findings by calculating the product of the probabilities for each pathway (presented in parentheses at right of tree) and summing the products as follows:

PV+

$$p \text{ (Disease given both findings)} = \frac{(1)}{(1) + (5)} = \frac{.0039}{.0039 + .0064} = .38$$

$$p \text{ (Disease given either finding)} = \frac{(2) + (3)}{(2) + (3) + (6) + (7)}$$

$$= \frac{.0087 + .0054}{.0087 + .0054 + .1003 + .0518} = .08$$

$$p \text{ (Disease given neither finding)} = \frac{(4)}{(4) + (8)} = \frac{.0120}{.0120 + .8115} = .01$$

PV−

$$p \text{ (No disease given neither findings)} = \frac{(8)}{(4) + (8)} = \frac{.8115}{.0120 + .8115} = .99$$

Notice that the positive predictive value for disease given that both findings are positive (38%) is two to three times greater than the positive predictive value for a hard nodule only (11%) or for a fixed nodule only 14%.

In practice, multiple signs, symptoms, and test findings are typically not independent, because the presence of one finding increases the probability of the presence of another finding. Of course, the opposite is also possible, in that the second finding may be less likely in the presence of the first. Either way, the assumption of independence is violated, and the practice of calculating products of sensitivities in compound Bayesian trees (e.g., .42 × .31 in first pathway) does not produce accurate predictive values. Instead, the sensitivity and specificity for the actual compound finding must be known, such as the probability of the combined findings of hard and fixed nodule. At present, this information is limited in the clinical research literature, but studies of compound findings with their sensitivities and specificities are increasing with the hope that this information will be available for clinical practice in the foreseeable future.

Decision Analysis

Diagnostic reasoning is only the first step in clinical decision-making. After reaching a decision about diagnosis, the physician must decide on a plan for treatment and management of the problem for the particular patient. These decisions must take into account the probability and utility (i.e., worth or value) of each possible outcome of the treatment or management plan given the patient's population (gender, age, ethnicity, inpatient, outpatient, etc.). Similarly, the physician may need to decide whether to order laboratory tests to confirm a diagnosis only suggested by the signs and symptoms elicited with the clinical examination. These test-ordering decisions must be based on the probability and utility of the possible outcomes of the test (possibly invasive and costly), again taking into account the patient's population. The purpose of this section is to extend the discussion of clinical decision-making to include making decisions about test ordering, treatment, and management.

Typically, a decision tree is used to represent the various alternatives, with probabilities assigned to the alternatives and utilities attached to the possible outcomes. Sackett and colleagues present an excellent, detailed discussion of clinical decision-making that is strongly recommended for reference. The author of this book relies on their test-ordering, decision-making example in the following discussion.

Their example involves "a 35-year-old man with 'heartburn' for several years, no coronary risk factors, and a 6-week history of nonexertional, squeezing chest pain deep in his lower sternum and epigastrium, usually radiating straight through to his back and most likely to occur when he lies down after a heavy meal. He has a negative physical exam."

The clinician in the example concludes that esophageal spasm is the best diagnosis and that significant coronary stenosis is very unlikely, perhaps 5% at most for this patient's population. To address the latter possibility (serious, though unlikely), the clinician considers an exercise electrocardiogram (E-ECG) just to be on the safe side, knowing that for greater than 70% stenosis the sensitivity and specificity of the E-ECG are 60% and 91%, respectively. Using this information and Bayes' theorem or the nomogram, PV+ = .26 and PV− = .98.

■ Construct Decision Tree

To decide whether to test with the E-ECG, the physician performs a decision analysis, first by constructing the decision tree in Figure 25–5, which depicts the decision-making situation. The physician will decide whether to order an E-ECG, as indicated on the left by the branching at the box-shaped "decision" node. If the physician orders the E-ECG, the results can be positive or negative, as shown by the next branching from the circular "chance" node; in either case, the patient may or may not have coronary stenosis, as shown by the branchings at the next two "chance" nodes. If the clinician decides not to order the E-ECG, the patient may or may not have the disease as shown by the branching at the lower right "chance" node.

■ Assign Probabilities

Next, a probability is assigned to each branch in the tree, as shown in Figure 25–6. Ideally, probabilities should be based on strong clinical research studies. The proportions of patients with positive and negative E-ECGs are known to be 12% and 88%, respectively. Of those with positive results, 26% have stenosis, 74% do not. Notice tht this first probability is PV+, the positive predictive value, which shows the proportion of individuals with a positive test, who in fact have stenosis; the second proportion is 1 − PV+. Of those with negative results, the probabilities are 2% and 98%. The second probability here is PV−, the negative predictive value, and the first is 1 − PV−. In the general population not given an E-ECG, 5% have stenosis, 95% do not.

■ Attach Utilities

A utility is then attached to each of the possible outcomes, which are represented by the pathways through the tree. The utility refers to the worth or value of the outcome. Utilities may be objective, stated in monetary terms or expected years of life, or subjective, stated in relative terms of anticipated value to the patient or society. In the example, there are six outcomes (pathways through the tree), with a description or label for each outcome at the right of the pathway. A positive E-ECG for a patient with stenosis, for example, is labeled "stenosis diagnosed." To the right of these labels are the utilities assigned by Sackett and colleagues. These utilities are subjective, but they

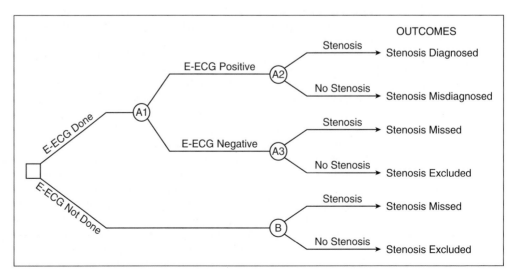

Figure 25–5

A decision tree for exercise electrocardiography.

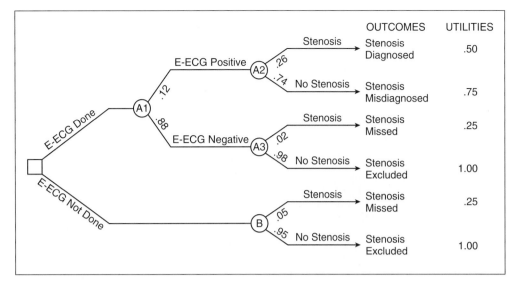

OUTCOMES   UTILITIES

Figure 25–6

A decision tree for exercise electrocardiography with probabilities and utilities added.

clearly show the relative worth of each of the outcomes, from stenosis excluded (1.00, most valuable), stenosis misdiagnosed (.75), and stenosis diagnosed (.50), to stenosis missed (.25, least valuable). The exact numerical value of each subjective utility is arbitrary, but the ordering of outcomes given by the utilities is not. That is, the same decision would be reached had the utilities been, say, 4, 3, 2, and 1, respectively. Of course, if the value of one outcome is much greater than that of a second, which is similar to those of a third and fourth, the difference between the utilities for the first and second outcomes should be much greater than that between the second and the third and fourth outcomes, such as, say, 1.00, .50, .45, and .40. And this assignment of utilities could affect the decision reached.

▪ Compute Expected Values

The expected value for each pathway through the tree is equal to the product of the probabilities and the utility for that outcome. For the first pathway, the expected value is given by $.12 \times .26 \times .50 = .0156$. The expected values for all six pathways, then, are .0156, .0666, .0044, .8622, .0125, and .9500. The expected value for each decision node is computed by summing the expected values for the outcomes originating from that node. For the decision to order an E-ECG, the expected value is the sum of the expected values for the first four outcomes: $.0156 + .0666 + .0044 + .8624 = .949$. For the decision not to order an E-ECG, the expected value is the sum of the last two outcomes: $.0125 + .9500 = .962$.

▪ Make a Decision

The expected value of the decision not to order an E-ECG (.962) is greater than that for ordering one (.949). The decision analysis shows the "best" decision for this patient is not to test. The decision would have been the same had the utilities been 4, 3, 2, 1 rather than 1.00, .75, .50, .25: the expected values for testing versus not testing were 3.796 and 3.850. Had the utilities been 1.00, .50, .45, and .40, the expected values would have been .928 and .970.

Clearly, the utilities are the Achilles' heel of decision analysis, in particular subjective utilities, although even objective utilities can be somewhat arbitrary. The expected values of the decision are affected by the utilities chosen for the analysis, and different utilities may lead to different decisions. Also, the probabilities assigned to the branches of the tree will affect the outcome of the decision analysis, but the probabilities are typically less subjective than the utilities, being based on actual values such as sensitivities, specificities, and positive and negative predictive values obtained from the clinical research literature. Because the variability in the utilities and probabilities can affect the conclusion of the decision analysis, it has been suggested that the decision maker should systematically vary the utilities and probabilities within the range in which they could reasonably vary for the patient in question. This will test the vulnerability of the decision to reasonable variation in the utilities and probabilities. This is called a *sensitivity analysis* (although vulnerability analysis might be a better term to avoid confusion with conventional test sensitivity). If the decision to test or not to test is consistent over these variations in utilities and probabilities, the clinician can be more confident in the decision. Otherwise, the decision is reduced to a "toss-up" between the alternatives.

In the Sackett example, the expected values for the decisions to test or not were quite close (.949 and .962), but they seem informative, at least intuitively, possibly because they are surprising by showing a greater value for not testing. At the least, the decision analysis shows that testing with this patient is no better than not testing. But what if the results were reversed, with the expected values for testing or not equal to .962 and .949, or with expected values for surgery or not at .962 and .949? Close values like this are not uncommon in decision analysis, and they illustrate the need to think clearly about the subjective meaning of the utility scale, which is given in terms of the nature of the outcomes to which the utilities are attached. For example, consider a four-point scale where 4 represents stenosis excluded, 3 represents stenosis misdiagnosed, etc.; the expected values for test and not test of 3.796 and 3.850, respectively, differ by only .054 of the unit distance between stenosis excluded (4) and stenosis misdiagnosed (3). The two decisions are closely valued. Nevertheless, in the absence of any other information, the "best" decision would be not to test, meaning simply that in the long run with close-call decisions like this, a slight advantage should accrue by acting in accordance with the decision analysis.

The Rational Clinical Examination

In 1992 the *Journal of the American Medical Association* initiated a series of articles on the *rational clinical examination*. This series underscores the points made in this chapter, namely that signs and symptoms provide critical information in diagnostic reasoning and that the operating characteristics (sensitivity and specificity) of the signs and symptoms must be considered in the reasoning process as must the prevalence of the disease in question. In other words, the clinical examination can and should be more rational, based on empirical evidence for the predictive value of signs and symptoms used in diagnostic reasoning.

The rational clinical examination is part of a broader movement called *evidence-based medicine,* which "de-emphasizes intuition, unsystematic clinical experience, and pathophysiologic rationale as sufficient grounds for clinical decision making and stresses the examination of evidence from clinical research." The evidence-based approach to the practice of clinical medicine has its origins in clinical research generated within the relatively new field of *clinical epidemiology.* In the past, epidemiology has been concerned with the etiology of diseases and hence has been interested in establishing that exposure to certain risk factors are causes of certain diseases. Thus, classical epidemiology has been characterized as the study of the distribution of disease across time, place, and peoples. Clinical epidemiology has expanded this focus to encompass the study of the entire clinical process including diagnosis, treatment, prognosis, prevention, evaluation of health-care services, and risk-benefit analysis. It appears that evidence from clinical research in these areas will be sought to provide an empirical base for rational clinical practice, including diagnostic reasoning, as the "art" of clinical decision-making becomes more of a science.

Bibliography

Brorsson B, Wall S: Assessment of Medical Technology: Problems and Methods. Stockholm, Swedish Medical Research Council, 1985.

Cutler P: Problem Solving in Clinical Medicine: From Data to Diagnosis, 2nd ed. Baltimore, Williams & Wilkins, 1985.

Kassirer JP: Diagnostic reasoning. Ann Intern Med 110:893, 1989.

Sackett DL: A primer on the precision and accuracy of the clinical examination. JAMA 267:2638, 1992.

Sackett DL, Haynes RB, Guyatt GH, et al: Clinical Epidemiology: A Basic Science for Clinical Medicine, 2nd ed. Boston, Little, Brown and Co., 1991.

Weinstein MC: Clinical Decision Analysis. Philadelphia, W.B. Saunders, 1980.

CHAPTER 26

The Clinical Record

May I never forget that the patient is a fellow human creature in pain. May I never consider the patient merely a vessel of disease.

From *Oath of Maimonides*
1135–1204

Putting the History and Physical Examination Together

Until this point, we have dealt separately with the history and the physical examination. Chapters 1–4 give an in-depth analysis of the techniques of taking the history. Chapters 5–19 discuss the many elements of the physical examination, and Chapter 20 provides a suggested approach to performing the complete examination and its write-up. Chapters 21–24 discuss the evaluation of specific patients. Chapter 25 discusses data gathering and data analysis. This chapter discusses how the history and the physical examination can be integrated into one succinct statement about the patient.

In writing up the history and the physical examination, the examiner should follow several rules:

Record all pertinent data
Avoid extraneous data
Use common terms
Avoid nonstandard abbreviations
Be objective
Use diagrams where indicated

The patient's medical record is a legal document. Comments regarding the patient's behavior and attitudes should *not* be part of the record unless they are important from a medical or scientific standpoint. Describe all parts of the examination that you have performed and indicate those that you have not. A statement such as "the examination of the eye is normal" is much less accurate than "the fundus is normal." In the first case, it is not clear whether the examiner actually attempted to look at the fundus. If a part of the examination is not performed, state that it was "deferred" for whatever reason. Finally, it is not necessary to state all of the possible abnormalities if they are not present. It is acceptable to state that "the pharynx was normal" instead of "the pharynx was not injected, and there was no evidence of discharge, erosion, masses, or other lesions." It is clear from the first statement that the examiner inspected the pharynx and believed that it was normal.

We now return to our patient, Mr. John Doe, whose interview was recorded in Chapter 4, Putting the History Together. The following text describes the complete history and physical examination of this 42 year old lawyer.

Patient: John Doe
Date: August 19, 1997

■ History

Source

Self, reliable.

Chief Complaint

"Chest pain for the past six months."

History of Present Illness

This is the first Mount Hope admission for this 42 year old lawyer with atherosclerotic coronary artery disease. The patient's history of chest pain began 4 years before admission. He described the pain as a "dull ache" in the retrosternal area, with radiation to his left arm. The pain was provoked by exertion and emotions. On July 15, 1996, Mr. Doe suffered his first heart attack while playing tennis. He had an uneventful hospitalization in Kings Hospital in New York City. After 3 weeks in the hospital and 3 weeks at home, he returned to work. The patient suffered a second heart attack 6 months later, again while playing tennis. The patient was hospitalized in Kings Hospital, during which time he was told of an "irregularity" of his heart rate. Since then, the patient has not experienced any palpitations, nor has he been told of any further irregularities.

Over the past 6 months, Mr. Doe has noted an increase in the frequency of his chest pain. The pain occurs now four to five times a day and is relieved within 5 minutes with one or two nitroglycerin tablets under his tongue. The pain is produced by exercise, emotions, and sexual intercourse. The patient also describes one block dyspnea on exertion. The patient relates that 6 months ago he could walk two or three blocks before becoming short of breath.

Although the patient shows significant denial of his illness, he is anxious and depressed.

The patient has currently been admitted for elective cardiac catheterization.

Past Medical History

General. Good.

Past Illnesses. History of untreated hypertension for years (blood pressure not known); no history of measles, chickenpox, mumps, diphtheria, or whooping cough.

Injuries. None.

Hospitalizations. Appendectomy, age 15 years, Booth Hospital in Rochester, New York (Dr. Meyers, surgeon).

Surgery. See Hospitalizations.

Allergies. None.

Immunizations. Salk vaccine for polio, tetanus vaccine, both as a child; no adverse reactions remembered.

Substance Abuse. 40 pack-year (2 packs a day for 20 years) history of smoking; stopped smoking after first heart attack; marijuana on rare occasions in past; drinks alcohol "socially" but also admits to having the need to have a drink as the day goes on (CAGE score, 1); denies use of other street drugs.

Diet. Mostly red meat, with little fish in diet; 3 cups of coffee a day; recent decrease in appetite, with a 10 pound weight loss in past 3 months.

Sleep Patterns. Recently, falls asleep normally but awakens around 3 AM and cannot go back to sleep.

Current Medications

Inderal LA 120 mg once daily
Isordil 20 mg qid
Nitroglycerin 1/150 grains prn
Chlor-Trimeton for colds
Aspirin for headaches
Multivitamins with iron daily

Family History (Fig. 26–1)

Father, 75, diabetes, broken hip
Mother died, 64, stomach cancer
Brother, 45, heart attack at age 40
Sister, 37, alive and well

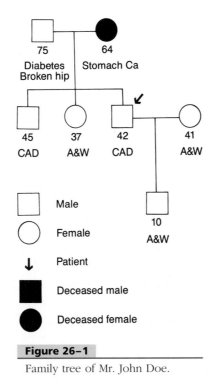

Figure 26-1

Family tree of Mr. John Doe.

Son, 10, alive and well
Wife, 41, alive and well

There is no family history of congenital disease. No other history of diabetes or cardiac disease. No history of renal, hepatic, or neurologic disease. No history of mental illness.

Psychosocial History

"Type A" personality; born and raised in Middletown, New York; family moved to Rochester, New York, when Mr. Doe was 13 years of age; patient moved to New York City after high school; college and law school in New York City; works as a senior partner of a law firm for the past 17 years; married to Emily for the past 13 years; was an active tennis player before second heart attack; before 6 months ago, enjoyed the theater and reading.

Sexual, Reproductive, and Gynecologic History

Patient is a male, exclusively heterosexual, with one partner, his wife. He has one son, age 10 years. Recently, because of angina, the patient has stopped having sexual relations.

Review of Systems

General. Depressed for the past 6 months as a result of his ill health.

Skin. No rashes or other changes.

Head. No history of head injury.

Eyes. Wears glasses for reading; no changes in vision recently; saw ophthalmologist 1 year ago for routine examination; no history of eye pain, tearing, discharge, or halos around lights.

Ears. Patient not aware of any problem hearing; no dizziness, discharge, or pain present.

Nose. Occasional upper respiratory infection, two or three times a year, lasting 3–5 days; no hay fever, sinus symptoms.

Mouth and Throat. Occasional sore throats and canker sores associated with colds; no difficulty in chewing or eating; brushes and flosses twice a day; sees dentist twice a year; no gingival bleeding.

Neck. No masses or tenderness.

Chest. History of occasional blood-tinged sputum and cough in the morning when patient was smoking, not recently; last chest x-ray 1 year ago, was told it was normal; one block dyspnea on exertion (as noted in History of Present Illness); no history of wheezing, asthma, bronchitis, or tuberculosis.

Breasts. No masses or nipple discharge noted.

Cardiac. As noted in History of Present Illness.

Vascular. No history of cerebrovascular accidents or claudication.

Gastrointestinal. Recent decrease in appetite with 10 pound weight loss in past few months; uses no laxatives; no history of diarrhea, constipation, nausea, or vomiting; no bleeding noted.

Genitourinary. Urinates four to five times a day; urine is light yellow in color, never red; nocturia ×1; no change in stream; no history of urinary infections; no sexual intercourse in past 6 months, owing to angina during sex; no history of venereal disease.

Musculoskeletal. No joint or bone symptoms; no weakness; no history of back problems or gout.

Neurologic. No history of seizures or difficulties in walking or balance; no history of motor or sensory symptoms.

Endocrine. No known thyroid nodules; no history of temperature intolerance; no hair changes; no history of polydipsia or polyuria.

Psychiatric. Depressed and very anxious about his ill health; also anxious about the results of the upcoming cardiac catheterization; asked, "What's going to happen to me?"

Physical Examination

General Appearance. The patient is a 42 year old, slightly obese white man, who is lying in bed. He appears slightly older than his stated age. He is in no acute distress but is very nervous. He is well-groomed, cooperative, and alert.

Vital Signs. Blood pressure (BP), 175/95/80 right arm (supine), 175/90/85 left arm (supine), 170/90/80 left arm (sitting), 185/95/85 right leg (prone); heart rate, 100 and regular; respirations, 14.

Skin. Pink; no cyanosis present; five to seven nevi (0.5–1.5 cm in diameter each) on back, most with hair; normal male escutcheon.

Head. Normocephalic, without signs of trauma.

Eyes. Visual acuity with reading glasses using near card: right eye (OD) 20/40, left eye (OS) 20/30; confrontation visual fields full bilaterally; extraocular movements (EOMs) intact; pupils are equal, round, and reactive to light and to accommodation (PERRLA); eyebrows normal; conjunctivae pink; discs sharp; marked arteriovenous (AV) nicking present bilaterally; copper wiring present bilaterally; a cotton-wool spot is present at 1 o'clock position (superior nasal) in the right eye and at 5 o'clock position (inferior temporal) in the left eye; no hemorrhages are present.

Ears. Normal position; no tenderness present; external canals normal; on Rinne's test, air conduction > bone conduction (AC > BC) bilaterally; on Weber's test, no lateralization; both tympanic membranes appear normal, with normal landmarks clearly seen.

Nose. Straight, without masses; patent bilaterally; mucosa pink, without discharge; inferior turbinates appear normal.

Sinuses. No tenderness present over frontal or maxillary sinuses.

Throat. Lips pink; buccal mucosa pink; all teeth in good condition, without obvious caries; gingivae normal, without bleeding; tongue midline and without masses; uvula elevates in midline; gag reflex intact; posterior pharynx normal.

Neck. Supple, with full range of motion; trachea midline and freely mobile; no adenopathy present; thyroid not felt; prominent "a" wave seen in neck veins while lying at 45°; neck veins flat while sitting upright.

Chest. Normal anteroposterior (AP) diameter; symmetric excursion bilaterally; normal tactile fremitus bilaterally; chest resonant bilaterally; clear on percussion and auscultation.

Breasts. Normal male, without masses, gynecomastia, or discharge.

Heart. Point of maximum impulse (PMI), 5th intercostal space, midclavicular line (5ICS-MCL); S_1 and S_2 normal; normal physiologic splitting present; a loud S_4 is present at the cardiac apex; no murmurs or rubs are heard (Fig. 26–2).

Vascular. Pulses are present and symmetric down to the dorsalis pedis bilaterally; no bruits are present over the carotid or femoral arteries; no abdominal bruits are present; no edema is present.

Abdomen. A well-healed appendectomy scar is present in the right lower quadrant (RLQ); the abdomen is slightly obese; no masses are present; no tenderness, guarding, rigidity, or rebound is present.

Rectal. Anal sphincter normal; no hemorrhoids present; prostate slightly enlarged and soft; no prostatic masses felt; no stool in ampulla.

Genitalia. Circumcised male with normal genitalia; penis normal without induration; testicles, $4 \times 3 \times 2$ cm (right) and $3 \times 6 \times 4$ cm (left) with normal consistency.

Lymphatic. No adenopathy noted.

Musculoskeletal. There are several stony hard, slightly yellowish, nontender masses over the extensor tendons on the patient's hands; normal range of motion of neck, spine, and major joints of upper and lower extremities.

Neurologic. Oriented to person, place, and time; cranial nerves II–XII intact (cranial nerve I not tested); cerebellar function normal; plantar reflexes down; gait normal; deep tendon reflexes as in Table 26–1.

Summary

Mr. Doe is a "type A" 42 year old man with a history of two myocardial infarctions, whose current admission is for elective cardiac catheterization. His risk factors for coronary artery disease are untreated hypertension and a long history of cigarette smoking. The patient also has a brother, who suffered a myocardial infarction at the age of 40.

Physical examination reveals a slightly obese man with hypertension and its associated early-to-intermediate funduscopic changes. Cardiac examination reveals a loud

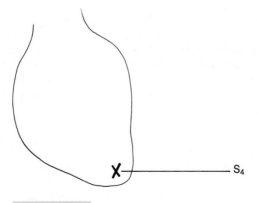

Figure 26–2

Diagram showing location of abnormal cardiac findings.

Table 26–1   Deep Tendon Reflexes of Patient John Doe

	Biceps	Triceps	Knee	Achilles
Right	2+	2+	2+	1+
Left	2+	2+	1+	1+

fourth heart sound, suggestive of a noncompliant (stiff) ventricle. This may be a manifestation of ischemic heart disease or ventricular hypertrophy secondary to the hypertension. Although the patient is not aware of any lipid abnormalities, numerous tendinous xanthomata are present, which are strongly suggestive of hypercholesterol-emia, an additional risk factor for premature coronary artery disease.

The problem list containing all the health problems identified with their dates of recognition and resolution for Mr. Doe might look like Table 26–2. The problems in the list are used each time the patient is seen and examined. For each problem, the student or physician should develop a strategy for its ultimate resolution. Each problem should have the following four components:

- *S*ubjective data
- *O*bjective data
- *A*ssessment
- *P*lan

This is the SOAP format (Weed, 1967), which contains an update of the subjective and objective data as well as the assessment of the problem and the plan for its resolution.

Table 26–2   Problem List for Patient John Doe

Problem	Date	Resolved
1. Chest pain	1996	
2. Myocardial infarction	July 15, 1996	2 weeks later
3. Myocardial infarction	January 1997	3 weeks later
4. Hypertension	Years	
5. Smoking	1976	July 15, 1996
6. Tendinous xanthomata	?	
7. S_4 gallop		
8. Dyspnea on exertion	6 months ago	
9. Depression Weight loss Sleeping abnormality	3 months ago	
10. Diet modification		

The Human Dimension

The practice of medicine is an extraordinary profession. The memory of the thrill of interviewing and examining our first patient should stay in our minds. We must always remember that even during the most trying times, we as students or physicians have been granted the enormous responsibility of caring for a patient. Common courtesy, kindness, respect, and attentiveness to the patient go a long way in establishing the so-called bedside manner, which has become less evident in the past few decades. Imagine yourself in the patient's situation. How would you like to be treated? Each student in medical school has the potential to develop into a devoted and compassionate physician.

Always strive for precision and accuracy. Be strict in your approach to the history and physical examination. Always follow the same basic routines. Do not take short-cuts. The development of the skills of inspection, palpation, percussion, and ausculta-tion takes time. Only with experience can the student or physician master physical diagnosis. This textbook is only the introduction to a lifetime of learning about patients and their problems and diseases. As students, you will learn much from your patients. Even seasoned diagnosticians learn daily from their patients. Just as no two individuals have the same face or body appearance, no two individuals will react the same way to the same disease. This is one of the major excitements about medicine: every day offers new patients, new problems, new solutions.

Bibliography

Weed LL: Medical records that guide and teach. N Engl J Med 278:593, 652, 1967.

Epilogue

I will use treatment to help the sick according to my ability and judgment, but never with a view to injury and wrongdoing.

And whatsoever I shall see or hear in the course of my profession in my discourse with others, . . . I will never divulge, holding such things to be holy secrets.

From *The Physician's Oath*, Hippocrates
460–377 BC

Over the last 30 years, there has been an increased awareness and interest in medical ethics. With the first human heart transplantation by Dr. Christiaan Barnard in 1967, the declaration by the U.S. Supreme Court in 1973 that state laws were unconstitutional in prohibiting abortions, and the issue of removing a respirator in a patient with irreversible brain damage in the case of Karen Ann Quinlan in 1975, modern medical ethics was born. Touching on three key issues—organ transplantation, abortion, and the standards of death—these landmark cases set the stage for current thoughts about the ethical dimensions of health care.

Since then, there have been many other ethical challenges to the health-care system. In 1978, Louise Brown became the first baby to be conceived in a test tube. In 1982, Dr. Barney Clark was the first person to receive a mechanical, artificial heart, the Jarvik-7. In 1984, the infant Baby Fae received a heart transplanted from a baboon. In 1988, the Baby M case involved the ethical issues of Mary Beth Whitehead's "surrogate motherhood" for William Stern.

As physicians in the 21st century, you will be faced with many ethical medical issues: standards of brain death, assisted voluntary death, in vitro fertilization, informed consent, surrogate motherhood, confidentiality, abortion, interracial transplantation, allocation of scarce medical resources, "blowing the whistle" on unethical colleagues, patients as research subjects, mandatory AIDS testing, and genetic engineering. One of the first potential ethical issues you may face is the use of patients as "teaching tools."

A current ethical issue is mandatory testing for human immunodeficiency virus (HIV). Should individuals be tested for HIV in premarital testing, preadmission to hospitals, preinsurance examinations, or pre-employment testing? There have been several arguments made in its favor, including a person's right to donate blood, the tracing of potential infected contacts, determination of the incidence and rate of spread of HIV, quarantine of the infected, and the tattooing of those infected. The arguments against mandatory testing include discrimination, "social purification," violation of a person's privacy, false-positives of the test, and health insurance difficulties.

An ethical problem is one in which two or more norms or principles create a challenge about what to do. There are many types of ethical problems. These problems can be divided into four main groups:

Ethical distress: An individual knows the course of action, but a barrier prevents the ability to accomplish it.

Ethical dilemma: Two or more courses of action exist, each of which is right or wrong, and selecting one will compromise the end result.

Distributive justice: Benefits are given to several individuals, not everyone; on what basis should the distribution be made?

Locus of authority: There are two or more authorities, all believing that they know what outcome will benefit the patient best, but only one will prevail.

Consider the following examples of contemporary issues in medical ethics:

Avia and Michael are newlyweds. They want to have children, but each is from a family with a known inherited illness. Any or all of their children may be affected. Genetic alteration may be an option. Is it right for such couples to endeavor to change their future children's genetic makeup? Is modification of natural biology a human right?

Florence is 31 years of age. When Florence became pregnant, she was overjoyed. She is now in her second month of pregnancy. Recently, she developed fever, a rash, and a sore throat. She was diagnosed with rubella. Although she dreads the thought of giving birth to a retarded, blind, or congenitally malformed child, she knows her religion will not allow abortion. On the other hand, she questions is it right to bear a child whom she knows will live a life of suffering?

Ted, a major benefactor to the hospital, is 76 years of age with Parkinson's disease and diabetes mellitus who is in the emergency room complaining of severe chest pain. Emily is a 41 year old nurse with a history of angina who is also in the emergency room complaining of severe chest pain. There is only one bed left in the coronary intensive care unit. Who should get the bed?

Rosy is 20 years of age and is the single mother of two children. She is in her 1st trimester of her third pregnancy. Recent symptoms of severe weakness and gingival bleeding brought her to medical attention. A work-up revealed acute myelocytic leukemia and an anemia of 7.8 grams of hemoglobin. The therapy for her leukemia would be a great risk to the life of the fetus, but the patient refuses termination of her pregnancy. To complicate the issue, her fiancé, a Jehovah's Witness, has convinced the patient to refuse any transfusion of blood or blood products. How do you, as her physician, handle this situation?

One of the significant problems currently seen in health care is the unethical labeling of patients. Terms such as "gomer" ("*get out of my emergency room*"), "albatross," "turkey," and "slug" are examples of disrespect. Health-care providers who use such terms are often reacting negatively to certain social and personal traits of their patients as well as to certain medical conditions. This is particularly evident in those medical illnesses that are usually incurable, self-inflicted, or challenge the provider's faith in the "science" of medicine. Often, these patients may have an illness that defies medical interventions, thus frustrating the health-care provider. A patient who is of low social class, has an illness engendering fear or disgust, is uncooperative, or is psychologically dysfunctional is at the greatest risk of being labeled in this derogatory fashion. Health-care providers may use these negative terms as "safety valves" for the emotionally charged environment in which they work, but this only serves to further distance them from their patients. Each provider must come to grips with his or her anxieties about illness and treating patients, recognize them, and not allow these destructive attitudes to interfere with the care of the sick. Remember the quote from Peabody that introduces this book, "*. . . the secret in the care **of** the patient is in caring **for** the patient.*"

As a health-care professional, you will be faced with many types of problems that involve complex decision-making. Treatment of your patients and colleagues must always be provided with fairness, respect, and dignity. The care for the aged, poor, handicapped, and terminally ill must be the same as for all other patients. Most individuals who enter the profession strive to be compassionate healers; unfortunately, the educational medical environment can often dampen such enthusiasm. Dedicate your life with honesty and compassion to caring for the sick.

Bibliography

Napodano RJ: Values in Medical Practice: A Statement of Philosophy for Physicians and a Model for Teaching a Healing Science. New York, Human Sciences Press, Inc., 1986.

Papper S: Doing Right: Everyday Medical Ethics. Boston, Little, Brown and Co., 1983.

Pellegrino ED, Thomasma DC: The Virtues in Medical Practice. New York, Oxford University Press, 1993.

Pence GE: Classic Cases in Medical Ethics: Accounts of the Cases That Have Shaped Medical Ethics, with Philosophical, Legal, and Historical Backgrounds. New York, McGraw-Hill Publishing Co., 1990.

Petrinovich L: Living and Dying Well. New York, Plenum Press, 1996.

Purtilo R: Ethical Dimensions in the Health Professions, 2nd ed. Philadelphia, W.B. Saunders Co., 1993.

Rosner F (ed): Medicine and Jewish Law. Northvale, Jason Aronson, Inc., 1990.

Rosner F: Modern Medicine and Jewish Ethics, 2nd ed. New York, Yeshiva University Press, 1991.

Seedhouse D, Lovett L: Practical Medical Ethics. Chichester, John Wiley & Sons, 1992.

Weiss AE: Bioethics: Dilemmas in Modern Medicine. Hillside, Enslow Publishers, Inc., 1985.

APPENDIX A

Commonly Abused Drugs

Drug	Street Name	How Used	Symptoms and Signs
Marijuana Hashish	*Pot, grass, reefer, weed, hash, sinsemilla, joint*	Smoked Ingested	Loss of interest Recent memory loss Dry mouth and throat Mood changes Increased appetite
Alcohol	*Booze, brew, hooch*	Ingested	Impaired coordination Impaired judgment
Nicotine	*Smoke, butt, coffin nail*	Smoked Chewed	Tobacco smell Stained teeth
Amphetamines	*Speed, uppers, pep pills, bennies, dexies, black beauties, meth, crystal*	Ingested Injected Sniffed	Dilated pupils Increased energy Irritability Nervousness Needle marks
Cocaine	*Coke, crack, snow, white lady, toot*	Snorted Injected Ingested Smoked	Dilated pupils Increased energy Restlessness Intense anxiety Paranoid behavior Needle marks
Barbiturates	*Downers, barbs, yellow jackets, red devils, blue devils, double trouble*	Injected Ingested	Constricted pupils Confusion Impaired judgment Drowsiness Slurring of speech Needle marks
Methaqualone	*Ludes, sopors, quaaludes*	Ingested	Slurring of speech Drowsiness Impaired judgment Euphoria Seizures
Heroin Morphine	*Junk, scag, dope, horse, smack, dreamer*	Injected Smoked Sniffed Skin popped	Constricted pupils Needle marks Drowsiness Mental clouding
Codeine	*School boy*	Ingested Sniffed	Constricted pupils Drowsiness
Demerol Methadone Percodan Pentazocine		Ingested Injected	Constricted pupils Drowsiness Mental clouding Needle marks
PCP (phencyclidine)	*Angel dust, hog, killer weed, supergrass*	Smoked Snorted Injected Ingested	Dilated pupils Slurring of speech Hallucinations Blurring of vision Uncoordination Agitation Confusion Aggressive behavior

Table continued on following page

continued

Drug	Street Name	How Used	Symptoms and Signs
LSD (lysergic acid diethylamide)	*Acid, cubes, purple haze*	Ingested Injected	Dilated pupils Hallucinations Mood swings Increased alertness Acute panic reactions
Mescaline	*Mesc, cactus*	Ingested	Dilated pupils Hallucinations Mood swings
Psilocybine	*Magic mushrooms*	Ingested	Dilated pupils Hallucinations Mood swings
Airplane glue* Paint thinner*		Inhaled Sniffed	Poor motor coordination Impaired vision Violent behavior
Nitrous oxide	*Laughing gas, whippets*	Inhaled Sniffed	Hilarity Euphoria Lightheadedness
Amyl nitrate	*Poppers, rush, locker room, snappers, amies*	Inhaled Sniffed	Hilarity Dizziness Headache Impaired thought

* The active agent in airplane glue and paint thinner is toluene. Naphtha, methyl ethyl ketone, and gasoline may produce similar symptoms.

Signs and Symptoms in Deficiency States

Deficiency	Signs	Symptoms
Vitamin A	Hyperkeratinization of the skin Keratinizing metaplasia in the linings of the respiratory, gastrointestinal, and genito-urinary tracts Metaplasia of the endocrine, salivary, sebaceous, and lacrimal glands	Night blindness Retarded growth (children) Xerophthalmia Xeroderma
Vitamin D (rickets, osteomalacia)	Craniotabes Rachitic rosary* Bowing of the legs Knock-knee Pigeon chest deformity Harrison's grooves† Scoliosis Compression of affected vertebrae Carpopedal spasms Generalized spasticity Convulsive seizures	Irritability Restlessness Dental problems Coughing Pulmonary infections Seizures
Thiamine (beriberi)	Bilateral, symmetric peripheral neuropathy (distal parts of lower extremities first) Decreased perception to light touch Calf muscle tenderness Loss of vibratory sense Loss of normal reflexes Motor weakness Secondary muscle atrophy Cardiac enlargement Congestive heart failure Wide pulse pressure Arrhythmias Polyneuropathy	Lack of initiative Anorexia Mental depression Irritability Poor memory Easy fatigability Inability to concentrate Vague abdominal problems Paresthesias of the toes Burning of the lower extremities Dyspnea Palpitations Peripheral edema
Niacin (pellagra)	Extensive dermatitis (commonly on parts of body exposed to sunlight or mechanical trauma; often bilateral and symmetric) Glossitis Stomatitis Chronic hypertrophy with induration of the skin Pigmentation on pressure points	Skin rashes Swollen tongue Increased salivation Burning sensation in the mouth Poor digestion Diarrhea (often foul-smelling; sometimes bloody) Gaseous distention Eructation Vomiting

* Beading of the ribs at the costochondral junction.
† Lateral thoracic depressions at the sites of attachment of the diaphragm.

Table continued on following page

continued

Deficiency	Signs	Symptoms
Niacin (pellagra) *(continued)*	Skin fissuring Atrophic skin changes Scaling of skin	Disorientation Confusion Hallucinations Delirium Paranoia Depression
Riboflavin	Cheilosis Angular stomatitis Glossitis Seborrheic dermatitis, especially in the nasolabial region, around the eyes, behind the ears, and on the scrotum Ocular manifestations	Photophobia Burning of eyes Itching of eyes Skin rashes Fissuring of mouth
Vitamin C (scurvy)	Defective collagen formation Ecchymoses Subperiosteal hematomas Follicular hyperkeratoses Petechial hemorrhages (lower extremities) Gingival hemorrhages Hemarthroses Hemorrhages Anemia Scorbutic rosary‡	Impaired wound healing Failure to thrive, irritability, and frequent crying (children) Bleeding tendencies Painful joints Weight loss Nonspecific aches and pains Brown pigmentation Curling of hair Keratoconjunctivitis sicca§ Emotional changes
Protein-calorie (kwashiorkor)	Retarded growth Edema Hyperpigmentation of skin Depigmentation of skin Hepatomegaly Severe tissue wasting Loss of subcutaneous fat Functional dehydration	Apathy Anorexia Edema Changes in hair color and consistency Changes in skin color Abdominal enlargement Diarrhea Steatorrhea
Calcium	Osteoporosis Osteomalacia	Bone fractures
Iron	Anemia Koilonychia ‖ Glossitis	Pallor Weakness Fatigability Dyspnea on exertion Headache Palpitations Fissuring at corners of mouth Painful tongue
Iodine	Goiter	Swelling of neck Hypothyroid symptoms (see Chapter 7, The Head and Neck)
Zinc	Growth retardation Hypogonadism Delayed sexual maturation Seborrheic dermatitis	Loss of taste Anorexia Behavioral problems Skin rashes Hair loss Decreased libido Decreased fertility Diarrhea

‡ Beading of the ribs at the costochondral junction.
§ A condition of marked hyperemia of the conjunctiva, lacrimal deficiency, thickening of the corneal epithelium, itching and burning of the eye, and reduced visual acuity.
‖ Spoon nail (koilonychia).

continued

Deficiency	Signs	Symptoms
Magnesium	Vertical nystagmus	Muscle tremor Choreiform movements Convulsions Weakness Paralysis Dysphagia
Potassium	Arrhythmias	Diarrhea Weakness Nervous irritability Disorientation Palpitations
Sodium	Dehydration signs	Confusion Coma Vomiting Lethargy Anorexia Nausea Headache Obtundation Seizures

Conversion Tables*

Temperature

Centigrade	Fahrenheit	Centigrade	Fahrenheit
33.0	91.4	37.8	100.0
33.2	91.8	38.0	100.4
33.4	92.1	38.2	100.7
33.6	92.5	38.4	101.1
33.8	92.8	38.6	101.4
34.0	93.2	38.8	101.8
34.2	93.6	39.0	102.2
34.4	93.9	39.2	102.5
34.6	94.3	39.4	102.9
34.8	94.6	39.6	103.2
35.0	95.0	39.8	103.6
35.2	95.4	40.0	104.0
35.4	95.7	40.2	104.3
35.6	96.1	40.4	104.7
35.8	96.4	40.6	105.1
36.0	96.8	40.8	105.4
36.2	97.1	41.0	105.8
36.4	97.5	41.2	106.1
36.6	97.8	41.4	106.5
36.8	98.2	41.6	106.8
37.0	98.6	41.8	107.2
37.2	98.9	42.0	107.6
37.4	99.3	42.2	108.0
37.6	99.6	42.4	108.3

* To convert Centigrade to Fahrenheit: $(9/5 \times \text{Centigrade Temperature}) + 32$
To convert Fahrenheit to Centigrade: $5/9 \times (\text{Fahrenheit Temperature} - 32)$

Weight†

Pound	Kilogram	Kilogram	Pound
1	0.5	1	2.2
2	0.9	2	4.4
4	1.8	3	6.6
6	2.7	4	8.8
8	3.6	5	11.0
10	4.5	6	13.2
20	9.1	8	17.6
30	13.6	10	22
40	18.2	20	44
50	22.7	30	66
60	27.3	40	88
70	31.8	50	110
80	36.4	60	132
90	40.9	70	154
100	45.4	80	176
150	66.2	90	198
200	90.8	100	220

† To convert pounds to kilograms: pounds × 0.454 kilogram
  To convert kilograms to pounds: kilograms × 2.204 pounds

Length‡

Inch	Centimeter	Centimeter	Inch
1	2.54	1	0.4
2	5.08	2	0.8
4	10.16	3	1.2
6	15.24	4	1.6
8	20.32	5	2.0
10	25.40	6	2.4
20	50.80	8	3.1
30	76.20	10	3.9
40	101.60	20	7.9
50	127.00	30	11.8
60	152.40	40	15.7
70	177.80	50	19.7
80	203.20	60	23.6
90	228.60	70	27.6
100	254.00	80	31.5
150	381.00	90	34.4
200	508.00	100	39.4

‡ To convert inches to centimeters: inches × 2.54 centimeters
  To convert centimeters to inches: centimeters × 0.3937 inch

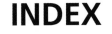

INDEX

Note: Page numbers in italics refer to illustrations, page numbers followed by a t refer to tables.

A

A wave, of jugular venous pulse, 283, *283*
ABCD warning signs, of malignant melanoma, 98
Abdomen, 354–388
　areas of, 354, *355*
　auscultation of, *370,* 370–371, *371*
　disease of, clinicopathologic correlations of, 386–387, 386t, 387t
　　symptoms of, 356–362, *358, 358*t
　　vocabulary of, 388
　enlargement of, in pregnancy, 570
　examination of, 363–386
　　in acutely ill patient, 660
　　in adolescent, 635
　　in geriatric patient, 652
　　in infant, 620
　　in newborn, 606
　　in older child, 629
　　in pregnant patient, 576, *576, 577*
　　in young child, 625
　　with patient supine, 553–554
　　writing up, 388
　inspection of, *363–369,* 364–369
　mass in, 362
　palpation of, 375–380, *375–380*
　　deep, 376, *376*
　　light, *375,* 375–376
　percussion of, 371–375, *372–374,* 374t
　protuberant, 366–367, *367*
　quadrants of, 354, *355*
　　structures in, 355t
　scaphoid, 366
　skin of, examination of, 102
　striae of, 367, *367*
　structure/physiology of, 354–356, *355,* 355t
　surgical scars of, 368, *368*
　xanthomata of, 292–293, *293*
Abdominal aneurysm, 321
　signs of, 327, 328t
Abdominal angina, 357
Abdominal aorta, palpation of, in peripheral vascular disease, 327–328, *328,* 328t
Abdominal bruits, evaluation of, 328, *328*
Abdominal compression, in jugular venous pressure assessment, 302–303
Abdominal distention, 361–362
Abdominal pain, 356–357, *358,* 358t
　amelioration of, maneuvers for, 358t
　in gynecologic disease, 426
　location of, 358t
Abdominal superficial reflex, 532
Abducens nerve, 516
　function of, 514t
　paralysis of, 186, *188*
Abduction, definition of, 452t
　of arms, testing of, 522, *522*

Abduction *(Continued)*
　of fingers, *456*
　　testing of, 524, *525*
　of hip, *457*
　　testing of, 526, *526*
　of shoulder, *453*
Abetalipoproteinemia, geographic distribution of, 47t
Abortion, complete, 580
　incomplete, 580
　inevitable, 580
　threatened, 580
Abruptio placentae, 581
Abscess(es), Bartholin's gland, 432, *433*
　skin, *105*
Abstraction, assessment of, 512
Abuse, child, history of, 21
　elder, history of, 21
　sexual, of children, 592
Accessory muscles, use of, in airway obstruction, 259
Accessory nipple, 339, *340*
Accommodation, of eye, 153
Acetone odor, in infant, 610
Acetylcholine, cardiac effects of, 277
Achilles tendon reflex, 532, *533*
Acne, 118, *118*
Acne rosacea, 210, *210*
Acne vulgaris, distribution of, *131*
Acoustic nerve, 194
Acquired immunodeficiency syndrome (AIDS), cutaneous manifestations of, 130, *130*
　oral candidiasis in, 234, *234*
　oral hairy leukoplakia in, 234, *234*
Acrocyanosis, in newborn, 598
Acromegaly, 22, *24*
Acromioclavicular joint, 470
Activities of daily living (ADL), in geriatric patient, 647
Acupressure, 67
Acupuncture, 65, *66*
　ear, 65, *66*
Acutely ill patient, 40, 655–662
　Cardiopulmonary Resuscitation Survey in, 655, *656,* 656–657
　Key Vital Functions Assessment Survey in, *657,* 657–658
　pediatric, 661–662, 661t, 662t
　secondary survey in, 658–661, 659t, *660*
Adam's apple, 224
Adduction, definition of, 452t
　of fingers, *456*
　　testing of, 524, *525*
　of hip, *457*
　　testing of, 526, *526*
　of shoulder, *453*
　of thumb, testing of, 524, *525*
Adenoids, 223

Adenoma sebaceum, 486
Adenopathy, cervical, 141, *142*
Adiadochokinesia, 542
Adie's tonic pupil, 169, 169t
ADL (activities of daily living), in geriatric patient, 647
Adnexa, 422
　palpation of, 438–441, *440*
Adolescent(s), abdomen of, 635
　breasts of, 635
　examination of, 634–635
　general assessment of, 634–635
　genitalia of, 635
　interview of, 591–592
　musculoskeletal system of, 635
　skin of, 635
Adult respiratory distress syndrome (ARDS), physical manifestations of, 273t
Adventitious sounds, 271, 271t
Aerophagia, 361
Affect, assessment of, 512
Affective disorders, in geriatric patient, screening for, 647–648
　voice disorders in, 228
Afferent limb, of pupillary light reflex, 152
African-Americans, home remedies of, 55
　illness in, cultural response to, 54–55
　malignant melanoma in, 111, *112*
　morbidity/mortality rates in, 51
AGA (appropriate for gestational age), 593, *597*
Age, gestational, determination of, 593, *594, 595,* 596t, *597*
　external criteria of, scoring system for, 596t
　in obstetric risk, 572
　in patient response, 33–37
Aged patient, 34. See also *Geriatric patient.*
Aggressive patient, 32
Aging, impact of, on patient, 650
Agnosia, 513
　tactile, 513
　visual, 513
AIDS (acquired immunodeficiency syndrome), cutaneous manifestations of, 130, *130*
　oral candidiasis in, 234, *234*
　oral hairy leukoplakia in, 234, *234*
AIDS patient, 38
Air conduction, of sound, 194
Air-conducting passages, 249, *249*
Airplane glue, abuse of, 690t
Airway obstruction, accessory muscle use in, 259
Alcohol, abuse of, 689t
　use of, history of, 16
　　in obstetric risk, 573
　　questions about, in mock interview, 78
Alcoholic patient, 40

Turgor, of skin, 99
in infant, 617
Turner's syndrome, 294, 605
Two-point discrimination, testing of, 540, *540*
Tympanic membrane, bulging of, 208
examination of, in infant, 620
in young child, 627
otoscopic, 207–209, *208, 209*
mobility of, testing of, 209
perforation of, *214,* 214–215, *215*
retraction of, 208, *209*
structure/physiology of, 192–193, *193*
Tympanosclerosis, 208, *209*
Tympanostomy tube, *216,* 216–217

U

Ulcer(s), aphthous, 238
in human immunodeficiency virus infection, 246t
signs/symptoms of, 244t
solitary (giant), 239, *239*
corneal, 168, *169*
in geriatric patient, 643
decubitus, in geriatric patient, 643, *643,* 653
stages of, 653
duodenal, stenosing, geographic distribution of, 47t
genital, features of, 444t
in peripheral vascular disease, 323, *323*
oral, 226
herpetic, signs/symptoms of, 244t
multiple, 239–240
traumatic, 238
signs/symptoms of, 245t
rodent, 109, *110*
skin, *105*
Ulcerative colitis, Crohn's disease vs., 386t
Ulnar nerve, testing of, 524, *525*
Umbilical cord stump, 606
Umbilical granuloma, 620
Umbilical hernia, 606
ascites with, *369*
Umbilicus, eversion of, 367
of infant, 620
of young child, 625
Umbo, 193, *193*
Unconscious bias, in physical examination, 89
Underbite, 628
Understanding, in patient interview, 5
Upper extremity(ies), anatomic terms for, 450t
arterial supply in, evaluation of, 331
strength of, evaluation of, 468, *469*
symmetry of, inspection of, 522
tone of, assessment of, 526
Upper motor neuron lesion, effects of, 547t
Upset stomach (empacho), in Latino culture, 59
Urethra, male, *391,* 392
palpation of, 406, *407*
Urethral meatus, 419, *419*
examination of, 432
in infant, 620
in newborn, 607
in young child, 626
Urinary bladder, stones of, geographic distribution of, 47t
Urinary incontinence, in geriatric patient, 653
male, 397
Urinary tract, evaluation of, in patient history, 23t

Urination, disturbances in, during pregnancy, 570–571
pattern of, changes in, in females, 427–428
in males, 397–398
Urine, red, in male, 398
Urticaria, 120, *121*
Uterine bleeding, dysfunctional, 424
types of, *443*
Uterine body, palpation of, 438
Uterine descent, pelvic relaxation and, *443*
Uterus, 420, *420*
growth of, 420, *421*
positions of, 442, *442*
size of, in pregnant patient, 576, *577, 578*
Utility, attachment of, in decision analysis, 678–679
Uvula, 221, *221,* 222
bifid, 604

V

V wave, of jugular venous pulse, 283, *283*
Vaccine, *Haemophilus influenzae* type B, 16
hepatitis B, 16
influenza, 15
measles, mumps, rubella (MMR), 16
pneumococcal polysaccharide, 16
Vagina, 420, *420*
bleeding from, abnormal, 424
examination of, in young child, 626
itching of, 426
walls of, speculum examination of, 437
Vaginal discharge, 425, 426t
in infant, 620
in pregnancy, 571
in young child, 626
Vaginal introitus, 419, *419*
Vaginal orifice, of female newborn, examination of, 607
Vaginismus, 427
in female infertility, 430
Vaginitis, 442–444
nonspecific, 426t
Vagus nerve, 225, 519
function of, 514t
Valgus, 451
Value, expected, computation of, in decision analysis, 679
Varicella, 639t
Varicocele, 408, *408,* 412
differential diagnosis of, 413t
Varicose veins (varicosities), geographic distribution of, 47t
inspection for, in peripheral vascular disease, 325, *326*
Varus, 451
Vas deferens, *393,* 393–394
palpation of, 408, *408*
Vasa previa, 581
Vascular nevi, in newborn, 599
Vascular system, peripheral. See *Peripheral vascular system.*
Vasomotor rhinitis, 200
Vasovagal syncope, 288, 289t
Vein(s), 276. See also names of specific veins.
of abdomen, examination of, 369, *369*
Venous hum, characteristics of, 317t
in pediatric patient, 638t
Venous stasis, chronic, *325*
Venous system, 321. See also *Peripheral vascular system.*
insufficiency of, skin changes in, 322
Venous thrombosis, geographic distribution of, 47t

Ventral, definition of, 450, *450*
Ventral corticospinal tract, 500
Ventral spinothalamic tract, 500
Ventral suspension, in newborn, *594, 595*
Ventricular septal defect, in pediatric patient, 638t
murmur in, characteristics of, 317t
Vertebra prominens, 251
Vertex presentation, 566–567, *567*
Vertical strip (grid) technique, of breast examination, 348–349
Vertigo, 198–199, 505
Vesicle, *104*
Vesicobullous diseases, differential diagnosis of, 132t
Vesicular breath sounds, 267, *268*
Vestibular nerve, 194
Vestibule, 194, 419, *419*
Vestibulocochlear nerve, 518
function of, 514t
Vibration, sense of, testing of, 538, *539*
Vibrissae, 196
Vietnamese, illness in, cultural response to, 60
Vincent's disease, 241, *242*
Violence, domestic, history of, 21
Virilization, 427
Visceral pericardium, 276
Visceral pleura, 249
Viscus, obstruction of, 370
Vision, binocular, 155
disturbances in, 506–507
double, 155–156
impairment of, patient with, 38
loss of, 155
poor, evaluation of, 159
tunnel, 161
Visual acuity, 159
of infant, 618–619
of newborn, 603
of older child, 629
of young child, 626
Visual acuity card, pocket, 159
Visual agnosia, 513
Visual cortex, 495
Visual fibers, 152, *153*
Visual fields, 159–162, *160, 161*
abnormalities of, 161, *161*
assessment of, confrontation testing in, 160, *160*
in young child, 626
Visualization, in relaxation, for patient interview, 25
Vital signs, assessment of, 551
in acutely ill patient, 661
in geriatric patient, 651
Vitamin A deficiency, 691t
Vitamin C deficiency, 692t
Vitamin D deficiency, 691t
Vitiligo, 120, *120*
Vitreous humor, 153
Vocabulary, assessment of, 512
of abdominal disease, 388
of breast disease, 352
of chest disease, 272
of ear disease, 218
of eye disease, 188–189
of gynecologic disease, 445
of head/neck disease, 147
of heart disease, 317
of male urologic disease, 415
of medicine, 90–91
of musculoskeletal disease, 493
of neurologic disease, 548
of nose disease, 218
of oral cavity disease, 246

ISBN 0-7216-7514-X

9 780721 675145

90071